Dance Injuries

Reducing Risk and Maximizing Performance

Jeffrey A. Russell, PhD, ATC
Ohio University
Editor

HUMAN KINETICS

Library of Congress Cataloging-in-Publication Data

Names: Russell, Jeffrey A., 1959- editor.
Title: Dance injuries : reducing risk and maximizing performance / edited by Jeffrey A. Russell.
Description: Champaign, IL : Human Kinetics, 2025. | Includes bibliographical references and index.
Identifiers: LCCN 2023043730 (print) | LCCN 2023043731 (ebook) | ISBN 9781718211865 (paperback) | ISBN 9781718211872 (epub) | ISBN 9781718211889 (pdf)
Subjects: LCSH: Dancing injuries. | Dancing injuries--Prevention. | Dancers--Health and hygiene.
Classification: LCC RC1220.D35 D35 2025 (print) | LCC RC1220.D35 (ebook) | DDC 617.1/0275--dc23/eng/20240119
LC record available at https://lccn.loc.gov/2023043730
LC ebook record available at https://lccn.loc.gov/2023043731

ISBN: 978-1-7182-1186-5 (print)

The web addresses cited in this text were current as of November 2023, unless otherwise noted.

Acquisitions Editor: Bethany J. Bentley; **Senior Managing Editor:** Anne E. Mrozek; **Copyeditor:** Joanna Hatzopoulos; **Proofreader:** Leigh Keylock; **Indexer:** Rebecca McCorkle; **Permissions Manager:** Laurel Mitchell; **Senior Graphic Designer:** Joe Buck; **Cover Designer:** Keri Evans; **Cover Design Specialist:** Susan Rothermel Allen; **Photographs:** © Human Kinetics, unless otherwise noted; **Photo Asset Manager:** Laura Fitch; **Photo Production Manager:** Jason Allen; **Senior Art Manager:** Kelly Hendren; **Illustrations (cover):** Kamila Baimukasheva / iStock (tap dance image); VectorMine/ iStock (ballroom dance image); Tetiana Garkusha/ iStock (ballet and modern dance images); taylan_ozgur/ iStock (ethnic dance image); Viktor Kostenko / iStock (hip hop dance image); **Illustrations (interior):** © Human Kinetics, unless otherwise noted; **Printer:** Sheridan Kentucky

Printed in the United States of America

10 9 8 7 6 5 4 3 2 1

The paper in this book is certified under a sustainable forestry program.

Human Kinetics
1607 N. Market Street
Champaign, IL 61820
USA

United States and International
Website: **US.HumanKinetics.com**
Email: info@hkusa.com
Phone: 1-800-747-4457

Canada
Website: **Canada.HumanKinetics.com**
Email: info@hkcanada.com

E8544

To my colleagues on the dance faculty and the dancers of Belhaven University from 2001 through 2005. During those years when I was on the Belhaven sports medicine and exercise science faculty, they welcomed me into their world of dance, patiently taught me, and collaboratively worked with me to launch my career change from sports medicine to dance medicine and performing arts medicine. Were it not for them investing in me then, this book would not have been created now. To this day, their dance department and dance medicine program thrive. I may have left, but I have never forgotten.

Contents

Foreword

In June 2023 I received the crushing news that my dear friend Ruth Solomon had passed away unexpectedly. What a shock to the dance medicine and science world, and especially to those of us who had known and worked closely with Ruth and her husband John for many years. Then, while preparing the final edits for this book, I got word from one of their children that John passed away in October 2023. I am beyond thrilled that Ruth and John both were willing and able to write this foreword together before Ruth passed. They authored two editions of a dance injuries book for Human Kinetics that were precursors to this textbook, just one reason why I invited them to take up this assignment. Though they are now gone, both of them remain pioneers in our field. They tirelessly compiled and edited the seminal resource *Dance Medicine & Science Bibliography* through nine editions. And in 2017, as but one measure of their substantial contributions, they were awarded the International Association for Dance Medicine & Science's Lifetime Achievement Award. I remember and honor my friends here for their lasting investment in all of us.

—Dr. Jeff Russell

Our longtime colleague Jeff Russell opens his preface to this book with the seemingly audacious statement that this book is "a unique resource." *Come on, Jeff*, we are prone to think, *by now an abundance of books must exist in the dance medicine and science lexicon; surely yours can't be all that unique*. Well, in some important respects, Jeff is right! Primarily, this book is unlike any other because it is the first book of its kind to so explicitly address dancers. That statement requires some historical perspective.

Our *Dance Medicine & Science Bibliography* (Solomon & Solomon, 2023) demonstrates that book-length treatments of the subject began to appear in 1982 with the publication in Denmark of E. Thomasen's *Diseases and Injuries of Ballet Dancers*. That book was written by one doctor addressing other doctors on a wide range of medical issues. It was quickly followed by Caroline Shell's *The Dancer as Athlete (The 1984 Olympic Scientific Conference Proceedings, Volume 8)*, which is more important for our purposes because (1) it was published in the United States—as were all of the similarly themed books that followed—and (2) it established the format on which most of them were modeled. The subtitle of Shell's book identifies it as proceedings from one in a series of congresses; that information in itself indicates what went into its compilation; namely, Shell, seizing an opportunity to elevate dance medicine and science to a prominence it had never before enjoyed, went to her friends (and friends of her friends) to provide her with studies from which she could cobble together the requisite number of floor presentations for the Congress and eventually a book. We can assure you that is exactly how Ryan and Stevens' *Dance Medicine* (1987), Clarkson and Skrinar's *Science of Dance Training* (1988), and our own *Preventing Dance Injuries* (1990, 2005)—as well as our latest endeavor in the field, *Prevention of Injuries in the Young Dancer* (2018)—came about.

Not that there was anything wrong with the way we early pioneers went about gathering material for our books. The point is that we knew we were on to something new and well worth pursuing, and were trying to determine how and where it should go. Specifically, we knew that there were already numerous top-notch researchers out there who had in one way or another been attracted to the field, and we sensed that one way to move the field forward would be to collect their work between the covers of a book. (It should be noted that at this same time, the International Association for Dance Medicine

& Science [IADMS] was being created to explore another way.) Those early books were the product of a search for direction, but they are not without a sense of where they would like to see things go. Nor are they outdated; you can find a multitude of references to the studies they contain in today's scholarly research. Above all, they sought to appeal to all aspects of the disparate worlds of dance and medicine in order to establish a sense of community.

Now, the book you hold in your hands has the same basic appearance as those earlier books (it is a series of topics grouped by subject matter), but if you take the long view, you will see that those topics—and those groupings—have greater continuity and are more narrowly focused. It is easy to envision Jeff approaching prospective contributors with a pitch that went something like this: "I would like to have you add your area of expertise to a book I am editing about reducing the risk of dance injuries that will specifically target dancers." That is far more narrowly focused than any directive we could offer our people. Incidentally, here is a word about that "reducing the risk of" rather than "preventing" dance injuries: At first glance, it seems to be mere hair-splitting; however, in fact, Jeff's way does put the onus for minimizing injuries more directly on the people who are actively involved in the activity—in this case the dancers themselves.

A secondary way in which this book is distinguished from virtually all others is that it is defined as a textbook. One predecessor shares that same nomenclature, the ground-breaking *Textbook of Performing Arts Medicine*, edited by Robert J. Sataloff, Alice Brandfonbrener, and Richard Lederman (1990). However, the use of the term is very different in these two cases. As its title suggests, a performing arts medicine book takes a sweeping look at some medical problems experienced by performers in a wide range of art genres. Thus, on the one hand, it can be considered a textbook only in that, taken as a whole, it is unified around the theme that all performing artists are vulnerable to what we commonly call overuse injuries. It makes a universal statement. On the other hand, the book's wide scope limits its attention on dancers to just three chapters, which focus on such diverse subjects as psychological issues, the foot and ankle, and reproductive disorders (another example of the early practice of picking up studies that are available and somehow suitable to the book's purpose).

Jeff's use of "textbook" is more classical in nature. His book is so practical that it cries out to be taken into the classroom (or dance studio) to help shed light on the subject matter at hand. It is explicitly the student's (dancer's) friend. Furthermore, it has all the trappings we might expect to find in a textbook: learning objectives, discussion questions, sidebars, and so on. Yes, it is truly a textbook; and yes, it has that narrow focus we have praised so highly as its distinguishing characteristic. However, it would be a mistake to think of it as useful only for dancers. It is totally applicable for dance teachers, the flip side of the student–teacher dyad. One can easily imagine it becoming assigned reading for dance classes at all levels of dance education and training. Perhaps it is not even too far-fetched to hope that the medical personnel who oversee the health of dancers might discover the benefit of having it around.

Finally, we commend you for having bought this book, and we leave you with the assurance that you will not regret having done so. As editors of the first generation compilations of dance medicine and science research, we are truly pleased to welcome this new addition into the fold. It is a clear indicator of how far we have come.

Ruth Solomon, Professor Emerita
University of California, Santa Cruz
Honorary Fellow, Division of Sports Medicine, Harvard Medical School

John Solomon, PhD
Freelance Editor

Preface

Dance Injuries is a unique resource for all students of dance. Whether you are pursuing a dance degree at a college or university, you are enrolled in a conservatory, or you are studying dance on your own, this book will benefit you. It was created primarily to help you access the wealth of information necessary to stay well and keep dancing as long as it is in your heart to do so. If you are a health care professional who currently does or wants to work with dancers or you are a dance educator, this book will yield great dividends for you, too.

A great strength of this textbook is that many of my most treasured colleagues agreed to contribute to it. These authors include experts in reducing the risk of dance injuries and in managing such injuries when they occur. They are physicians, athletic trainers, physical therapists, researchers, and dance educators who have devoted countless hours to serving dancers. In the pages of this book, they serve you, too; they share their breadth of expertise so you can gain valuable insights about dance injuries.

You may have noticed that the word *prevention* does not appear in the title of this book. This omission acknowledges the fact that pain and injuries will happen; they are part of dancing. However, to sustain yourself as a dancer, you need to have a plan to reduce the risk of injury and to care for injuries when they occur. The information in this text can help you with both parts of that plan.

Attention to reducing injury risk will improve your chances of staying where you want to be—in classes, rehearsals, and performances. Although pain and injuries are expected in dance, there are right ways and wrong ways to deal with them when they occur. For example, dancing through pain is never a wise idea because that can lead to extended difficulties and even shorten your dance career. A better approach is to properly train yourself technically, physically, and mentally so you can dance at your peak of ability. You should care for your entire self, learn what pain's signal is designed to tell you, and find trusted and qualified professionals to assist you. In addition, dancing in a supportive environment as well as establishing open communication with teachers, choreographers, directors, and health care professionals are essential. This book helps you address all these important factors of dealing with dance injuries.

Another strength of this text is that it is grounded in a whole-person—or whole-dancer—approach to wellness. One can neither compartmentalize the physical component of dance nor group only the physical and emotional dimensions together; humans are more complex than those categories suggest. You have many facets, so you need a multidimensional approach to your wellness. Chapter 1 explains this approach, offering detailed definitions that set the stage for the rest of the book.

The book is divided into four parts, Part I: Setting the Stage for Reducing Injuries (chapters 1-4), Part II: Care Inside and Out (chapters 5-10), Part III: Common Dance Injuries (chapters 11-14), and Part IV: Coordinated Safety and Wellness (chapters 15-16). The first of these focuses on helping you understand wellness, injury risk, your body, and the principles necessary to keep yourself well. After the framework for whole-dancer wellness and injury risk is established in chapter 1, notably in chapter 2 we lay the foundation for this recurring theme: Dance is more than just ballet and modern or contemporary dance. As beautiful as those well-established genres are, they get nearly all of the attention in dance literature, especially in dance medicine and science research. However, dance is much richer and broader than two genres.

Throughout the book, science-based evidence underpins all recommendations for improving your wellness. Chapter 3 takes that scientific focus a step further by helping you learn how to find, read, and evaluate scientific research literature yourself. Research forms the basis for what is known about safe dancing. Like dance, this knowledge is constantly evolving, so your ability to access and keep current on research findings is essential to your success. There is no need to be afraid of or put off by science and research; this chapter teaches you how to make these tools your friends. Closing the first part, chapter 4 presents the crucial information you need about how your body works under the physical load of dance.

The next section, *Care Inside and Out*, unpacks the best ways to keep yourself working as optimally as possible in dance. Chapters 5 through 7 cover conditioning; flexibility training; and nutrition, hydration, and rest. Following those foundational topics, chapter 8 discusses mental health challenges that are common in dancers—an extremely important topic for today's dancer. Next, you'll find chapters 9 and 10 explaining the basics of different types of injuries and what to do about them, including how to manage first aid and emergency situations in a dance studio or performance space.

From this general information you'll move to the *Common Dance Injuries* portion of the book, chapters 11 through 14, to explore injuries and their care in all parts of the body, including the upper and lower extremities, the lumbar spine, the core, the pelvic floor, and the head. None of these is unimportant! Some of the world's most esteemed dance medicine specialists will lead you through well described, superbly illustrated chapters that unlock many of the common injuries dancers encounter. In case one of these besets you, you will be well equipped to manage it!

Coordinated Safety and Wellness concludes the main body of the text with two chapters about topics that are rarely (if ever) found in a dance textbook. Chapter 15 addresses one of the most difficult aspects any injured dancer must face: how to work with health care providers to receive needed care. This will be a gold mine of information to help you successfully navigate a sometimes scary profession. Next, chapter 16 makes sure that all the information provided to you has a way to get into the studio and helps you, your fellow dancers, and your instructors create a safe environment for everyone. This information will not only be helpful for your dance practice as a student, it will also prepare you for the day when you may be a dance teacher yourself. It is intended to help dancers and teachers work together for their mutual benefit as well as promote the artistic advancement of dance.

The book closes with several appendixes, and do not neglect to consult other supplemental content included in the HK*Propel* online resource. These short pieces have been specially curated to present content that is important for you as a dancer but that did not fit neatly into one of the main chapters of this book. The various fascinating topics include takeaway messages, practical resources, and additional insights. Other supplemental contributions are included in the online resources that accompany several chapters, including 3, 6, and 9. All of this information is offered with the goal of helping you look toward your future career in dance, whether it be as a professional dancer, a dance teacher, a dance studio owner, or another passion that strikes your fancy. Think of these resources as letters of encouragement to you from experts who want you to succeed as a dancer.

Throughout the book, you will find special features to help you embrace the subject matter. Each chapter opens with learning objectives to show you what you will gain, and it concludes with discussion questions to test your newly obtained knowledge. Within the chapters are sidebars and other elements that emphasize important pearls of wisdom and help you apply the material to your dancing. We acknowledge that dancers like to move and do things. Therefore, activities are included for the pieces of information that are best learned through experience. Finally, for your instructor, additional resources accompany each chapter, including presentation slides from which to teach.

Are you ready to embark on a journey to understanding your body, dance injuries, and wellness? The contributors and I have created a path to support you in your quest for a healthier, longer, well-lived dance career. We are excited to share the knowledge in this book with you so you can apply it to your whole dance life. We hope that as you read and learn, you will dance with not only new understanding but also with new passion. Make this journey an adventure and enjoy it!

Dr. Jeff Russell
Athens, Ohio, USA

About the Student and Instructor Ancillaries

Student Resources

The HK*Propel* learning content contains key term flash cards and downloadable resources to enhance your learning experience.

Introduction

- International Dance Medicine and Science Resources, by Robin Kish, MFA
- Interactive key term flash cards by chapter

Chapter 1

- Discussion questions

Chapter 2

- A Window Into Ballroom Dance, by Katherine Nicole Noakes, LAT, ATC, and Amanda Donahue, MS, ATC
- Components of Hip-Hop Dance, by Nefeli Tsiouti, PT, MA, MSc
- Hearing Loss in Dance: Occupational Hazard, by Steven Karageanes, DO, FAOASM
- Discussion questions

Chapter 3

- Common Search Engines and Databases table
- Reading Guide for Primary Research Articles, by Jeffrey A. Russell, PhD, ATC
- Primary Research Article Reading Assignment
- Discussion questions

Chapter 4

- Discussion questions

Chapter 5

- Physical Activity Goals and Tracking spreadsheet
- Discussion questions

Chapter 6

- Video using a blood orange to demonstrate how fasciae work
- Nerve gliding activity
- Special Considerations for Hypermobile Dancers, by Linda Bluestein, MD
- Discussion questions

Chapter 7

- Discussion questions

Chapter 8

- Common Mental Health Challenges
- International Mental Health Resources
- Blank Eisenhower matrix
- Discussion questions

Chapter 9

- Emergency Action Plan template
- Discussion questions

Chapter 10

- Discussion questions

Chapter 11

- Inside Views of the Ankle and Foot en Pointe, by Jeffrey A. Russell, PhD, ATC
- Evaluating Readiness for Dancing en Pointe, by Selina Shah, MD, FACP, FAMSSM
- Discussion questions

Chapter 12

- Discussion questions

Chapter 13

- Discussion questions

Chapter 14

- Discussion questions

Chapter 15

- Figure 15.5 The process of evaluating, diagnosing, and establishing a plan of care for a dance injury
- Pain Diary Template
- Discussion questions

Chapter 16

- Discussion questions

Instructor Resources

Instructors will find an array of useful ancillary materials in HK*Propel,* including those listed above. To supplement the chapter material and discussion questions, the *instructor guide* includes an overview and sample syllabuses, as well as chapter objectives, suggested readings, and instructional activity ideas for each chapter.

The *test package* is a bank of over 300 questions that include true-false, fill-in-the-blank, short-answer, multiple-response, and multiple-choice formats. The files may be downloaded for integration with a learning management system or printed for use as paper-based tests. Instructors may also create their own customized quizzes or tests from the test bank questions to assign to students directly through HK*Propel.* Multiple-choice and true-false questions are graded automatically, and instructors can easily review student scores in the platform.

The *presentation package* includes a series of PowerPoint slides for each chapter. The slides highlight the most important concepts from the book. Depending on the particular emphasis an instructor wants to give the chapter—or on the background and expertise of the students—instructors may want to delete some slides or embellish others.

These ancillary materials may be accessed in HK*Propel.* See the card at the front of the print book for your unique HK*Propel* access code. For ebook users, reference the HK*Propel* access code instructions on the page immediately following the book cover.

Acknowledgments

Harkening to the African proverb, if it takes a village to raise a child, what does it take to raise a book? I can tell you now, it's three villages. Trust me, a book is no small project.

Village 1 is my author team. In describing them, *wow* is about the only word that comes to mind. What a group of dance medicine and science rock stars. The fact that they willingly joined this project and then gave everything they had to creating a unique product speaks volumes about their character. My deepest gratitude to each of them for getting important words out of their minds and into a word processor.

Village 2 is the team at Human Kinetics. Bethany Bentley, my acquisitions editor, had the vision to get this project off the ground after talking to my Human Kinetics sales representative, Merry Blakey. What a privilege to be invited to produce something of this magnitude. It can only happen, however, when each uniquely talented person applies their craft to their piece of the work. Anne Mrozek, my managing editor at Human Kinetics, made an enormous project seem doable and ensured that I always knew what was going on and what I was supposed to do next. I'm afraid I do not have any idea who the rest of the talented people in this village are individually, but I can say that they are a fabulous team to work alongside.

Village 3 is a one-person village: My wife, Ruth, is ever my encourager. She has been by my side for more than 40 years; thus, she has seen it all and been through it all. I would not have a career in dance medicine and performing arts medicine were it not for her. This book would not exist, either, because it was her blessing that opened the door to me taking up the project. Yes, she's incredible, and I owe her more than I could ever pay.

Part I

Setting the Stage for Reducing Injuries

1

Introduction to Injury Risk Reduction and Performance

Caroline Bolling, PT, PhD
Robin Kish, MS, MFA
Jeffrey A. Russell, PhD, ATC

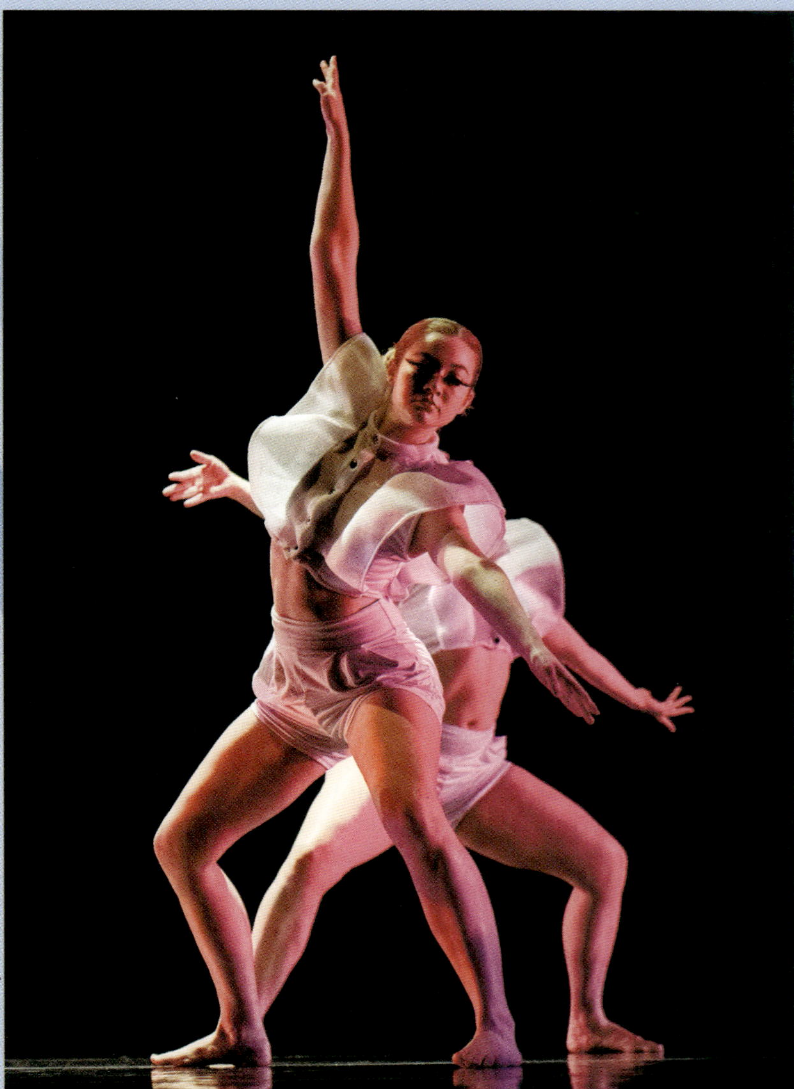

Ohio University School of Dance, Athens, Ohio. Photo by Laura Bilson/Courtesy of Ohio University; Dancer: Erica Lewis

Key Terms

- extrinsic motivation
- health
- holistic
- incidence
- intrinsic motivation
- prevalence
- risk reduction
- signs
- symptoms
- wellness

Being a dancer comes with many risk factors; indeed, injuries are common in dance. To reduce your risk of injury and maximize your performance, you must learn to care for yourself from a whole-person perspective and understand the importance of making wise decisions that support your dancing.

LEARNING OBJECTIVES

After completing this chapter, you will be able to do the following:

- Distinguish between health and wellness.
- Define the six primary dimensions of whole-person wellness.
- Explain how the dimensions of wellness interconnect and how they affect a dancer's performance and overall well-being.
- Differentiate between intrinsic and extrinsic motivation.
- Articulate the mindset of a university dancer and their relationship with health and wellness choices.
- Discuss the concepts of exposure and inherent risk of injuries.
- Defend *risk reduction* as a preferred term over *prevention* in the context of dance injury occurrence.
- Outline key scientific research related to reduction of injury risk.
- Describe dancer risk reduction while considering the complexity of the dance context and the full system around the dancer.

Reducing the risk of injuries and maximizing one's performance in dance are both logical and worthy goals for any dancer. After all, you cannot dance or perform at an optimal level physically or artistically if an injury compromises your ability to execute choreography. This textbook centers on helping you dance all out with artistic passion while dancing all in with holistic wellness. Sustaining zero injuries during a dance career is not a realistic expectation; however, getting as close to zero as possible is a worthwhile target. This chapter lays the groundwork for the rest of the book while it introduces a new way of thinking about wellness, injuries, and your role in injury risk reduction and care. It offers the base of support for you as you aim at the lowest possible likelihood of sustaining an injury.

Health and Wellness

The terms *health* and *wellness* may seem similar if not synonymous. Traditionally, **health** is more focused on attaining the absence of disease (and ill-health on the presence of disease), while **wellness** seeks to establish an optimum quality of life across the several dimensions of humanness. In the preamble to its constitution, the World Health Organization (WHO, 1946) defines health this way: "Health is a state of complete physical, mental and social well-being and not merely the absence of disease or infirmity" (p. 1). However, while they admirably try to extend the definition of health beyond a simple disease-based construct, a proper concept of whole-person wellness suggests that considering only physical, mental, and social well-being leaves some holes in one's whole.

Wellness, on the other hand, is defined by the National Wellness Institute (NWI) (n.d.) as "an active process through which people become aware of, and make choices toward, a more successful existence" (p. 6). Other authors confirm that wellness relates to the overarching ability of a person to successfully navigate through life (Johnson, 1986; Swarbrick, 2006). These definitions imply that in order to successfully exist, a person's entire being must receive adequate development and nurture. Moreover, Johnson (1986) summarized and agreed with others who suggest that wellness requires personal responsibility. All these interpretations form the foundation for a model of wellness comprising six dimensions. The next section explores this model.

Holistic Wellness

In the context of human wellness, the term **holistic** is often misapplied, misconstrued, or misunderstood. It comes from the Greek word *hólos*, which means "whole." In order to operate from a truly holistic view, one must understand the full complement of domains that blend to make an individual both unique and alive.

What Is a Fit Dancer?

Helen Laws is an authoritative source who speaks on behalf of, about, and to dancers in *Fit to Dance 2: Report of Dance UK's Second National Inquiry Into Dancers' Health and Injury in the UK* (2005). She offers 10 recommendations for dancer fitness that are based on the results of this inquiry. These recommendations largely coincide with many principles of dancer wellness offered in this textbook. Laws states them as follows (pp. 95-105):

1. Dancers should be physically fit.
2. Dancers should warm up and cool down properly.
3. Dancers should eat and drink properly.
4. Dancers should not smoke.
5. Dancers should never have to work in unsuitable environments.
6. Dancers, teachers, choreographers, and directors should know more about how the body works.
7. Dancers should receive immediate, high quality treatment for injury.
8. Special consideration should be given to the menstrual status of female dancers.
9. Dancers should know how to, and be enabled to, relax, pace themselves, [and] combat staleness.
10. Dancers' psychological needs should always be considered alongside their physical ones.

The term *whole person* is a way to express *holistic* specifically in terms of human beings. When *holistic* is used properly as an adjective, the terms *holistic wellness* and *whole-person wellness* are synonymous. William Hettler, a physician who cofounded the NWI in 1976, developed a model of wellness (NWI, n.d.) that helps explain the complexities of whole-person humanness (figure 1.1). Hettler's model comprises six dimensions of wellness: occupational, physical, social, intellectual, spiritual, and emotional. A person could have a level of reduced health in their life (e.g., the presence of a chronic disease) and still foster a level of wellness that is as close to optimal as possible across the spectrum of dimensions. Overall, then, your goal as a dancer and as a human being should be to manage and preserve all six of your dimensions at as high a level of wellness as possible. Each of the six dimensions is defined next.

Occupational Dimension

The occupational dimension of wellness encompasses aspects related to the primary area where they spend their time in a typical day. For many people, this area is an occupation—such as a full-time job—tied to the financial necessities of life. In general, students are not full-time employees. Instead, with classes and other academic and extracurricular activities related to education, the occupational dimension for students usually relates to their studies at their school, university, or similar institution. For students who also work a part-time job to pay some or all of their bills, this job is included in the occupational dimension. Optimal wellness in this dimension suggests a dancer is either employed in a dance environment that matches their skills and interests or enrolled in a program of study leading to employment that aligns with their career goal and is able to meet their financial obligations without undue stress.

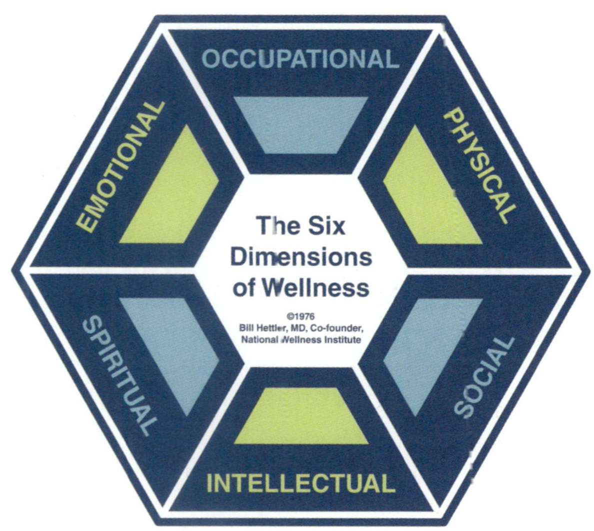

Figure 1.1 The six dimensions of human wellness as described by Dr. Bill Hettler.

Content has been reprinted with permission from the National Wellness Institute, Inc., NationalWellness.org

Physical Dimension

The physical dimension of wellness is typically the easiest for people to understand. Physical bodies are visible, and they provide people with the ability to function in activities of daily living. Wellness in the physical realm means that an individual's physical body functions at a capacity that is optimal for the activities of their life. For example, an Olympic swimmer would need higher physical capacities (e.g., cardiorespiratory function; muscular strength and endurance; and flexibility) than a recreational swimmer who swims laps for enjoyment and general fitness. However, both of these individuals can be considered well if physically they are able to function appropriately at the level of activity in which they engage. Likewise, a university student majoring in dance—with all the demands that the major entails—must have higher physical capacities than another student who participates in biweekly activities of the university's social dance club. Both of these students can be optimally well in their physical dimension as long as they can accomplish physically what is necessary for them in their lives.

Social Dimension

Wellness in the social dimension depends on success in interacting with others. You may associate with a wide variety of groups that contribute to your social wellness. Most people have a family and a circle of friends in this dimension. Social groups in the university dance environment include dancers in a particular dance piece, students taking the same course, participation with a professor in an independent study or research project, or participation in clubs (e.g., fraternities, sororities, and extracurricular interests).

Intellectual Dimension

The intellectual dimension of wellness relates to using one's mind. For example, you are applying your intellect as you read this book. You make decisions all day long, such as what to wear when you get dressed; whether you want a bagel, a bowl of cereal, or a fried egg for breakfast; which path across campus you will take to get to class; what words to use when texting your friend; and other choices necessary to get through a day. In dance, converting choreography into a performance, learning the history of ballet, and evaluating music to match a set of steps also require a well mind. Furthermore, throughout life, you have many opportunities to learn apart from traditional academics. Overall, the intellectual dimension pertains to what cognitively carries you through your time on Earth.

Spiritual Dimension

Of the six dimensions of wellness, the spiritual dimension may be the most misunderstood and difficult to manage; it is not widely taught, and it is very personal. At its core, your spiritual dimension relates to your purpose for being a human during the span of your life in the place on the planet where you are. In other words, it relates to finding meaning in your life. While it sometimes relates to religious practice, religion is not necessarily a factor of the spiritual dimension. However, this dimension tends to be connected to a transcendent purpose because otherwise your purpose is wound up in yourself, by yourself—a state that leaves people feeling undervalued and empty because their search for meaning does not extend beyond their own confines. Other words used for *purpose* in this context include *life meaning* and *reason for living*. Research clearly supports that a heightened sense of knowing one's purpose is associated with lower levels of negative behaviors, including in students. For example, students with greater addiction to their smartphones show lower scores of meaning and purpose in life (Çevik et al., 2020). This finding is just one piece of evidence for how the spiritual dimension intersects with other dimensions in Hettler's model.

Emotional Dimension

The emotional dimension of wellness pertains to how one feels. This dimension may be the most interactive with the other five because people are emotional beings. For example, your feelings can be drastically affected by an injury (physical), how you are treated by friends or family (social), the extent to which you can manage decisions in your life (intellectual), a sense of being lost in the world (spiritual), and whether or not you end up in a fulfilling career (occupational). Your mental health is heavily associated with both the emotional and intellectual dimensions. Moreover, social media use—a ubiquitous part of life, especially with young people—can negatively impact the emotions. A short-term social media fast was associated with reduced body shame and body surveillance in 10- to 19-year-old female dancers (Roberts et al., 2022). In general, the emotions are greatly assisted by rejecting stigmatization, pursuing self-care, and seeking appropriate health care or counseling when necessary. These issues are discussed in detail in chapter 8.

Applying the Holistic Wellness Model

You may be starting to see how the six dimensions of wellness overlap and interrelate. The hexagonal shape of Hettler's diagram is important; it indicates that the dimensions are connected to compose the whole. To emphasize this point even more, one can draw lines between each dimension and all the others. Within one person, no dimension operates solo; think of your own wellness dimensions as a six-person dance piece where each dancer is integral to the choreography. If one of those dancers is not able to perform at maximum capacity, or perhaps cannot perform at all, the entire performance suffers.

Imagine a simple, commonly occurring scenario in which a dance student experiences an injury, such as a sprained ankle or a persistent overuse injury. The condition is a physical problem, but clearly its repercussions extend well beyond the physical realm. If an injured dancer is unable to participate in classes, rehearsals, and performances, consider what may be disrupted. Because a student's occupational dimension consists of primarily the academic environment, the occupational dimension is affected. The injured dance student is used to the social dimension of dancing with their classmates and teacher; however, this dimension will be negatively affected during the injury recuperation period, especially if the student is relegated to sitting at the side of the studio and watching everyone else participate.

Next, consider how the negative impacts in the occupational and social dimensions can also adversely affect the emotions as the injured dancer tries to deal with the void left by not being able to engage in their customary activities. In addition, the intellectual dimension is compromised because the dancer is not able to participate at a level that would allow complete learning of movements, steps, choreography, and other knowledge offered in class. Finally, in the case of an injury that is severe enough to warrant an extended time away from dance (or, worse, the end of a dance career), even the spiritual dimension may be influenced. Thus, no dimension of wellness may be left untouched by what on the surface seems to be an injury affecting the physical dimension.

Another example relates to the way instructors think of their students. Some teachers are concerned with only the intellectual dimension of wellness in their students. For example, they may adopt a misguided, uncompassionate view such as *After all, these students are in school to learn, and by now they should know how to rise above their problems and perform well academically*. Instructors with that perspective will miss the negative, intertwined, multidimensional fallout of any of a variety of challenges that students encounter. These instructors only see the final product: the dancer in full costume, under lighting, and performing for an audience (figure 1.2). They cannot see the occupational dimension of student wellness as tied to the academic program. They will not understand a failed exam or assignment brought about by a physical injury that causes a student to miss class sessions. They will not be able to appreciate a student's declining semester performance that is caused by a difficult family situation creating havoc in that student's social and emotional dimensions. They will not be able to intervene when a student shows signs of addictive or self-harm behaviors that are associated with dysfunction and dire consequences in the emotional, intellectual, physical, and spiritual dimensions. Thus, without a full understanding of and commitment to whole-person wellness, neither dancers nor anyone else are able to achieve their full potential.

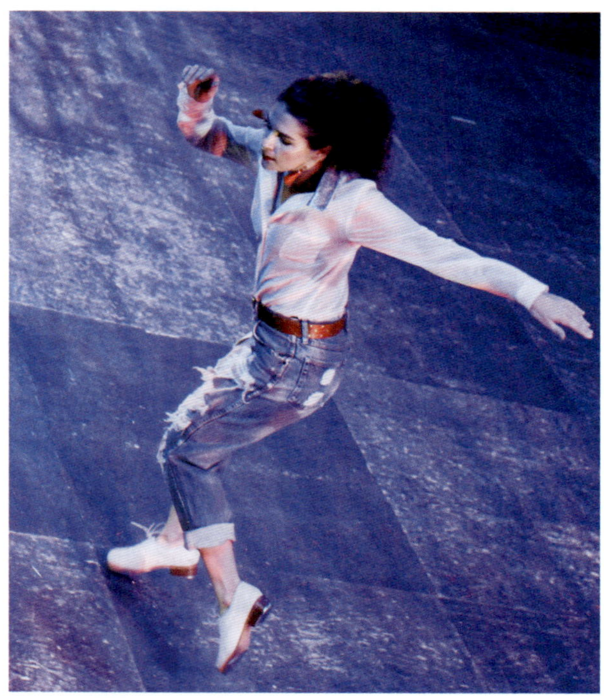

Figure 1.2 A tap dancer is an example of someone with high dance skill whose occupation creates multiple demands on wellness.

Azuki Umeda

Intrinsic and Extrinsic Motivation

As you enter your collegiate or preprofessional years, it is likely that you have spent countless hours training in the dance studio; performed in numerous recitals, conventions, and competitions; and skipped over chunks of a typical childhood—all for the sake of your art. Dancers find their way into dance through various paths. You may have started in a recreational dance class for fun, your parents might have put you in dance classes to burn off energy, or maybe you followed an older sibling into the studio. Regardless of the entry point, dance eventually became your primary focus and way of life. As you read the rest of this chapter and the rest of this book, remember that you are a whole dancer—and a whole person—who is made up of many dimensions. Understanding this principle is key to your success in dance and in life.

As a serious student of dance, you approach life with an artist's mindset, which means you are driven by and focused on your future career in dance. It is best when that drive comes from an **intrinsic motivation**, where the pure joy for dance originates within you and is connected to a holistic view of yourself. Unfortunately, often **extrinsic motivation**—where the drive for success is external—can continually push dancers too hard. Extrinsic factors include pressure from parents, teachers, or peers as well as academic and financial stresses related to completing a college degree with an uncertain future. Without a strong intrinsic reason for dancing, a dancer may also lose their individual identity and identify only as a dancer. If a dancer faces an injury that prevents them from dancing for an extended period, this loss of the individual outside of dance can create a rude awakening. With so much at stake, a collegiate dancer may not slow down or consider carefully enough opportunities to audition or join a dance ensemble. Unfortunately, this mentality of *Push, no matter what* can have significant physical and mental consequences. Thus, the intertwined nature of a dancer's identity, career, and motivation requires that successful treatment of any injury include the entire dancer and their environment; in other words, it must consider whole-person wellness.

University Dance Training

The life of a university dance student is multifaceted. While other students may be going to class, doing homework, and enjoying social time, a dancer also spends endless hours in the studio preparing for their next performance. Dancers are notorious for not saying no to an opportunity that comes their way. With the burden of academics, training, working, and multiple performance opportunities on and off campus, downtime is rare for a dancer in college. Being a dance major is challenging; it can feel like being in a pressure cooker for the duration of the program. The intensity of dance training, along with the academic work both inside and outside the dance department, is at a higher level than what a dancer will experience outside of college. In addition, dancers in a collegiate dance program may not have much choice regarding types of choreography, technique styles, and approaches to dance.

After completing their university training, dancers are free to explore the real world. At this stage, they can be more selective; they can gravitate toward the type of work, choreographers, and physical demands that best serve not only their artistry but also their body. If you are a dancer in the university setting, focus not only on the work you are doing now but also keep your eyes on the big picture: life after college. As demonstrated in figure 1.3, the artistic, environmental, and technical demands can vary depending on the project and this will continue as you pursue your career. Having this balanced outlook is extremely important in helping you get through this intense time.

The high intensity of a collegiate dance program can lead to many positive outcomes; however, if pushed to the breaking point in college, a dancer's career can end before it ever starts. You only have one body; it must last not only for the duration of your dance career but for your entire life! When a string breaks on a cello, a musician can quickly replace it and keep playing without affecting their own body; however, a dancer cannot quickly replace an injured muscle, tendon, or bone and simply move on without consequence. In the collegiate setting, it is important to pace yourself, find safe ways to supplement your training with conditioning techniques, and become educated about your body. This advice is not a justification for laziness or for giving less than your best effort. Rather, it is a recommendation to establish a process of using your intelligence, respecting your limits, and applying careful planning to ensure that you are able to dance as well as possible for as long as possible. Knowledge allows for ownership of what is going on in your body and the ability to find the help you need. Securing credible health and wellness information, finding a reliable network of health

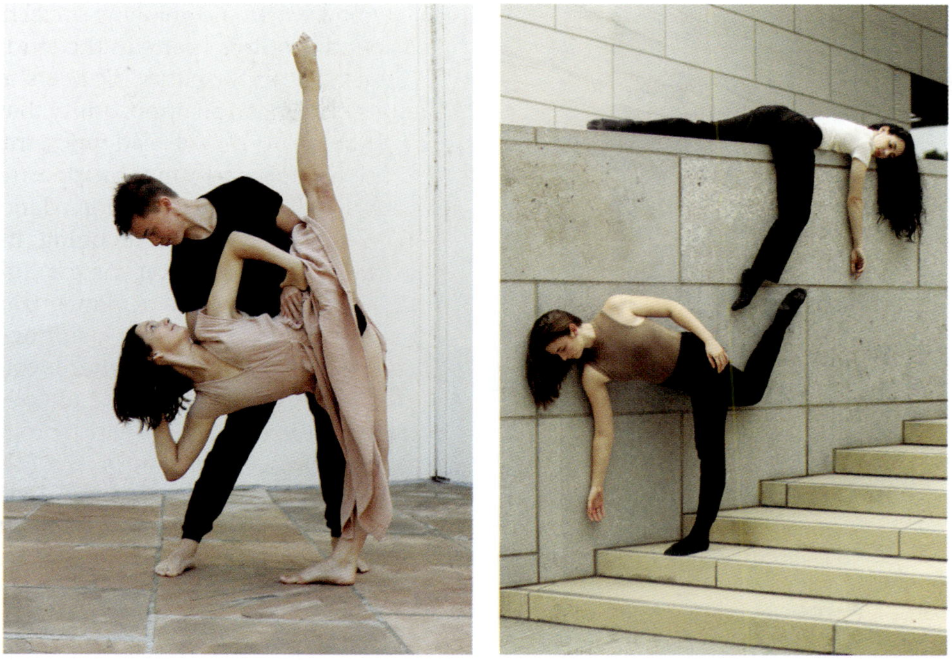

Figure 1.3 Modern dance, a common genre of dance in university dance departments, requires a well-trained set of multidimensional capacities that are suitable to its demands.

(a) Azuki Umeda ; *(b)* Jericho Trim

care providers, and maintaining a healthy mindset that is focused on whole-person wellness support the primary purpose of this textbook: to equip you for longevity as a dancer.

Wellness Mindset

Dancers are in a unique position as artists because their own bodies are their primary tools for expression. Therefore, injuries to their bodies affect both art and life. Unfortunately, sometimes the opportunity to perform overrides their instincts for self-preservation. Dancers tend to hold the mindset that they will have a short career because their bodies will give out sometime in their twenties. This assumption creates an attitude of dancing all out and at all costs; they know they cannot dance forever, and they are satisfied (at least at the moment) to deal with the repercussions later when their body suffers the consequences. The demands of various dance genres create increased injury risks such as those in the hip-hop dancer depicted in figure 1.4. (A more in-depth review of injuries in different genres is presented in chapter 2.) Although a dance career does require dedication and a certain amount of sacrifice, it does not require taking a fatalistic approach; a preferable strategy is to adopt a wellness mindset. This mindset assumes a more positive, caring relationship with the body, and it may reduce or prevent the regret that often results from deciding to pay a high price now and deal with the aftermath later.

A wellness mindset is essential to the longevity of every dancer no matter what dance style or career path they choose. Nevertheless, it is common for all dancers to experience the following thoughts—which are counter to this mindset—at some point in time:

- *If I slow down, I might miss an opportunity.*
- *If I get injured, someone else will seize the opportunity to take my place.*
- *I need to do this now because my body won't last forever, and a dance career is short.*
- *If I let anyone know I am in pain, I will be seen as weak.*
- *Dancing with an injury is like a badge of honor.*
- *If my choreographer knows I have an injury, they won't want to keep working with me.*
- *I'll take care of myself at the next break.*
- *I am in pain, but it isn't an injury.*
- *My choreographer/director/teacher said I am exaggerating, and I need to keep performing so I don't let everyone down.*

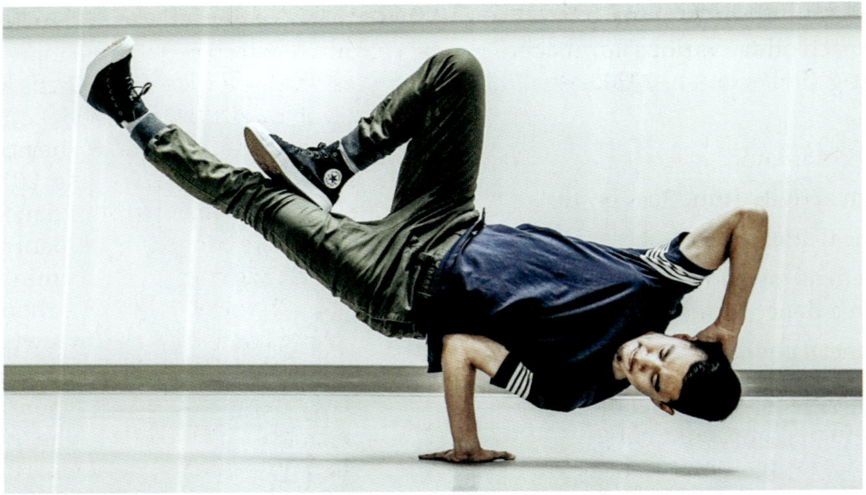

Figure 1.4 The unique, freestyle nature of hip-hop and its urban or street performance setting present challenges to maintaining wellness and to accessing health care if an injury occurs.

Megan Kyle Allen

In addition to having these thoughts, many dancers may have had difficulty working with medical professionals. Chapter 15 offers an overview of the medical profession and how to get along with its practitioners, but for now we will acknowledge that prior adverse experiences negatively affect a dancer's motivation to obtain appropriate health care. Do any of the following statements sound familiar?

- *My doctor said, "Just stop dancing and rest." That wasn't really an option, so I kept dancing.*
- *I have tried physical therapy, but they just didn't understand what I needed my body to be able to do.*
- *No one can give me a real reason for my pain, so it must not be an injury.*
- *I don't understand why they keep giving me exercises to do. I just need someone to fix what is hurting.*

Dealing with pain or injury is not enjoyable; it can be annoying, distracting, or worse. However, pretending the pain or injury doesn't exist can be harmful. This response risks cutting your career short, and it potentially increases the complications from whatever your condition may be. This book addresses many helpful methods of reducing the risks of dance injuries, and it offers a comprehensive understanding of injuries and their management. Educating yourself about your body, how to keep it well, and how to deal with injuries will help you find your voice to advocate for yourself.

Some of the statements listed previously exemplify how dancers struggle with speaking up about their needs to choreographers, directors, and teachers out of fear of negative consequences. They reinforce common narratives such as *No pain, no gain*; *You are choosing to be a starving artist*; *If you are not hurting, you don't want it enough*; and *You must sacrifice for your art*. All dancers require a supportive environment, and all dancers deserve clear communication that balances both artistic and medical needs. When this type of environment is available to dancers, the narratives change, becoming more consistent with a wellness mindset.

Dance Injuries

The idea of inherent risk and the complex nature of an injury are big challenges in dance; however, defining the term *injury* is an even bigger, if more basic, challenge. What exactly is a dance injury? Epidemiological studies use definitions based on research guidelines. The International Association for Dance Medicine & Science (IADMS) Standard Measures Consensus Initiative recommends that the concept of *time loss* be part of the definition of injury (Liederbach et al., 2012). Therefore, an injury is said to occur when a dancer is unable to participate in dance; in other words, when dancing time is lost, it is clear that an injury has occurred. For example, one could say that a dancer does not sustain an injury unless they miss at least one day of class, rehearsal, or performance after the incident that created the injury (Liederbach et al., 2008; Liederbach et al., 2012). Using a specific definition in this way is beneficial when data are compared among different research studies. Unfortunately, however, most studies apply definitions of injury that are not consistent with each other. Various approaches include the following (Fuller et al., 2020; Allen et al., 2014):

- Any physical complaint
- Time lost from activity (time-loss injury)
- Seeking medical attention
- Visiting a medical provider and having an entry made in a dancer's medical record
- Making a financial payment for receiving care

Different definitions of injury influence the rates and estimations of injury burden among dancers (Kenny et al., 2017). Consider the situation of using time loss as the basis, where an injury is said to occur only if a dancer misses one or more days of dance activity after the day the injury occurred. If a dancer sustained a painful episode on Monday, but that dancer is dancing in classes and rehearsals on Tuesday, one presumes that no injury occurred, even though pain was felt and the dancer had to stop participating on Monday. It is clear, then, that this type of definition has constraints. The other definitions of injury shown above likewise have deficiencies.

A more comprehensive definition of injury that includes pain and performance limitations might be more useful, allowing for early detection of health problems and potential injuries (Bronner & Wood, 2017; Lee et al., 2017). The Oslo Sports Trauma Research Center Questionnaire (OSTRCQ; Clarsen et al., 2013; Clarsen et al., 2014) allows monitoring of multiple outcomes, such as pain, performance limitation, and training modification, thus providing a comprehensive view of health problems. In addition, the OSTRCQ can be applied to monitor dancers' health progressively in time (van Seters et al., 2020). Applying some of the constructs of the OSTRCQ, such as dance performance and pain, presents an opportunity for early recognition of potential injuries.

Another injury definition might rely on whether or not a dancer visited a health care professional for care (Anand Prakash, 2017). In this instance, an injury will not be counted unless a health care visit is undertaken. However, what if a dancer does not report pain and reduced function to anyone? What if a dancer refuses to go to a medical professional even if it is obvious that they should? When you consider the gamut of perspectives and experiences of dancers, *injury* is not a clear-cut concept; it can assume different meanings.

Professional dancers present an especially wide spectrum for which to define an injury (Bolling et al., 2021), as do elite athletes and circus artists (Bolling, Barboza, et al., 2019; Bolling, Mellette, et al., 2019). Previous studies also describe the normalization of pain in dance (McEwen & Young, 2011) by identifying the idea that pain is part of a dancer's life. Injury is, in this sense, a context-dependent concept, which should be considered when examining injury risk.

It is clear that when thinking about reducing the risk of injury, context determines what is perceived as an injury. For example, a young dance student may sense a painful condition differently than a professional dancer would, even if the two cases exhibit the same **signs** and **symptoms**. The context also dictates the variety of risk factors and the dynamic relationships between such factors. Once again, the importance of understanding a whole-person, multidimensional view of wellness is evident. Many factors, including different dance styles or genres; different footwear, wardrobes, and facilities; different abilities and levels; different organizations, schools, and policies; and different teachers must be considered in understanding injuries. In addition, these factors should be viewed as variables that can contribute to injuries or to reduction in injury risk. Bolling and colleagues (2018) illustrate this idea of context in the socioecological framework depicted in figure 1.5. In this model, the injured dancer is at center stage, and the context around the dancer

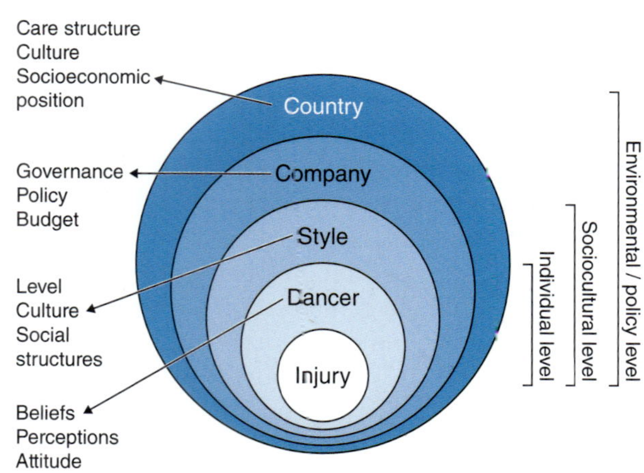

Figure 1.5 Dance injury as represented in the socio-ecological framework.

creates dynamic relationships between physical, biological, sociocultural, environmental, political or organizational, and other aspects. It is necessary to adopt a solid understanding of the dance context and injuries as complex phenomena before developing strategies to reduce the risk of dance injuries.

Prevalence of Dance Injuries

Because dance has high physical demands, dancers are sometimes compared to high-performance athletes. In addition to being athletes, dancers are performers, artists, and workers (in the case of professional dance). Dancers' injuries have a high **incidence** and **prevalence** (Jacobs et al., 2012; Kenny et al., 2016; Allen et al., 2014). Injury details can be reported in studies in a number of ways, including incidence, prevalence, injuries per dancer, or total number of injuries (Allen et al., 2014). For example, based on a systematic review (Hincapié et al., 2008), lifetime prevalence estimates for injury (the percentage of dancers affected by injury sometime in their lifetime) in professional ballet dancers ranged between 40 percent and 84 percent, while the point prevalence of minor injury (the percentage of dancers affected by injury at one point in time) in a diverse group of university and professional ballet and modern dancers was 74 percent (Jacobs et al., 2012). However, those numbers arguably are underestimated (Kenny et al., 2016).

At the time of this book's publication, the majority of available dance injury studies are related to ballet and modern or contemporary dance. Studies about other dance styles are limited, although they are increasing in number (many of these are discussed in the next chapter). The results of a systematic review show that compared with preprofessional ballet dancers, professional ballet dancers have largely similar injury patterns, with foot and ankle and spinal pathologies being predominant (Smith et al., 2016). In general, most dancers' injuries are mild or minor, and they require minimal time off (Jacobs et al., 2012). Occasionally, however, they can have a huge effect on a dancer's life. Depending on their severity, they can interrupt a class, a season, or an entire career. More than time off, it is already clear how significant injuries can affect a dancer's life in different ways, with consequences extending across the dimensions of wellness.

Dance Injury Risk

A fundamental truth about dance is that risk of injury is part of participating. In other words, if you dance, you risk getting injured. From an epidemiological perspective, when a dancer dances, there is an exposure to injury; with that exposure comes risk. For example, if you cross the street, there is a risk that you will be run over by a car. You are exposed to injury potential as soon as you place a foot on the street. Of course, you can create strategies to reduce the chance of being run over. You can respect the traffic lights, use the crosswalk, look before you cross, and so on. All of these methods reduce the risk of an accident. However, even if you follow your strategies to reduce the risk, the risk still exists because of the exposure. The fact that you cross the street creates the possibility that you will be hit by a vehicle even if you take precautions.

In the same way, dancing comes with a risk of injury. If you dance more, you are exposed to risk more often; consequently, you might sustain more injuries. To frame this risk, some research studies use number of injuries per 1,000 hours of dancing to link injury occurrence to amount of exposure. Given that dancing means putting yourself at risk, the best way to avoid injuries is to not dance at all, which brings your exposure to zero and therefore eliminates the risk. Of course, not dancing is an impossible option for a dancer! However, you can find and use strategies to reduce the risk of injuries while you dance, just as you do when you cross the street. Many of these strategies are presented throughout this book.

Risk Reduction Versus Injury Prevention

The idea of **risk reduction** (decreasing the likelihood of a problem by altering risk factors) is not new, but the concept of **prevention** (creating prophylaxis or safeguards to keep a problem from happening) has an ancient origin. The old saying *An ounce of prevention is worth a pound of cure* was first recorded in Latin in Henry de Bracton's *De Legibus et consuetudinibus Angliae* [The Laws and Customs of England] in about 1240 (Ammer, 2003). The simple concept behind this axiom is to avoid a problem before it happens. Today, preventive health care has innumerable measures that exemplify this principle, such as using condoms to reduce risk of contracting sexually transmitted diseases, increasing physical activity to prevent obesity, or wearing a lead apron when undergoing an X-ray to prevent the negative effects of radiation exposure. When applying this concept to dance, you may wonder what strategies function effectively as the ounce of prevention—a good diet, enough sleep, or a proper warm-up? In actuality, a focus on reducing risk is more beneficial overall.

Scientific literature has long focused on prevention of injuries. Sports medicine has actively evolved the concept of injury prevention for more than 20 years, while dance medicine has been following a similar path, albeit for a shorter period of time. Traditionally, sport injury prevention approaches have followed the sequence of prevention, which was originally proposed by van Mechelen and colleagues (1992). This four-step model uses systematic logic, moving from injury problem assessment to the design of an evidence-based solution for preventing injuries (figure 1.6).

The first step aims to describe the extent of the injury problem, and the second step aims to investigate etiological factors and injury mechanisms (the way an injury occurs). The goal of the third step is to develop science-informed injury prevention measures, and the fourth step assesses whether the developed measures actually work to solve the problem. This four-step framework has guided research and practice toward injury prevention strategies since it was first proposed. The model has also been applied to dance injury prevention where many studies describe injury incidence (Allen et al., 2013; Hincapié et al., 2008; Lee et al., 2017), risk factors (Kenny et al., 2016; Biernacki et al., 2018; van Seters et al., 2020), preventive interventions (Allen et al., 2013; Vera et al., 2020), and outcomes regarding injury reduction (Fuller et al., 2020; Ojofeitimi & Bronner, 2011; Vera et al., 2020).

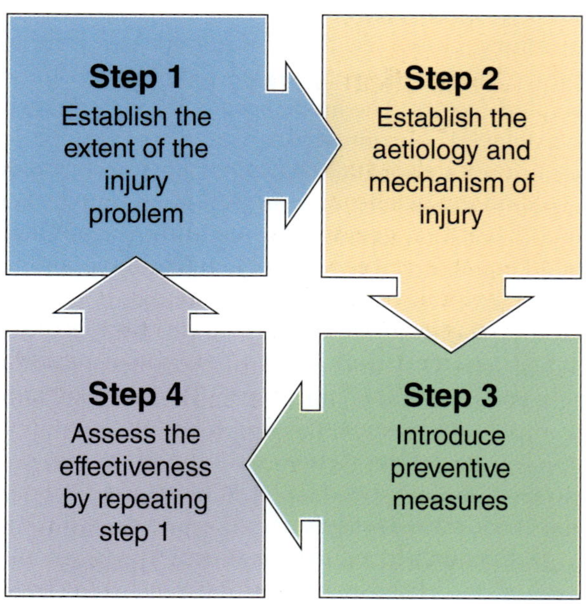

Figure 1.6 The sequence of prevention of sport injuries.

Reprinted by permission from C. Bolling, W. van Mechelen, H.R. Pasman, and E. Verhagen, "Context Matters: Revisiting the First Step of the 'Sequence of Prevention' of Sports Injuries," *Sports Medicine* 48, no. 10 (2018): 2227-2234. https://doi.org/10.1007/s40279-018-0953-x. Distributed under the terms of the Creative Commons CC BY License (https://creativecommons.org/licenses/by/4.0/).

Despite the attention given to prevention and its common usage as a term, all possible safeguards—except for not participating in dance at all—are unlikely to help you avoid every injury. On the other hand, reducing the risk of dance injuries, and therefore their frequency, is possible, even though this is a relatively new topic in dance science. Keep in mind, however, that research evidence of efficacy of a risk reducing measure does not necessarily equal effectiveness in practice or effective implementation (Finch & Donaldson, 2010). In other words, the fact that something works under ideal conditions in a controlled study does not mean it has the same effect in the real world.

To account for this, implementation of evidence has been presented as a key process to bring controlled research findings into actual practice (McGlashan & Finch, 2010; O'Brien et al., 2016). Finch (2006) proposed the TRIPP (translating research into injury prevention practice) model, which added two steps to the sequence of prevention model. These two additional steps are related to (1) the understanding of the implementation context and (2) the evaluation of the implementation process of preventive measures; these provide an improved framework for reducing injury risk.

All current studies that present the concept of injury prevention and its challenges are theoretically trying to reduce injury risk. Once again, we assert that prevention is not the ideal term when discussing dance injuries because the word implies that there is a complete avoidance of injuries. Clearly this is not feasible. Consider the concept of exposure discussed earlier. In actuality, the main idea behind so-called preventive measures is to reduce the risk of injury occurrence, even though it is not possible to completely avoid sustaining all injuries. The primary reason for this is exposure; participating in dancing is associated with inherent injury risk. This explains why the phrase injury risk reduction is more accurate than injury prevention.

Considering this information, the best plan for you as a dancer is to continue dancing while simultaneously reducing your risk of injuries. To do so, you must know about likely injuries and their potential causes, as outlined by van Mechelen's sequence of prevention. The next challenge is knowing how to measure dance injuries and how to explore the causes of these injuries.

Research Into Practice

When examining injury prevention research to reduce ankle sprains, evidence shows that introducing neuromuscular exercises into training helps reduce the risk of reinjury (Vriend et al., 2016). To build this type of evidence, researchers provided participants who had prior ankle sprains with neuromuscular training in a controlled environment (regular training sessions with supervision) during a specific period, while another group of participants did not receive exercises. The researchers then measured the number of injuries sustained by participants in both groups. The group that performed exercises had significantly fewer injuries, thus making it reasonable to conclude that the intervention of providing exercises was effective at reducing risk of reinjury in individuals who sustain an ankle sprain.

However, when this intervention is applied in a real-world environment (without regular exercise sessions and supervision by researchers), most people do not perform the exercises correctly nor do they modify the exercises according to their ability level and rehabilitation progress. Therefore, an implementation strategy is needed to ensure that the intervention shown to be effective in a research setting will also be effective in a specific real-world context.

Such an approach needs to follow the two additional steps of the TRIPP model, considering the implementation context and evaluating the implementation process. For example, some researchers have developed different ways to deliver exercises, such as preparing booklets, videos, and mobile phone apps to guide their participants (Vriend et al., 2015). Then researchers evaluate the processes of how the exercise-based measures are delivered along with how the participants implement the instructional materials to determine whether participants benefited and risk of reinjury truly was reduced.

This book presents common dance injuries and the factors that contribute to them. However, dance injuries have multiple components, and they are dynamic. Even with a broad description of risk factors or injury mechanisms, one will never be able to completely explain injury occurrence. To understand that limitation, it is necessary to examine the complexity of dance injuries. Assuming that an injury is complex, Bittencourt and colleagues (2016) imply acceptance of the unpredictability of injuries. Injuries cannot be seen as isolated events. Every injury is unique and complex (Bekker & Clark, 2016; Hulme et al., 2018). A combination of many injury risk factors of different levels, interacting in a dynamic arrangement, is what leads to injury. Sometimes, present circumstances are similar to those associated with a prior injury, but an injury will not occur because of the emergence of a new factor. Again, it may not be possible to predict an injury, but an injury's underlying risk factors and the interrelated aspects of the event that caused it can eventually be uncovered.

Risk Factors and Reducing Injury Risk

Another reason why it is preferable to focus on reducing injury risk versus injury prevention is because it typically addresses a broader set of variables. To reduce your risk of injury as a dancer, you must recognize potential risk factors. For example, demi-pointe is a position of the ankle and foot that can lead to an ankle sprain. Performing on an uneven floor surface may also contribute to such an injury. However, to truly understand how to reduce injury risk, you need to look beyond these isolated factors. The ankle sprain could be related to a delayed neuromuscular response of your body because of a poor night's sleep. Using an old pair of pointe shoes because you forgot yours that day or did not have enough money to buy new ones could also contribute to such an injury. In addition, those factors may interact with considerations such as being in the demi-pointe position, fatigue at the end of rehearsal, and a lack of focus because of a fight you had with your friend the night before. This example underscores the complexity of any injury scenario, its dynamic interactions, and its equifinality (the same outcome from different paths). Notice that it also integrates with the understanding of multidimensional holistic wellness. Therefore, the goal is to try to reduce the risk of injury to the extent possible by mitigating as many factors as you can.

In light of the discussion so far, dance injury prevention sounds impossible—and it is! As mentioned in the previous section, in the pure sense of preventing (completely avoiding) injuries, you are powerless. However, you can manage the risk to which you are exposed, and that task is fully within your power. You can reduce risk by knowing the main factors related to injuries and how to control them. This topic is the heart of reducing the risk of injury in dance, and it is explored across dance genres in chapter 2.

Ultimately, strategies that are incorporated as preventive measures in dance have as their end goal to modulate injury risk factors. Demographic, biomechanical, and environmental risk factors have been identified in different dance settings and at different levels (Hincapié et al., 2008; Kenny et al., 2016; Russell, 2013; van Seters et al., 2020). Some risk factors presented in the literature are age, sex, years of dance experience, performance level, style of dance, hours of training each day, dance setting (e.g., performance, rehearsal, dance class), prior injury, personality traits, work dissatisfaction, menstrual dysfunction, muscular tension before performing, joint hypermobility, sensorimotor control, choreography demands, stretching and flexibility training, and performing on a raked or angled stage (Hincapié et al., 2008). Overall, these reported associations are preliminary in nature. Psychosocial and psychological issues such as stress and coping strategies also have been described as factors that affect injury frequency and duration (Hincapié et al., 2008; Jacobs et al., 2012). Overall, scientific literature reviews suggest inconclusive or divergent results, which brings into question the quality of research evidence regarding dance injury risk factors (Hincapié et al., 2008; Kenny et al., 2016). Chapter 3 provides an excellent opportunity for you to learn to interact effectively with scientific research—to become a consumer of science and an applier of that science to your artistic endeavors with the goal of keeping your risk of injury as low as possible.

Many risk factors, such as age, are not modifiable. Other risk factors can be modulated; to some extent, they can also reduce the risk of injury. Some studies report reductions in dance injuries over time (Allen et al., 2013; Bronner et al., 2003; Ojofeitimi & Bronner, 2011; Vera et al., 2020). Most of the strategies center on altering a dancer's individual risk factors, mostly through exercise-based interventions. Several of these strategies are presented in subsequent chapters.

However, when observing the big picture of injury through holistic and socioecological frameworks as presented earlier, injury risk reduction should extend beyond an individual dancer. Contemporary studies in sports medicine show that leadership, communication, and teamwork all are essential to reducing the risk of injuries (Ekstrand et al., 2019; Ekstrand et al., 2018; King et al., 2018). Considering this finding, a dancer cannot be the only one responsible to mitigate the risk of their injuries; it is a shared responsibility where a variety of stakeholders play an active part.

For example, if you experience pain or discomfort as a dancer, you should report your symptoms and request rest or health care attention before the situation worsens and an injury takes hold. Appropriate care is likely to minimize or eliminate your time loss while decreasing the likelihood that the problem will continue. However, to increase the odds that you will report your pain, you understandably want verification that open and trustworthy communication among faculty, staff, and dancers is well established. Consider the concept of the wellness mindset introduced earlier in this chapter. It would be most helpful to everyone involved if university dance departments, conservatory training programs, professional dance companies, and even summer intensives adopted this mindset alongside individual dancers.

Broadly, injury risk reduction should not be restricted only to stakeholders who deal directly with artists. Multiple individuals and departments can influence risk factors because of the interconnectedness and complexities of dance injuries. For example, in a study with artists from Cirque du Soleil, Bolling and colleagues (Bolling, Mellette, et al., 2019) identified a wide variety of actors and other professionals who were related to the company's artists and their injury occurrences; they are depicted in figure 1.7. Although it is a large, international, professional artistic company, the principle still applies in a university setting. Many of the individuals and groups shown in levels A through D are also integral to universities' dance productions. The potential impact (either positive or negative) of a wide swath of a university on the well-being of the institution's dancers is striking. Influencing factors can include nutrition, food quality, and food safety in dining halls; facility maintenance and cleanliness, including inhibition of potential infections in dance studios (Unsworth & Russell, 2013); the accessibility of student services, especially those related to physical health, mental health, and transportation; environmental control; public safety; and generally proactive attention to a variety of health and safety-related campus concerns.

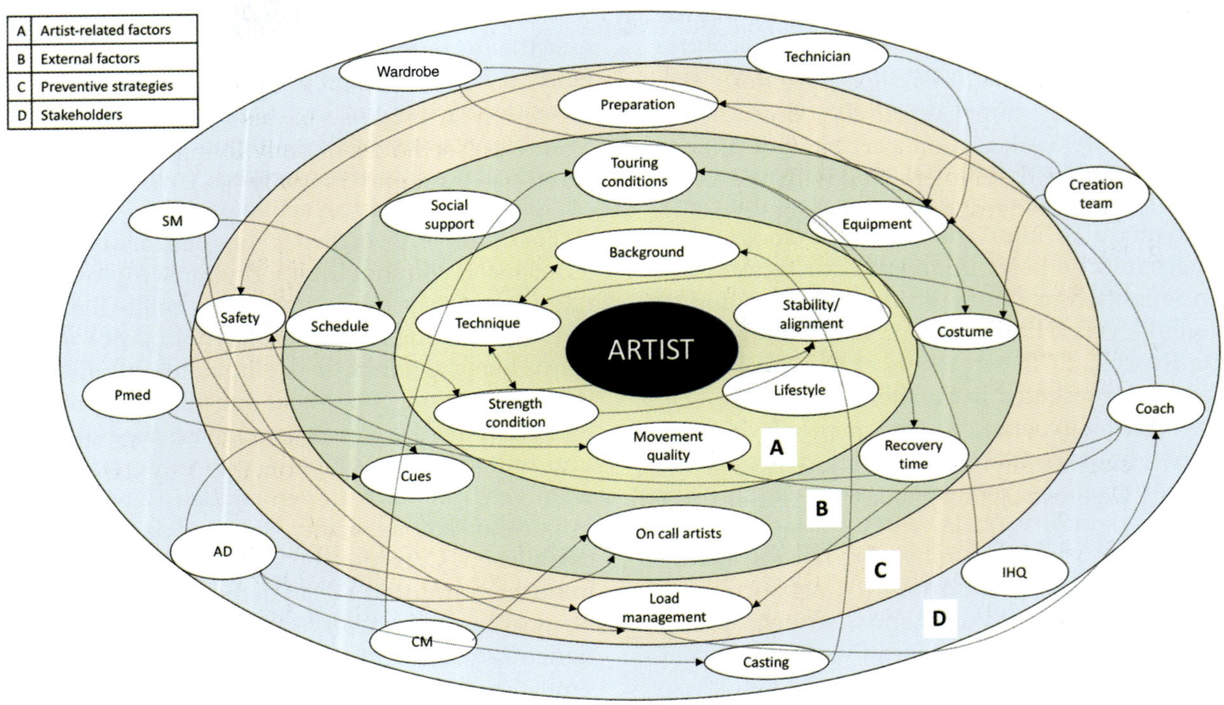

Figure 1.7 A multilevel system map with factors, strategies, and stakeholders in relation to injuries and their prevention. Starting at the center of the map (the artist) and moving outward, circle A entails artist-related intrinsic injury factors; circle B presents external injury factors; circle C describes the main preventive strategies (e.g., load management, safety, and preparation), which are driven by the factors from the inner two circles; and circle D represents the stakeholders in the system as well as how they connect to the strategies and factors across the multiple levels. (SM: Stage Management; Pmed: Performance Medicine; AD: Artistic Director; CM: Company Manager; IHQ: International Headquarters of Cirque du Soleil).

Reprinted by permission from C. Bolling, J. Mellette, H.R. Pasman, W. van Mechelen, and E. Verhagen, "From the Safety Net to the Injury Prevention Web: Applying Systems Thinking to Unravel Injury Prevention Challenges and Opportunities in Cirque du Soleil," *BMJ Open Sport and Exercise Medicine* 5, no. 1 (2019b); e000492, with permission from BMJ Publishing Group Ltd. https://doi.org/10.1136/bmjsem-2018-000492.

Conclusions and Practical Relevance

Dance is a multifaceted, highly physical artistic activity. Dancers are talented, driven, and reticent to stop or even slow their pursuit of their art form. No isolated approach, limited view of health, or simplistic paradigm can possibly be enough to understand and deal with dance injuries or with the efforts to reduce the risk of injury. Chapter 2 will present a matrix to also illustrate this approach considering not only physical factors, but also emotional, cognitive, social, and environmental factors, including their potential negative and positive effects. With the ultimate goal of keeping dancers dancing—and keeping them optimally well across all of their dimensions in the process—only a holistic (whole-person) view of these artists can enable understanding of the totality of each dancer and dance environment. This approach underscores the complexity and unique challenge of attaining wellness and injury risk reduction. When dancers and those who work with them (influencing them either directly or indirectly) mutually achieve this goal, the art form is elevated and the ability of dance to interact with and affect society is maximized.

Discussion Questions

1. To what extent have you previously considered your life as a dancer to be composed of multiple dimensions? How does each of the six dimensions outlined in this chapter inform your work as a dancer? How do they inform your other activities of daily living? How do you see them interacting with one another as you move through your daily life (as a dancer and in the rest of your activities)?
2. Describe some situations where you (or a dancer you know) experienced an injury and that physical circumstance affected other dimensions of your (or their) wellness. In what ways were you (or they) able to manage the situation effectively? In what ways did the situation create difficulties? How could you (or they) have handled it better by incorporating the six dimensions of wellness?
3. Consider what motivates you to continue to train and pursue a career in dance. Are you extrinsically or intrinsically driven? What are the factors that take away from the joy of dance? Do these factors increase your daily stress?
4. Take a moment to recognize how you define yourself and your life. If you couldn't dance for an extended period, what does your human, nondancer identity look like? Can you define yourself, your activities, and how you interact with the world without dance as part of that definition?
5. Consider the inherent risk of injury of any dance-related activity. Try to think beyond the within-dancer factors. What is around you that can play a role in injury occurrence?
6. As proposed in this chapter, injury risk management should be part of the daily life of dancers and anyone working with them. How would you in your role (as a dancer, teacher, choreographer, health care professional) reduce dance injury risk in your practice? Which measures will be most helpful to mitigate injury risk?

WWW Go to HK*Propel* to access supplemental information and activities connected to chapter content.

2

Injuries Across Dance Genres

Róisín Cahalan, PhD, PT
Kelli Sharp, DPT
Rose Schmieg, DHSc, PT, ATC, CISSN, CSCS

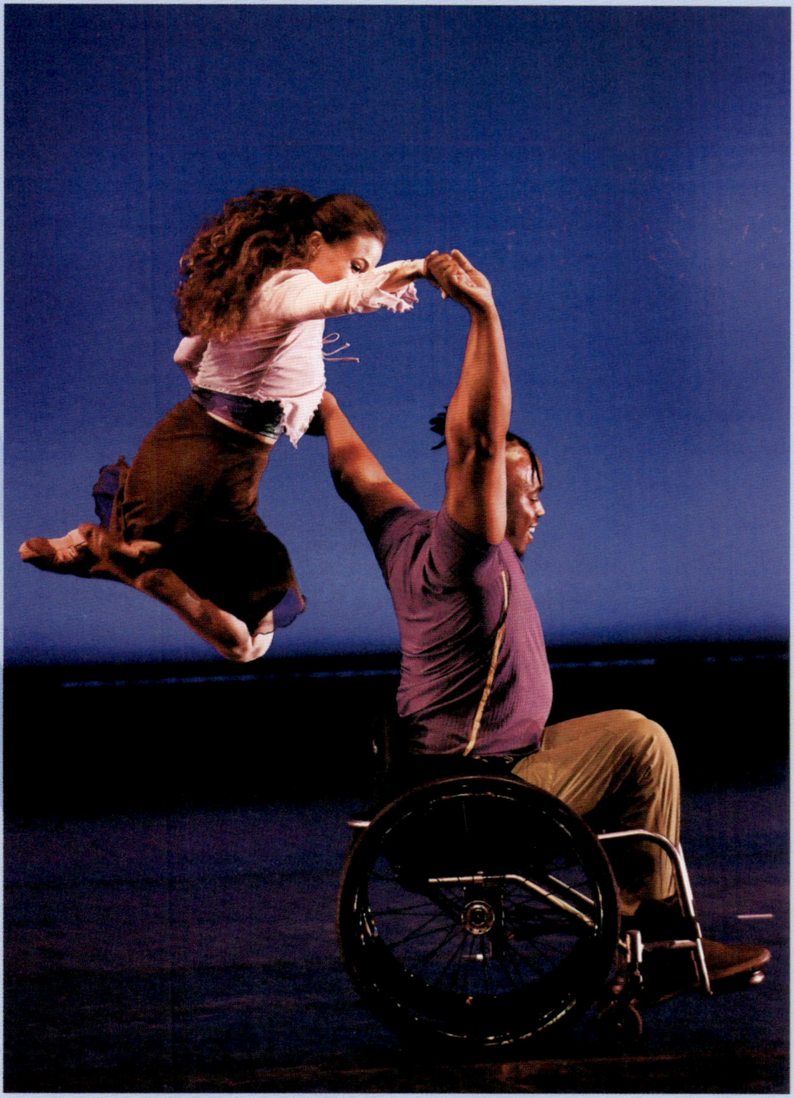

Stand-up dancer Celina Naima Speck and sit-down down dancer DeMarco Sleeper of the Dancing Wheels Company partner in a duet from "An Ella Encounter," choreographed by Laura Ann Smyth. Photo: Mark Horning (2023). Photo courtesy Dancing Wheels Company & School, Cleveland, Ohio, Mary Verdi-Fletcher, Artistic Director.

Key Terms

- aerobic
- amenorrhea
- anaerobic
- bone mineral density
- catastrophizing
- cross-training
- dysmenorrhea
- genotype
- in vivo
- lumbopelvic
- mechanism of injury (MOI)
- menarche
- motor control
- periodization
- plyometrics
- rating of perceived exertion (RPE)
- restorative sleep

Dance has a multitude of genres, each with its own interesting movements, music, and physicality. Until recently, most research was focused on ballet and modern dance with a smattering of studies on other styles. However, that trend has been changing quickly, and this chapter reflects that change. Thus, the chapter will acquaint you with dance injuries in general while also providing a breadth of available information about injuries in different styles of dance.

LEARNING OBJECTIVES

After completing this chapter, you will be able to do the following:

- Describe a dance injury in terms of medical attention and time loss from class, rehearsal, or performance.
- Classify dance injuries as acute, chronic recurring, or chronic overuse.
- Describe dance injury risks through the lens of the biopsychosocial approach using the Cahalan-Schmieg-Sharp injury risk model.
- Differentiate between modifiable and nonmodifiable dance injury risk factors.
- Apply the Cahalan-Schmieg-Sharp injury risk model to the landscape and injury profile of the various dance genres.

The majority of scientific evidence on dance injuries began with a focus on ballet and then modern dance. For many years, those two dance genres received virtually all the research attention devoted to understanding mechanisms, risk factors, and prevention strategies for injuries in dance. However, since the decade of the 2010s, research has become more inclusive of many different dance genres, implementing more complex investigations to further elucidate the various intricacies of injuries in these genres. You have probably participated in more than just one genre of dance. This chapter teaches you about the multifaceted factors of dance injuries, which affect genres of dance that are familiar to you as well as some you may have yet to try.

What Is Injury?

Dance injuries are best classified in terms of medical attention and time loss (Liederbach et al., 2012). In the sports medicine arena, a medical attention injury requires treatment by a team physician, whether or not time is lost from competition (Fuller et al., 2006). A medical attention injury for professional ballet and contemporary dancers has been defined as an anatomical tissue-level impairment that results in a dancer seeking care from a medical practitioner (Kenny et al., 2016). A sports time-loss injury has been defined as a loss in time from competition or training (Fuller et al., 2006). In dance, a time-loss injury results in a dancer not being able to complete a present or subsequent class, rehearsal, or performance 1 or more days beyond the day of the onset of injury (Kenny et al., 2016). A study on managing injury incidence and cost in a modern dance company defined injury as any physical insult that required financial outlay (workers compensation or self-insurance) or caused a dancer to cease dancing beyond the day of injury (a time-loss injury) (Ojofeitimi & Bronner, 2011). University dance programs and professional companies have a vested interest in tracking dance injuries along with surveying injury time loss. These data can be used for developing programs to reduce injury risk.

Dance injuries should also be classified in terms of severity. Orthopedic injuries are categorized as acute, chronic recurring, and chronic overuse (Knight, 2008), as shown in figure 2.1. Acute injuries are sudden in nature. They result from high-intensity external forces (e.g., a contact injury from a dancer colliding with a prop or another dancer) or high-intensity internal forces (e.g., a dancer landing a jump awkwardly that causes an ankle sprain).

A chronic recurring injury is an acute injury that happens more than once (usually several times). For example, chronic ankle instability (CAI) is a condition in which one has recurring ankle sprains after the first acute injury; this condition yields an inability of the ankle ligaments to properly stabilize the ankle joint. A study of university dance majors found that of 81 dancers surveyed, 41 (53.2%) had CAI (Simon et al., 2014). A chronic overuse injury differs from acute and recurring injuries in that the injury mechanism is usually of low intensity, and the symptoms may linger for a long duration (Knight, 2008). Tendinopathy of the flexor hallucis longus (FHL)—known as dancer's tendinopathy—is a chronic overuse injury of low force (the foot moves from the floor to demi-plié to pointe and back again) and high repetition (performing this movement in multiple classes and rehearsals daily) (Berglund, 2006).

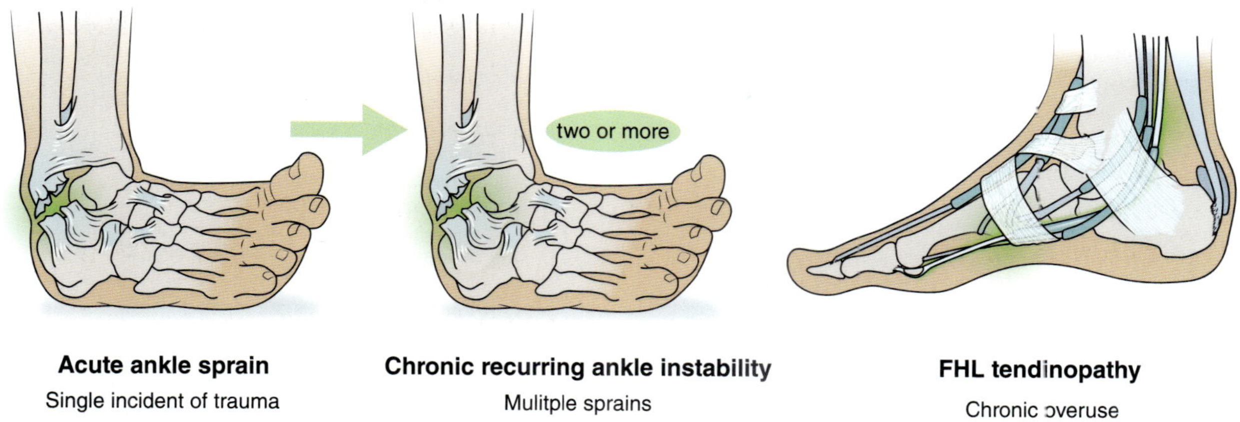

Figure 2.1 Different types of injuries have different characteristics. An acute injury may occur only once. However, an acute sprain (e.g., in the ankle) that occurs more than once becomes a chronic, recurring injury, usually with instability in the joint where the ligaments are located. Repeated activity while neglecting pain signals and appropriate care (e.g., in the flexor hallucis longus [FHL] tendon that controls flexion of the great toe) may lead to a chronic overuse injury.

Injury and Pain

The International Association for the Study of Pain defines pain as "an unpleasant sensory and emotional experience associated with, or resembling that associated with, actual or potential tissue damage" (Raja et al., 2020, p. 1980). Pain is always personal, and it is influenced to varying degrees by biopsychosocial—biological, psychological, and social—factors. In practice, this means that two dancers who sustain identical tissue damage from an ankle sprain could have two entirely different responses to the pain based on characteristics of their current life situations.

Imagine the various biopsychosocial factors involved in two dancers with this injury. Dancer 1 is in a professional ballet company and may fear losing a starring role; the injury may have financial implications. This dancer is part of a ballet culture that rewards a principal dancer who pushes through the pain. Dancer 2 is a first-year college student who has access to a physical therapist or athletic trainer for injury care. This dancer has support and communication with dance faculty to decrease workload, thus allowing the ankle to heal.

Dancers must separate injury pain from performance pain. A study on professional dancers found that dancers termed performance pain as *good pain* and injury pain as *bad pain* (Harrison & Ruddock-Hudson, 2017). In addition, dancers and athletes have been reported to have higher pain tolerance than nonathletes (Pettersen et al., 2020; Tajet-Foxell & Rose, 1995). It is imperative that dancers be well-educated about normal pain associated with intense training and about not crossing the line into pain that increases injury risk or suggests an injury is present.

Injury Risk Factors

Injury risk in dance is multidimensional; it has physical, emotional, cognitive, social, lifestyle, environmental, general health, and training aspects. A dancer should be educated, supported, and committed to improving modifiable risk factors. Studios, universities, and companies can minimize injury risk by providing safe instruction, safe choreography, and safe facilities.

When considering risk factors that may predispose a dancer to injury, an individualized approach is necessary. No two dancers are the same, and each will have a unique profile of modifiable and nonmodifiable traits that must be considered to ensure optimal resilience and performance (figure 2.2). Pain and injury in dance are occupational hazards, and sometimes even the most robust dancer can fall prey to bad luck or an accident. However, much can be done to anticipate and address potential areas of weakness and vulnerability in dancers. The Cahalan-Schmieg-Sharp model of injury risk draws on evidence from various genres of dance and sport, and it applies to a lesser or greater degree to all forms of dance. The model adopts a biopsychosocial approach to injury, and it explores the balance between the resilience and vulnerabilities of the dancer while considering modifiable, partially modifiable, and nonmodifiable factors.

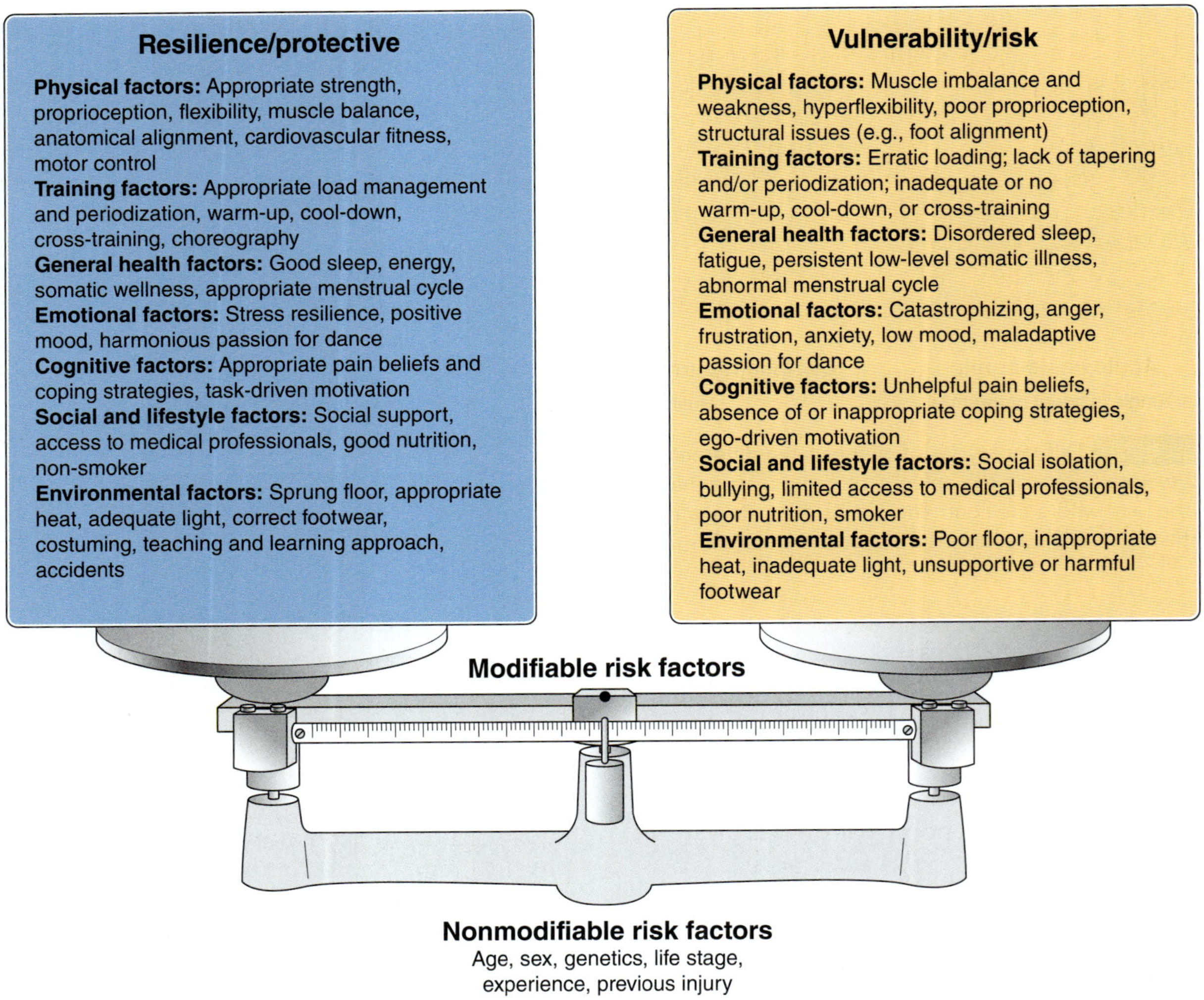

Figure 2.2 The Cahalan-Schmieg-Sharp model of injury risk. Modifiable risk factors on both sides of the balance must be carefully monitored and adjusted as necessary to reduce injury risk. At the same time, nonmodifiable risk factors affect a dancer's susceptibility to injury. The modifiable factors must be maintained optimally to counteract the factors that cannot be changed.

Adapted from R. Cahalan et al., *Complete Irish Dancer: Optimization of Health and Performance in Irish Dancers* (Hauppauge, NY: Nova Publishers, 2020).

Nonmodifiable Risk Factors

Nonmodifiable factors are intrinsic traits or characteristics that cannot be changed and which may increase the risk of injury at different stages or under various circumstances. For instance, previous injury—in particular, severe injury—is known to predispose dancers to future injury in many genres (van Rijn & Stubbe, 2021). Likewise, a dancer's sex may influence the nature and likelihood of injury, depending on the dance genre. For instance, some research suggests that elite male ballet dancers are more predisposed to back injury due to lifting and carrying a partner; however, this predisposition is not common to all dance genres (Wanke et al., 2013). Stage of life is another important and often transient risk factor that dancers and teachers must consider.

Adolescence, a maturational stage typically marked by rapid periods of physical growth and emotional change, has been associated with an increased risk of injury in many dance cohorts, including modern, ballet, jazz, and Irish dancing (Bowerman et al., 2014; Cahalan et al., 2018; Steinberg et al., 2011). The impact of menopause on bone health and muscle strength is a period of increased vulnerability (Rizzoli et al., 2014), and dancers should be particularly mindful of their health and well-being at this time. Nonetheless, the specific role of age is less clear; one study shows increased age to be associated with higher levels of injury in jazz and contemporary dance but not in classical ballet, folk dance, or tap (Soares Campoy et al., 2011). Some authors argue that the experience of older dancers leads to lower injury rates than in younger dancers, who may have lower pain thresholds and have less to lose than their older, more prolific counterparts (Novosel et al., 2019). However, this finding is not consistent; other research failed to find differences in injury rates across genres among elite student, recreational, and professional dancers (Vassallo et al., 2019).

Finally, a dancer's genetic composition may work either for or against them. For instance, research in ballet has found that **genotype** is associated with flexibility, body composition, and performance capacity. Given that dance is an aesthetic pursuit, one's inherent musculoskeletal structure (including factors such as bony alignment, height, collagen protein distribution, and so on) may impact the potential of the dancer as a performer and their possible predisposition to injury. As an example, joint hypermobility syndrome, a strongly genetically mediated condition, allows for flexibility and range of motion inherent in many genres, but is also associated with a high incidence of injury in dancers with this condition (Armstrong & Greig, 2018).

Modifiable Risk Factors

Modifiable risk factors are aspects of the dancer and dance environment that one can change (at least partially), depending on the circumstances. As such, it is often possible to turn a perceived weakness into a helpful strength by applying appropriate knowledge and interventions.

Physical Factors

Much of the existing research in dance medicine explores the physical characteristics of the dancer, including strength, flexibility, balance, cardiovascular fitness, and motor control. All of these characteristics are key components of robust dancer screening programs (Southwick & Crupi, 2017). Intuitively, these elements are understood to be very important; it may be challenging to effectively execute certain dance steps without addressing the requirements of these factors. However, the extent to which they affect different dance genres may vary. For example, flexibility and range of motion are fundamentally important to ballet choreography. A systematic review of risk factors for injury in the lower limb of elite and recreational ballet dancers identified a plethora of associated issues, including poor **lumbopelvic** control, decreased muscle strength (especially in the lower limbs), suboptimal **aerobic** fitness, and hypermobility at the hip and ankle (Biernacki et al., 2021).

Greater functional hip turnout has been identified as an issue in ballet (Armstrong & Greig, 2018), thus indicating the importance of motor control coupled with flexibility in this genre. Hypermobility also is a risk factor for injury in modern dancers, and likewise for limited flexibility and muscle tightness (Bronner & Bauer, 2018), despite the research about this being inconsistent (van Rijn & Stubbe, 2021). A study of factors screened by dance companies and dance schools showed that while flexibility was measured by over 95 percent of institutions, cardiovascular fitness was assessed by only 21 percent (Armstrong, 2019).

In addition to fitness screening, Armstrong (2019) further advocated for evaluation of muscle strength and speed. Female dancers typically exhibit poorer baseline fitness than other female power-endurance athletes (Sanders et al., 2021), and they may benefit from appropriate supplemental training to address this facet of performance. For some genres, where a dancer's performance duration lasts for less than approximately 2 minutes, the activity is predominantly anaerobic; any assessment of fitness must consider this fact. Genres such as flamenco and Irish dancing are largely **anaerobic** at the elite level (Forczek et al., 2017). Chapter 4 discusses the physiology of different types of physical activity and chapter 5 discusses conditioning in detail.

Given the high level of foot and ankle injury across multiple dance genres, excellent **proprioception** and balance are key requisites, particularly for dancers in styles that emphasize **plyometrics**. Research in several genres (hip-hop, urban dance, rock and roll, and standard or Latin dance genres) have identified increased risk of injury due to poor dynamic balance (Sekulic et al., 2020; Ursej et al., 2019). Additionally, having sufficient strength and being physically robust enough to carry out choreography is critically important. As with many areas of dance science, rigorous research in this area is lacking, but a 2017 systematic review confirmed the association between low muscle strength and dance injury (Moita et al., 2017). (The importance of systematic reviews to health and wellness in dance is discussed in chapter 3.) Appropriate strength and conditioning allow effective and efficient performance of choreography, like a finely tuned machine. Without this optimal mix of muscle strength and fitness, performance is compromised and musculoskeletal overload can occur, leading to injury.

A professional familiar with the requirements of the genre should lead strength and conditioning programs designed to improve dance performance. This approach will ensure optimal benefits and prevent potential harm that can result from overloading already hard-worked muscle groups.

Governing all facets of physical performance is **motor control**, which refers to the manner in which the brain and nervous system control posture and motion to perform all movement tasks, including dance. With repetitive practice, motor patterns become embedded and movements are consistently performed in the same manner. Therefore, it is key that as dancers learn a new skill, the skill is repeated accurately; each repetition is a means of reducing the likelihood of problems that may lead to injury. The use of verbal and (especially) visual feedback is important in ensuring optimal motor control for dancers.

Training Factors

Research indicates that dancers generally recognize the importance of a good warm-up before dancing and that most dancers engage in this practice. According to Riding McCabe and colleagues (2014), the 2011 Fit to Dance study provided a snapshot of practices across multiple dance genres, revealing that 88 percent of dancers regularly perform a warm-up in comparison to 46 percent who engage in a postperformance or postclass cool-down. Sound evidence shows that the performance of an appropriate warm-up helps to mitigate the risk of injury (Cahalan et al., 2019). Similarly, performance of a cool-down has been found to reduce risk of injury and limit next-day muscle soreness (Herbert et al., 2011; Malliou et al., 2007).

A key tenet of injury risk reduction is the idea of progressive loading and **periodization**. In other words, the amount of workload undertaken must build progressively and be monitored to ensure that it does not become excessive. This premise is particularly pertinent during times of transition, such as when returning to dance (following injury or a vacation) or prior to key examinations or performances (Fuller et al., 2020). A related issue is tissue loading, which refers to the ability of the body's tissues to withstand the physical load placed on them by the movements involved in choreography or other physical activity. How tissues withstand these stresses depends on many factors.

Periodization is a planned program of activity that allows a dancer to build their physical capacities gradually to full performance through successive periods (Surgenor et al., 2020). Load management must consider not only the amount of work performed (external load) but also the difficulty of the work (internal load). This load is sometimes measured using a **rating of perceived exertion (RPE)**, where an exercising individual selects a number from 0 to 10 that corresponds to the difficulty of the session; 10 is the maximal effort possible (Shaw et al., 2020). It is important to record the load value for each session and monitor total load over time to identify sudden spikes in activity. Using periods for training without appropriate rest has been shown across numerous cohorts to predispose dancers to injury (Cahalan et al., 2019; Kenny et al., 2016; Lee et al., 2017). Dancers must recognize that rest is an important and integral part of their training week and that it is critical for allowing their bodies to heal and their brains to assimilate and embed newly learned patterns. Therefore, rest must be planned into each week of a training program, and it must be adhered to diligently.

Cross-training is an essential consideration to factor into any load prescription. It is recommended for dancers to improve strength, fitness, and career longevity (Bronner et al., 2016). Striking a balance by identifying a training regimen that adds benefits without overloading the dancer is the correct way to accomplish this. For instance, non-weight-bearing exercise (e.g., swimming) may be appropriate to aid fitness, or nonplyometric strengthening work may be appropriate for muscle development. Dancer preference and available resources should be considered to support compliance with cross-training.

Of course, one of the most important training factors is choreography. Steps that are unfamiliar, too difficult, or repeated too often have been identified as a source of injury (Malkogeorgos et al., 2011). In some genres, such as ballet, the dancer follows specific pathways on the way to safely attempting a new movement; going *en pointe* is one example. In other genres, such as Irish dancing, age is the determining factor for attempting to achieve a movement. However, an age-based approach does not ensure that the dancer has the requisite strength or control to attempt the movement; therefore, this approach increases their risk of injury.

A further consideration is appropriately modifying choreography to facilitate a dancer who is returning from injury or managing an injury while continuing to dance at a reduced level. For instance, a lower-extremity tendinopathy would benefit from reduced loading from plyometric elements (e.g., jumping, bounding) while still allowing some relative loading to assist the tendon's controlled repair process. Finally, overuse injuries abound in dance (Murgia, 2013), and they may be exacerbated by repeating the same movement over and over for prolonged periods. Dancers and teachers must be mindful to avoid this practice without careful attention to any pain signals; these signals may be early indicators of an injury that would eventually derail the artistic excellence being pursued.

General Health Factors

A number of issues are related to general health factors. **Restorative sleep**—particularly in a highly active athletic population such as dancers—is key to ensuring good health and reducing the risk of injury. Poor sleep has been found to negatively impact several performance domains, including endurance and execution, attention and recall, and parameters of physical wellness such as illness and injury (Simpson et al., 2017). It is startling to learn from research that of the main reasons professional dancers visit primary care and mental health centers, psychological fatigue and sleep deprivation are associated with 35 percent of the visits (Alimena et al., 2016).

Early research identified how fatigue and ill-health are closely linked with burnout in dancers, which can be addressed in part by beneficial sleep (Koutedakis, 2000). Other research in ballet cohorts identified an association between injury and daytime sleepiness or sleep disturbances. While not entirely mitigated by improved sleep, this association did support the need for better planning and coping strategies for affected dancers (Adam et al., 2004). Studies of Irish dancers also report a link between suboptimal sleep and injury as well as consistent findings of associations between poor general health and injury (Cahalan et al., 2019; Cahalan et al., 2016).

In comparison to injury, little consideration is given to illness in the literature. Nonetheless, more recent findings by Jeffries and colleagues (2020) suggest that rates of both injury and illness are high in dance cohorts. Of equal concern is their finding that dancers continue to train when ill or injured even though it may predispose them to adverse events, including further injury. Keep in mind that illness may include low-level complaints such as colds or stomach bugs that persist or recur frequently. Dancers should seek medical help and cease dancing while unwell.

Menstrual status in females is another important indicator of health. Any significant delay to **menarche** or disruption or cessation of menstrual periods (**dysmenorrhea** or **amenorrhea**) should be investigated by a health care professional. Menstrual disorders have been recorded in many dance investigations. One systematic review reported that 32 percent of university-level dancers developed a menstrual disturbance in their first year of intensive dance training (Hincapié & Cassidy, 2010). An established relationship exists between disordered eating, menstrual disturbances, and low **bone mineral density** (known previously as the female athlete triad) (Doyle-Lucas et al., 2010). More recently, relative energy deficiency in sport (REDs) has been defined as a syndrome that arises "when insufficient calories are consumed to support exercise energy expenditure, resulting in compromised physiological processes, such as menstrual irregularities in active females" (Logue et al., 2020, p. 1). More information about nutrition and REDs is available in chapter 7. Overall, the implications of this syndrome are serious and far reaching; the circumstances of any dancer experiencing persistent menstrual disturbances should be investigated.

> WWW Another general health factor that is underappreciated in the dance environment is noise-induced hearing loss. A discussion of how it applies to dance is included in this book's HK*Propel* online resource.

Emotional and Cognitive Factors

Taken together, emotional and cognitive factors reflect the psychological health of a dancer. Just as physical wellness affects an injury, so does a dancer's psychological well-being. This area is receiving increasing attention from dance teachers, academics, and researchers as recognition of the role of psychological wellness grows. A 2017 systematic review found that psychological variables can affect both the incidence and outcome of dance injuries (Mainwaring & Finney, 2017). Variables of note include stress, psychological distress (defined as a negative mood state), personality, coping, sleep quantity and quality, disordered eating, and social support.

Stress in dance can arise from several sources that are both external and internal to a dancer (Adam et al., 2004; Anderson & Hanrahan, 2008). External sources include the competitive dance environment; pressures from teachers, parents, or peers; and trying to balance dance and other life responsibilities. Internal stress comes from within the dancer; it is often related to one's motivation for dance. Seminal work by Rip and colleagues (2006) identified two types of passion for dance: obsessive and harmonious. Obsessive passion is hallmarked by a drive for perfection where a dancer continues to dance—even when injured—and is slow to seek help, which often results in chronic injury. Harmonious passion for dance, on the other hand, promotes healthy coping strategies through which the dancer takes appropriate measures to address injury and moderate dance practice, resulting in fewer difficult injuries and a greater likelihood of a long and healthy dance career. Other authors have extended and confirmed these concepts (Akehurst & Oliver, 2014; Padham & Aujla, 2014). Dancers should reflect on passion in themselves, and teachers should evaluate this characteristic in their students.

The relationship between stress and injury is inconsistently reported in research literature; some studies have found no relationship between the two (Byhring & Bø, 2002; Cahalan et al., 2015). This discrepancy is likely due to the influence of other factors, including coping strategies, personality, and mood. Evidence suggests that positive coping strategies help moderate the impact of injury, while absent or poor coping strategies render a dancer more vulnerable to injury (van Winden et al., 2020). Personality factors such as negative mood (including a tension/anxiety combination and anger) and catastrophizing have also been associated with injury in dancers participating in Irish dance, a genre where these factors have been extensively studied (Cahalan et al., 2015; Cahalan et al., 2016).

Catastrophizing refers to an expectation that the worst possible outcome will occur in any given scenario. It may also encompass dwelling on pain or perceptions of one's inability to cope. Earlier research identified higher levels of catastrophizing coupled with poor coping skills in ballet dancers (Mainwaring et al., 2001). Some later work in professional ballet and contemporary dancers found that where dancers viewed pain as a threat, they would catastrophize their pain and use avoidance coping strategies (Anderson & Hanrahan, 2008).

An additional area of interest in emotional and cognitive factors is one's motivation for dance. Motivation may be broadly categorized into performance (ego) or mastery (task) motivation, where the former is driven by perfectionism, achievement, and external plaudits while the latter focuses on learning as an end in itself (Andrzejewski et al., 2013). In the case of performance motivation, failure to achieve one's goals may lead to shame and a loss of self-esteem (Ellison & Partridge, 2012). Striving for perfection can also lead to maladaptive practices and resultant vulnerability to injury. It is widely accepted that a mastery-motivated climate is more beneficial for dancer health and well-being than a performance-motivated climate (Quested & Duda, 2009); teachers should foster such a climate as much as possible. See chapter 8 for further insights about dancers' mental health.

Social and Lifestyle Factors

The importance of a healthy lifestyle in reducing the risk of injuries and managing them is intuitively obvious to most dancers. For example, smoking or overindulging in alcohol or illegal drugs may affect a dancer's body in a way that is harmful to health and performance. Cigarette smoking in particular has detrimental effects on the lung capacity and fitness of a dancer, slows tissue healing, and may cause a plethora of lifelong health issues. Cigarette smoking has been directly linked to increased injury rates in female ballet dancers, while drinking alcohol has been associated in females with absence from dance (Novosel et al., 2019).

Appropriate nutritional choices also are key to reducing the risk of injuries and supporting health. Nutrition is especially important when dance is pursued as both an aesthetic and athletic activity. Researchers have discovered that nutrition knowledge across many different dance cohorts at the university level is poor (Challis et al., 2020; Hanna et al., 2017). This news is not surprising given the well-documented challenges that disordered eating creates in many dancers (Kalyva et al., 2021).

Another important consideration is recognition of social support in the management of injury. Research has shown that dancers with strong social networks of family, friends, and dance peers cope better with the effects of injury than dancers without such networks (Noh et al., 2005; Patterson et al., 1998). More recent qualitative research confirms the perceived value of social support in helping dancers manage their injury journeys (Higginbotham & Cahalan, 2020). Other factors include access to appropriate medical providers and other professionals who can help reduce the risk of injuries and manage the injuries when they do occur. Dancers are reticent to consult a practitioner who is not knowledgeable in their dance genre for fear that the caregiver will not understand the physical demands or be familiar with the associated terminology (Pollard-Smith & Thomson, 2017; Wang & Russell, 2018). Dancers clearly benefit when they can identify a clinician who is either well versed in a dancer's genre or is willing to learn. Chapter 15 discusses various types of health care professionals and how to work with them.

Environmental Factors

The environment of dance is the physical space in which a dancer works, as well as the equipment and accessories of the trade, including footwear, costuming, props, and even partners. Inappropriate flooring or stages are acknowledged sources of injury (Wanke et al., 2012), but other factors to consider include the lighting, heating, and ventilation of the studio or room where dancers work. Industry guidelines can assist teachers and dancers in optimizing their dance space (One Dance UK, 2011). Anecdotal reports of collisions with props, dropping partners, and tripping over unseen obstacles abound. One study attributed 14.6 percent of injuries to accidents (Cahalan et al., 2015); however, it is difficult to establish how much other factors such as fatigue or the environment may have contributed to this figure.

For those dancers who use shoes, footwear requires careful attention. Shoes must be fit for purpose and replaced when they become too worn or broken, no matter how tedious and painful the process of "breaking-in" a new pair might be. A systematic review of research articles confirmed the association between footwear and injury across several dance genres and highlighted how ill-fitting or restrictive shoes can impede a dancer's movement (Fong Yan et al., 2011).

Costuming can also lead to injury due to trips, tangles, malfunctioning fasteners, and the like. Thus, care should be taken to ensure that one's costume does not present a risk. Accidents in general are an unfortunate and unavoidable source of injury, no matter how robust, fit, and healthy a dancer may be.

As mentioned previously, the role of the teacher in reducing injury risk in dance classes, rehearsals, performances, and the environment cannot be overemphasized. The motivational climate has already been discussed, but other factors, such as the teaching and learning style of teachers and students, must be considered. It is an unfortunate reality borne out by research that many dance teachers provide more negative than positive feedback during practice sessions (Klockare et al., 2011), and they often use punishment rather than positive and specific feedback (Lakes, 2005). The implications of these practices may lead to overdancing in pursuit of perfection or to avoidance behaviors. Positive and specific feedback may help to create a healthier environment for both dancers and teachers. Peer feedback is also helpful (Quinn et al., 2017).

Additionally, interactions between members of the dancer–teacher–parent triad (where relevant) can support dancer health. Communication that keeps all parties abreast of the ethos and expectations for classes is critically important. Although it is an emerging area of study in dance, a robust body of evidence in sport indicates that parental influence (for better or worse) is key to a young athlete's participation, experience, and accomplishment (Knight et al., 2017).

A final fundamental issue is the culture inherent within many dance genres—particularly at the elite and professional levels—that the show must go on, regardless of the cost (McEwen & Young, 2011). This culture underpins a practice of injury concealment where dancers resist seeking help and continue to dance while injured for fear of appearing weak or losing a key role (Aujla & Farrer, 2015). Such practices are almost certain to exacerbate and prolong injury (with obvious detrimental implications for dancers), and they should be rebuffed clearly and consistently by senior leadership and all other stakeholders in positions of authority.

Mechanisms of Injury

Traditionally, **mechanism of injury (MOI)** is defined as the manner in which force or forces produce particular trauma when those forces are applied to the human body, specifically focusing on the type of force and subsequent tissue response (Toney-Butler & Varacallo, 2021). Identifying MOIs in dancers is complex (Bahr & Krosshaug, 2005), and a multitude of variants must be considered beyond dancers' flexibility, fitness, strength, balance, and biomechanics of repetitive movements and landings (Costa et al., 2016). Although these components play an active role in properly identifying MOIs, it is necessary to investigate various contributing systems and the interdependence between these systems.

Many different methodological approaches have been used to investigate MOIs in dance, including extensive analysis of self-reporting across various genres, comprehensive clinical evaluations, biomechanical analysis, radiography, magnetic resonance imaging (MRI), computed tomography (CT), and **in vivo** studies to identify tissue property changes (Campoy et al., 2011; Krosshaug et al., 2005). Musculoskeletal-based investigations are extremely valuable, but the prime focus should be on intrinsic and extrinsic factors (Campbell et al., 2019; Steinberg et al., 2012) as well as the varying degrees of vulnerability and resilience inherent to an individual dancer (Arbinaga, 2018).

In general, intrinsic factors are defined as internal personal factors that can be broken down into modifiable and nonmodifiable factors. Examples of intrinsic nonmodifiable factors for dancers are anatomical characteristics, dance experience, and biological functions such as menstrual history (Aujla & Farrer, 2015; Campbell et al., 2019). Hypermobility, fatigue, overuse, some types of neuromuscular dysfunction, weakness of core musculature, and some lower-extremity range of motion (ROM) discrepancies are examples of modifiable intrinsic factors (Campbell et al., 2019). Time spent dancing and practicing technique skills are considered environment-related, or extrinsic factors (Steinberg et al., 2012). These factors combined are key components of the scaffold that defines a MOI in a dancer.

Injuries in Different Dance Genres

Dance comes in many forms, and injuries occur in all of them. Injuries in one genre of dance may differ from injuries in others; it largely depends on how a given style of dance is executed and under what conditions. Thus, the environment of the genre's performance as well as the biomechanics and other physical aspects of the body while a dancer performs the genre are necessary considerations. The following sections present what is known from the scientific literature about the specialized characteristics of different genres of dance. They summarize the injuries that may be sustained in these genres using the framework of landscape, injury profile, and mechanism of injury (MOI) for each genre.

Ballet

Ballet (figure 2.3) is perhaps the best-known and most widely practiced dance form internationally. Its origins date back to the 15th century and the Italian Renaissance, during which the nobility were treated to spectacular ballet performances (Homans, 2013). Later, the French aristocracy embraced ballet, which emerged as an independent and unique art form. The Russian dance masters of the 19th century were the pioneers of classical ballet technique, emphasizing pointe work, precision of movement, and turnout (Vaganova, 1969). The ballet tutu known today dates from this period. Ballet has inspired and influenced numerous other genres, even while it continues to evolve and grow itself.

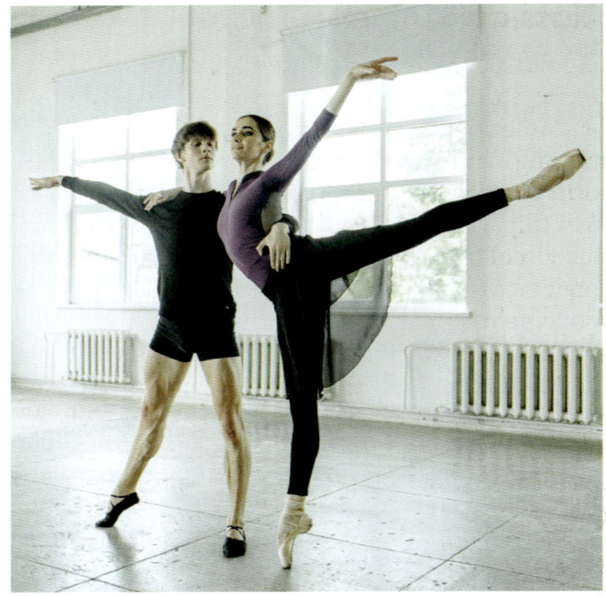

Figure 2.3 An example of classical ballet.
Mart Production on Pexels

Landscape

Ballet is a globally recognized dance genre with established companies worldwide. Due to the demanding nature of the genre, elite dancers typically have a relatively short career; they tend to retire before age 30 (Pollard-Smith & Thomson, 2017). Grade exams are widely used to monitor the progress of students, and ballet competitions are popular in many countries. Of these, the prestigious Prix de Lausanne for elite dancers is possibly the most celebrated.

Injury Profile

Injury is common in ballet. Incidence rates vary from 1.4 to 4.4 injuries per 1,000 dance hours in professional dance (Allen et al., 2012; Novosel et al., 2019) and from 0.8 to 1.4 injuries per 1,000 dance hours in young student and preprofessional dancers (Ekegren et al., 2014; Leanderson et al., 2011). Injuries most commonly affect the foot and ankle as well as the lumbar spine (Ramkumar et al., 2016). Due to the repetitive nature of the technical aspects of the genre, overuse injuries are more common than traumatic injuries in ballet, though traumatic ballet injuries tend to be more severe than overuse ballet injuries (Allen et al., 2012; Ekegren et al., 2014).

Mechanisms of Injury

Research to date has focused predominantly on physical risk factors, and it has identified causes such as hypermobility, inadequate strength and control, and poor aerobic fitness (Biernacki et al., 2021). However, the importance of other factors (e.g., sleep, personality, and social support) in injury risk for ballet has also been recognized (Mainwaring & Finney, 2017).

Classical Chinese Dance

Classical Chinese dance (figure 2.4) dates to 220 BCE during the Quin Dynasty; it was derived from the principles of Confucian etiquette (a form of moral training) and ritual dances (Wang, 1985). The art form comprises three main components: technical skill (flips, aerial skills, and spins), form (continuous circular pathway of movement with distinct movement patterns), and bearing (inner spirit of movement) (Shen Yun Performing Arts, n.d.). This art form is very distinct from Western forms of dance due to its focus on these three components, the inclusion of the similar movements used in fighting in martial arts, and the usual distinctiveness of the female role with its rapid heel–toe stepping pattern (Wang, 1985; Dang et al., 2020).

Landscape

Classical Chinese dance is performed for ceremonies, theater stages, genre-specific dance competitions, and in public spaces (e.g., gardens, town plazas). There are children's training programs that focus on this genre beginning as early as 5 years old. In addition, many dance companies continue the heritage of this art form.

Injury Profile

Injury incidence data for this population is limited, but one unique study reported a rate of 3.9 injuries per dancer in a 12-month period, with the majority of these injuries occurring during classes (Dang et al., 2020). This study also highlighted that both males and females indicated the highest prevalence of pain occurred in the knees, followed by the ankles, arms, and shoulders (Dang et al., 2020).

Mechanisms of Injury

The main MOIs in classical Chinese dance are fatigue, overwork, insufficient warm-up, incorrect technique training, and recurrence of old injuries (Dang et al., 2020). Additional research is needed to further elucidate the injury mechanisms and appropriate injury risk reduction strategies.

Indian Classical Dance

Originating during the Middle Ages or medieval period, Indian classical dance forms hold vital aspects of sacred rituals (Chatterjea, 1996; Paul & Kapoor, 1998; Royo, 2010). The original form was derived from the *Bharata Natya Shastra* (a Sanskrit treatise on the performing arts), which includes dance, drama, and emotion drawn from Indian mythology and epics (Chatterjea, 1996; Royo, 2010). The art form combines rhythmic movement, melody, expression, musical theater, storytelling, and emotions. Many of the forms include the use of special costuming (figure 2.5), including head dresses, jewelry, ankle bells (with bare feet), elaborate face masks, and other props that should be considered when addressing injury risk reduction and treatment (Lalli, 2004).

Landscape

A majority of the classical Indian dance forms originated with worship practices in Hindu temples (Mickeviciene, 2004). Various regions in India

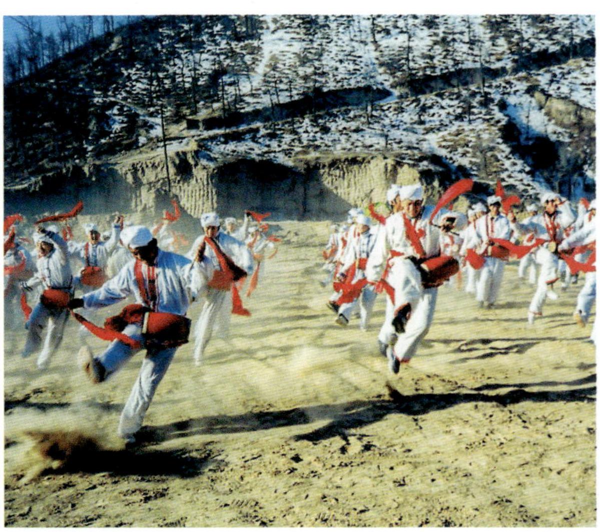

Figure 2.4 An example of classical Chinese dance.
Shih-Ming Li Chang

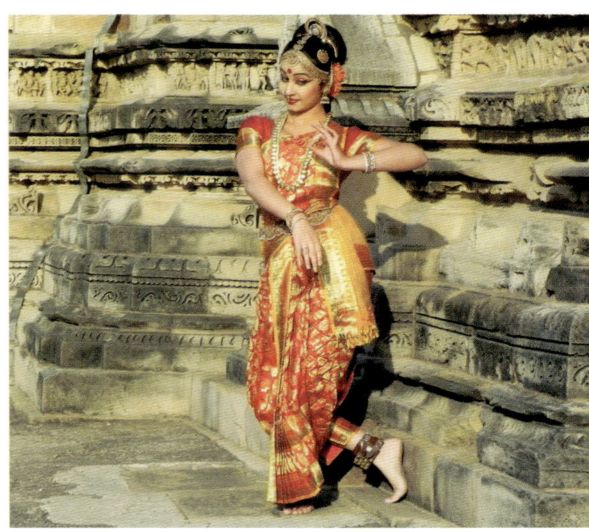

Figure 2.5 An example of Indian classical dance by dancer and physician Dr. Pranamya Suri.
Pranamya Suri

developed their own styles of dance based on the *Bharata Natya Shastra*. It serves as the foundation for these nine styles that originated from different geographical regions (Ministry of Culture, Government of India, n.d.):

- *Bharata natya* from Tamil Nadu
- *Chauu* from Eastern India
- *Kuchipudi* from Andhra Pradesh
- *Kathak* from Northern India
- *Kathakali* from Kerala
- *Manipuri* from Manipur
- *Mohiniattam* from Kerala
- *Odissi* from Orissa
- *Sattriya* from Assam

Dancers start extensive dance training as early as age 5, and some continue performing into their 80s. Dance training in India typically occurs in a residential gurukulam format (where students stay in the institution to learn the ancient arts that are passed down). The rigorous training includes total body conditioning; lifestyle, Ayurveda, and yoga practice; music; *nattuvangam* (art of rhythmic cycles); and dance theory (Pandya, 2014). In the United States, dancers usually attend weekly academies or dance schools specializing in Indian classical dance. A graduation ceremony (called *arrangetram*) celebrates the completion of their basic dance studies (Kopytko, 2011).

Injury Profile

Although research is becoming more abundant for this art form, there is still a dearth of inclusive longitudinal investigations across the various forms. Studies to date have reported on the prevalence of pain in specific body regions of bharata natya dancers; the highest incidences occur in the back, followed by the ankle, knee, neck, and shoulder (Nair et al., 2018; Panhale et al., 2020).

Mechanisms of Injury

Injuries in the dance forms of bharata natya and kathak consist of repetitive rhythmic tapping that cause changes in the medial longitudinal arch resulting in pes planus (flatfeet). Sustained poses requiring excessive lumbar lordosis and anterior pelvic tilt have been associated with increased back, knee, ankle, and foot injuries (Andhare et al., 2018; Chandan et al., 2018; Jacobs et al., 2012; Masal & Borkar, 2021).

DanceSport

DanceSport is competitive ballroom dancing that consists of individuals dancing together as a pair (figure 2.6) or in formations (multiple sets of pairs). In wheelchair DanceSport, at least one of the pair is in a wheelchair (USA Dance, n.d.; International Dance Federation, n.d.; McCabe et al., 2013). The first unofficial ballroom competition took place in 1909 in Paris, and the first live broadcast of a competition was in 1960 (World DanceSport Federation, 2022). The name DanceSport was developed to aid ballroom dancing in becoming an Olympic sport (World DanceSport Federation, 2024b).

DanceSport has two major styles that are based on traditional ballroom dances: the international style (10 dances) and the American style (9 dances). As seen in tables 2.1 and 2.2, each style is broken down into two subgroups (USA Dance, n.d.;

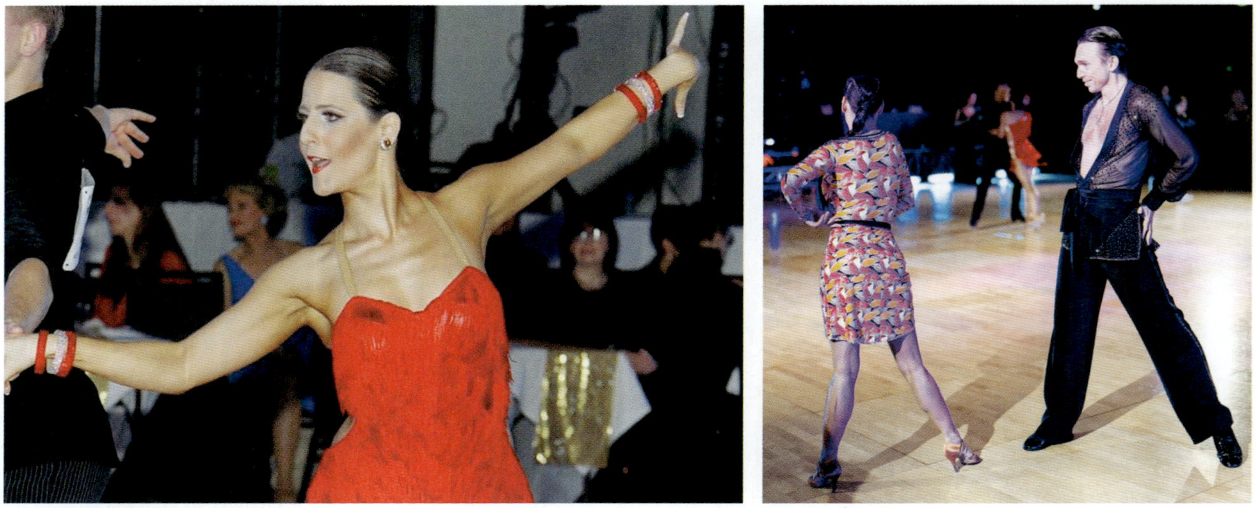

Figure 2.6 Examples of competitive ballroom dance, otherwise known as DanceSport.

A: Photo: Curtis Donahue; Dancer: Amanda Donahue. B: Photo: David Outevsky; Dancers: David Outevsky and Sophie Cazeneuve.

Table 2.1 **Dances Used in the International DanceSport Style**

International standard or international modern	International Latin
Waltz	Cha-cha
Tango	Rumba
Slow foxtrot	Samba
Viennese waltz	Paso doble
Quickstep	Jive

Table 2.2 **Dances Used in the American DanceSport Style**

American smooth	American rhythm
Waltz	Cha-cha
Tango	Rumba
Foxtrot	Samba
Viennese waltz	Mambo
	Bolero

International Dance Federation, n.d.; McCabe et al., 2013). This form combines sport and ballroom dance, allowing the participants to improve physical fitness and mental well-being as well as to create social relationships while competing at all levels (Miller & Hoffman, 2009).

Landscape

DanceSport is governed by organizations such as the National Dance Council of America, World Dance Council (WDC), World DanceSport Federation (WDSF), and country-specific DanceSport associations (National Dance Council of America, 2021; World Dance Council, 2023; World DanceSport Federation, 2024a). Approximately 71 countries participate in competitions worldwide, and the 15 DanceSport competition classifications range from professional to pre-teen (McCabe et al., 2013). While traditionally ballroom and DanceSport are performed with male and female dancers as partners, same-sex partnerships are becoming more common.

WWW HK*Propel* online resources for chapter 2 provide additional information about ballroom dancing and DanceSport.

Injury Profile

This dance form challenges both the aerobic and anaerobic energy systems. The research literature suggests there is a higher demand for intensity of females compared to males due to the unique hold patterns of the upper extremities and trunk (Bria et al., 2011; McCabe et al., 2013; Vaczi et al., 2016). According to Eberman and colleagues (2011), female DanceSport dancers most commonly report pain in the toe region, followed by the upper back, lower back, knee, ankle, and foot. They also have a lower incidence of hip and calf pain than males. In male dancers, pain is most prevalent in the upper back region, followed by the knee, hip, ankle, calf, and toe.

Mechanisms of Injury

Female DanceSport dancers perform in 2.5- to 3.5-inch (6-9 cm) high heels with very little shock absorption. They jump, turn, and perform for prolonged periods in these shoes. They maintain a rigorous training and competition schedule requiring sustained hyperextension and lateral flexion of the trunk and neck for aesthetic enhancement; this posture creates an increased risk of injuries (Banio, 2016; Eberman et al., 2011; Miletic et al., 2015). The art form requires male dancers to perform quick, rhythmic movements at high amplitudes and with jumps, turns, and lifts. These movements heighten the risk of injuries in the lower back, pelvic, and knee regions, and they increase the incidence of injury as a male DanceSport dancer ages (Bria et al., 2011; DeMann, 1997; Miletic et al., 2015).

Modern and Contemporary Dance

Although these genres often are viewed synonymously, modern dance is codified with clearly defined techniques in comparison to the broader and less prescriptive genre of contemporary dance.

Modern dance preceded and greatly influenced contemporary dance, which also borrowed from jazz, ballet, and other classical formats. However, modern and contemporary dance have marked similarities, including the expansive range of movements available to the dancer; the flexibility in pace and length of dances; the freedom to dance solo, in pairs, or in larger groups; and the techniques used during jumping and landing (figure 2.7).

Landscape

These combined genres represent some of the most popular and widely practiced dance forms internationally, particularly in the United States and Europe. Educational opportunities to study them at the university level are expanding globally. Although previously limited primarily to established dance organizations and schools, competitions in contemporary and modern dance are now gaining popularity in the United States and across the world. Due to the great flexibility these genres offer, many dancers continue to engage in them throughout their life span. Indeed, renowned modern dancer Martha Graham documented her last performance at 76 years of age!

Injury Profile

A study of injury in a modern dance company recorded an incidence of 0.41 injuries per 1,000 hours, with 60 percent of these affecting the lower limb—predominantly the foot, ankle, and knee (Ojofeitimi & Bronner, 2011). A similar rate (0.44 injuries per 1,000 hours) was recorded in a touring modern dance company (Bronner & Wood, 2017), with injury incidence for a cohort of full-time contemporary dance students reported at 1.9 injuries per 1,000 hours (van Winden et al., 2019). In this latter group, the foot, ankle, lower back, and knee were most affected.

Mechanisms of Injury

The literature reports multiple injury risk factors in these genres, including (in contemporary dance) age, psychological coping skills, limited ankle ROM (Kenny et al., 2019; van Seters et al., 2020), and (in modern dance) hypermobility, technique, muscle tightness, and prior injury (Bronner & Bauer, 2018).

Hip-Hop

Hip-hop dance (figure 2.8) originated in the Bronx of New York City in the early 1970s with African American and Latino youth (Ojofeitimi et al., 2012; Icon Collective, LLC, 2024). Although the art form has become very popular and enjoys a large international presence, true hip-hop dancers are very protective of their dance practice and the purity of the style. For example, *breaking* is the correct term for one of the core styles (as opposed to the often misused term *breakdancing*).

WWW See HK*Propel* online resources for chapter 2 for further insights into the hip-hop genre.

Hip-hop dance has two main styles. Old school dance styles consist of breaking, popping, and locking, while new school dance styles include house, krumping, Harlem shake, and street jazz (Ojofeitimi et al., 2012; Ursej et al., 2019). Each style possesses unique and complex movement patterns that rely on a wide range of physical abilities (Ojofeitimi et

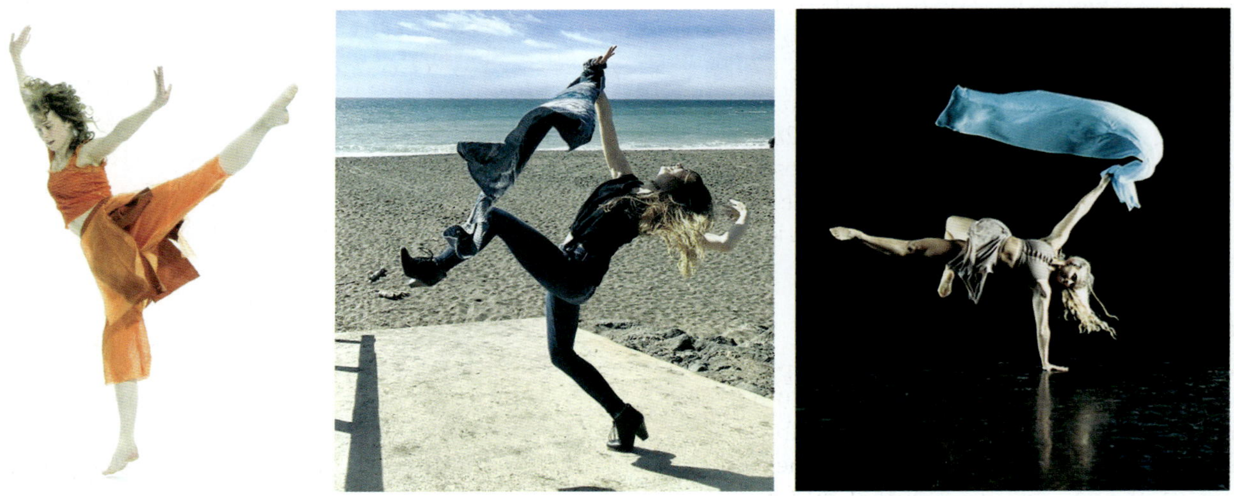

Figure 2.7 Modern and contemporary dancers.

A: Photo: Tom Caravaglia; Dancer: Lindsay Gilmour. B: Photo: Evan Redel; Dancer: Kaylyn Redel. C: Photo: www.FotosByFranco.com; Dancer: Cara Thomas.

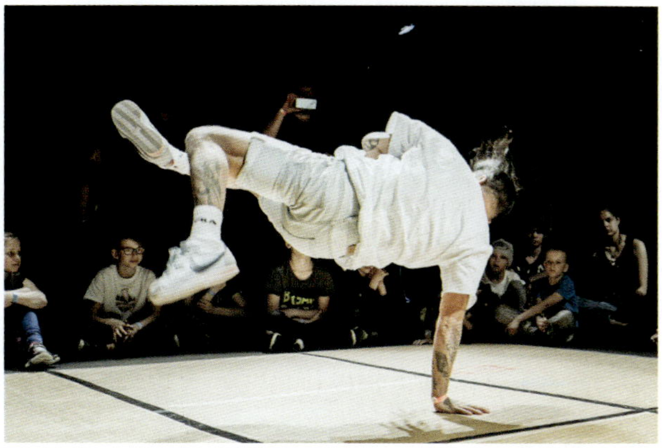

Figure 2.8 An example of hip-hop dance.
Ilja Tulit on Unsplash

al., 2012; Russell, 2013). The complex movements place a high demand on the aerobic and anaerobic systems, muscular strength, agility, coordination, and proprioception (Grčić et al., 2015; Kim & Kim, 2007; Ursej et al., 2019).

Landscape

Hip-hop is performed by individuals of all ages. In addition, it has a vast presence in commercial settings, including music videos, theater stages, clubs, street performances, dance battles, competitive dance venues, and film. In 2024, competitive breaking became an Olympic sport (International Olympic Committee, 2020).

Injury Profile

The reported incidence of injury in hip-hop is 3.1 musculoskeletal injuries or problems per dancer per year (Ursej et al., 2019). A descriptive study found the most frequently injured body location in female hip-hop dancers was the knee (42%), followed by the back region (32%) and the ankle (15%) (Ursej et al., 2019). Hip-hop dancers responding to a survey about their injuries experienced 1.156 injuries per 1,000 hours of dance during the year prior to completing the survey (Tjukov et al., 2020). Of these dancers, breakers sustained the highest incidence of injury, which was more than twice that of the average for all the dancers—2.456 injuries per 1,000 hours of dance over the prior year.

Mechanisms of Injury

Due to the repetitive nature of hip-hop movement vocabulary, research indicates that 50 percent of hip-hop dancers most commonly attribute injuries to overuse (Ojofeitimi et al., 2012). The high prevalence of knee injuries reported by females may be related to the fast and complex footwork, deep squats, twists hitting the ground with high impact, landings from jumps with extended knees, and quick directional changes (Ursej et al., 2019).

Additionally, hip-hop gives rise to some rather interesting injuries described in the medical literature, including one called headspin hole (Kauther et al., 2009), which occurs when a breaker spins on the crown of the head. This dance move eventually produces a patch of hair loss and an altered contour and tissue appearance on top of the head seen on magnetic resonance imaging and called the conehead sign (Korczynski et al., 2020).

Irish Step Dancing

Irish dancing is a traditional dance form with a documented history going back to the early 18th century. It is a broad term that includes *ceilí* (pronounced kay-lee) dancing, or group dancing similar to Scottish *ceilidh* dancing, and solo *sean-nós* (pronounced shan-nose) dancing, where the dancer performs rhythmic, low-to-the-ground choreography with a relaxed body posture. Irish step dancing, where dancers individually perform bespoke choreography, is the most demanding form of the genre. Dancers perform using techniques termed either *light shoe* (with a focus on elevation, movement, and tricks performed on the tips of the toes) or *heavy shoe* (where their dancing is characterized by rhythm, power, and stamina). Unique features of the genre include the stationary torso and arms held firmly by the sides of the body (figure 2.9).

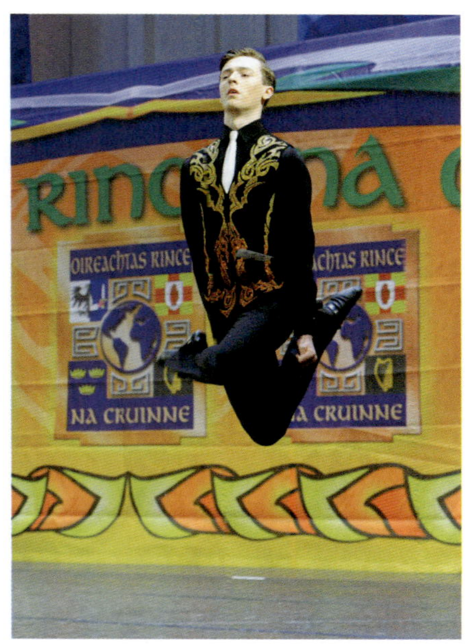

Figure 2.9 An example of Irish step dancing by two-time world champion David Pyke.
Feis.photos

Landscape

Irish step dancing is largely a competitive pursuit, culminating in the annual World Irish Dancing Championships. Many dancers also take grade-based exams for beginner through elite levels. These exams are now required by some Irish dancing governing bodies (of which many exist) to become a qualified Irish dancing teacher. Established Irish dancing academies exist in over 40 countries worldwide, and dancers range in age from as young as 3 or 4 up to adults in their 60s and 70s who dance for fun and fitness.

Injury Profile

The incidence of time-loss injuries in elite adolescent Irish dancers has been recorded as 4.5 injuries per 1,000 hours of dance (Cahalan et al., 2019). Areas of the lower limb—in particular the foot, ankle, knee, and hip—are the body parts most often injured in Irish dancing (Cahalan et al., 2016).

Mechanisms of Injury

The MOIs among Irish dancers are varied and include poor general and psychological health, catastrophizing, low mood, inadequate sleep, inappropriate footwear, and failure to complete an adequate warm-up or cool-down (Cahalan et al., 2019; Cahalan et al., 2015; McGuinness & Doody, 2006).

Tap Dancing

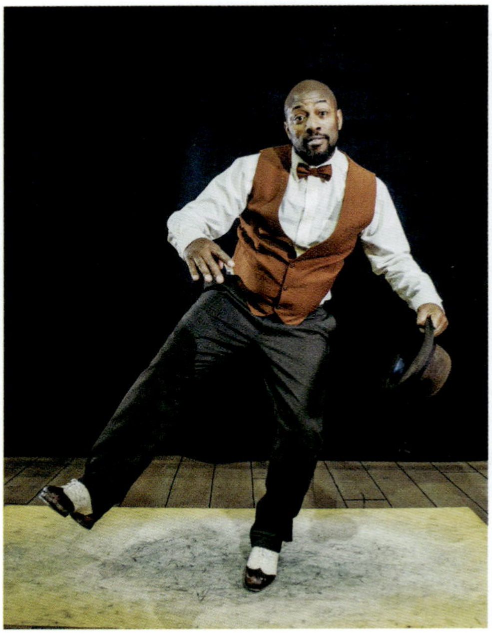

Figure 2.10 Tap dancer Lee Payne.

Anja Poehlmann Photo and Film

Tap dancing (figure 2.10) originated in the United States, but it is a confluence of West African sacred and secular step dances (*gioube*) and Scottish, Irish, and English clog dances, hornpipes, and jigs. Until the last part of the twentieth century, tap was commonly thought to have arisen from enslaved Africans and Irish indentured servants observing and adopting each other's dance forms. However, historians now report that tap was nurtured in urban melting pots such as the Five Points District in New York City. This unique percussive art form has seen many evolutions, including the minstrel shows of the 1830s to 1850s; the vaudeville performances of the late 19th century; the golden age of Hollywood with Shirley Temple, Fred Astaire, and Ginger Rogers; and onward to modern masters such as Gregory Hines and Savion Glover (Hill, 2014).

Landscape

Tap dancing was initially practiced on the margins of society—in urban areas of large cities in the United States. The genre declined in popularity after World War II, but it saw a resurgence in the 1980s through Broadway shows such as *42nd Street* and *The Tap Dance Kid*. These productions and those that succeeded them brought the genre to a global audience once again, and it now enjoys its status as a dance form practiced by dancers of all ages around the world.

Injury Profile

Although research is sparse for this genre, tap dancers do appear to experience fewer injuries than other percussive dance genres. One study estimated injury rates per 1,000 dance exposures at 0.21 injuries for males and 0.34 injuries for females. Minor joint sprains and muscle strains to the lower limb, back, and neck account for the majority of injuries. Unlike in ballet, most tap injuries (71%) are traumatic in nature (Mayers et al., 2003).

Mechanisms of Injury

Compared to other more ballistic genres, tap dancers experience small ground reaction forces (forces of the ground that react to forces exerted against the ground by the feet) and joint forces (forces exerted in joints by body weight, anatomical configurations, muscle contractions, and movements). This factor may explain their relatively low injury incidence (Mayers et al., 2010). In addition, greater experience provides biomechanical ability to dance with greater control and coordination (Rocha et al., 2017). Research to specifically identify possible risk factors for injury in tap dancers is lacking, but these factors likely include a combination of intrinsic and extrinsic modifiable and nonmodifiable factors.

Jazz

Jazz dance (figure 2.11) is an American art form with its origins in West African culture, where music was combined with dance to express the joy and strife of life's everyday passage. In the United States, vernacular jazz started on plantations and moved into social settings such as house parties and juke joints in the early 20th century (Hubbard, 2008). Early dances included the cakewalk, Charleston, and Lindy hop. Jazz incorporates a lowered center of gravity, a forward inclined torso, bent support leg(s), flatfeet, and a mobile spine with articulated limbs (Guarino & Oliver, 2014; Hubbard, 2008). A defining jazz feature is its grounded swing movement with syncopation and polyrhythm (Emery, 1981). Jack Cole led development of the modern theater jazz movement of the 1950s as jazz became infused with elements of ballet, modern, tap, and other forms.

Landscape

Jazz dance as a commercial art form is performed in film, theater, cabaret, and lounge shows as well as in music videos and competitive dance television series. Jazz dance companies abound in variety from those grounded in jazz's authentic roots to those that show off its fusions.

Injury Profile

Injury incidence is not established in this genre. A descriptive study showed that female jazz dancers have an injury frequency pattern in which the ankle and knee are most commonly injured, and these dancers have greater frequency of elbow and hand injuries than ballet and modern dancers (Reynolds et al., 2013). A survey of female and male festival dancers found that 27.92 percent of the total injuries occurred in jazz and contemporary dancers, with the thigh and leg most affected (Soares Campoy et al., 2011).

Mechanisms of Injury

In jazz dancers, older age, heavier weight, and greater weekly frequency of practice are linked to higher injury risk (Soares Campoy et al., 2011). A typical jazz shoe is rubber with a split sole. A biomechanical analysis showed jazz shoe design may increase knee flexion angles while reducing frontal plane ankle and midfoot motion during sauté landings, thus decreasing shock absorption of the lower extremities and potentially adding to injury risk (Fong Yan et al., 2014).

Flamenco Dance

Flamenco is an expressive art form combining song (*cante*), musicianship (*toque*), and dance (*baile*) (figure 2.12). *Baile* is an essential part of Spanish culture originating in Andalusia, gaining importance in dance schools by 1765, and recently being named a World Heritage Treasure in 2010 (Cuellar-Moreno, 2016). *Baile* has many styles (*palos*) in which the flamenco dancer (*bailaor* or *bailaora*) performs with great passion and emotion using repetitive percussive footwork and heel work that produce sounds from stomping the floor (*zapateados*). Male and female bailaors and bailaoras wear flamenco dance shoes with rigid soles and metal tacks on the heel and sole for sound production. The heel heights range from 1.5 to 2.75 inches (4.0-7.5 cm) (Cuellar-Moreno, 2016). Male dancers perform with heavy foot percussion, whereas female dancers move more softly and sensually.

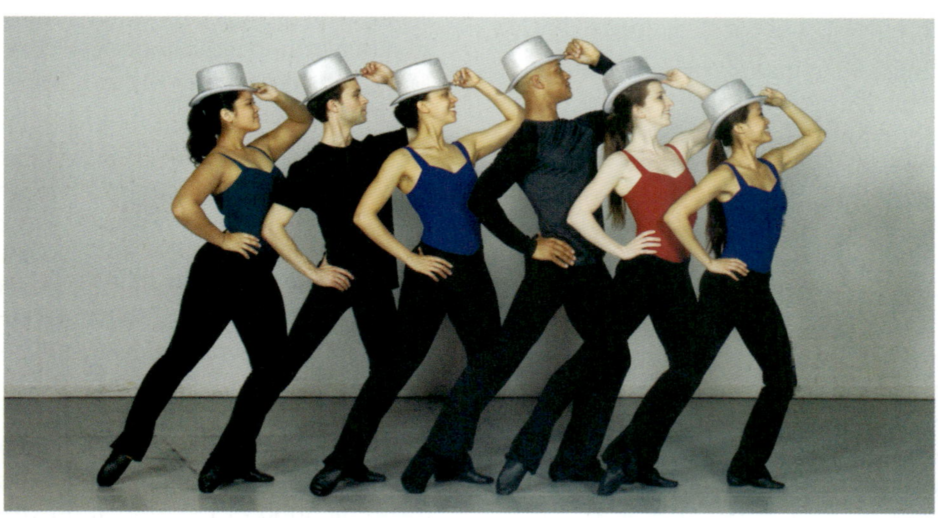

Figure 2.11 An example of jazz dancers.

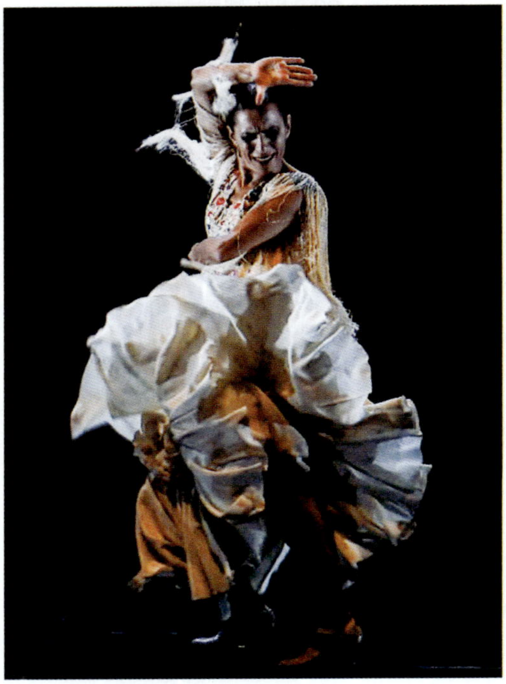

Figure 2.12 Flamenco dancer Yolanda Gonzales Sobrado.

Photo: Belén de Benito; Dancer: Yolanda Gonzales Sobrado.

Landscape

An estimated 300 academies, conservatories, and centers teach flamenco dance in Spain (Forczek et al., 2017). Mexico and Japan follow Spain in embracing this art form. Historically, the intense emotion of *baile* was akin to a form of protest performed in backyards, selling fairs, private salons, and schools (Cuellar-Moreno, 2016). Contemporary *baile* performances in theaters and universities may hold to the original form, or its elements may be blended with other dance forms such as Latino or American style ballroom dancing.

Injury Profile

Incidence and time loss of injuries in flamenco dancers is not yet reported. Injuries occur in the lower extremity, mainly within the foot (Castillo-López et al., 2014). Spinal injuries are also reported (Castillo-López et al., 2016). Using a case study approach with a female flamenco dancer, Vargas-Macías and colleagues (2021) suggested that the biomechanics and impact of the heel strike in this genre may increase the likelihood of knee injuries. It is clear that flamenco dance should receive substantially increased research attention to more fully appreciate how its physicality affects its participants.

Mechanisms of Injury

The flamenco shoe lacks shock absorption. This factor, combined with a typical flamenco performance having an average of 240 *zapateados* (foot impacts) per minute and an average of 1,400 *zapateados* within a standard dance, leaves the foot at risk for injury; moreover, the neck and lower back are at risk from the repetitive vibration (Bejjani et al., 1988; Castillo-López et al., 2016).

Lyrical Dance and Musical Theater

Lyrical dance expresses the lyrics and emotions of a song and emphasizes the dancer's individual style while pulling from jazz and ballet. In the late 1990s, Netting (1998) defined lyrical jazz as an expression of emotional sentiment through the use of the balletic line as a counterbalance to jazz rhythm. Lyrical dance may even incorporate acrobatics, such as in Cirque du Soleil productions. With storytelling at the heart of lyrical dance, it has shared elements with dance in musical theater (figure 2.13) as the dancer brings emotion, style, and their own personality to choreography set to show tunes.

Landscape

Lyrical dance is growing in popularity in studios for children through adults because it allows the dancer to express individual style through a wide range of music. Lyrical dance is a common style performed in dance competitions as solo, duet, or group performances. Many musical theater productions make use of lyrical dance.

Injury Profile

Injury incidence specific to lyrical dance is not reported. One could consider injury risks seen in jazz and ballet as relatable to lyrical dance. In terms of musical theater, one study reported male dancers sustaining 0.44 injuries and females 0.33 injuries per 1,000 hours (Wanke et al., 2014). More than half of a sample of 37 musical theater students reported at least one orthopaedic injury per year (Wanke et al., 2012). Musical theater injuries appear to be most common in the lower extremity, which is similar to trends seen in other dance genres.

Mechanisms of Injury

An injury surveillance questionnaire of West End Performers found that 72 percent of injuries occurred during performances, and 50 percent of those injuries were to the lower extremity (James & Lazarczuk, 2019). In this study, intrinsic risk factors included jumps, landings, lifts, tripping, falling, costume changes, and collisions with part of the set. High-heeled shoes and a raked stage were contributing extrinsic factors.

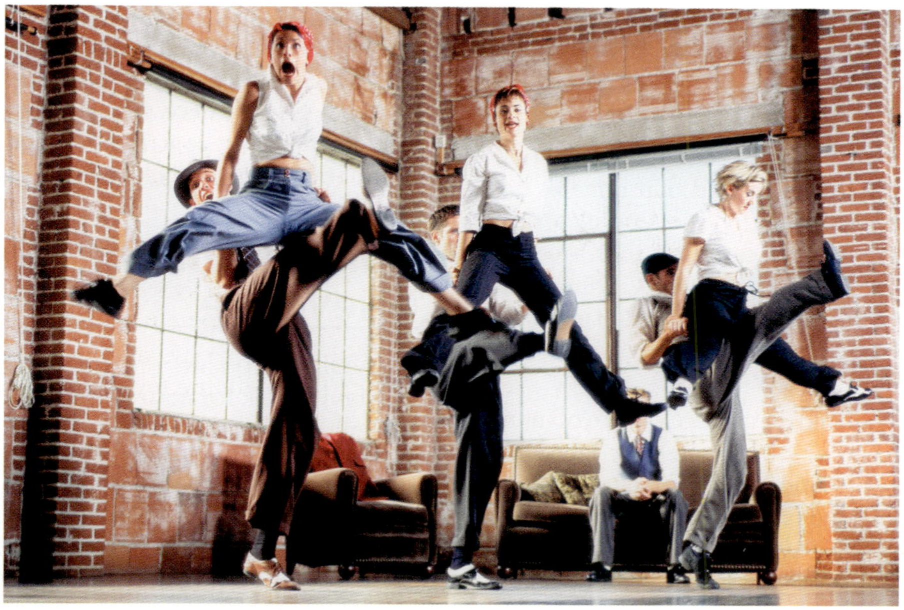

Figure 2.13 An example of lyrical dance and musical theater.
Stephen Simpson/Stone/Getty Images

Tango and Latin Dance

The Argentine tango originated in the late 19th century in Buenos Aires. In 1902, tango emerged in the balls of the Teatro Opera. The history of tango is a story of immigration. Tango's rhythm has Andalusian and African roots, whereas its melody is a European fusion. Tango is a complex genre involving dance, music, poetry, song, narrative, gesture, and drama (Azzi, 1996). Historically, the tango expressed passionate *sentimentos* (feelings) between a man and woman, but it now also has a home in the LGBTQ community. Argentine tango (figure 2.14*a*) is improvised, whereas the more modern ballroom tango (figure 2.14*b*)—as seen on film, stage, and television—is choreographed.

Landscape

In 2009, Argentine tango was recognized by the United Nations as part of the world's intangible heritage (Toyoda, 2012). Argentine tango is danced worldwide. In Asia, Japan leads the continent in numbers of tango schools, dance halls, and tango dancers (Toyoda, 2012). Tango enhances specific brain activity because its music evokes emotional reactions that are strengthened by dance, making it an effective dance therapy intervention for healthy elderly individuals and patients with Parkinson's disease as well as for health and wellness promotion in women (Hackney et al., 2007; Witkoś & Hartman-Petrycka, 2021).

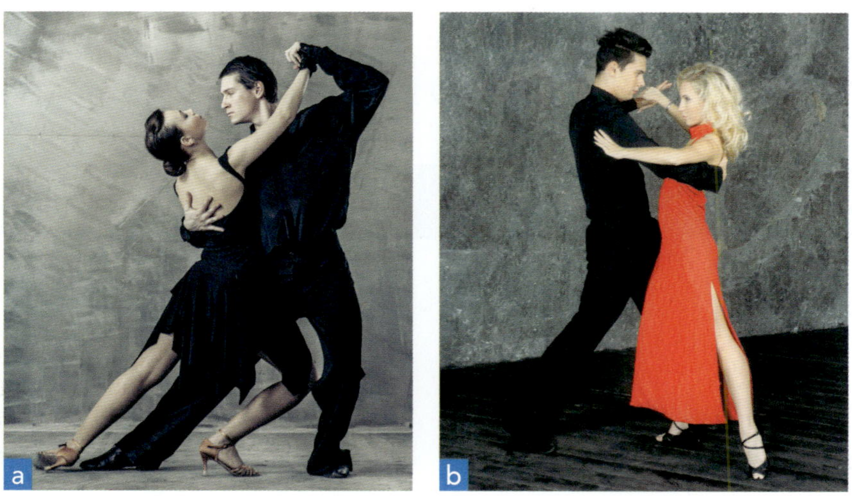

Figure 2.14 Examples of *(a)* Argentine tango and *(b)* modern ballroom tango.
A: Oleg66/E+/Getty Images. B: Anton Leonardovich Varfolomeev on Pexels.

Injury Profile

There are no known injury data for Argentine tango. However, it is one of several genres comprising the realm of DanceSport. A study on age and gender differences in DanceSport found that females had a higher median injury incidence over males; traumatic injuries were more common than overuse injuries; and injuries most frequently occurred in the neck, lower back, and knee (Premelč et al., 2019).

Mechanisms of Injury

There is limited research on the mechanism of injury specific to tango as its own genre. As one of the components of DanceSport, a retrospective investigation on age and gender differences with regard to injury (Premelč et al., 2019) found that females had a significantly higher injury incidence than males and that 61.5% of all injuries were reported as traumatic. While the mechanisms of these injuries are not yet fully established, it is thought that females may be more at risk for traumatic injury over their male counterparts in tango due to having more extreme spinal extension range-of-motion demands, along with a higher volume of rotations while performing in high heels. The necessity of performing explosive movements may contribute to the higher rate of traumatic injury over chronic overuse.

Conclusions and Practical Relevance

As a dancer, you are a highly trained athlete with substantial risk for injuries due to a complex array of elements that can be classified as nonmodifiable and modifiable risk factors. The majority of these factors are similar across genres of dance; however, unique factors exist for each genre, and they must be addressed to maintain your wellness. Your training plan requires a multidimensional approach that includes all the modifiable risk factors so that you can make small changes that enhance your overall wellness.

Discussion Questions

1. Consider your most recent injury. How would you categorize this event using the terms presented in this chapter?
2. Do you distinguish between pain and injury? If so, what parameters do you use to make this distinction?
3. Considering the nonmodifiable risk factors for injury as presented in the Cahalan-Schmieg-Sharp model, what factors affect you most?
4. Considering the model more broadly, are any factors surprising to you, or are any factors missing from the model?
5. Has this chapter inspired you to make any changes to your approach to dance health and wellness? If so, what are those changes?
6. How do your experiences with the dance genres in which you participate relate to what you've read in this chapter? Do you have any insights to add to what has been presented here?

WWW Go to HK*Propel* to access supplemental information and activities connected to chapter content.

3

Using Scientific Research to Reduce Injury Risk and Maximize Performance

Danielle N. Jarvis, PhD, ATC
Sheyi Ojofeitimi, PT, DPT, OCS, CFMT
Jatin Ambegaonkar, PhD, ATC, OT, CSCS, FIADMS

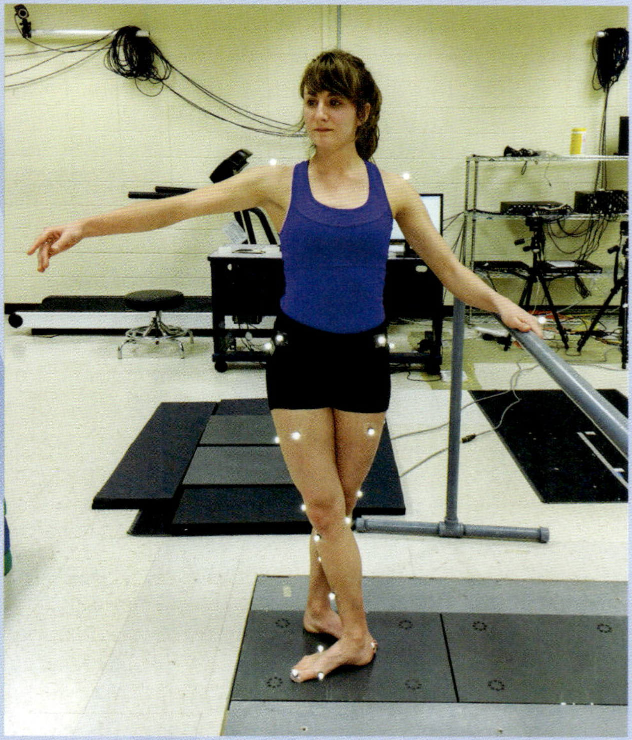

University of Wyoming Department of Theatre and Dance, Laramie, Wyoming. Photo: Rachael Greenwell; Dancer: Scarlett Barnes.

Key Terms

analysis of variance (ANOVA)
chi-square statistic
confidence interval (CI)
correlation coefficient (r)
empirical rule
evidence-based practice
hypothesis
Mann-Whitney U test
mean
median
mode
odds ratio
open access
peer review
primary sources
probability value (P value)
qualitative research
quantitative research
randomized controlled trial
secondary sources
standard deviation
statistics
study design
systematic review
t-test
z-score (Z value)

A great deal of knowledge about dancer wellness, training, and injury care stems from scientific research, which is published in scientific journals. Although as a dance practitioner (dancer, teacher, or choreographer) you may not necessarily conduct scientific research yourself, staying current in your field requires that you become an educated consumer of research. So, you must know how to access, evaluate, and use scientific research. Initially, some dance practitioners may find this task scary. It is helpful to remember that science and research are not your enemies; they exist to inform and support you on your dance journey. This chapter will set you on a path to confidently explore scientific research to help reduce injury risk and maximize dance performance.

LEARNING OBJECTIVES

After completing this chapter, you will be able to do the following:

- Discuss the importance of scientific research.
- Demonstrate how to access scientific research.
- Explain the typical sections in a research article.
- Evaluate the quality of scientific research articles.
- Describe how scientific research presented in the literature can help reduce injury risk and maximize performance.

As a dancer, you are aware of the rigorous physical and mental demands of dance, including what it takes to allow you to dance successfully while not getting injured. Therefore, you know that keeping your mind and body healthy is a priority. Consider your dance classes. Your training focuses on learning technique and building the skills necessary to perform at your best. In addition to learning actual dance techniques and choreography, you likely perform warm-ups, cool-downs, and other strategies to increase your abilities when dancing. Certainly, you want to do these tasks as well as possible.

Along with physical training, reading and applying research can help enhance your dance abilities. Research enables you to choose best practices as a dancer. Practitioners and researchers working in the broad multidisciplinary field of dance medicine and science aim to answer questions that are important for keeping dancers healthy. If you think that research is too formal or complicated, or you think that scientific writing is too dense for your day-to-day practice as a dancer, this chapter is for you. It is designed to help make research more accessible. It will enable you to use evidence to determine best practices for training, dance education, reducing injury risk, and other topics that are relevant to you as a dancer, choreographer, or dance educator. Developing this ability will help you become a better and healthier dancer. To read research or other pieces of scientific literature, you must first understand how researchers use the scientific method to generate information.

The Scientific Method

In simple words, all research using the scientific method begins with a question. This question may be a direct question (e.g., *How are they able to do all those pirouettes without falling over?*) or an indirect one (e.g., *Does Pilates training improve dance performance?*). You may have wondered about one of these or similar kinds of questions.

In **quantitative research**, researchers use this kind of questioning to develop one (or more) research question(s). Then, they develop a possible explanation by creating a **hypothesis**. Next, they design an experiment to test that hypothesis. On the other hand, in **qualitative research**, the researchers may not have a hypothesis; instead, they want to examine a phenomenon (e.g., the lived experiences of a principal dancer in a professional dance company). Regardless of the type of research, researchers create methods that are appropriate to answer the research question(s). Then, they analyze the data, generate results, interpret the results, and discuss the findings. The discussion section of a good research report (often published in a scientific journal) presents the results of the study in the context of prior research. It suggests how the new findings support or refute the hypothesis, or it describes qualitative themes that emerge from the data. Then, it compares the results to results from other researchers, and it provides information about the relevance or applicability of the research.

For example, if researchers have a question about injury risk in contemporary dancers, they may hypothesize that a strength and conditioning program would reduce injury risk in the dancers. They could then design a study where such a program is implemented using a group of dancers who are given an exercise regimen to follow; those dancers would be monitored over time for injury occurrence. Researchers could then compare the injury numbers in this group to those of a group of dancers who did not participate in the exercise program. This analysis would help determine whether the exercise program was effective in reducing injury risk. After finishing the study, the researchers would publish and share the results in the form of an article in a peer-reviewed scientific research journal. **Peer review** is a process by which other experts in the field (peers of the researchers) review the proposed article for proper methods, accuracy of results, and importance of conclusions before it is accepted for publication.

Journals publish several types of research articles. The most common type is the **primary source** article. In this type of article, authors describe original research where they have used the scientific method to examine and describe a phenomenon, test a hypothesis, or make some inferences from their observations.

Typical Sections in a Primary Source Research Article

Generally, most research journals use a standard way of presenting a primary source (original) research study. The acronym for the basic form is IMRaD—Introduction, Methods (or Materials and Methods), Results, and Discussion. Sometimes an A (abstract) is added at the beginning, making the acronym AIMRaD.

Abstract

The abstract provides a summary of the study; it is the first place where you get a big picture perspective of the investigation that was performed. The abstract may be structured (using multiple paragraphs or including subheadings) or not; either way, it should contain enough information to describe the study. While the length may differ across journals, generally an abstract is between 150 and 400 words.

Introduction

The introduction section begins the main body of the article. While research articles usually display the AIMRaD headings of Abstract, Methods, Results, and Discussion, the section title "Introduction" may or may not appear; it depends on the preference of the journal. However, the descriptive section that begins the main part of the article after the abstract is consistently known as the introduction, even without the heading. In this section, researchers provide the background and significance of the study. Researchers should also describe the gap in the body of knowledge about the topic and establish the need for the study. Then, they should provide the purpose of their research investigation. The purpose may include hypotheses for a quantitative study or a rationale for a qualitative study. A good purpose statement directly leads to the next section of the study, where researchers describe their methods.

Methods

In this section, researchers clearly describe what they did in the study. Often this section has subsections, which may include subheadings such as Research Design, Participants, Setting, Equipment, Procedures, and Data Analysis. These subsections should provide any reader with enough information to replicate the methods in a follow-up study. In the Research Design subsection, researchers typically describe how they chose to design their study. This design should provide a guide for the other Methods subsections.

The Participants, Setting, and Equipment subsections include information about the individuals who are studied; the setting where the study was conducted; and any equipment (e.g., measurement devices, training systems), software, and other testing materials (e.g., surveys) that were used to complete the study. If the study included human participants, the authors should provide information about obtaining approval from a research ethics committee, which may be called an institutional review board (IRB) or something similar. Authors should indicate that the participants signed an informed consent document (when the research participants are minors, under the age of 18, they sign an assent form and their parent or guardian signs the informed consent) acknowledging any risks of the study and stating that they willingly chose to participate. In this section, the researchers also explain their inclusion and exclusion criteria. These criteria clarify who was and who was not included as a participant in the study and why researchers made those decisions.

Next, the researchers describe their procedures. They include the step-by-step process of how they performed the study from the participants' point of view. Then, the researchers explain the variables and outcome measures evaluated in the study. Variables include independent variables that the researchers created for the study (e.g., dancers vs nondancers, dance genres participated in, age) and dependent variables that are the outcome measures they assessed (e.g., lower-leg strength, jump height, flexibility, nutritional intake).

After the Procedures subsection, researchers explain their analyses; they describe how they extracted the raw data and how they analyzed the data. For example, in quantitative parametric research, the authors should describe whether or not they examined if their data were normally distributed (indicated by a normal bell-shaped curve when the results are plotted on a graph), what statistical tests they used based on the research design, and other important statistical measures for their study. For qualitative studies (which are very different from quantitative research because qualitative researchers do not analyze numbers from measurements), they should explain their coding and analysis techniques.

Results

In this next section, the researchers present their results. They often use a combination of written and visual graphical display formats (e.g., tables, charts, graphs, photographs, or illustrations) to showcase what they found. In this section, the researchers do not explain the reasons for the results; they only state the results in an objective and unbiased manner.

Discussion

Next, researchers provide a comprehensive discussion of their results. They explain why the results are important, how they compare to prior research, what value they offer to the field's knowledge, possible shortcomings of their study, recommendations for further research, and their conclusions and take-home points.

Depending on the style used by the journal in which an article is published, some discussion sections use subsections with subheadings while others do not. Regardless of the subheadings, the information follows a typical pattern. Ideally, the discussion should be a review of the study's purpose and how the results inform its hypothesis (or multiple hypotheses). The first part includes the primary findings where the readers can clearly see the study's main observations. In the next part, the researchers compare and contrast their results with other published research, and they describe how their results support or refute this prior research. They also offer explanations for their findings. Thereafter, researchers explain how and why they believe their hypothesis or hypotheses (for quantitative studies) or their interpretations of the data (for qualitative studies) were or were not supported.

Then, the researchers discuss their study's limitations or reasons for possible errors. No study is perfect; they all have limitations. In this section, researchers describe only those limitations they could not address or control for when conducting their study as well as the possible effects these limitations may have had on their study. Following this description, researchers offer recommendations for further research, using the study's findings as a stepping stone for additional work in the topic area. Following this subsection, they explain the practical implications or clinical applications of their study, and they provide clear information about how the study helps advance the field. In the final part of the article (the conclusion section), the researchers summarize their study in a few short sentences, including take-home points that give the reader a final understanding of the study's usefulness.

Keep in mind that while the previously described sections represent the typical format of a research article, they may differ depending on a journal's specific requirements, the questions asked by the researchers, and the intended audience. Nevertheless, all studies should leave you with a final impression of the value of the research that is reported. After reading the study, ask yourself questions such as *What new and useful knowledge did I gain?* and *How can this knowledge advance my own understanding and work in the field?* Asking these questions can help you gather a final takeaway from any research article or other research resource.

Research Resources

When a piece of information comes to your attention, you should assess its source; in other words, consider the question *What is the origin of this information, and who produced it?* Research evidence can be found in many places, and some of those places are more reliable than others. The most rigorous (and thus most believable) types of research evidence are found in peer-reviewed journal articles, which are typically published in a reputable scientific journal. For example, the *Journal of Dance Medicine & Science* (*JDMS*), an international journal for research related to dance medicine and science, is a peer-reviewed journal. A number of dance medicine and science-related articles also appear in the journal *Medical Problems in Performing Artists*. In addition, it is common to find articles on dance injuries, dance psychology, and other topics related to dance medicine and science in a wide array of journals that pertain to fields other than dance. Examples include the *American Journal of Sports Medicine*, the *Journal of Athletic Training*, the *Journal of Sports Sciences*, the *Journal of Strength and Conditioning Research*, *Medicine & Science in Sports and Exercise*, and the *Scandinavian Journal of Medicine and Science in Sports*.

When a peer-reviewed journal receives an article from an author to be considered for publication, the article is sent for evaluation to fellow researchers (peers). These reviewers provide their opinion to the journal editors about whether the article should be rejected, accepted as is, or revised before they can make a decision. If the general idea of the article falls within the area of research interest for the journal and its audience, and if the study has merit to serve the audience, the reviewers will work with the journal editors and provide constructive feedback to the authors to improve the clarity of the article's sections. Only when the article is deemed satisfactory by these reviewers is the article published in the journal for readers to access, hence the term *peer reviewed*. This designation does not automatically mean that an article is of high quality, but electing to read articles from peer-reviewed journals is a good first step toward obtaining expert information and using reputable evidence.

As you might imagine, many other sources offer good information that is not peer reviewed. Magazines, websites, blogs, and social media outlets can also provide material that you may find useful. Sometimes, these types of sources share information that is based on a peer-reviewed journal article. If possible, it is always best to refer to the original published article. Overall, though, if a resource is not reviewed by peers, you must critically evaluate the quality of its information. Later in this chapter, the section titled Reading Research to Evaluate Quality will guide you in this process.

Types of Research Literature

The two main types of research literature are primary sources and secondary sources. **Primary sources** are artifacts, documents, manuscripts, recordings, or any other sources of information that were created at the time under study. They serve as original sources of information about the topic. In research and scholarship, primary sources present original data that were collected by the researchers who wrote the article. Various types of primary sources include **randomized controlled trials**, descriptive research, cohort studies, and case studies.

On the other hand, **secondary sources** are documents or other forms of information that relate or discuss information originally presented elsewhere. These compile information from one or more primary sources. They can be extremely valuable because they pull together a large amount of evidence about a topic, and they are often published in scientific journals alongside primary sources. However, they do not present their own data. Secondary sources include articles such as **systematic reviews**, meta-analyses, narrative reviews, and clinical practice guidelines. You should evaluate both primary and secondary sources to ensure they are valid (accurate) and reliable (consistent) before you apply them in your own situation.

Approaches to Research

Approaches for answering a research question vary, and researchers may use different types of **study designs** based on the approach chosen. Qualitative research tends to address more theoretical questions, or it tries to describe a construct or experience. Qualitative research studies are often based on surveys or interviews with participants who explain experiences or ideas about a topic. For example, Pollard-Smith and Thomson (2017) investigated the experiences of dancers who sought health care for a dance injury. Quantitative research, on the other hand, uses specific measurements to examine a concept, reports the results numerically, and uses traditional **statistics** to draw conclusions about the data. For example, researchers used a quantitative approach to determine that dancers demonstrate changes in lower-extremity jumping mechanics after fatigue, thus indicating a potential deficit in eccentric muscle strength (Abergel et al., 2021).

Both qualitative and quantitative research can be conducted using different types of study designs, which depend on the research question. All of these different types of studies can provide useful results or evidence that may affect dance practice. The term **evidence-based practice** suggests that a particular action—whether it be a health care procedure, a physical training method, a psychological technique, a dance training practice, or something else—is performed in a way that uses research evidence to ensure that the action is done correctly, maximizing the chance that the desired effect of the action is achieved.

As explained earlier, all scientific research begins with a research question. The question determines what research study design should be used to answer it. Table 3.1 provides a list of common scientific research designs. While it is not a complete list, each study design provided can be very useful depending on the research question to be answered and whether it is interpreted in the context of the type of decision making it allows. While systematic reviews and randomized controlled trials are considered higher-level evidence and more reliable and valid than other types of research, they may not always be the best choice for providing information

A Scientific Abstract: The Whole Article at a Glance

In the AIMRaD system, the letter A stands for "Abstract," which is a short synopsis of a scientific article. Although an abstract is brief, it includes a wealth of information. For example, the abstract in figure 3.1 summarizes a research study about injuries, illnesses, and intensity of physical training in contemporary dancers. The full article was published in the *Journal of Athletic Training,* but the abstract was found using the PubMed database of the National Library of Medicine, pubmed.gov (Jeffries et al., 2020). Within the abstract, you can see the remaining IMRaD pieces along with additional important descriptors about the article; the boldface headings tell you that it is a structured abstract. Note that abstracts from different journals may be written slightly differently, but the order of the IMRaD pieces are essentially the same.

A B C D

J Athl Train. 2020 Sep 1;55(9):967-976. doi: 10.4085/1062-6050-477-19.

1 **Injury, Illness, and Training Load in a Professional Contemporary Dance Company: A Prospective Study**

Annie C Jeffries, Lee Wallace, Aaron J Coutts, Ashlea Mary Cohen, Alan McCall, Franco M Impellizzeri

Abstract

2 **Context:** Professional dance is a demanding physical activity with high injury rates. Currently, no epidemiologic data exist regarding the incidence of injury and illness together with training load (TL) over a long period of time.
Objective: To provide a detailed description of injury, illness, and TL occurring in professional contemporary dancers.

3 **Design:** Descriptive epidemiology study.
Setting: A single professional contemporary dance company during a 1-year period.
Patients or other participants: A total of 16 male and female professional contemporary dancers.
Main outcome measure(s): Injury data consisted of medical-attention injury (Med-Inj) and time-loss injury (Time-Inj). Illness was measured using the Wisconsin Upper Respiratory Tract Infection Survey. Training load was collected for each dance session using the session rating of perceived exertion and classified into 3 groups based on individual and group percentiles: low, medium, or high.

4 **Results:** Reported injuries totaled 79 (86.1% new, 6.3% reinjury, and 7.6% exacerbation). The Med-Inj incidence rate was 4.6 per 1000 hours (95% confidence interval [CI] = 3.8, 5.8), and the Time-Inj rate was 1.4 per 1000 hours (95% CI = 0.8, 2.1). The median time until injury for Med-Inj and Time-Inj was 3 months. The number of days dancers experienced illness symptoms was 39.9 ± 26.9 (range = 1-96), with an incidence rate of 9.1 per 1000 hours (95% CI = 7.7, 10.7). Mean weekly TL was 6685 ± 1605 (4641-10 391; arbitrary units). Inconsistent results were found for the incidence of injury and illness based on individual and group categorizations of TL.

5 **Conclusions:** Professional dancing is associated with high injury and illness rates. This is worrying from a health perspective and underlines the need for further studies to understand how to decrease the risk. The TL is higher than in other sport disciplines, but whether the high incidence of injuries and illnesses is related to high training demands needs additional investigation, possibly conducted as international, multicenter collaborative studies.

6 **Keywords:** individual differences; injury surveillance; rating of perceived exertion; upper respiratory tract infection.

Figure 3.1 A scientific abstract with many types of information, as depicted in the PubMed database of the National Library of Medicine (pubmed.gov). See the key at the end of this sidebar.

Adapted from Jeffries et al. (2020).

(continued)

Use this key to learn about the various pieces in the figure:

1: *Journal publication information.* The top line includes bibliographic information, such as the following:

A: Abbreviated journal title (an abbreviation for the *Journal of Athletic Training*)

B: Publication date (September 1, 2020)

C: The journal's volume number (55), the volume's issue number (9), and the page numbers where the article appears (967-976)

D: The digital object identifier (doi), a unique number given to any object that its creator wants to register (in this case, a journal article)

The lines that follow include the article's title and its authors.

2: *I—Introduction.* This section includes the context for the study and its objective, or purpose. Some abstracts may include the pertinent background for the study.

3: *M—Methods.* This section includes how the study is categorized according to its research design, what type of environment it was conducted in, and what was measured during the study.

4: *R—Results.* This section includes the findings of the study. Usually, limited space allows for only the primary results, those that are most important to advancing scientific knowledge, or those that have the greatest practical implications.

5: *D—Discussion.* This section includes the Conclusions portion of the discussion. Once again, because of space limitations in an abstract, researchers provide only the highlights of how their study can impact the field.

6: Although it is not part of the AIMRaD arrangement, this section offers keywords—words and phrases that categorize the research and can help you find related information by searching for other articles that contain those same words and phrases.

Table 3.1 **Common Types of Scientific Research Designs**

Study design	Description
Systematic review	Researchers use a systematic method to extract, compile, analyze, and review information from the existing literature about a specific research question.
Randomized controlled trial	Researchers study the effects of an intervention by randomly assigning participants to groups, where at least one group takes part in the intervention (intervention group; e.g., dancers taking part in Pilates) and another group (the control group; e.g., dancers not taking part in Pilates) does not take part in any intervention.
Cohort study	Researchers examine data for a single group at multiple time points, or they compare data between two or more predetermined groups (e.g., dancers and nondancers).
Case-control studies	Researchers compare groups—one group with a certain condition (e.g., Achilles tendinopathy) and a control group (e.g., healthy dancers); groups are matched on certain characteristics, such as age, activity level, weight, or type of dance.
Case series	Researchers provide detailed information about a small group of individuals with a similar background or who sustain a specific type of injury or have a specific condition.
Case study	Researchers provide detailed information about one individual with a specific background or who sustains a specific type of injury or has a specific condition.
Basic science	Researchers examine a question that pertains to the area but does not include human participants (e.g., examining the stiffness properties of a sprung dance floor, presence of the amount of pathological bacteria on dance surfaces).

about a certain research question. As you search for evidence related to topics of interest, keep in mind the different types and levels of study designs.

When designing and conducting research, researchers do as much as possible to eliminate the introduction of bias to the study results. Bias in a research setting is any factor that could influence the results of the study beyond what is being examined by the researchers or that could produce inaccuracy in the results. Minimizing bias is an important goal in research. However, while the best controlled studies may minimize bias, they may also eliminate factors that are relevant in the real world, making it harder to apply the results in the field. Therefore, researchers should balance these factors when designing studies. Different types of studies may have different levels of susceptibility to bias. The following section discusses some tools for assessing the quality of a study.

Accessing Research

Thanks to the Internet, research articles are much easier to access today than they used to be. You can find the abstracts of most articles by simply typing an author's name with their article's topic or its title and year of publication into any search engine. While multiple useful databases and search engines exist for gathering these articles, many require an institutional affiliation or paid journal subscription to acquire full-text articles. *Full text* denotes the complete document of an article rather than just the abstract. Table 3.2 provides a list of common databases and search engines that are useful in dance medicine and science. For an example of how to use these databases, see the sidebar titled A Simple Way to Find Dance Medicine and Science Research Articles.

When locating journal articles of interest, you may see the term **open access**. Open-access articles are those where the authors, their institution, or (occasionally) a journal publisher have paid a fee to cover the costs of producing their published journal article. These fees usually range from US$1,000 to US$4,000 per article. The advantage of open-access articles is that they are made available for free to anyone who wishes to access them worldwide. Therefore, a reader (or their institution) does not need to purchase a subscription to the journal in order to read an open-access article.

WWW Go to HK*Propel* to download table 3.2.

Performing Arts and Non–Performing Arts Sources

Information on dance medicine and science is available in a myriad of periodicals, books, magazines, and blogs; table 3.3 includes samples of resources that are wholly or partially devoted to it. Within the decade from 2011 to 2021, the number of publications in this topic area notably increased and that trend continues. To refine searches in PubMed, a system called Medical Subject Headings (MeSH) is used. MeSH terms are simply consistent, finite sets of words and phrases by which scientific articles are classified. One of these sets is *dance injury*. To demonstrate the expansion of dance medicine and science literature over two decades, a MeSH query for *dance injury* in PubMed to find articles published between 2000 and 2010 yields 180 results. The same query for the period of 2011 to 2021 yields 402 results, which is more than double the number of articles from the prior decade.

The *Journal of Dance Medicine & Science* and *Medical Problems of Performing Artists* are the only two international journals devoted specifically to the health, medical, and scientific aspects of performing arts. Between them, they published nearly one-third of the peer-reviewed journal articles on dance injury in the query for articles between 2011 and 2021. This means the remaining 70 percent of peer-reviewed dance injury articles were published in non–dance science journals. Thus, do not limit your search to dance-specific sites or journals. You should also look for information in journals and resources related to sports, nutrition, psychology, occupational health, and many other disciplines.

Reading Research to Evaluate Quality

Now that you have a general understanding of where to find information about dance injuries and related topics, the next step is to be able to read research and evaluate the quality of the available information. The first two decades of the 21st century and beyond have been a golden age of information; during this time, more information became available than ever, and its production pace continues to accelerate. For any consumer of information, the sources from which information originates are almost limitless. These sources include scholarly journals, newspapers, television, magazines, websites, blogs, podcasts, and social media outlets.

There are almost 30,000 journals that publish close to 2 million scientific research papers yearly (Altbach & de Wit, 2018). With so much information available, you may often feel as if you were drinking it from a fire hose. In addition, it can be challenging to choose which information to believe when making decisions for yourself or for dancers with whom you are working. As mentioned earlier, research is evidence with which to make evidence-based decisions. To use it, you need a

Table 3.2 **Common Search Engines and Databases**

Database	Details	Link and access to full-text articles
PubMed	Free-to-use database containing more than 34 million items in the U.S. National Library of Medicine (citations come from a bibliographic database called MEDLINE) Also includes other types of article resources	www.pubmed.gov Contains abstracts only, with links to obtain full-text articles (some access may require a fee) Possible subscriptions available to university libraries with full-text access for students and faculty
PubMed Central (PMC)	Free-to-use search engine accessing primarily the MEDLINE database of references as well as abstracts on life sciences and biomedical topics that appear in articles with full-text copies available	www.ncbi.nlm.nih.gov/pmc Provides links to full-text content from publishers' websites May charge a fee for access
BioMed Central	Provides access to more than 290 peer-reviewed journals in the fields of biology, clinical medicine, and health	www.biomedcentral.com/journals Open access available
Dimensions	Contains a variety of more than 100 million publications, ranging from articles published in scholarly journals and books to preprints and conference proceedings	https://app.dimensions.ai/discover/publication Open access available
Google Scholar	Free search engine that indexes the full text or metadata of scholarly literature across an array of publishing formats and disciplines	https://scholar.google.com Provides links to full-text content from publishers' websites (which may charge a fee for access)
JSTOR	Provides access to academic journals and books covering a wide range of disciplines Also includes some limited primary source collections	www.jstor.org Limited open content and free access to read online Requires institutional or individual subscription
Paperity	Multidisciplinary aggregator of open-access journals and papers	https://paperity.org Open access available
Public Library of Science (PLOS)	A nonprofit, open-access science, technology, and medicine publisher	https://plos.org Open access available
Science Open	Offers open access to more than 28 million articles in all areas of science	www.scienceopen.com Open access with a free registered account
ScienceDirect	Provides access to a large bibliographic database of scientific and medical publications of the Dutch publisher Elsevier	www.sciencedirect.com Mix of open-access materials and resources requiring an institutional subscription
Scopus	Commercial bibliographic database that covers scholarly literature from almost any discipline; provides academic journal rankings and author profiles	www.scopus.com/home.uri Limited free previews; full access by institutional subscription only

so-called smell test to find out if it's good or if it stinks; in other words, you must examine evidence as you would anything else you consume. When deciding what research deserves your attention, you need a filter to support your critical thinking.

One such filter is a method for conducting a quality assessment that is aptly named the CRAAP test; CRAAP stands for currency, relevance, authority, accuracy, and purpose (Blakeslee, 2004). The CRAAP test was created by Sarah Blakeslee of the Meriam Library at California State University, Chico. While the CRAAP test can be used in any field, this chapter provides an adapted version for dance medicine and science (see table 3.4).

Use the CRAAP test to assess how valid and reliable a resource is, whether it be a scholarly article, an

A Simple Way to Find Dance Medicine and Science Research Articles

Do not be afraid of scientific research! Research articles can be very enlightening and helpful for improving many aspects of dancing. The process of finding research articles is very straightforward, so use this hands-on example to jump in.

First, visit the website for PubMed, the database of the U.S. National Library of Medicine (pubmed.gov). An easy way to start is simply to enter the words *dance injuries* into the search box. Figure 3.2*a* shows the results of this search, including links to two articles. Clicking on the first of the two articles yields the article information and abstract (figure 3.2*b*). There are several places you can click to obtain further information, including the option to download the full article if the abstract piques your interest. Keep in mind that your college or university library probably has subscription packages that will allow you to obtain the complete articles from some journals but not for others. Check with your librarian for further information about obtaining specific articles.

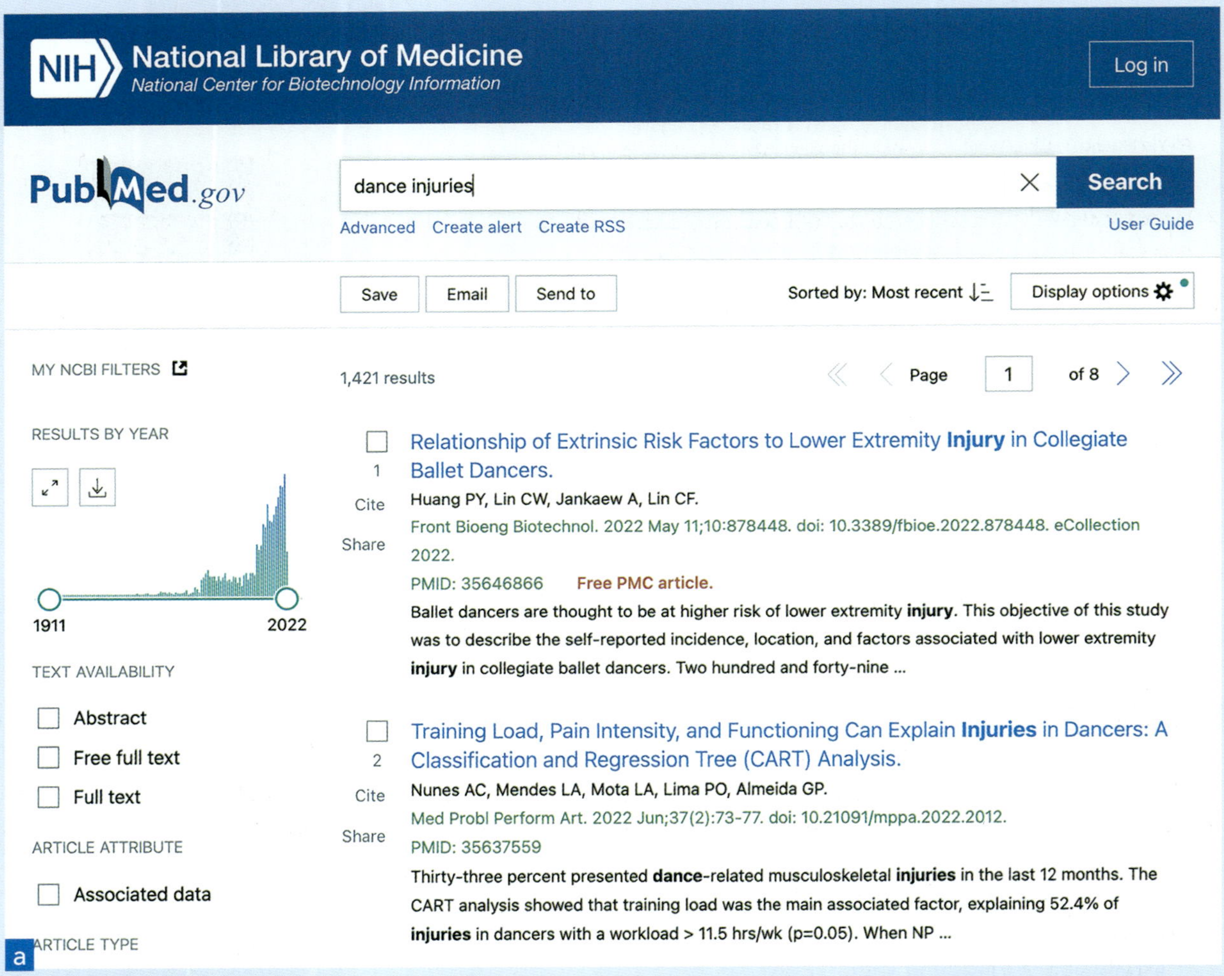

Figure 3.2 *(a)* The beginning of the results from a sample search using the key words *dance injuries* at pubmed.gov. *(b) continued*

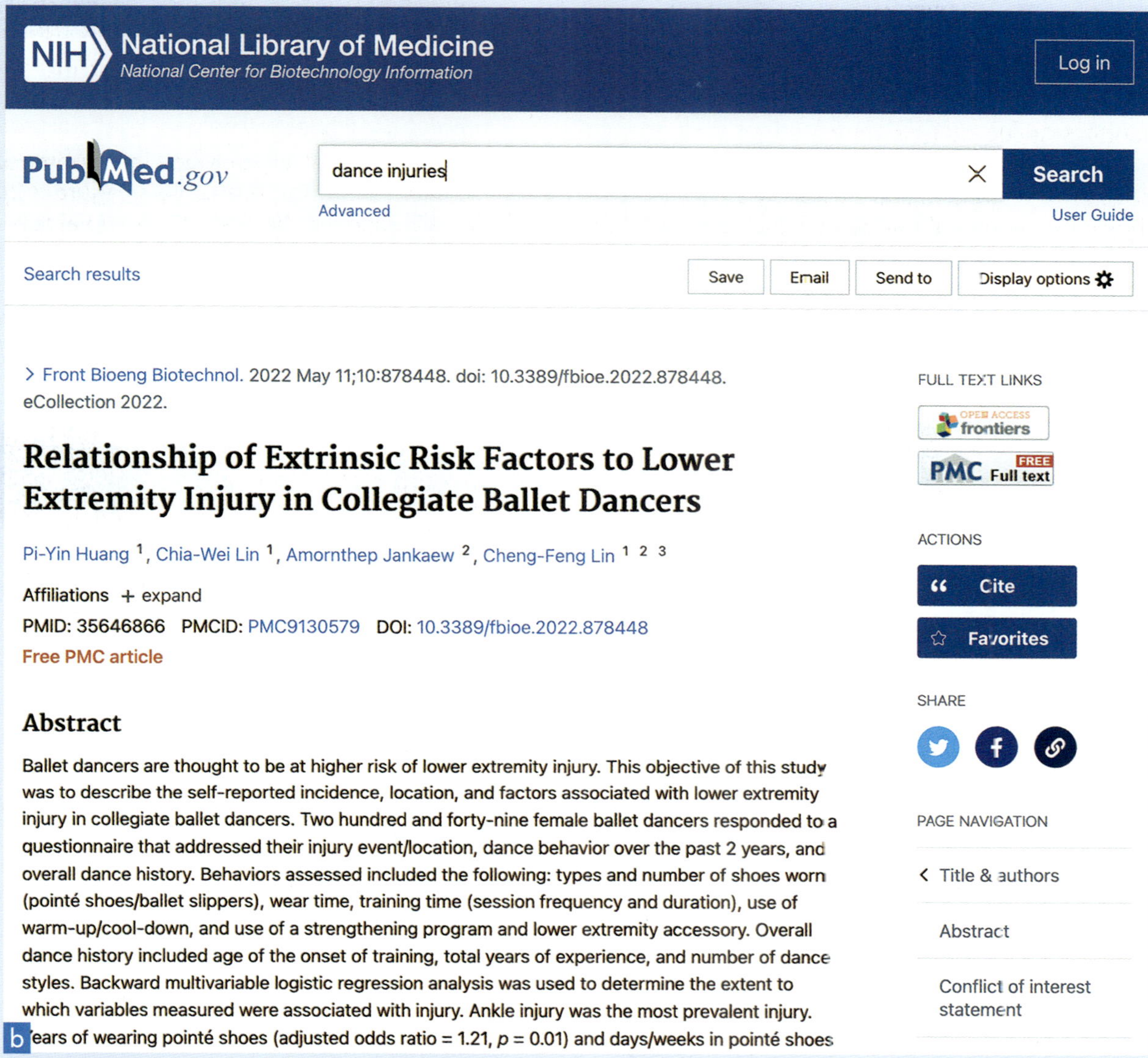

Figure 3.2 *(b)* The information produced when you click on the first article retrieved by the search. (Note that only part of the article's abstract is shown here.)

To find more specifically oriented articles, you can enter certain text strings such as those shown in **bold** in the following list. Be sure to type them exactly as shown (e.g., no space between a word and a command in square brackets).

- Enter **dance** to find articles with the word *dance* anywhere in the article's record.
- Enter **dance AND psychology** to find articles with both *dance* and *psychology* anywhere in the article's record.
- Enter **dance[ti]** to find articles with the word *dance* in the title.
- Enter **danc*[ti]** to find articles with any words that begin with *dance* in the title, such as *dance, dances, dancer, dancing*, and so on.
- Enter **ballet[ti] OR modern[ti]** to find articles that have only the word *ballet*, only the word *modern*, or both words in the title.
- Enter **Smith[au]** to find articles by all authors with the last name or surname of Smith.
- Enter **Smith AB[au]** to find articles by the author A.B. Smith.
- Enter **Smith AB[au] AND dance[ti]** to find all articles written by A.B. Smith and that have the word *dance* in the title.

(continued)

A Simple Way to Find Dance Medicine and Science Research Articles *(continued)*

Although many other combinations exist, trying these commonly used ones will help you get started. Remember that a database is a computer, and a computer cannot think the same way you do. Thus, it is likely that during any search, you will find several articles that have nothing to do with what you are looking for, and maybe they will not even be related to dance. Just continue to refine your search until you find articles that are relevant to your interests.

Now, take your own exploratory journey through the PubMed database to find fascinating scientific literature. Try searching with some of the other databases mentioned in table 3.2 too.

Table 3.3 **Sample Resources With Dance Medicine and Science Topics**

Peer-reviewed journals*	Books	Magazines, blogs, and other resources
Journal of Dance Medicine & Science	*Dance Anatomy*, Second Edition by Jacqui Greene Haas (2016)	*Dance Magazine*
Medical Problems of Performing Artists	*Dance Anatomy and Kinesiology*, Third Edition by Karen Clippinger (2023)	*Pointe*
Medicine and Science in Sports and Exercise	*Safe Dance Practice* by Edel Quin, Sonia Rafferty, and Charlotte Tomlinson (2015)	*Dance Teacher*
International Journal of Sports Medicine	*Injury Prevention and Management for Dancers* by Nick Allen (2019)	*Dance Spirit*
BMJ Open Sport & Exercise Medicine	*Dance Medicine in Practice: Anatomy, Injury Prevention, Training* by Liane Simmel (2014)	4dancers.org (science-based resource center for dancers)
Clinical Journal of Sport Medicine	*Dancing Longer, Dancing Stronger*, Second Edition by Robin Kish and Jennie Morton (2019)	https://iadms.org/resources/blog (blog of the International Association for Dance Medicine and Science [IADMS])

*Note that the word *journal* does not appear in many journals' titles.

article on a website, a piece shared on social media, a news program, a blog, or another source. Each component of the test offers insight for evaluating the research by examining the currency, relevance, authority, accuracy, and purpose (CRAAP) of the resource. Table 3.4 provides an easy-to-use scheme to implement the test. Table 3.5 shows the scale used to evaluate the CRAAP score for a resource.

After you determine the quality of the source and decide that you want to use it, the next step is to read through the details of the article. When reading peer-reviewed articles that report quantitative research, you will note that researchers use numerical values and statistical calculations to describe their results, determine whether their hypotheses were supported or refuted, and make predictions. The following sections include tips and information to help you more easily interpret this information.

Interpreting Statistical Information

Interpreting statistical information may make your heart, breathing, and sweat rates increase just as they do in a challenging dance class. However, once you learn a few approachable terms and concepts, research articles will be much more understandable. While **mean**, probability value (P value), **odds ratio**, **analysis of variance (ANOVA)**, and other common tests may sound like a foreign language, do not skip this section of a research article to go straight to the researchers' conclusions. The accuracy component of the CRAAP test asks how reliable, truthful, and correct information is. Therefore, a basic understanding of statistics is central to answering the accuracy questions. The purpose of this section

Table 3.4 **Grading Rubric for Conducting the CRAAP Test**

CRAAP test component	Yes (2 points)	Maybe (1 point)	No/cannot assess (0 points)	Score: ___/2
Currency: How timely is the information?				
How long ago was the information published or posted?	0-5 years (2 points)	6-9 years (1 point)	10+ years (0 points)	
Is the information still current for your topic?				
Does the source cite current facts, opinions, and studies?				
Does it discuss other current studies or articles?				
Has the information been revised or updated?				
				Currency: ___/10
Relevance: How important is the information to you?				
Does the information relate to your topic?				
Do you know the intended audience?				
Is the information presented at an appropriate level?				
Have the authors looked at a variety of sources before writing?				
Would you use this source to change your health care or dance practice?				
				Relevance: ___/10
Authority: What is the source of the information?				
Is the author, publisher, source, or sponsor named?				
Does the work list contact information, a publisher name, or an e-mail address?				
Are the author's credentials and affiliations given?				
Could you find the credentials easily?				
Is the author qualified to write about the topic?				
				Authority: ___/10
Accuracy: How reliable, truthful, and correct is the information?				
Has the information been reviewed or refereed by other peers or experts?				
Is the information supported by evidence?				
Can you verify any of the information in another source?				
Is the language or tone unbiased and free of emotion?				
Is the information free of spelling, grammar, or other kinds of typographical errors?				
				Accuracy: ___/10

(continued)

Table 3.4 *(continued)*

CRAAP test component	Yes (2 points)	Maybe (1 point)	No/cannot assess (0 points)	Score: ___/2
Purpose: Is the reason why the information exists clear?				
Do the authors make their intentions or purpose clear?				
Does the point of view appear objective and impartial?				
Is the information free of political, ideological, cultural, or religious biases?				
Does the resource include supporting evidence and not just personal opinion?				
Does the resource use rhetorical appeals* (ethos, pathos, logos) equally?				
				Purpose:___/10
			Total score:	**___/50**

*Rhetorical appeals originated with Aristotle as he described the persuasiveness of arguments. *Ethos* is the communicator's ability to persuade an audience based on the personal character of the communicator; *pathos* is the communicator's ability to draw an emotional response from the audience; and *logos* is the communicator's ability to use facts, logic, and reasoning to persuade the audience.

Adapted from S. Blakeslee, "The CRAAP Test," *LOEX Quarterly* 31, no. 3 (2004), 6-7.

Table 3.5 **CRAAP Test Score Interpretation**

Score	Letter	Meaning
45-50	A	Source is excellent; it is current, reliable, authoritative, accurate, and purposeful.
40-44	B	Source is mostly current, reliable, authoritative, accurate, and purposeful.
35-39	C	Source is lacking in two or more core areas; it should be used with caution.
30-34	D	Source is severely lacking; it should be used only if another source is found to confirm it.
0-29	F	Source should not be used.

Adapted from S. Blakeslee, "The CRAAP Test," *LOEX Quarterly* 31, no. 3 (2004), 6-7.

is to help you understand statistical results commonly presented in quantitative research articles. Detailed descriptions of statistical analyses or tests are beyond the scope of this chapter; if you are interested in learning more, consult statistical textbooks and the myriad of other available resources on statistics.

There are two main types of statistical methods: descriptive and inferential. Both are important for different reasons. Descriptive statistics (e.g., frequencies, percentages, averages, and ranges) summarize the data and are reported numerically or graphically. They can also provide information about relationships among different variables. Inferential statistics, on the other hand, make an inference, suggestion, or judgment about the described data and the associated variables. They may also provide information about cause-and-effect relationships. Figure 3.3 offers a list of common statistical analyses under each method. Definitions for them are provided in the glossary.

Descriptive and inferential statistics are often used in combination. That is, more than one of each type of analysis often are employed in a single research study. We are now going to work with an example of one such study. Novosel and colleagues (2019) examined sex-specific correlates of injury occurrence and time off due to injury in professional ballet dancers. They considered the relationship between injury occurrence rate and factors that could affect injury risk. The differences between sexes were examined by the **Mann-Whitney U test** (for number of injuries) and the **chi-square statistic** (for injury occurrence). Figure 3.4 contains excerpts from the Methods and Results sections of their published article. As previously mentioned,

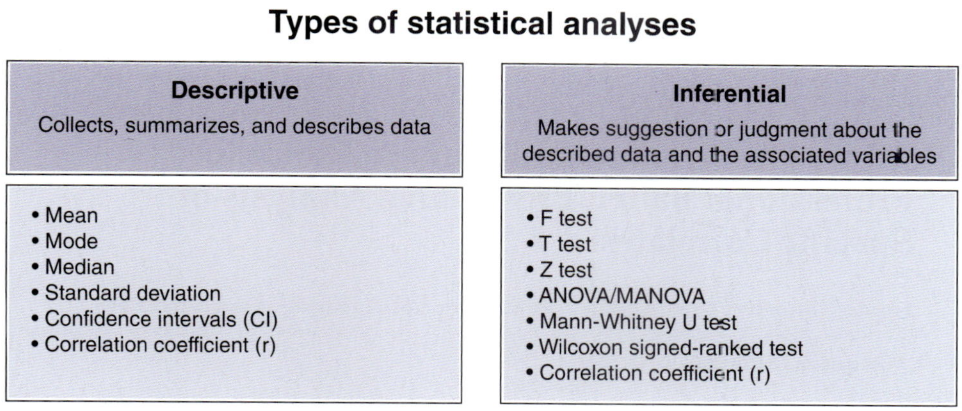

Figure 3.3 Common statistical analyses used in descriptive and inferential methods.

this section does not discuss the tests themselves in any detail but focuses on how to interpret the results presented. You are encouraged to access and read the entire article to gain a full understanding of the study.

Before we go further, it is important to note that the example we are using is an excellent study for learning practical statistical principles. However, there is one flaw in the article, and it is a common error seen in current scientific literature. The research abstract speaks of gender when it discusses examining differences between females and males. Gender is a social construct with several possible choices; an individual can select a gender identity with which they are most comfortable. However, when we conduct research with females and males—using these as labels for individuals with specific biological traits—we are really examining differences between sexes. Thus, while the Novosel et al. (2019) abstract in figure 3.4 uses "gender," we will use the appropriate terminology of "sex" in the following section where we discuss research on females and males.

First, read through the text in figure 3.4. Do not be concerned if some of it seems mysterious at first; the text explains it later. The researchers studied 99 dancers over a one-year period. Their results indicate that a total of 196 injuries occurred in the 99 dancers; dividing the number of injuries by number of dancers results in 1.9 injuries per dancer during the year. Males had a higher frequency of injuries than females did; males had 2.4 injuries per dancer (95% CI: 1.7-3.1), and females had 1.59 injuries per dancer (95% CI: 1.1-2.1). The percentage of dancers who reported no injury was similar across sexes (23.7% and 25.42% for males and females, respectively), with no significant difference between sexes (chi-square: 0.20, p = 0.66; odds ratio: 1.5 [95% CI: 0.81-2.94]). Also, there was no statistically significant difference in number of injuries (Mann-Whitney Z value: 1.11, p = 0.26) nor severity of injuries (Mann-Whitney Z value: 0.44, p = 0.65) by sex. The following paragraphs explain each of the results presented.

From the descriptive statistics results in figure 3.4, it is evident that the overall **mean** (average of all the values) number of injuries per dancer is 1.9 (letter A). The **median** (middle value of all the values) number of injuries is not reported, and the **mode** (most frequently occurring value) is not applicable in the discussion of the excerpt provided. However, table 1 of the full article lists the injury locations, of which the ankle was the most frequently injured.

In the excerpt, the mean number of injuries is immediately followed by the **confidence interval (CI)** (letter B). The CI indicates the possible range around the mean value (which is actually an estimate) and how accurate that mean's estimate is. The most common CI used in research is the 95 percent CI, which means that one can be 95 percent confident that the real value of a measurement is within the given CI range. A narrow CI indicates that the results are more precisely known. A wide CI suggests the results are somewhere in a wide range of possible values (du Prel et al., 2009). In this case, the estimate is the mean number of injuries per dancer. For males, it is 2.4, with a 95 percent CI of 1.7 to 3.1, which translates to 95 percent certainty that the real average is somewhere between 1.7 and 3.1 injuries per dancer. Note that the CI range includes the mean number of injuries (2.4 per dancer) in this dancer population that was studied by Novosel's (2019) research team.

International Journal of
Environmental Research and Public Health

MDPI

Article

Injury Occurrence and Return to Dance in Professional Ballet: Prospective Analysis of Specific Correlates

Bozidar Novosel [1,2], Damir Sekulic [3,*], Mia Peric [3], Miran Kondric [4] and Petra Zaletel [4]

. . . .

2. Materials and Methods

. . . .

2.3. Statistics

The statistics were reported as frequencies (number of observations) and percentage (Table S1). Injury rates were calculated as the ratio of injuries per 1000 h of dance (HD) with corresponding 95% confidence intervals (95% CI). The differences between genders were evidenced by Mann-Whitney test (for number of injuries), and Chi square test (injury occurrence). Additionally, to establish the difference in injury rates between genders the Odds Ratio (OR) with corresponding 95% CI were calculated.

To establish the associations between AUDIT, cigarette smoking (smokers vs. non-smokers) and consumption of illicit drugs (users vs. non-users), and criteria, logistic regression analyses were performed for binomial outcomes (injury occurrence: injured vs. non-injured; time-off from injury: absent vs. non-absent). To establish the association between remaining predictors (age, educational level, ballet related factors (experience, performance level, number of training hours), cigarette smoking (observed at ordinal scale), and binge drinking), and two outcomes (injury occurrence, time-off from injury) we calculated Mann-Whitney test. A value of $p < 0.05$ was considered statistically significant. Statistical analyses were performed using Statistica ver 13.3 (Tibco Software Inc., Palo Alto, CA, USA).

3. Results

During the one-year period, a total of 196 injuries occurred, equating to an injury rate of 1.9 injuries per dancer per year (95% CI: 1.6–2.3). The higher frequency is founded in males than in females (2.4 (95% CI: 1.7–3.1) and 1.59 (95% CI: 1.1–2.1) injuries per dancer per year in males and females, respectively). It altogether corresponds with 1.4 (95% CI: 1.1–1.7) injuries per 1000 dance hours (1.7 (95% CI: 1.2–2.2) and 1.1 (95% CI: 0.7–1.5) injuries per 1000 HD in males and females, respectively).

The percentage of dancers who reported no injury was similar across genders (23.7% and 25.42% for males and females, respectively), with no significant difference between genders (Chi square: 0.20, $p = 0.66$; OR: 1.55 (95% CI: 0.81–2.94)). Also, there was no significant difference between genders when number of injuries was observed on an ordinal scale (Mann-Whitney Z value: 1.11, $p = 0.26$).

The ankle was the most common injured location in females, accounting for 36.5% of all injuries, followed by calf (14.6% of all injuries), foot and knee (both accounting for 12.5% of all injuries in females). Male dancers most commonly injured lower back (20% of all reported injuries) followed by ankle (14%), knee (11%) and foot (10% of all reported injuries in males) (Table 1).

. . . .

In females, cigarette smoking was associated with injury occurrence with a higher likelihood of injury in those dancers who smoke (OR: 4.33, 95% CI: 1.05–17.85). Alcohol drinking observed by the AUDIT scale was a significant predictor of absence from dance in females (OR: 1.29, 95% CI: 1.01–4.21) and males (OR: 1.21, 95% CI: 1.05–3.41) (Table 2).

. . . .

Mann-Whitney test revealed significant differences between injured and non-injured female dancers for cigarette smoking status observed at ordinal scale (Z: 2.05, $p = 0.04$), with higher rates of smoking in injured dancers (55% and 41% of non-smokers among non-injured and injured dancers, respectively). Finally, less experienced dancers were more likely to be absent from dance as a result of injury than their more experienced peers (Z: 2.02, $p < 0.04$; with 39% and 30% of dancers with >25 years of experience in ballet among non-absent and absent, respectively) (Table 3).

Int. J. Environ. Res. Public Health **2019**, *16*, 765; doi:10.3390/ijerph16050765 www.mdpi.com/journal/ijerph

Figure 3.4 These excerpts from a study by Novosel and colleagues (2019) show important components of a real research article. Each letter is keyed to a description in the accompanying text.

One descriptive statistic that is not reported in the Novosel (2019) article—but warrants mentioning—is the standard deviation. **Standard deviation (SD)** is a descriptive statistic that tells how far the measurements are spread out from the mean value. A low standard deviation means that most of the numbers are close to the average, while a high standard deviation means that the numbers are more spread out. A convention called the **empirical rule** predicts that 68 percent of the values in a group of data fall in the range between one SD below the mean and one SD above the mean, 95 percent of the values fall within two SDs, and 99.7 percent fall within three SDs above and below. Figure 3.5 depicts this rule graphically.

Examining the inferential statistics in figure 3.4, it is evident that the chi-square statistic [letter C] is 0.20 and the Mann-Whitney Z value [letter D] is 1.11. What do these numbers mean? Do they support the author's statement that no significant difference existed between males and females in the number and severity of their injuries? Why use two different types of tests? For now, do not concern yourself with why a test was used. A statistics course is a good place to learn more about that question. Instead, focus on understanding the numbers. Here are some key points to remember:

- The chi-square statistic compares the injury occurrence actually observed in these dancers to what would be expected in a group of dancers like this one. Greater differences between expected and actual data produce a larger chi-square value. The larger the chi-square value, the greater the probability that there really is a significant difference between expected and observed values. If the expected and observed injury occurrences were identical, then the chi-square value would be 0.
- The Mann-Whitney U is a test used here to compare whether a difference exists in the dependent variable (number of injuries) for two independent groups (in this study, males and females). The **Z value** reported is related to a **probability value (P value)**. The farther a Mann-Whitney Z value is from 0, the lower the P value will be (McLeod, 2019).
- Neither of these tests is ever reported without a P value. This value tells you whether the results are significant. For example, in Novosel's (2019) study, are males and females truly different in the number of injuries they experience, or are they essentially the same even if it looks like they have a slight difference? If males and females are not significantly different when their data are tested using statistics, then you can assume they are the same for the value measured (number of injuries, in our example).

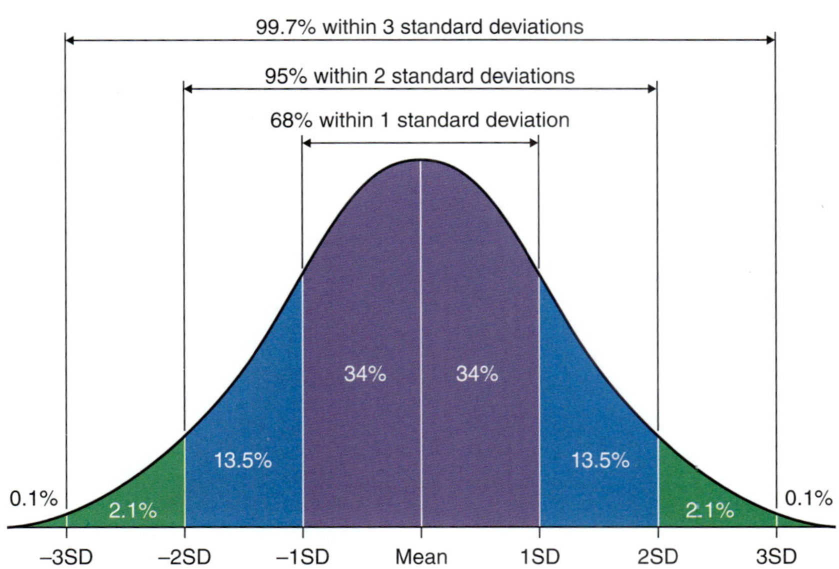

Figure 3.5 Visual depiction of a bell-shaped spread of data; data arranged in this shape are considered normally distributed. The mean (average) value occurs in the center, and plus or minus 1, 2, or 3 standard deviations (SD) extend on both sides from the mean.

The concept of a P value is very important for interpreting research. A P value is a probability (a number between 0 and 1) that indicates the likelihood that the results observed in research were due to chance. A P value of less than 5 percent (< 0.05) is often used as the threshold for statistical significance. In common language, this number means that if the experiment were repeated 100 times, the results would be similar at least 95 times and different less than 5 times. The implication is that the researchers will accept that there may be an error or some type of random variation in their measurements no more than these 5 times.

Clearly, then, the lower the observed P value, the more confident you would be as a researcher (and as a reader of research) that differences exist between the measured variables. For example, if the P value reported in an article is $p < 0.01$, then the experiment will show a true difference more than 99 out of 100 times, and you would expect that a measurement error or random variation exists that makes the results different less than one time out of 100. A probability of $p < 0.001$ suggests that you would see incorrect or random results less than 1 time in 1,000. P values should be considered in conjunction with other measures that are outside the scope of this chapter to determine clinical and meaningful importance. However, knowing the basics of P values will greatly assist you in understanding and applying research evidence to your dance and training practices.

Returning to the results in Novosel's (2019) article, the two P values reported in the excerpt in figure 3.4, 0.66 [letter E] and 0.26 [letter F], are both greater than 0.05. These values indicate there were no significant differences in any of the variables examined by the study.

The final statistic provided in the example is the **odds ratio (OR).** The OR is a measure of the strength of association between an exposure and an outcome. An odds ratio greater than 1 means that the exposure creates greater odds of the outcome occurring; in other words, there is a stronger association between the two. When OR equals 1, the exposure has no effect on the odds of the outcome. When OR is less than 1, the exposure produces lower odds of the outcome occurring. One important point to note is that if the 95 percent confidence interval (CI) for the OR includes 1, the results are not statistically significant, but there still may be some association between the exposure and the outcome (Szumilas, 2010).

Now, apply this information about OR to the Novosel (2019) study (figure 3.4). First, look at the *exposure* of sex (M or F) and the *outcome* of number of injuries. The OR is relatively small (relatively close to 1.0) at 1.55 (letter G), so it helps confirm that there was no association between number of injuries and sex of the dancer. Next, consider the exposure of smoking and the outcome of number of injuries. The OR for those factors is relatively large, at 4.33 (letter H), which suggests that smoking and sustaining more injuries were highly related. In other words, being a smoker increases a dancer's odds of experiencing an injury. This relationship also is confirmed by the statistically significant P value of 0.04 (letter I) from the Mann-Whitney U test showing that there were more uninjured dancers who did not smoke (55% of uninjured dancers were non-smokers) than there were injured dancers who did not smoke (41% of injured dancers were non-smokers).

These examples should provide you with a better understanding of how to interpret statistical results in a research article. Again, while descriptions of advanced statistics is beyond the scope of this chapter, the information offered in this chapter is good preparation to help you make sound decisions about training, injuries, and a variety of other topics where evidence-based practice is important. Try using PubMed that we introduced earlier to find some other research articles with which you can put these techniques to use.

Application of Research

Now that you understand the importance of scientific research and how to access it, evaluate its quality, and interpret its statistics, you can learn how to use research information to reduce injury risk and maximize performance; in other words, you can begin applying research. The first step is to find a research article that addresses a question in which you are interested. Since this book is about reducing injury risk and maximizing performance, let's turn this topic into your question and examine it in two parts.

In part 1, your question could be *How can I reduce my risk of injury and enhance my dance performance?* You do your literature search (for this example, in the PubMed database, pubmed.gov) by typing the term *dance injury* into the PubMed search box and you end up with more than 1,500 articles that cover injury patterns, rates, locations, risk factors, and so on. To have a chance of obtaining the information you are looking for, you need to whittle this list down to 10 articles or fewer. Next, you will narrow your search by placing quotation marks around the words *"dance injury"*—this finds articles containing that exact phrase. You will see the number of available articles decrease dramatically here; when we wrote this chapter our search dropped from 1,564 articles to 39 articles by adding the quote marks. Keep in mind that the National Library of Medicine and all other information repositories continuously add resources, so the numbers you obtain when you try this will be different than ours. The process is the same, however.

Since your question is about reducing risk of injury, you must first learn the most common injury risk factors in dancers, so you are going to add to your search. To do so, you change your search query to *"dance injury" AND "risk factors"* to further trim the number of articles. When we did this, we found 12 articles—much more manageable, but still a lot of articles to read. Next, use the PubMed search engine to filter your results. You'll find several ways to filter the resources in PubMed, but try filtering to obtain articles within the last 5 years. When we did this, the process netted us 6 articles out of the original 1,564, all of which have the phrases *dance injuries* and *risk factors*. If you followed the procedure, you've retrieved a very reasonably sized stack of information to review.

In part 2 of your quest, after reviewing the articles from part 1 and thinking about your dance experience, you realize fatigue is something that always seems to give you a struggle. Therefore, you change your PubMed search terms to *dance injury AND fatigue* and then filter the results for the last 5 years. (Leave off the quotation marks this time; that will help you find more articles because the database will look for *dance*, *injury*, *dance injury*, plus *fatigue*.) When we did this we got a list of 28 articles. Looking down the list of articles you just created, you find 6 that have the word *fatigue* in the title. You hone in on one from the journal *Sports Biomechanics* titled "Dancers exhibit decreases in postural control after fatigue" (Bulkley and Jarvis, 2023). This sounds particularly intriguing to you because you know how challenging it has been to maintain your posture during your late afternoon dance classes and evening rehearsals. Additionally, this article passes the CRAAP test and meets all the other criteria discussed in this chapter, so you really feel like you hit the jackpot!

From the abstract of the research you see in PubMed, you learn that when the dancers in the study were fatigued, their postural control in a *passé* stance made them sway more and some of their lower-extremity joints moved more than when they weren't fatigued. This could conceivably lead to an increase in falls while dancing and may increase the likelihood of overuse injury as a fatigued dancer's body must work extra hard to maintain its balance. While the dancers in the study had fewer fatigue problems in their dominant limb compared to their non-dominant limb, the researchers suggest that postural stability training to the point of fatigue will help dancers with their balance (Jarvis and Bulkley, 2023). With this information, you can now apply the research findings to your own training. Your goal in doing so is to reduce the effects of fatigue on your dancing, thus potentially reducing your injury risk and also improving your performance. You are encouraged to obtain the full article by Bulkley and Jarvis. You can use the reference list of this article to find similar articles. You also can repeat these steps to practice the process outlined above, locate other articles of interest, and help you incorporate the tools described in this chapter.

Conclusions and Practical Relevance

Overall, you do not need to be a researcher to read, understand, and benefit from research. This chapter encourages you to become a research-savvy practitioner; in other words, you can be a critical consumer of research who knows where to find evidence, how to assess the quality of that evidence, and how to use it to improve your practice. Whether you are a dancer, educator, choreographer, health care professional, or someone else with an interest in dance, these tools will assist you in determining current best practices. An enormous world of new information is accessible to you. You can use it to reduce your injury risk and maximize your performance.

Discussion Questions

1. What exposure to scientific research have you had up to this point in your dance career? What are some ways that research affects the way you train in dance or explains how your body works to allow you to dance?
2. How has the content in this chapter changed your understanding of how research can be applied to dance practice? Discuss this question with other dancers and with your dance teachers. Is there room for using this new understanding to guide you in rethinking or changing certain approaches to dance?
3. Propose some questions about improving your dance performance or reducing your injury risk. (For example, *What would happen if . . . ?* or *Why does this occur when . . . ?* or *Why* is . . . *better than . . . ?*) Select the question that is most interesting or urgent for you, then do the following:
    a. Identify which type of study design you would use to answer this question.
    b. Outline a research study you could use to answer your question.
    c. Suggest the results that, if they occurred in the research project, would cause you to make changes in your dance practice.

WWW Go to HK*Propel* to access supplemental information and activities connected to chapter content.

4

Physiology of Dance Training and Performance

Emma Redding, PhD, FIADMS
Sarah Needham-Beck, PhD

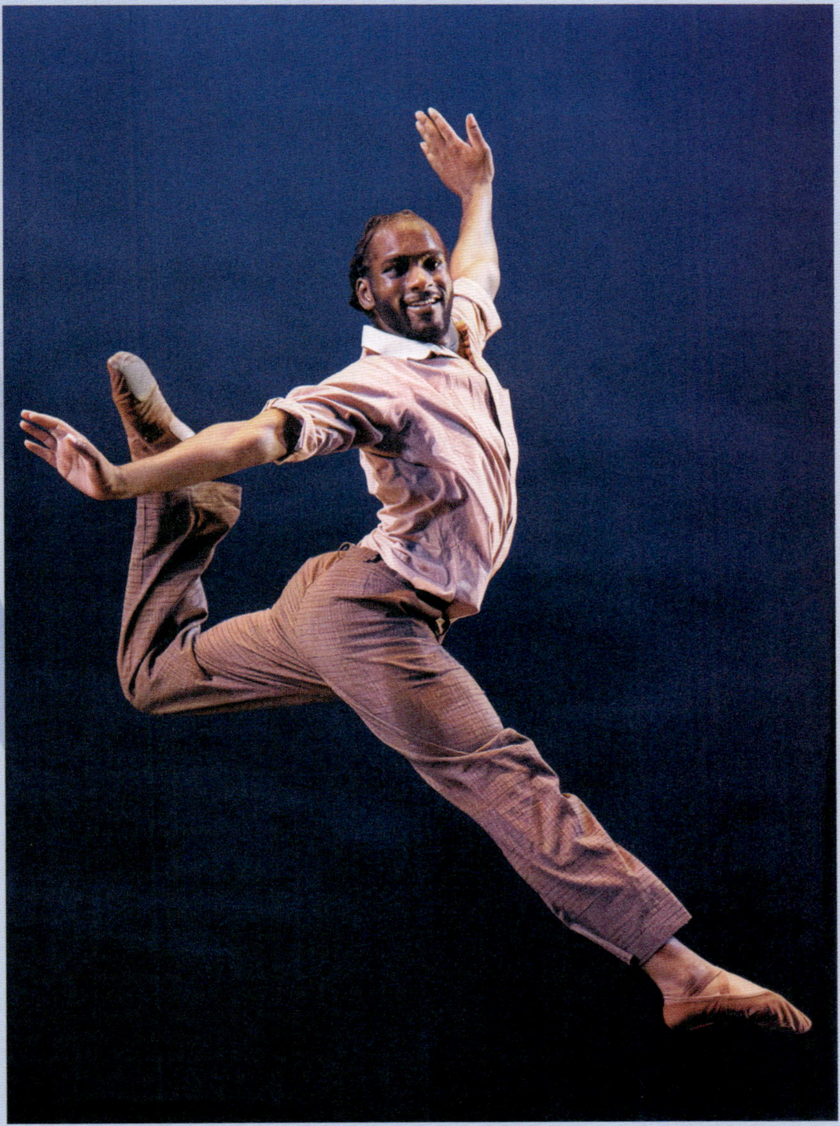

University of South Carolina, Betsy Blackmon Dance Program, Columbia, South Carolina. *The Legend of the Hatfields and McCoys* (2023) choreographed by Peter Powlus. Photo: Sadie Whitehead; Dancer: T.J. Warren.

Physiology is a science that describes the way the body functions. The body cannot dance unless physiological processes (which can be trained and optimized) are operating. As a dancer, understanding the cardiovascular, respiratory, and muscular systems will enable you to test and train your body to meet the physiological demands of dance.

Key Terms

- adenosine triphosphate (ATP)
- aorta
- autonomic nervous system
- cardiac output
- cardiorespiratory fitness
- glycolytic energy system
- intensity
- muscle fascicle
- muscle fiber
- myocardium
- myofibril
- oxidative energy system
- oxygen uptake
- parasympathetic nervous system
- phosphagen energy system
- positive adaptation
- stroke volume
- sympathetic nervous system
- thoracic cavity
- tidal volume
- vascular

LEARNING OBJECTIVES

After completing this chapter, you will be able to do the following:

- Explain the structure and function of the cardiovascular and respiratory systems.
- Describe the structural organization of skeletal muscle and the mechanisms of muscle contraction.
- Classify the body's responses to exercise and how the body adapts to exercise over time.
- Differentiate between the energy systems utilized in dance.
- Identify the various energy demands of dance class, rehearsal, and performance.
- Distinguish between different methods of measuring the physiological demands of dance and the physiological capacities of dancers.

Exercise physiology is the study of the body's response and adaptation to exercise, which involves acute and sustained metabolic and circulatory changes in the heart, lungs, blood, and skeletal muscles. Understanding how best to approach dance training requires an appreciation of the key principles of exercise physiology, including how the body works as well as how it responds and adapts to the training stimulus placed on it. Learning how muscle contraction occurs and how the inner processes of the body adapt through exercise to improve one's ability to cope with future physical demands allows a dancer to build stamina, recover more quickly from intense bouts of dancing, and focus more intently on the artistic and qualitative aspects of movement. Thus, the knowledge you acquire throughout this chapter will help empower you as a dancer to optimize your training and performance practices.

Cardiovascular System

The cardiovascular system serves to supply nutrients and oxygen to the working muscles and other organs as well as to transport waste products away from the muscles and organs. The cardiovascular system comprises the heart (cardio), which acts as a pump to distribute blood and its components to the tissues, as well as vessels (**vascular**), the arteries, veins, and capillaries through which substances pass. In other words, the cardiovascular system is the pressure distribution circuit serving to physically move (push) substances around the body.

The Heart and Blood Flow

Situated in the chest cavity slightly to the left of the midline of the body, the heart (also known as the **myocardium**) contains four chambers that are made of cardiac muscle. The striated (striped) muscle tissue of the heart is similar to slow-twitch skeletal muscle; it is rich in capillaries and mitochondria, the energy compartments of the heart's cells. Functionally, the heart works as two pumps, each of which has two chambers: an atrium and a ventricle. On the right side, the heart receives blood returning from the body in the right atrium, and it sends the blood out to the lungs from the right ventricle. The left side of the heart receives oxygenated blood from the lungs into the left atrium, and it pumps this blood out from the left ventricle through the thick-walled vessel called the **aorta** for distribution around the body (figure 4.1). Several important valves allow the blood to pass from chamber to chamber in the heart so that its direction and volume are effectively controlled. These valves repeatedly opening and closing are what gives the heart its characteristic *lub-dub* heartbeat sound.

Arteries, Veins, and Capillaries

Once oxygenated blood enters the left atrium, it moves to the left ventricle and subsequently is expelled into the aorta by a forceful contraction of the heart muscle. From there, the aorta pumps the blood into high-pressure vessels (arteries) that carry the blood to the tissues of the body. Artery walls contain smooth muscle tissue that pumps

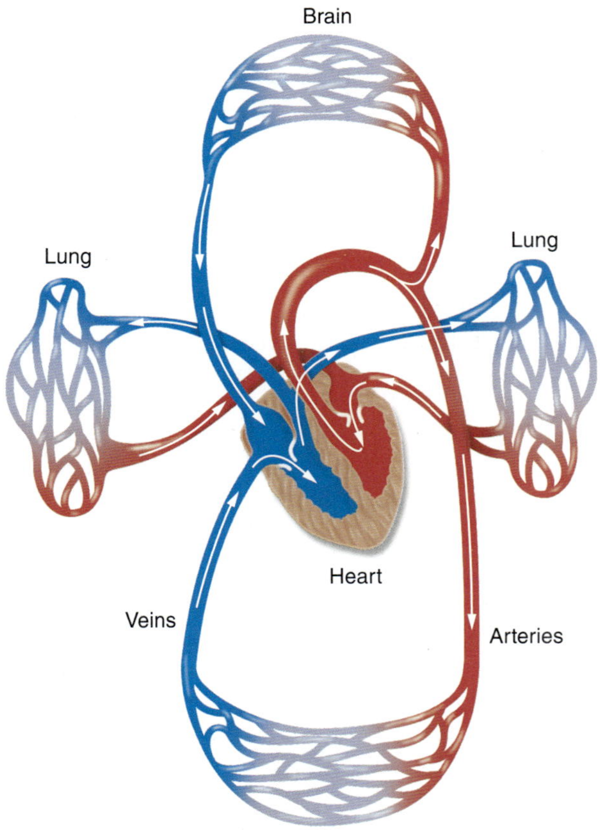

Figure 4.1 Schematic view of the cardiovascular system showing the heart and vascular circuits.

the blood onward. Blood vessels decrease in size as they travel away from the heart. All of the blood vessels together—arteries, veins, and capillaries—are known as the vascular system.

From the arteries, smaller arterial branches (arterioles) regulate blood flow by repeatedly constricting (contracting) and dilating (expanding) their diameters. During exercise, the body redirects concentrations of blood from the organs to the skeletal muscles to meet the muscles' increased demand for oxygen. From the arterioles, blood travels to the tiniest vessels, the capillaries; from there, it begins its return to the heart via the venous vessels.

The venous system comprises vessels that carry this deoxygenated blood back from the tissues, initially through the small capillaries in tissues and then through the slightly larger venules. The venules empty into veins; eventually, veins carry blood back toward the heart by sending it through the inferior vena cava (the largest vein in the body) from the lower extremities and abdomen or through the superior vena cava, which serves the upper body. Unlike muscular-walled arteries, the veins have thin, nonmuscular walls. Therefore, they require skeletal muscle activity in the extremities to pump their blood.

Both venae cavae deposit blood into the right atrium of the heart; the blood then moves to the right ventricle. From the right ventricle, blood is directed to the lungs via the pulmonary arteries to undergo gas exchange. In the lungs, carbon dioxide is released from the red blood cells, and oxygen attaches to the red blood cells. The blood then returns to the left atrium of the heart through the pulmonary veins, and the cycle of blood flow repeats.

Regulation of Heart Rate and Circulation

During physical activity, heart rate and blood flow increase to supply the exercising muscles with all they need to continue their contractions. The body alters its resting state and distribution of blood to accommodate its altered needs while exercising (figure 4.2). Blood vessels quickly constrict or dilate to distribute blood where necessary to aid metabolism. The maintenance of heart rate, blood flow, and blood pressure require careful regulation. Blood pressure controls the flow of blood around the body, and it reflects **cardiac output** (amount of blood pumped by the heart per minute) and the total peripheral resistance to blood flow. Total peripheral resistance is the amount of resistance to blood flow that occurs throughout the body's blood vessels. Thus, if the resistance is higher, blood pressure must be higher to overcome the resistance; and if the resistance is lower, blood pressure will be lower.

Heart rate changes constantly because of continuous messages sent through nerves to the myocardium to signal an increase or decrease in accordance with the activity (or anticipation of activity) of the body. The **autonomic nervous system** is divided into the **sympathetic nervous system** and **parasympathetic nervous system**. These divisions act in parallel with one another to regulate the cardiovascular system as well as other systems in the body (figure 4.3). Generally speaking, the sympathetic nervous system speeds things up, and the parasympathetic system slows things down. These divisions are

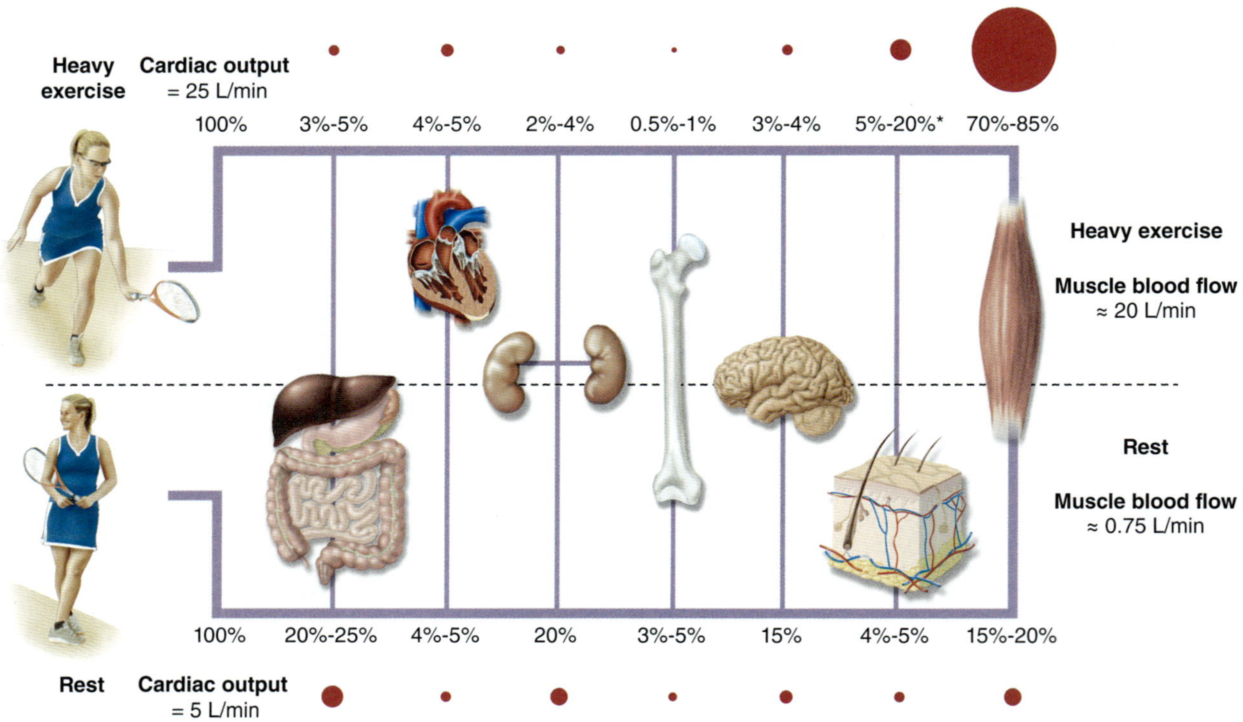

Figure 4.2 Blood distribution throughout the body changes as needed from rest to strenuous exercise.

Reprinted by permission from P.O. Åstrand et al., *Textbook of Work Physiology: Physiological Bases of Exercise*, 4th ed. (Champaign, IL: Human Kinetics, 2003), 143.

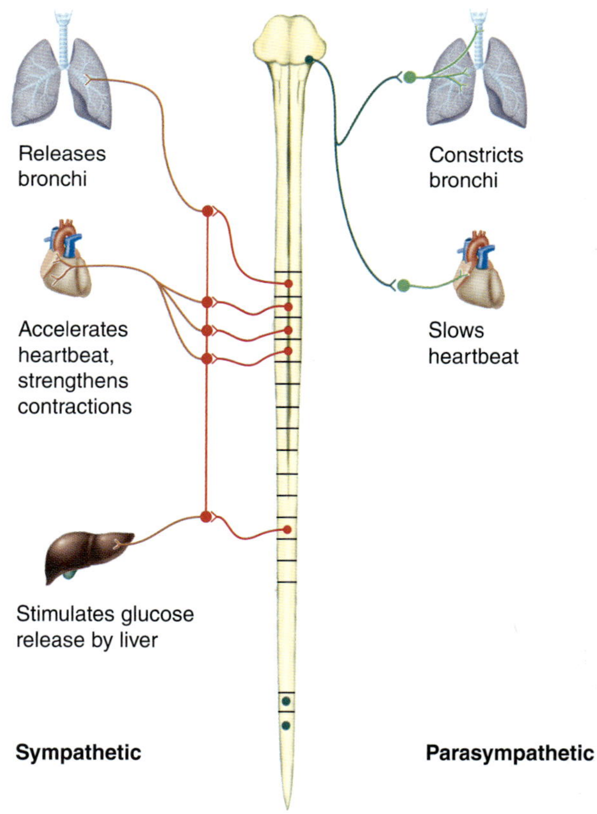

Figure 4.3 The sympathetic and parasympathetic portions of the autonomic nervous system have different roles, as summarized here. Note that only the portions of the autonomic nervous system directly related to exercise are included here.

sometimes called the *fight-or-flight* (sympathetic) system and the *rest-and-digest* (parasympathetic) system. As the body becomes more accustomed to exercising regularly, a number of positive changes occur within the cardiovascular system that increase its efficiency and its ability to perform well. For example, cardiac output and **stroke volume** values increase, as does the body's ability to take up and utilize oxygen when exercising.

Respiratory System

The respiratory system serves to transport air from outside the body to the lungs and back again. The air you breathe enters the nose and mouth, then flows through the ventilatory structures that include the trachea, the two bronchi that enter the lungs, and the smaller bronchioles (figure 4.4). The average volume of air in the lungs is 5 liters, which is similar to the volume of air contained in a basketball.

Mechanics of Breathing

When we breathe in (inhalation), the ribs lift upward because of the activation of the intercostal muscles that lie between them (*intercostal* means "between the ribs"). At the same time, the diaphragm muscle contracts and moves downward to allow the **thoracic cavity** to expand. This enlargement of the thoracic cavity decreases its pressure, and the corresponding higher pressure of the atmosphere outside the body moves air into the lungs. The opposite occurs when we breathe out (exhalation). The diaphragm relaxes and rises, the intercostal muscles relax, and the thoracic cavity shrinks. This shrinking increases the thoracic cavity's pressure, which is now higher than the atmospheric pressure, and thus it forces air out of the lungs.

Lung Capacities and Gas Exchange

At rest, breathing remains constant, and the adult body takes an average of 12 breaths per minute. As you begin to exercise, the body's demand for oxygen to supply the muscles increases. Therefore, the amount of air you inhale and exhale increases through more frequent and deeper breathing. The body uses its inspiratory reserve volume, which is the additional air taken up from inhaling more fully. It also uses its expiratory reserve volume to breathe out more air than usual. This deeper breathing increases the body's **tidal volume**—the volume of air inspired (inhaled) or expired (exhaled) per breath. Figure 4.5 shows these important lung volumes.

In addition to inhalation and exhalation, the lungs have another important function during exercise. They provide surfaces for gas exchange, whereby oxygen transfers from inhaled air to the blood, and carbon dioxide transfers from the blood to the air for exhalation. The lungs are spongelike, relatively solid organs; they are not open spaces like balloons. Once air travels through the trachea, bronchi, and bronchioles, inside the lungs it reaches the alveoli. These saclike structures, which are arranged like bunches of grapes, are where gas (oxygen and carbon dioxide) exchange occurs (figure 4.6).

Muscle Physiology

The human body has these three types of muscle: skeletal (attached to bones), cardiac (heart), and smooth (e.g., muscle lining the walls of arteries and intestines). Each type of muscle is distinct in terms of structure and function. Cardiac and smooth muscle activity occurs involuntarily, whereas skeletal muscle operates mostly under voluntary control. In other words, the rate at which the heart beats or food travels through the digestive system is not consciously controlled, while the moving of body segments during a dance phrase is the result of conscious decision making.

Architectural Structure of Muscle and Muscle Fibers

The human body has more than 600 skeletal muscles. Each muscle is wrapped in a connective tissue called the epimysium. A muscle contains bundles of **muscle fibers** that are grouped together; these bundles are called **muscle fascicles**. Each fascicle is surrounded by a connective tissue called the perimysium, which holds the bundles together. Each fiber in a fascicle is wrapped by a thin layer of connective tissue called the endomysium (figure 4.7).

Muscle fibers vary in length and size, and each muscle contains a different number of fibers. For example, the eyelid has many small fibers, and the quadriceps muscle has longer fibers, some of which measure more than 10 centimeters (4 in.). However, no fibers run along the entire length of a muscle. The alignment of the muscle fibers and the number

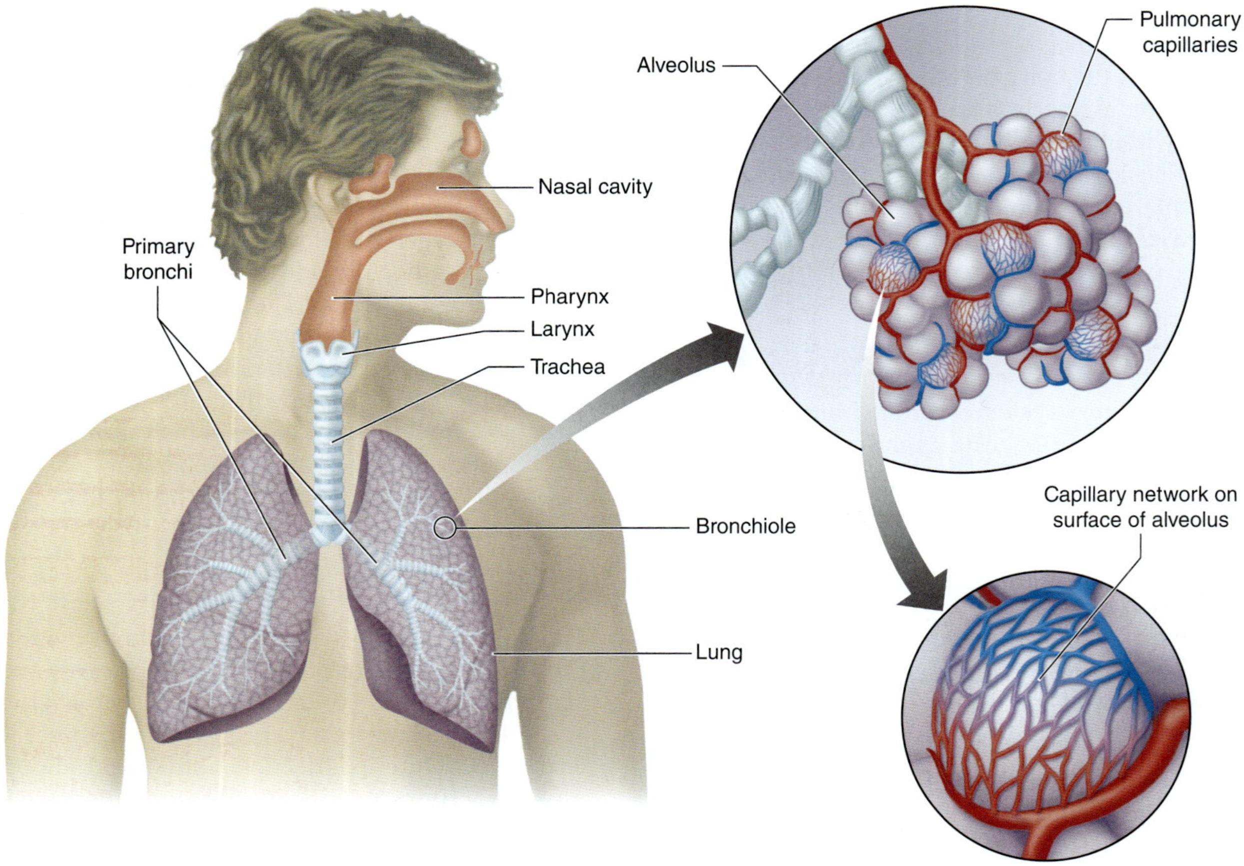

Figure 4.4 The anatomy of the breathing passages.

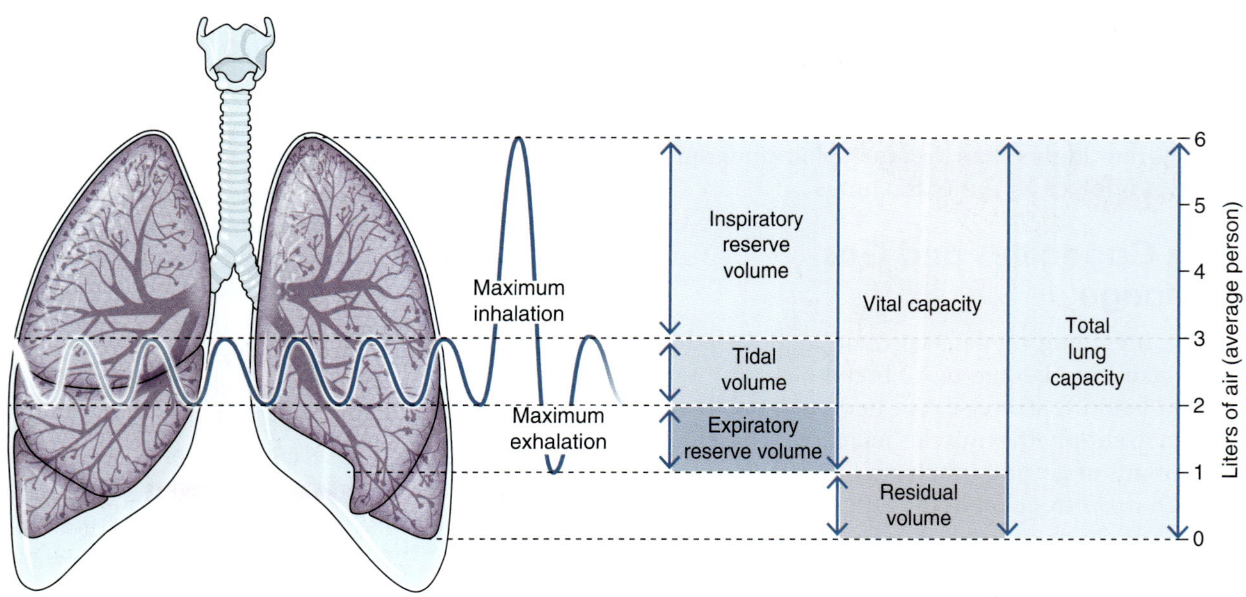

Figure 4.5 Lung volumes associated with normal breathing and physical activity.

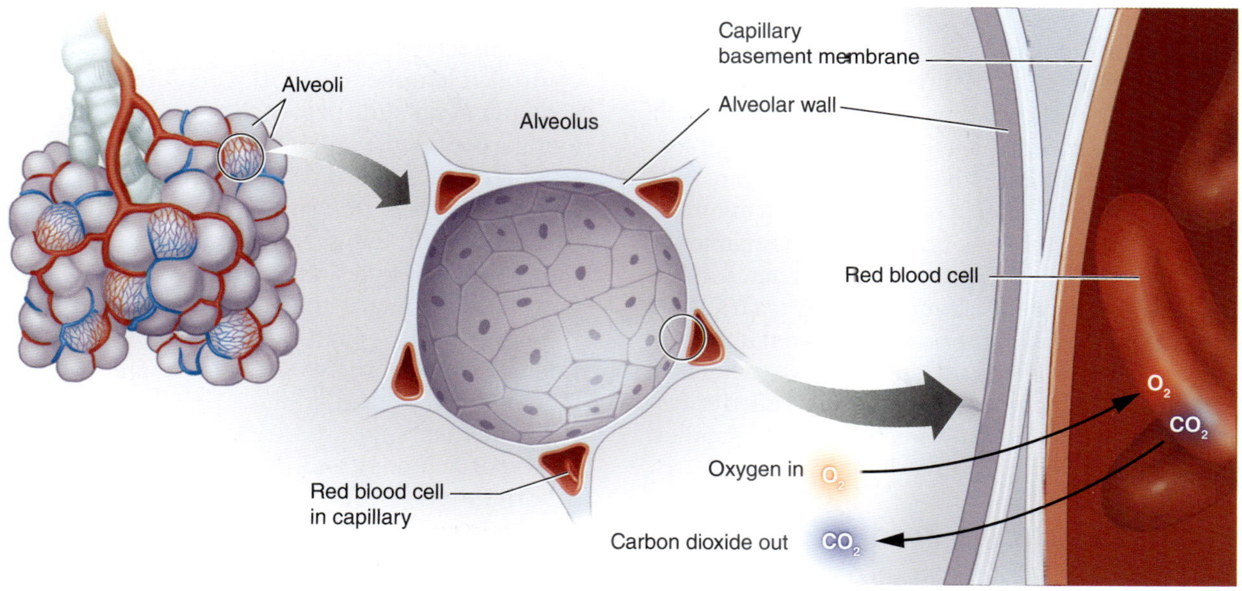

Figure 4.6 Oxygen and carbon dioxide are exchanged at the alveoli (plural of alveolus) of the lungs.

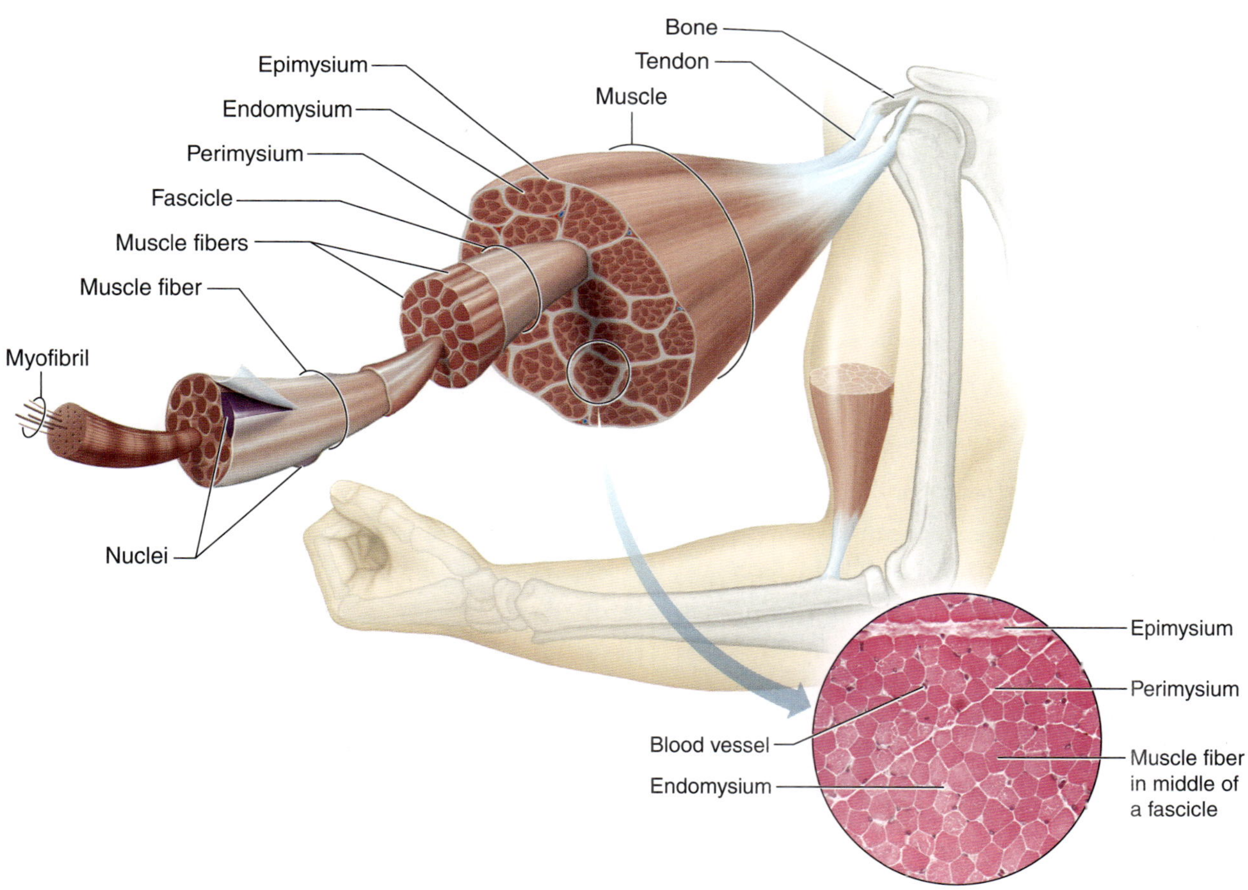

Figure 4.7 The anatomical structure of a typical skeletal muscle.

of fibers contained in a muscle affect the muscle's power-generating capacity and its range of motion.

Looking closer, each muscle fiber is made up of small structures known as **myofibrils** (figure 4.8). They are the contractile elements of a muscle, containing even smaller, functional subunits (myofilaments) that lie parallel to each other. Each myofibril consists of the proteins actin (thin myofilaments) and myosin (thick myofilaments). When viewed under a microscope, the muscle fiber is striped in appearance; it has light bands (I bands) and dark bands (A bands) along its length. Arrangements of these bands are divided into sections called sarcomeres along the fiber; a sarcomere is the smallest functional element of a muscle fiber.

Basic Contractile Process

The exact process of muscle contraction is still under investigation; however, the sliding filament model provides the best explanation for how movement occurs in the muscles. The model proposes that muscles contract (either to shorten a muscle or to allow controlled lengthening of it) when the myosin and actin filaments slide past each other. A sarcomere is a single contractile unit in a muscle comprising one section of a myofibril. Many sarcomeres arranged end to end form one complete myofibril. Within each myofibril, the crossbridges (globular heads) of myosin molecules attach to the actin molecules and ratchet toward the center of the sarcomere (figure 4.9). Movement of the crossbridges in this ratchetlike motion creates tension in each sarcomere, which, in turn, initiates tension throughout a muscle fiber.

The attachment and detachment between the myofilaments occur with energy provided by **adenosine triphosphate (ATP)** hydrolysis (the breakdown of ATP). The process begins when an electrochemical message is received from the brain telling contraction to occur. An electrical discharge

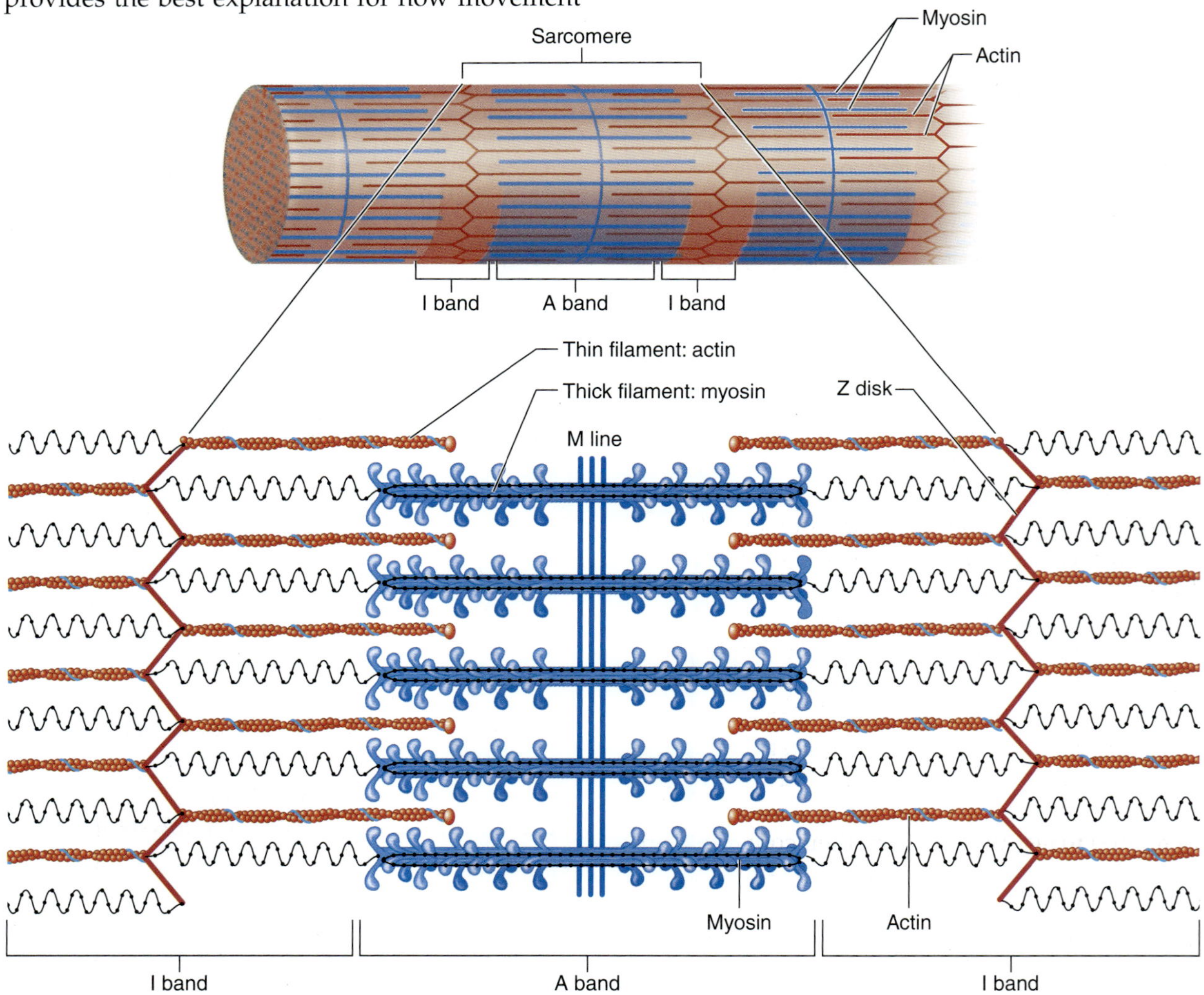

Figure 4.8 The microscopic structure of a muscle's myofibril.

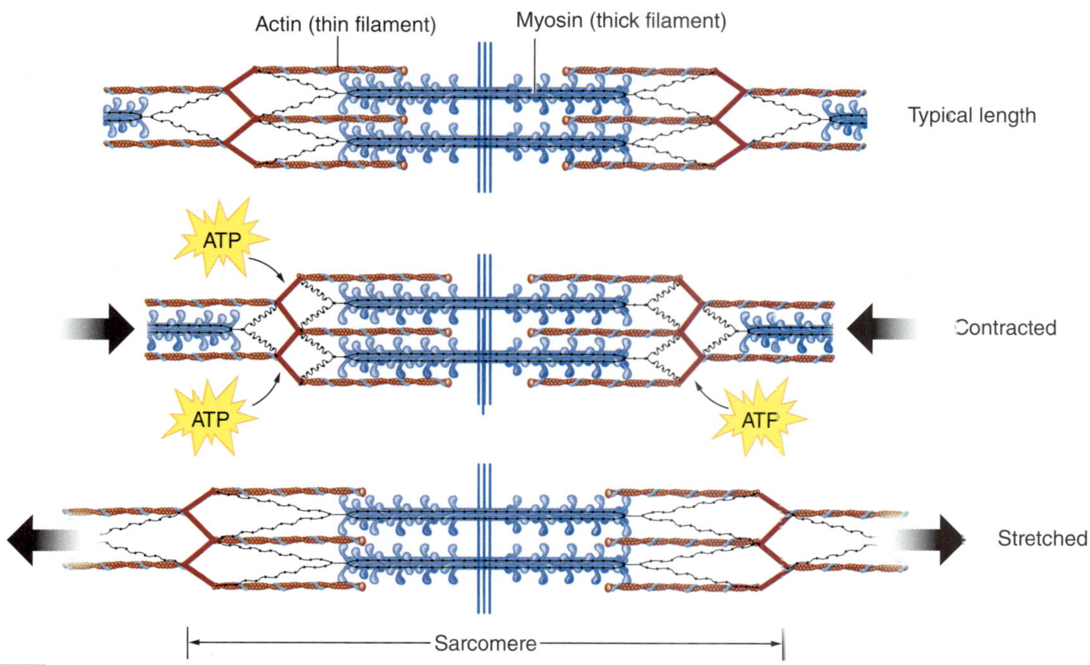

Figure 4.9 A single sarcomere, the fundamental contractile unit of a muscle. The interaction of myosin crossbridges with actin myofilaments inside this myofibril are powered by energy from hydrolysis (breakdown) of adenosine triphosphate (ATP) to produce tension in a muscle, thus initiating muscle contraction that causes movement.

at the muscle initiates the release of calcium into the contractile portion of the muscle. In the presence of calcium, the coupling and uncoupling of actin and myosin occurs. Once a signal to stop contracting is received, the contraction ceases, the calcium is pumped back to its original storage location, and the muscle relaxes because the myosin and actin myofilaments no longer interact.

Muscle Fiber Types

Muscles do not contain one type of fiber. Different types of muscle fibers have different metabolic and contractile characteristics. The two main types of fibers in skeletal muscle are type I and type II fibers. Type II fibers have several subtypes, each with slightly different characteristics (table 4.1). Type I fibers are slow-twitch fibers, and type II fibers are fast-twitch fibers, which relates to their relative speed of contraction; both types are important for dance.

Slow-twitch fibers are best suited for long-duration, sustained effort because they resist fatigue. Compared to fast-twitch fibers, their contractile process is slower, hence their name. Slow-twitch fibers are more dependent on the oxidative energy system (outlined later in this chapter) than are fast-twitch fibers. In addition, they have more capillaries, so they receive more blood flow to provide oxygen for their energy needs. They also tend to produce a lower amount of force than fast-twitch fibers.

Fast-twitch (type II) fibers are adept at rapidly dealing with the electrochemical signals that elicit contraction. They are divided into these three subgroups: type IIa, type IIx, and type IIb. Type IIa fibers are able to utilize a range of energy systems to replenish energy for muscular contraction. Type IIx fibers' characteristics lie essentially between those of types IIa and IIb. Type IIb fibers have a higher potential to shorten very quickly by utilizing energy systems that yield small quantities of ATP quickly (phosphagen and glycolytic systems) than do types IIa or IIx.

Fast-twitch fibers contain a higher level of the enzyme ATPase than slow-twitch fibers. This enzyme assists the process of breaking down ATP, thus making energy for contraction more readily available. The release of calcium needed to start a contraction happens quickly, and the result is a high rate of myosin crossbridge activity as the crossbridges interact with actin. In general, fast-twitch fibers contract more quickly than slow-twitch fibers, and they are used for movements that require a lot of force immediately, such as jumping or moving very quickly.

Different skeletal muscles contain different ratios of fast- and slow-twitch fibers. In addition, distinctive ratios of muscle fibers are found within

Table 4.1 **Characteristics of Slow-Twitch and Fast-Twitch Muscle Fibers**

Characteristic	Slow-twitch (type I)	Fast-twitch (type IIa)	Fast-twitch (type IIx)	Fast-twitch (type IIb)
Contraction speed	Slow	Somewhat fast	Fast	Very fast
Contraction force	Low	Medium	High	Very high
Type of activity	Aerobic	Long-duration anaerobic	Short-duration anaerobic	Short-duration anaerobic
Duration of activity	High	Relatively high	Medium	Low
Resistance to fatigue	High	Relatively high	Medium	Low
Capillary quantity	High	Medium	Low	Low
Mitochondrial density	High	High	Medium	Low

specific muscles of elite athletes. For example, the calf muscles of sprinters are more likely to have a higher proportion of fast-twitch fibers than those of long-distance endurance runners, who are more likely to possess a higher number of slow-twitch fibers (McArdle et al., 2023). Limited research exists about the muscle fiber composition needs of dancers. Nevertheless, when considering the physiological demands of dance, it is likely that dancers generally need a combination of fast-twitch and slow-twitch fibers.

Energy Systems

Energy is what allows a task to be performed. It is categorized as either potential energy or kinetic energy. The term *potential energy* refers to the energy's structure or position and what it can do once released as kinetic energy. Essentially it is stored energy that is ready for release. *Kinetic energy* creates motion or action. Energy in the human body contributes to the biosynthesis of cellular molecules, the mechanical aspects of muscle contraction, and the transportation of substances within and between tissues.

Humans need a constant supply of energy to function and undertake everyday tasks. The demand for energy increases further when people engage in exercise, including dance. Potential energy is mainly derived from food (carbohydrates, lipids, proteins); calories from food are simply a measure of the energy the food provides (see chapter 7 for more detailed information on nutrition). The splitting of chemical bonds in the food molecules begins the process of turning this potential energy into kinetic energy. The processes by which the body obtains the energy needed for its biological work involve energy-rich adenosine triphosphate (ATP). ATP is required for all muscular contractions to occur.

ATP molecules consist of three inorganic phosphates (hence the word *triphosphate*). They are adenosine diphosphate (ADP), a molecule with two inorganic phosphates (hence the word *diphosphate*), plus one spare phosphate bound to it. The process of breaking this phosphate bond in the molecule releases approximately 7.3 kilocalories of free energy, which is what subsequently stimulates the contraction of muscle fibers (McArdle et al., 2023). Small amounts of ATP are available in the muscle, but they are quickly depleted and require resynthesis for continued muscle contraction. Thus, different pathways provide phosphates for the resynthesis of ATP from ADP. These pathways are known as energy systems.

Three energy systems contain the metabolic processes for resynthesizing ATP: the phosphagen, glycolytic, and oxidative systems. It is important to note that all three of these systems work simultaneously in a dynamic energy continuum to support muscular contraction and the energy demand of an activity. Nonetheless, one system may be dominant at a given time depending on the characteristics of the activity. These characteristics include **intensity** (difficulty), duration (time), and factors such as availability of oxygen at the cellular level (figure 4.10).

Given the highly varied and dynamic nature of dance activity, where powerful movements (e.g., jumps, lifts, and explosive level changes) are interspersed among more continuous, transitional movements, it is important to view these energy systems as working together to meet the energy demands of dance rather than as separate, exclusive

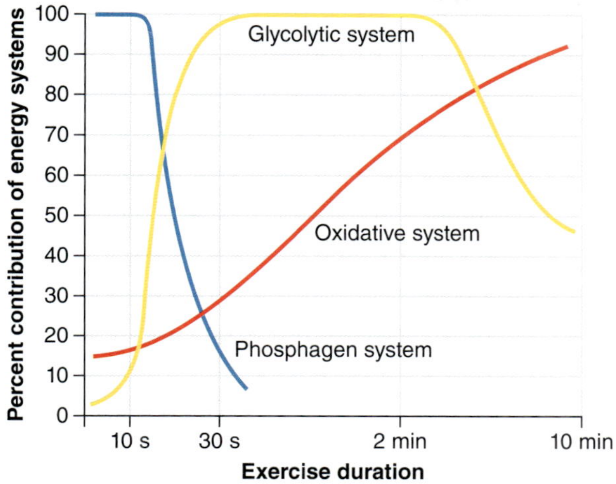

Figure 4.10 The contributions of the body's three energy systems when exercising over time. Note that each system offers differing amounts of energy for activity throughout an activity bout.

systems. Previous research has classified dance as an intermittent exercise form that requires the use of all energy systems interchangeably (Redding & Wyon, 2003) in a dynamic response to meet its varying demands.

Phosphagen Energy System

One way that ATP is resynthesized is through the splitting of another intracellular high-energy phosphate known as phosphocreatine (PCr) (figure 4.11). Physical activity that requires short, explosive bursts of energy (e.g., a short jump sequence in a dance class) is likely to be served by the **phosphagen energy system**. This system supplies short-term energy for maximal effort of up to 8 seconds. This system does not rely on a supply of oxygen (therefore, it is often called an anaerobic system), and it can replenish ATP more or less instantly. The most effective way of training this system is through repeated short bouts (6-10 s) of high-intensity explosive exercises (e.g., fast sprints or large jumps).

Glycolytic Energy System

If intense effort continues beyond the short time that limited PCr stores can support ATP resynthesis, the body must draw on other energy systems to continue resynthesis of ATP from ADP. *Glycolysis* refers to the breakdown of glucose molecules that are obtained from food into another molecule called pyruvate, which also results in the resynthesis of a small amount of ATP (2 molecules). Physical activity that requires up to approximately 2 minutes of effort (e.g., a short sequence at the end of a class or a single round in a hip-hop battle format) is likely to be served by the **glycolytic energy system**.

Like the phosphagen energy system, the process of glycolysis on its own does not rely on a supply of oxygen (therefore, it is also an anaerobic system), but it can replenish ATP relatively quickly. However, if sufficient oxygen is available at the cellular level (supplied through increased blood flow to the muscles during exercise, as explained earlier) then the pyruvate produced by glycolysis will undergo further metabolic processes to allow resynthesis of larger quantities of ATP and enable sustained activity (as further detailed in the next section, Oxidative Energy System).

If insufficient oxygen is available to match the rate of glycolysis, pyruvate instead binds temporarily with excess hydrogen to form lactate (commonly known as lactic acid). Lactate accumulates with continued exercise under these conditions; however, once sufficient oxygen is available, lactate can be fully oxidized again in the muscle cells to reform pyruvate, which is used in further metabolic processes. This process is one of the reasons (among many others) that you breathe heavily immediately after finishing a short duration of intense exercise, such as a challenging 60- to 90-second sequence in a class. Therefore, the boost of oxygen to working muscles facilitates oxidation of accumulated lactate.

The most effective way of training the glycolytic energy system is through interval training, such as high-intensity interval training (HIIT), or through circuit training (where work and rest periods

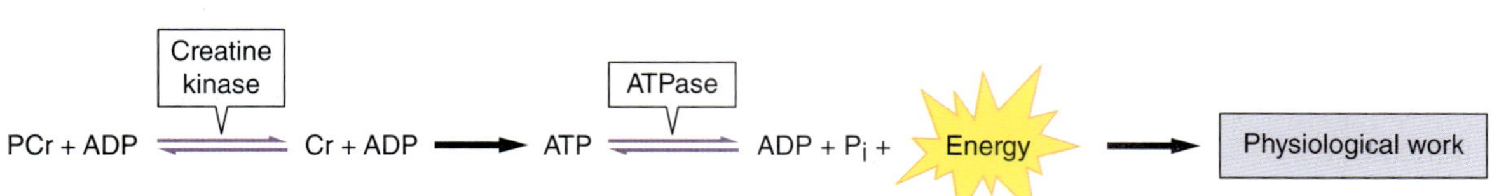

Figure 4.11 The mechanism of ATP resynthesis for energy from the phosphagen energy system that utilizes phosphocreatine (PCr). Since ADP needs another phosphate to become ATP, that phosphate is gained by splitting it from PCr. These biochemical processes are accomplished by the enzymes creatine kinase and ATPase, respectively.

are manipulated). These training methods may include sprints, jumps, and rolls onto and off of the floor for 30 to 90 seconds at a time; rest periods or lower-intensity intervals are interspersed with the higher-intensity portions.

Oxidative Energy System

When activity continues beyond a few minutes, ATP is primarily resynthesized through the **oxidative energy system**. It is the most complex of the systems by which the body resynthesizes ATP; it involves three biochemical subprocesses (figure 4.12). Here, this complex system is presented as simply as possible to help outline the very important method of your body getting the energy it needs to dance, exercise, and participate in other long-term physical activities.

The first subprocess of the oxidative system is glycolysis (described in the previous section). Following glycolysis, if sufficient oxygen is available, pyruvate is then converted to 2 molecules of a compound called acetyl-coenzyme A (acetyl CoA, for short). Acetyl CoA is used in the second biochemical subprocess, called the Krebs cycle, which releases hydrogen, carbon dioxide (CO_2), and 2 more ATP molecules. Hydrogen released by the first two subprocesses plus oxygen (O_2) then enters the third subprocess, the electron transport chain. This portion of the oxidative system leads to synthesis of much more ATP—28 molecules—than the first two subprocesses, and it produces 12 molecules of water (H_2O). Overall, this series of biochemical mechanisms results in the full oxidation of glucose, giving a high yield of 32 ATP molecules per glucose molecule (Kenney et al., 2021).

An effective way of training the oxidative energy system is by exercising using large muscle groups repeatedly (e.g., jogging, elliptical training, stationary cycling, doing lunges, moving the arms above the head) for 10 minutes or more. Because the oxidative mechanism is the energy system used by the body under these circumstances, this type of exercise is typically labeled aerobic.

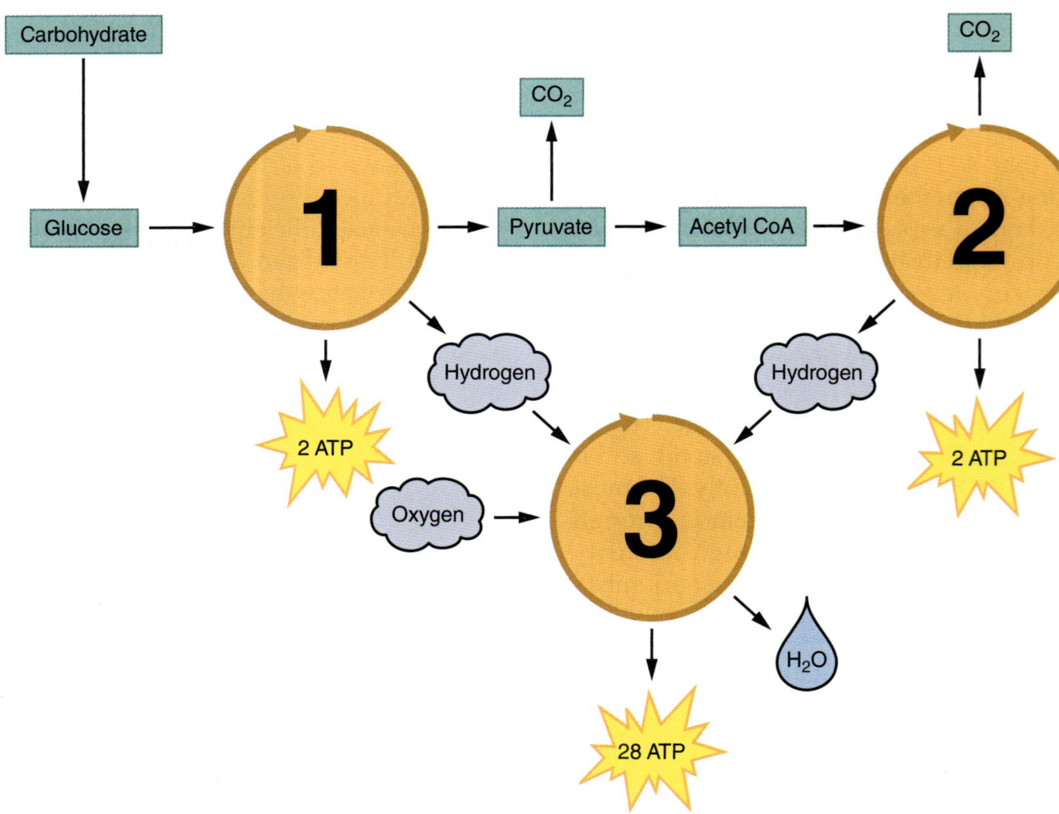

Figure 4.12 ATP is resynthesized by the oxidative system that includes these three subprocesses: (1) glycolysis, (2) Krebs cycle, and (3) electron transport chain. Note the quantities of ATP resynthesized by each part.

Physiological Demands of Dance

As outlined previously, the body responds to the onset of any physical activity through a complex series of integrated systems that work to ensure the energy demand of the activity is met. The energy demand of a particular dance activity, be it a single exercise or sequence or an entire piece of performance repertoire, is determined by factors of both time (how long) and intensity (how hard). However, the extent to which an individual dancer finds a particular activity demanding to perform is influenced by their own fitness level (both physiological and metabolic factors) as well as by other components relating to economy of movement. These factors include anthropometric (height, body mass, limb lengths, etc.), biomechanical (alignment, joint movements, etc.), and technical skill and proficiency, which are central in dance (Jones & Carter, 2000). Therefore, two individual dancers will experience different physiological intensities or demands from the same set of movements, depending on their individual characteristics and level of fitness conditioning.

Given the intermittent (stop, start) nature of dance, the ability to do repeated bouts of activity without a drop in performance quality is crucial. Movement sequences and phrases given in class are often broken up by moments of teaching and learning, whereas performances can consist of moments of both heavy and light intensity with fewer moments of rest between them. A dancer's ability to cope with these varying demands is largely determined by their ability to recover between bouts of activity so they are ready for the next episode and can avoid cumulative fatigue.

Demands of Class, Rehearsal, and Performance

Dance activity—regardless of genre or style—is commonly described in the literature as complex, diverse, non–steady state, intermittent, of moderate to high intensity, and possessing notable differences between training and performance intensities and durations (Cohen et al., 1982; Redding & Wyon, 2003; Schantz & Astrand, 1984; Twitchett, Koutedakis, et al., 2009; Wyon et al., 2004; Wyon et al., 2011). *Intensity* refers to how hard someone is exercising physically; it is often evaluated by measurement of heart rate (HR), by rate of **oxygen uptake** ($\dot{V}O_2$), or by a percentage of an individual's maximum capacity on these variables (%HRmax and %$\dot{V}O_2$max). As noted earlier in the discussion on body systems, the harder the intensity of exercise, the higher the HR and $\dot{V}O_2$ values will be because the body puts forth substantial effort to supply the working muscles with oxygen and other required substances to sustain muscular contraction. Beck and colleagues (2015) summarized typical values measured in dancers across different genres; some sample HR values were recorded during class, rehearsal, and performance, and they are presented in table 4.2.

Invariably, dance class is divided into preparatory (e.g., barre) and execution (e.g., center) work sections. Overall, the physiological demand of class is relatively low, with low work-to-rest ratios, particularly at the beginning. Somewhat higher intensities are seen when working in the center or traveling sections of class. The overall low intensity of class is probably due to the focus being on technical skill development as well as on teaching and feedback between movements.

The intensity of rehearsals largely depends on the state of a piece of choreography in the rehearsal process. In the early stages of creating and practicing material, rest periods tend to be longer. In addition, the dancing is invariably lower in intensity compared to the later stages of rehearsal, when pieces are being run from start to finish. These later stages more closely mimic the physiological demands of performance. Performance has generally been found to require higher physiological intensity than class or rehearsal; it is not uncommon for dancers to reach intensities of approximately 80 to 90 percent (Cohen et al., 1982; Blanksby & Reidy, 1988) of their individual maximum capacity as well as a greater work-to-rest ratio.

An issue highlighted in previous research relates to this apparent discrepancy between the demands of dance training (class and rehearsal) and performance (Wyon et al., 2004). It raises questions about the extent to which these forms of training provide adequate physical preparation for the demands of performance. It is important to note that dance class serves a crucial role in developing technical skill and artistry; therefore, it should not be expected to also serve as the place for physical training. That said, it is important to consider where physical training should occur because dancers must engage in appropriate conditioning that helps them meet the demands of performance repertoire.

Cross-Training for Dancers

Imagine you are in a ballet class. An allegro exercise is set toward the end of the class. Two of your dancer colleagues complete the sequence at the same time; both performed it fully and received positive feedback from the teacher. In the moments immediately after the exercise, one dancer is visibly out of breath and the other is not. In this scenario, both dancers are able to perform the required movements, but one has found them less physiologically demanding than the other. The dancer who found the sequence less physiologically demanding is likely to have a higher individual fitness level, is more able to cope with the demands of the dance class, and is more likely to be able to repeat the exercise again immediately if the teacher requests it. On the other hand, the less fit dancer may feel winded or fatigued after the allegro activity, and they may experience a performance drop in subsequent attempts.

This example underscores why it is important to participate in cross-training—physical conditioning other than dancing (figure 4.13)—that is purposefully designed to improve your fitness level, including **cardiorespiratory endurance** (endurance that depends on both the cardiovascular and respiratory systems or, together, the cardiorespiratory system). Research suggests that participating in dance class alone (as a physical activity by itself) may not be sufficient to increase your fitness levels high enough for optimum performance in dance (Needham-Beck et al., 2019; Stephens & Wyon, 2020; Twitchett, Koutedakis, et al., 2009; Wyon et al., 2004).

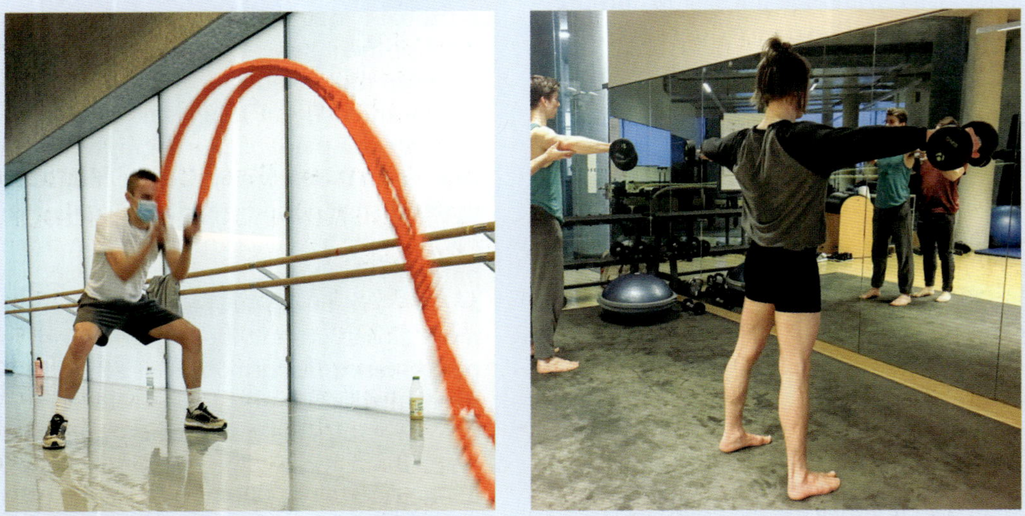

Figure 4.13 Cross-training for dancers incorporates physical training methods other than dance that prepare a dancer's body to perform with greater fitness. Ropes training and weight training are two examples of a wide variety of possible activities.
Emma Redding

It is important to consider whether your personal level of conditioning is appropriate for your current training and performance demands and whether it is suitable in preparation for the demands of your upcoming schedule. Do you take time over your summer break to work on your cardiorespiratory fitness in preparation for the beginning of your next semester or term of classes, or in preparation for approaching training and performance season? Remember, a fitter dancer is better able to cope with the physiological demands of dancing than one who is less fit.

Here are two significant questions for monitoring your current level of conditioning:

- Can you complete all movements fully, even toward the end of class, rehearsal, or the last session of the day?
- Do you think that you adequately recover between exercise sessions, classes, rehearsals, and performances, such that you feel fresh and prepared for the next session or exercise?

If the honest answer to either of these questions is no, you are empowered to improve. Chapter 5 contains helpful guidelines for engaging in additional physical exercise programs.

Table 4.2 **Sample Heart Rate (HR) Values Showing Activity Intensity as Recorded in Published Studies**

		Sample Intensity Data	
Activity	Genre	Mean HR (beats per minute)	Peak HR (beats per minute)
Class	Ballet	117-153 (Cohen et al., 1982)	158-178 (Cohen et al., 1982)
	Contemporary	107-126 (Wyon et al., 2004)	–
Rehearsal	Ballet	–	–
	Contemporary	108-134 (Wyon et al., 2004)	–
Performance	Ballet	160 (Cohen et al., 1982)	178 (Cohen et al., 1982)
	Contemporary	101 (Redding et al., 2009)	187 (Redding et al., 2009)

Data from Beck et al. (2015).

– indicates no data available; mean HR is the average heart rate (beats per minute) recorded during the activity; peak HR is the highest heart rate value (beats per minute) achieved during the activity

Differences Based on Technical or Stylistic Elements of Different Dance Genres

Dance activity of various genres includes jumps, lifts, turns, pace transitions, level transitions, and moments of controlled holds sustained throughout performance repertoire pieces of varying lengths (Wyon et al., 2011). However, there is much variation between genres in the stylistic and technical performance of these movements, and differences exist in the frequencies with which they are performed. This leads to differences in physical demands. For example, Wyon and colleagues (2011) conducted video analysis of 45 contemporary dance performances and 48 classical ballet performances. On average, ballet performances contained significantly more jumps than contemporary performances (about 5 per min vs about 2 per min). Overall, some dancers had many more and some had fewer, but clearly there was a difference between the two genres. This fact is important to understand when discussing physical demands and intensity.

An additional variation is found in the time-related characteristics of dance genres. For example, ballet and contemporary dance are relatively continuous with varying intensities as well as relatively long in duration (Wyon et al., 2011). By contrast, musical theater shows such as *Cats* or *Newsies* or theatrical dance productions such as *Riverdance* tend to involve shorter 2- to 3-minute pieces that are high in intensity with rests in between, repeated at varying intervals throughout the show's total duration. It is worth considering these elements of structure and the resultant demands of pieces you are performing in order to help you to identify appropriate ways to physically prepare yourself to meet those demands.

Differences Based on Variation of Repertoire and Individual Roles in a Genre

Considerable variation also exists within any given dance depending on individual dancers' roles. This variation is particularly apparent in genres such as classical ballet, where the principals, artists, soloists, and corps de ballet dancers have different roles and movement materials; therefore, they have different physiological demands placed on them (Wyon et al., 2007). Previous research (Twitchett, Angioi et al., 2009) has reported that principal dancers spent a higher percentage of total show time working at moderate intensities than soloists and artists, and they spent a lower percentage of the total show time resting (not onstage or not dancing). This variation is also evident in other dance styles, but it is less clearly defined. In any dance piece, there are moments where all or most dancers onstage are doing different movements; thus, each individual role within the piece has its own unique profile of demands.

Just as variation between dance genres exists (e.g., between hip-hop and classical ballet, figure 4.14), so does variation between different choreographies within a particular style (e.g., in contemporary dance, the requirements of a Cunningham piece are different from the requirements of a Limón piece). This variation can lead to highly varied

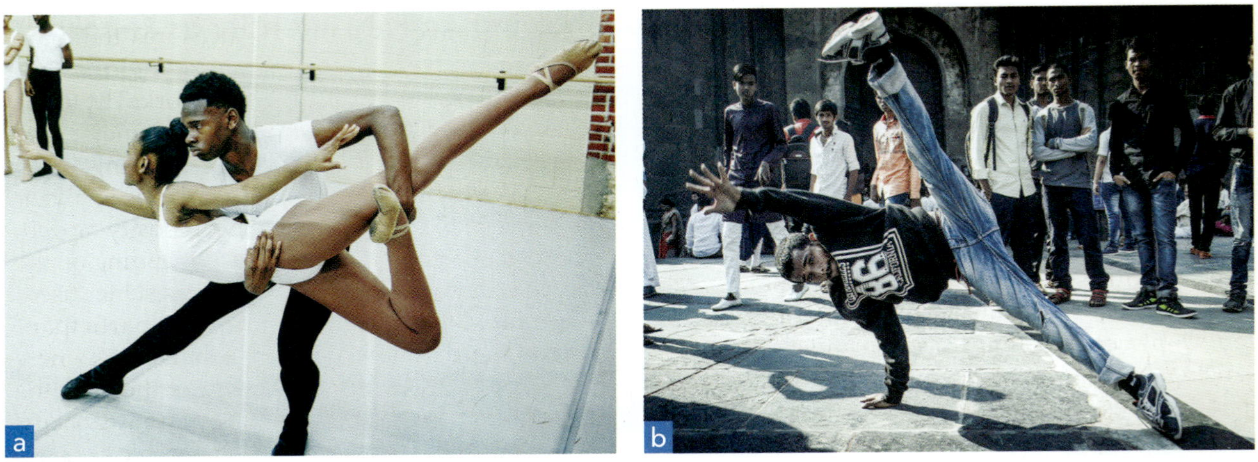

Figure 4.14 Different genres of dance require different physical abilities from dancers because their physiological demands are different.

A: Thomas Barwick/Stone RF/Getty Images; B: Atharva Tulsi on Unsplash

physiological demands. Some differences may be related to use and frequency of certain discrete skills that are known to greatly increase demands (such as jumping, as discussed in Differences Based on Technical or Stylistic Elements of Different Dance Genres). Other differences may stem from variations in tempo, intention, movement quality, and other elements (even for similar movements or discrete skills used).

Further variations in physical demands may be based on the time-related characteristics of dance genres. For example, the battle format in hip-hop competitions involves performing one to four rounds of 60 to 90 seconds each in a single battle; battles are then repeated multiple times within a day (a single competition), typically in round-robin and knockout style formats (World DanceSport Federation, 2023). This format is considerably different from a theatrical performance of hip-hop that may more closely mirror the time parameters of other theatrical dance performances.

Other Physical Demand Considerations

Dance activities, including performances, rarely occur as a one-off set of movements (with notable exceptions). The physiological effect of repeating performances over a long period (e.g., in a residential repertoire, long-running musical theater show, or touring company) is considerable. Performances can occur as frequently as 8 to 10 times a week. They can be even more frequent during holiday seasons and other times when extra shows are added to meet high-volume ticket sales.

In addition to the repetitive, high demands of this performance load, a touring show adds additional physical demands (Bronner & Wood, 2017), including travel, disturbed sleep routines, unfamiliarity with facilities (Hopper, Allen, et al., 2014), and limited access to quality nutrition (Cizek et al., 2016). Other external factors that may influence the physical demands of dance include climatic conditions (temperature, humidity, air pressure, etc.), the size of the dance space, flooring (Hopper, Wheeler, et al., 2014), and costumes or wardrobes (weight, fabric thickness, amount of a dancer's body surface they cover, etc.). It is always worth considering the whole picture when thinking about the demands of your upcoming schedule so that you can train and make necessary adjustments appropriately.

Adaptations to Training Cardiorespiratory Fitness

The term cardiorespiratory refers to the integration of the cardiovascular and respiratory systems. Thus, **cardiorespiratory fitness** relates to the ability of these systems to work together to supply oxygen to working muscles in response to the stimulus of undertaking physical activity. Cardiorespiratory fitness training is sometimes colloquially referred to as doing *cardio*, endurance, or stamina work. Various metabolic and cardiovascular adaptations take place as a result of regular cardiorespiratory fitness training. These adaptations can include increased heart size and volume that result in larger stroke volume and cardiac output, lower heart rate while exercising (relative to the exercise intensity), lower resting heart rate, and quicker recovery following exercise. **Positive adaptations** also include improved oxygen delivery and extraction from circulating blood at the muscle cell level, enhanced lung ventilation, and a more highly attuned ability of the muscle fibers to contract and work efficiently.

Importantly, performance gains are seen because of regular fitness training, so you will be able to do more physical work and recover more quickly if you adopt a cross-training regimen outside of your dancing. Improvements are typically greater at the start of a new training program, and they slow as the body adapts to continued exercise. Therefore, it is important to design an exercise plan specially tailored to each individual and their dance demands by applying the principles of training (e.g., the overload principle, as discussed in chapter 5 along with other concepts related to physical conditioning) to ensure that fitness gains continue. In general, fitness levels are increased by providing stimuli or stressors to the body's systems (as outlined earlier in this chapter) that are sufficient to elicit positive adaptations. In exercise prescription, training regimens are managed through carefully planned manipulation of four variables that are referred to by the acronym FITT: frequency (how often), intensity (how hard), time (how long), and type (mode) of exercise undertaken.

Testing Dancers' Physical Capacities

It is helpful to measure the physical attributes discussed so far; they are the capacities of your body to undergo the work required of being a dancer. Data such as these can identify your current fitness status and allow you to track changes (e.g., improvements) in your status over time. For example, your ability to perform a short bout of high-intensity exercise can be measured as a baseline. Then, after undertaking a cross-training fitness program, you can retest every 6 weeks using the same exercise bout as the baseline. Testing and tracking in this manner will provide a useful indicator of how your body is responding to your physical training. Your body's ability to sustain moderate-intensity exercise over incrementally longer periods of time can also be tracked.

Laboratory-Based Fitness Tests

The gold-standard measure of an individual's maximal aerobic capacity is the maximal oxygen uptake ($\dot{V}O_2max$) test, which measures the maximum volume of oxygen that an individual can absorb and utilize during physical work. The test is performed on a treadmill or a cycle ergometer (stationary exercise bike) while the person being tested wears a specialized breath-by-breath gas analyzer (figure 4.15). During this test, the intensity (speed, incline, or a combination of both, depending on the specific running protocol or cycling resistance used) is increased incrementally until the participant reaches the point of volitional exhaustion (where they cannot continue). This point is the sign the participant has reached their maximum capacity. Wyon (2006) recommends that an aerobic capacity test for dancers be performed on a treadmill, with speed increased by 1 kilometer per hour (0.62 mph) each minute until the point of volitional exhaustion. However, researchers have not specifically examined the effect of different protocols on test results in dance populations.

These fitness tests are widely conducted on a range of populations, including athletic and gen-

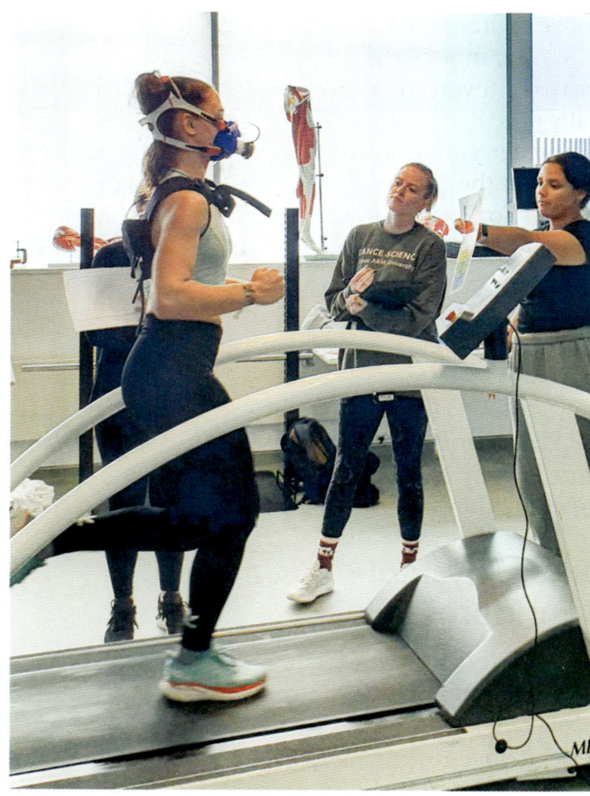

Figure 4.15 A typical exercise testing laboratory setup for collecting the data needed to calculate someone's maximum aerobic capacity. The dancer is wearing a breath-by-breath gas analyzer apparatus.

Emma Sng Ai Ming

eral populations, and they are often reported in published studies. A handful of studies have also reported mean values for various dance populations. However, be aware that these reports are mostly from small sample sizes (5-10 dancers from a single school or company), so they may not be generalizable to other dancers. Regardless, because of these available data, it is straightforward to compare your fitness level to the reference or normative (typical) values so you can see how your current fitness level ranks related to that of others (table 4.3).

According to the data in table 4.3, men typically exhibit higher $\dot{V}O_2max$ values than women, and $\dot{V}O_2max$ declines with age. However, high variations in fitness levels exist among all people depending on training status and other individual characteristics. Therefore, overlap exists in the fitness levels of different demographic groups within any given population. For example, not all younger dancers are fitter than all older dancers within a dance company.

Field Measurement of Dancers' Exercise Capacities

Individual fitness level or exercise capacity is most accurately measured by specific tests undertaken in an exercise science laboratory with specialized equipment, as described in the previous section. However, there are also field-based tests (tests conducted outside of a lab setting) and practical activities you can undertake to test your current cardiorespiratory fitness levels. These tests provide an expanded understanding of your preparedness to meet the demands of dance training and performance.

One simple example is testing yourself to see how far you can run in a set time (e.g., 12 min) or how quickly you can run a set distance (e.g., 2.5 km [1.5 mi]) on a treadmill, a track, or another suitable path. Another example is a multistage fitness test (sometimes called a beep test, bleep test or a shuttle run test), which consists of running continuous

Table 4.3 **Sample $\dot{V}O_2max$ Data From Available Studies**

Population	Mean reported $\dot{V}O_2max$ (mL·kg^{-1}·min^{-1})		Study reference
	Men	Women	
Ballet			Wyon et al., 2016
• Professionals: principals	50.5	45.9	
• Professionals: soloists	46.1	38.5	
• Professionals: artists	50.1	42.9	
Contemporary/Modern			
• Postgraduate students	52.7	47.5	Needham-Beck et al., 2019
Hip-hop			
• Elite breakers	64.8	–	Wyon et al., 2018
• Elite new style	–	45.9	
Musical theater			
• Vocational students	67.6	55.6	Stephens & Wyon, 2020
Ballroom			
• Elite competitive dancers	66.6	49.7	Liiv et al., 2013
Basketball players			Select values from Kenney et al., 2021 (p. 307)
• Age 18-30	40-60	43-60	
Gymnasts			
• Age 18-22	52-58	36-50	
Rowers			
• Age 20-35	60-72	58-65	
Nonathletes			
• Age 10-19	47-56	38-46	
• Age 20-29	43-52	33-42	
• Age 30-39	39-48	30-38	

– indicates no data available

20-meter (about 22 yd) shuttle distances in time with an audio track of beeps. The frequency of the beeps (thus, the speed of the test) increases periodically until you can no longer meet the required pace and you must withdraw. The audio track used for this test is accessible online and through various mobile applications. These field-based tests provide valid and reliable measurements that are frequently used in sports and occupational settings (e.g., military) to assess cardiorespiratory fitness quickly and easily on a regular basis.

Dance-Specific Fitness Tests

Field-based tests that are applicable to dance, while still allowing assessment of cardiorespiratory fitness, have also been developed. The dance aerobic fitness test (DAFT) (Wyon et al., 2003), the high intensity dance performance fitness test (Redding et al., 2009), and the ballet-specific aerobic fitness test (Twitchett et al., 2011) are examples of tests that dance companies and schools use to monitor levels of (and changes in) dancers' cardiorespiratory fitness. These tests allow the measurement of the relative physiological strain placed on participants during specific dance movements. They can provide a good marker of current preparedness for the demands of class and performance, and they afford the opportunity to track changes over time (e.g., if testing is repeated at the start and end of an academic year or season).

All dance-specific fitness tests involve relatively simple set dance phrases that are repeated for four or five stages. They can be undertaken in a group setting in a dance studio, with monitoring of heart rate (ideally through use of HR monitors) or individual ratings of perceived exertion (RPEs). Thus, they can be run in a class setting without the need for specialized staff, expensive equipment, and complex analysis, which are required for lab-based fitness testing.

Rating of Perceived Exertion (RPE)

A rating of perceived exertion (RPE) is another way to document the intensity of an exercise or fitness test. RPE evaluation does not require access to equipment to monitor HR or $\dot{V}O_2$. This method involves simply asking the person undertaking the activity to self-rate the intensity they are currently experiencing on a scale of either 6 to 20 or 1 to 10. These scales, originally devised by Gunnar Borg (1982), have been carefully validated by extensive research for use in various exercising contexts, including research on their use in dance (Shaw et al., 2020; Surgenor & Wyon, 2019; Jeffries et al., 2017). The scales include important anchors (descriptive words) to help you to choose the most appropriate number that represents how you rate your physiological response to an exercise. For example, on the 1-10 scale, a rating of 2 is described as "easy," while 4 is "somewhat hard," 7 is "very hard," and 9 is "nearly maximal."

Understanding Fitness Test Results

The primary purpose of completing a fitness test is to estimate your capacity to engage in physical work. As mentioned previously, test results can be examined against normative data from people with similar characteristics (e.g., sex, age, type of sport or dance activity, training status) and they can be compared with your own prior results to gauge your physical training progress. Improvement in cardiorespiratory fitness is usually indicated by an increase in $\dot{V}O_2$max, a decrease in $\dot{V}O_2$ or heart rate, or both, for a given movement phrase or other activity. These changes suggest you have an increased physical capacity to complete the phrases or activities of your dancing. They also mean that the relative strain of your physical work will be lower for you than it was previously. Therefore, you will be better able to cope with the demands of your dance training and performance schedule.

It is important to consider the timing of any fitness test, as this may affect the results. For example, on a Friday after a busy week, or at the end of a day of training, you may feel fatigued and not perform the test to the best of your ability. This consideration is especially important if you wish to compare results over two (or more) different time points to see how your fitness level has changed. Therefore, try to keep the conditions and timing of the test as consistent as possible each time you participate in a testing session to allow for an accurate comparison of the results.

Conclusions and Practical Relevance

This chapter covered a lot of detailed information about how the body responds to physical activity and supports your physical performance of that activity. Central to physical performance are the cardiovascular and respiratory systems, as well as the structure and function of skeletal muscle. Three energy systems contain the metabolic processes that ensure the regeneration of energy to support activity. The complex movement patterns and intermittent (stop, start) nature of dance activity require optimization of all three of these systems to consistently meet the varied demands of dancing. For these primary reasons, supplementary fitness training (cross-training) is recommended for dancers. It raises your personal fitness level to allow you to meet the demands of a busy training and performance schedule and avoid feeling too fatigued or overworked.

Typical dance classes and rehearsals may not provide all the physical conditioning you need for top-level performance. You are empowered to undertake your own supplementary training (following evidence-based guidance by appropriately qualified and experienced professionals) to ensure you are prepared for the demands of your dance schedule. A variety of methods are available to measure your personal cardiorespiratory fitness level so that you can track changes in this area over time.

Discussion Questions

1. Describe the changes you feel in your body as you go through a dance class in terms of your breathing, internal body temperature, and heart rate.
2. Imagine the first half hour of one of your dance classes. Then, compare it to the jumping and traveling sequences toward the end of class. How different are these two sections of the class, and in what ways do you physically feel either equipped or not equipped to participate at an optimal level?
3. Given that the focus of a typical dance technique class is on skill development and technique, what benefits do you envision if you would participate in regular supplementary fitness conditioning? If you already participate in this type of supplementary training, explain the advantages you feel compared to dancers who do not participate in it.

WWW Go to HK*Propel* to access supplemental information and activities connected to chapter content.

Part II

Care Inside and Out

5

Conditioning as an Injury Risk Reduction Measure

Elaine Winslow-Redmond, MS, ATC
Monica Lorenzo, MS, ATC
Diane Diefenderfer

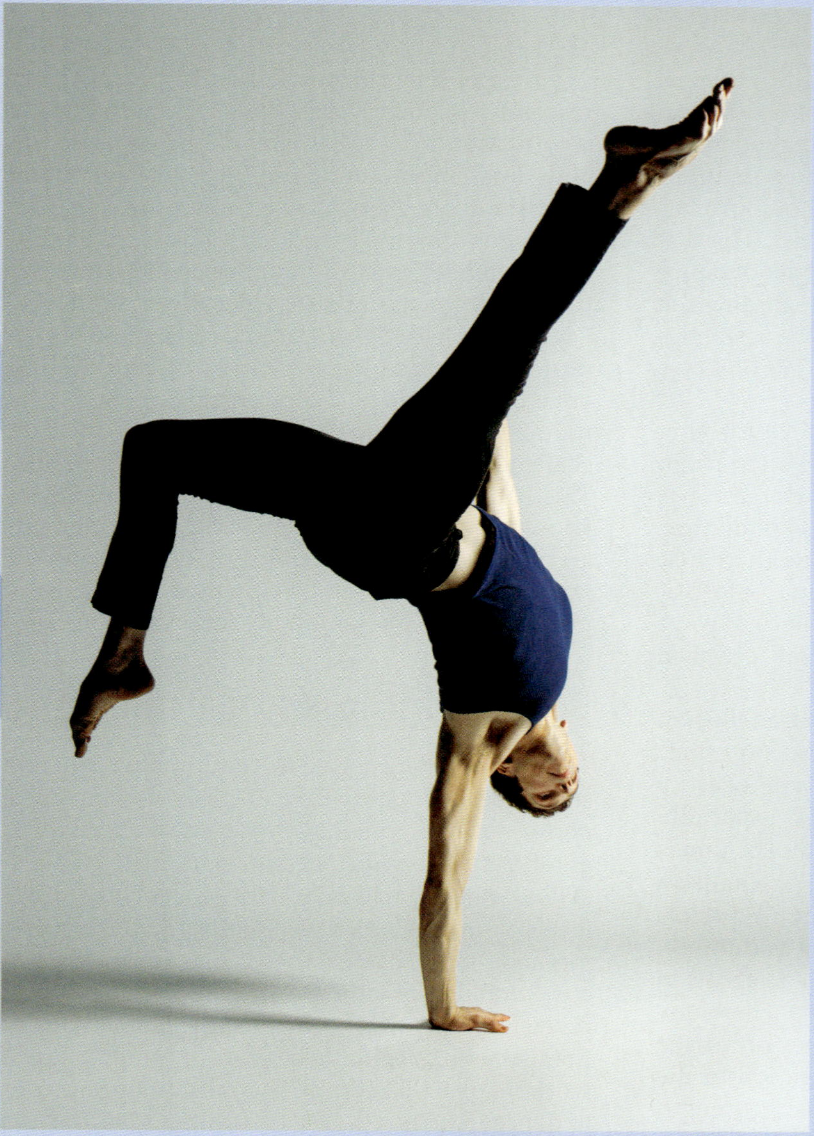

Belhaven University Dance Department; Jackson, Mississippi. Photo by Fluid Flames Dance Photography/Courtesy of Emily Roy; Dancer: Noah Smith.

Dance is a highly rigorous physical activity, and your body must be conditioned properly to meet its required demands. Therefore, understanding the basics of how to raise the physical condition of your body is integral to your success as a dancer.

Key Terms

aerobic training
anaerobic training
anterior chain system
concentric contraction
core muscles
eccentric contraction
endurance (muscular endurance)
fast-twitch (type II) muscle fiber
gluteals
hamstrings
hip external rotators
hypertrophy
iliac crest
lactate threshold
metatarsals
overload principle
pelvic floor
performance anxiety
posterior chain system
posterior tilt of the pelvis
power
prone
pubic bone
quadriceps
reversibility principle
sacrum
scapula
scapular depression
sit (or sitz) bones
slow-twitch (type I) muscle fiber
specificity principle
spinal extension
spinal forward flexion
spinal hyperextension
spinal lateral flexion
spinal rotation
strength
supine
supine tabletop position
thorax/thoracic
transversus abdominis (TA)

LEARNING OBJECTIVES

After completing this chapter, you will be able to do the following:

- Differentiate between anaerobic and aerobic training methods, and explain the benefits of each.
- Identify effective methods of muscular training and their benefits.
- Discuss how hormonal changes in the body affect physical conditioning.
- Describe the background of the Pilates Method as a conditioning technique for dancers.
- Perform basic conditioning exercises used in the Pilates Method.

Like many world-class athletes, dancers strive to achieve high levels of endurance, strength, power, and agility. Unfortunately, dancers are seldom afforded the same attention as other athletes with regard to physical conditioning, treatment of injuries, or reduction of injury risk. This discrepancy may exist because of the nature of dance training and how it evolved, myths regarding the effects of conditioning as it relates to the aesthetics of dance, or other barriers (e.g., lack of time or access to health care professionals).

Dance training typically begins at a very young age. Children as young as 3 years old often begin taking dance or creative movement classes once a week. For those who become truly committed, training intensifies to 5 or 6 days per week in their adolescent years. Rarely during this time of formative training are dancers offered guidance in ways to improve and maintain their overall physical conditioning or to resist injury.

The aesthetic nature of dance creates an illusion of ease, and it may also perpetuate misconceptions that it does not generate the same type of force or power as other physical activities, especially sports. However, researchers such as Dr. James A. Nicholas (1975) and Dr. William G. Hamilton (1992) established that when considering performance factors such as strength, agility, endurance, and coordination, dance is comparable to sports in terms of overall performance demands. Therefore, dancers are in fact performing athletes or artistic athletes who deserve equal consideration in the methods of injury risk reduction, muscle strength and endurance training, and cardiorespiratory conditioning. As a dancer, referring to yourself with the term *performing athlete* or *artistic athlete* may help you overcome mindset challenges and move you closer to embracing the true athleticism that is part of your artistic pursuit.

Dr. Carol Teitz (1986, p. 73) stated, "Dance is not seasonal." In other words, there is no such thing as an offseason in dance. There are seasonal productions, but dance training continues throughout the year. Therefore, many dance injuries are a result of overuse as opposed to sudden trauma, and finding time to rehabilitate an injury is challenging. The training regimen in dance resembles that of most Olympic athletes. When dance medicine and science professionals use the principles of conditioning offered in this chapter, they create comprehensive training programs that prepare dancers to meet the challenges of classes, rehearsals, and performances. This chapter is meant to empower you with the knowledge of these same conditioning methods and techniques. It also will provide you with the training tools necessary to help reduce your risk of injury and prepare your body for a lasting career.

Basic Principles of Training

The goal of a dance-specific conditioning program should be to reduce the risk of injury and maximize performance (figure 5.1). Uniting dancers' abilities as refined artists with the training methods of highly skilled athletes will help dancers achieve greater levels of success with fewer injuries. Sound training methods typically use the primary principles of conditioning, including overload, specificity, and reversibility. Within each principle lie methods of training with potential to be part of a comprehensive workout plan that addresses contributing variables to dance injuries.

Overload Principle

The **overload principle** involves challenging the body beyond its normal limits to achieve physical

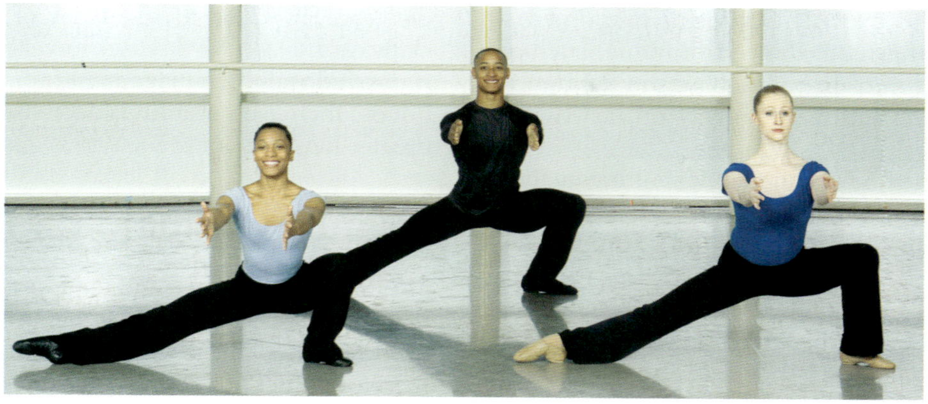

Figure 5.1 Physical conditioning should be a fundamental activity in the life of a dancer.

gains. It is well documented that fatigue is a contributing factor to injury risk (Jones et al., 2017). A conditioning program that increases the capacity of the primary energy systems used for different genres and intensities of dance will help you resist fatigue. Balancing strength and flexibility to complement training adaptations occurring in dance technique classes will prepare your body for the challenges of an intense rehearsal and performance schedule. These concepts (including anaerobic and aerobic conditioning as well as strength training) are discussed in later sections of this chapter.

Specificity Principle

The **specificity principle** of conditioning involves training the body consistently with the skills needed for the activity in which you are participating. Each exercise performed produces specific adaptations in the body; in turn, those adaptations produce specific training effects (McArdle et al., 2023) that help dancers meet the demands of their dancing. This principle is ideal for use when designing a program for performers because their unique athleticism is a significant part of their artistic identity. Somatic practices, such as Pilates, yoga, Alexander Technique, and the Feldenkrais Method, are excellent examples of training methods based on this principle. Including them in your conditioning program will be beneficial.

Reversibility Principle

The **reversibility principle** states that the training adaptations gained from a conditioning program will be reversed if the exercises are not performed consistently. The idiom *Use it or lose it* is a common way to express the reversibility principle. A balanced exercise program integrating different methods of conditioning should complement a dancer's technique training, and it should be performed on a regular basis. An ideal physical exercise program considers the level and type of dance and the frequency of technique training versus that of performance. Strategies to strengthen areas of weakness can be incorporated during periods when the dancer is primarily training and prior to beginning a new sequence of rehearsals and performances.

Anaerobic Training for Dance

As mentioned in chapter 4, anaerobic exercise is important in dance because it is the primary energy pathway used for activity that lasts approximately 2 minutes or less. That amount of time is typical of the intervals of effort in dance class and performances, and the stop-and-go format of dance naturally conditions the system without tapping into oxidative energy stores. **Anaerobic training** increases the **lactate threshold**, which is the point at which the muscles begin to experience fatigue. When training beyond this threshold, a dancer forces their body to work harder and longer to build resistance to fatigue. The probability of injury increases as fatigue becomes evident (Liederbach et al., 2013); thus, this type of conditioning increases a dancer's ability to resist fatigue and avoid injury (Wyon & Koutedakis, 2013).

Fast-twitch (type II) muscle fibers favor the anaerobic metabolic pathways, which do not require oxygen. These fibers are larger than **slow-twitch (type I) muscle fibers**, while they also produce greater force more quickly through short-term contractions to execute powerful movements. Movement patterns in dance technique, such as grand allegro jumps in ballet, wings in tap dance, or jackhammers in breaking, rely on fast-twitch muscle fibers.

Common methods of anaerobic training include weightlifting, high-intensity interval training (HIIT), plyometrics, and sprinting. Some of the equipment used in these activities are free weights, resistance bands, jump ropes, medicine balls, boxes, and benches. Specific benefits related to anaerobic training include increased muscle **power** (the ability to exert muscle force quickly or explosively), increased bone strength and density, increased lactate threshold, and resistance to muscular fatigue. Dance conditioning should primarily focus on accentuating anaerobic training to optimize risk reduction of injuries such as stress fractures and repetitive strain to soft tissues.

Aerobic Training for Dance

Aerobic training should also be included in any conditioning program for dancers. Aerobic exercise is important for improving dancers' endurance and sustainability during long rehearsals and performances. Regular aerobic exercise also provides many overall health benefits. Aerobic training consists of low- to moderate-intensity exercise that continues over relatively long periods (beyond 3 minutes) and utilizes the oxidative energy system (i.e., oxygen is required for energy production).

Slow-twitch (type I) muscle fibers are important for endurance exercise, and they favor the aerobic metabolic pathway. They produce less force and are slower to produce maximum tension than fast-twitch fibers. In addition, they can maintain longer contractions, and they are important for skeletal stabilization, including joint stability and posture, which are crucial for all types of dance.

Common methods of aerobic training include running, cycling, rowing, stair climbing, and swimming. Types of equipment used for aerobic training include bicycles, upper-body ergometer cycles, rowing machines, treadmills, elliptical trainers, stair climbers, and swimming pools. Aerobic training—also commonly called *cardio*—provides well-known benefits that include reduction in both resting and exercise blood pressure, resting and exercise heart rate, reduced insulin resistance, increased muscle tone, and increased lung capacity.

Both anaerobic and aerobic exercise also contribute to supporting the overall health and wellness of dancers. They lead to lower risk of disease (especially cardiovascular disease), lower blood pressure, improved weight management capability, stronger bones, increased stamina, decreased stress, and greater longevity of life.

Strength Training for Dance

Strength training is a pillar of cross-training for dancers. Dancers are comparable to traditional athletes in terms of the physical nature of their activity; therefore, their ability to sustain long durations of activity (endurance) and access sufficient power output must be developed in similar fashion to that of a soccer, basketball, or football athlete. Strength training has several benefits, including increased lean muscle mass, improved bone density, and—most importantly—injury risk mitigation. On a neurological level, strength training can improve sleep patterns, improve mood, and increase resilience to environmental and emotional stressors. The benefits of strength training go well beyond solely enhancing the musculoskeletal system (Thomas & Burns, 2016).

Benefits of Strength Training

First, strength training benefits the musculoskeletal system. When sufficient resistance is added to movement, the muscle tissue is stressed. (Recall the overload principle discussed earlier in the chapter.) The nerves in the muscle tissue sense this stress on the muscles and send a signal to the brain. The brain responds by sending messages to the bloodstream to transfer nutrients to the muscles that improve strength, vitality, and resilience against the stress. Over time, new tissue is produced, resulting in more lean muscle mass. More muscle mass does not necessarily mean that bulk is created in the muscles. Bulking of muscle, or **hypertrophy**, only occurs with a conscious training protocol that includes increased calories in one's diet in conjunction with high loads of weight resistance training conducted with specialized parameters. On the other hand, lean muscle mass is achieved by balancing the ratio of adipose (body fat) to muscle tissue. Each individual has their personal ratio embedded in their genetic coding. It can be enhanced with strength training, thus achieving the athletic output necessary to meet the strength demands of dance.

Strength training goes beyond strengthening only muscle tissue. Dancers who participate in strength training also benefit from increased strength of bones, tendons, and ligaments. This benefit helps reduce the chance of repetitive stress injuries that are common in dance, and it improves overall resistance to fatigue.

Performing strength training exercises that focus on muscles during controlled lengthening contractions (**eccentric contractions**) spurs improvement in the muscles' ability to decelerate the body against gravity. This ability affords dancers better control when landing jumps, which is a means of reducing injury risk (Haas, 2017).

Increased bone density is desirable for injury risk reduction and mitigation of early onset osteoporosis. Stress sensors in the musculoskeletal system gauge the stress of a muscle-tendon unit (the combination of a muscle and the tendons that attach it to bone) pulling against the bones as well as the gravitational load of body weight on the skeletal system. This stress is sensed by *osteocytes*, which are specialized bone cells embedded within the bone matrix. One type of osteocyte, *osteoblasts*, are bone-forming cells responsible for synthesizing new bone tissue. Mechanical loading during strength training activates osteoblasts, leading to increased bone formation. Osteoblasts produce collagen and other proteins that make up the matrix of new bone, a network packed with bone minerals that give bone its hard nature. Strength training affects *osteoclast* activity, as well. Osteoclasts are osteocytes responsible for breaking down old or damaged bone tissue. Strength training has been shown to inhibit the activity of osteoclasts, thus reducing bone breakdown and osteoporosis (Hong & Kim, 2018).

Strength training promotes adjustments in nerve receptors in muscle tissue. Refinement of the stress sensors and motor components in the musculoskeletal system has several positive effects. The body's awareness of itself in space is refined, and technique is better executed, thereby enhancing performance. This improvement assists in injury risk reduction because the musculoskeletal system is more adaptable to changes in environment and movement. Awareness of stress on musculoskeletal structures allows the body to assess when it reaches the limits of its capacity. For example, awareness of when the **hamstrings** are overloading during jumps or when a lift is being performed with too much weight provides the feedback needed to cease an action before an injury occurs or an existing injury worsens.

Strength training mitigates the risk of injury to ligaments by increasing stability around a joint through greater muscle tone and force of muscular contractions during activity. Moreover, strength training can stimulate the production of collagen, a key structural protein in ligaments and tendons. The mechanical loading during strength training may trigger *fibroblasts* (the cells responsible for collagen synthesis) to produce more collagen fibers in response to increased demand. The increase in tissue development is a response that improves joint stability (Brumitt & Cuddeford, 2015). This stability is important because many dancers exhibit a high degree of joint flexibility that can lead to ligamentous laxity (looser or hypermobile joints) or instability around the joints. In such a scenario, strengthening of muscles and their tendinous attachments counteracts the lax ligaments that cause the sensation of looseness. Therefore, dancers with hypermobile joints especially benefit from a carefully constructed strengthening program, even though all dancers will realize the positive effects of strength training.

Types of Strength Training

A variety of strength training methods exist. The only requirement for any method is to apply resistance to the lever systems of the body in such a way that the muscles receive resistance; based on the overload principle, the muscles have the opportunity to increase their force output, or strength. Common methods of developing muscular strength include the following:

1. *Weightlifting*. This method involves use of any of several types of weights in pushing, pulling, or lifting motions. Typically, each motion has a lifting portion and a lowering portion. The lifting portion is the concentric phase, during which the working muscles perform a **concentric contraction** (shorten). The lowering portion is the eccentric phase, during which the contracting muscles perform an eccentric contraction (lengthen in a controlled way). Barbells, dumbbells, kettlebells, and similar apparatus are ways to accomplish weightlifting.
2. *Resistance training with cables or bands*. This method involves using a system of cables, pulleys, and weights or resistance bands that provide resistance to the musculature. As with weightlifting, any given exercise usually involves both concentric (shortening or lifting) and eccentric (controlled lengthening or lowering) phases.

Contracting Does Not Always Mean Shortening

When speaking of muscle contractions, it is easy to imagine that a muscle is getting shorter. After all, in English grammar, a contraction forms when two words (e.g., *do* and *not*) are shortened into a single word (e.g., *don't*). The word *contract* indicates that something is getting shorter in other instances, too. However, in muscle physiology, *contraction* simply means that tension is generated by the proteins in the muscle. (Chapter 4 provides more detail on how muscles contract.) In strength training, muscle contraction is a practical consideration.

During a concentric contraction—when something is being lifted against gravity—a muscle's proteins generate tension, and the muscle gets shorter. This contraction is how an object is picked up, such as when lifting a bottle full of water from a table to your mouth with a concentric contraction of the biceps brachii muscle in your upper arm. However, during an eccentric contraction—when you lower that water bottle back down to the table—the biceps brachii gets longer, but it still creates tension (contracts). Try lifting and lowering a water bottle or something else with a bit of weight; as you lower the item, poke the biceps muscle with the fingers of your other hand, and feel the eccentric contraction occur. During an eccentric contraction, the body controls the muscle's lengthening by adjusting the amount of tension created by the proteins when the muscle lowers its load. The same process occurs when you lift and then lower a weight in a strength training exercise.

Here's another terminology caution related to muscle contractions. Don't say "flex" to describe a contracting muscle. Flex is a kinesiological term for a specific type of movement in certain joints or body regions, such as flexing your knee (bending it) or flexing your trunk (bending forward at the waist). When you want to talk about a muscle working to do its job, say "contract." For instance, you contract your hamstrings to flex your knee joint! And "flexing" your foot really is the motion of ankle dorsiflexion that happens when you contract your tibialis anterior muscle.

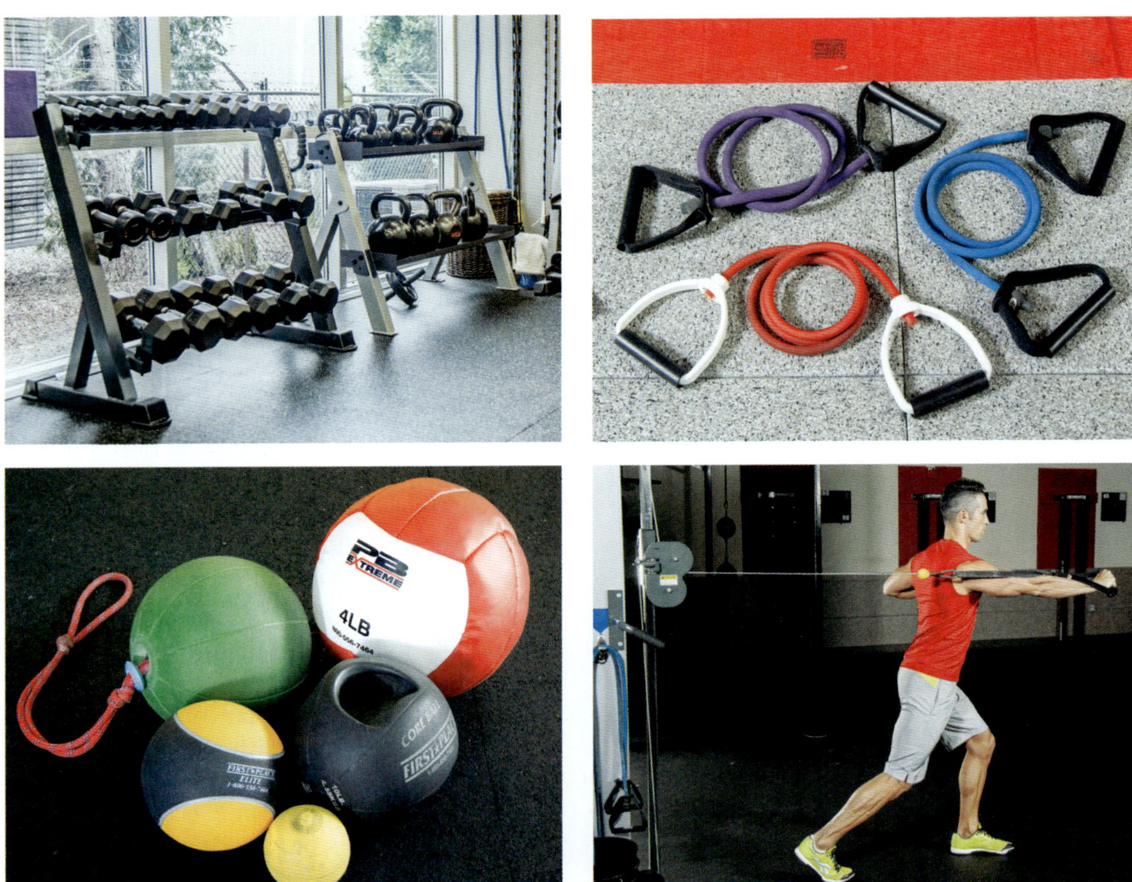

Figure 5.2 Dancers can choose from a variety of tools and equipment to augment their strength training.

A: Inti St Clair/Tetra images RF/Getty Images

3. *Body-weight exercises*. These exercises involve training that solely uses body weight against gravity as the resistance. Calisthenic exercises are a classic example, and many HIIT programs use only body weight. Body-weight training can involve supporting apparatus, such as inflatable balls, steps, bounding boxes, and the like.
4. *Suspension training*. This type of training requires the use of a suspension apparatus that allows one to perform pushing and pulling movements where body weight against gravity provides the resistance.

Apparatus for Strength Training

While some strength training can be conducted using only body weight as the resistance, a seemingly infinite number of devices are available to provide additional resistance (see figure 5.2 on previous page). Examples include the following:

1. Free weights (e.g., barbells and weight plates, dumbbells)
2. Resistance bands
3. Medicine balls
4. Cable columns or pulley systems

Building a Strength Training Program

When building a strength training program, the first step is taking a holistic inventory of your body's performance needs and current state of your muscular strength (and weakness). A main purpose is to establish your baseline—that point from where you will move forward by participating in training. Where you are headed from that baseline forms your goals. Here is an inventory to get you started:

1. What styles of cross-training have I practiced the past 6 months? (List the type, duration, and level of skill or intensity you achieved, if applicable. For example: *Running for 3 months; I can now run a 7-minute mile [1.6 km] and run 5 miles [8 km] without stopping* or *Strength training twice per week—both upper- and lower-extremity exercises—2 sets of 10 on cable equipment*.)
2. What injuries have I sustained, where am I in the rehabilitation process, and do any of these injuries still inhibit my full performance?
3. What are my personal goals for this performance or competitive season? How must I further develop my strength to meet these goals?
4. How long do I have from now until the start of my season to achieve these goals?
5. How can I improve other aspects of my health and wellness with nutrition, sleep quality and quantity, mental recovery, and physical recovery?

The answers about your weaknesses and injuries will provide a focal point for your strength training program in the initial phases. Mitigating future injury will be most successful if you can first apply corrective exercises to your movement; a qualified rehabilitation health care professional or health and fitness specialist can assist with implementing these exercises. Corrective exercises address increasing range of motion in a joint system that is limited or rebalancing opposing muscles around a joint or in the trunk that are affecting your technique. Common limitations in dancers are in **thoracic** spine extension, hip extension, hip external rotation, ankle dorsiflexion, and ankle plantar flexion (Storm et al., 2018).

WWW Go to HK*Propel* to download a physical activity and goals tracking spreadsheet.

Before beginning strength training exercises, performing mobility exercises in the initial phase of a program will help correct ranges of motion wherever necessary. Mobility exercises are slow-paced, active movements that contract and release muscles throughout a joint's range of motion. Some of these exercises may isolate certain joints, while others involve multijoint movement patterns. An example of a corrective mobility exercise is provided here:

MOBILITY WARM-UP FOR THE HIP: SUPINE HIP INTERNAL AND EXTERNAL ROTATION

1. Begin lying **supine** (on your back); bend both knees to plant your feet on the floor, about 8 to 10 inches (20-25 cm) apart (figure 5.3*a*).
2. Place both arms out to the sides to support the torso.
3. Slowly drop one knee outward, away from the center of the body (hip external rotation) and the opposite hip inward, toward and across the center (hip internal rotation) (figure 5.3*b*); hold the position for about 5 seconds.
4. Keep your glutes in contact with the floor, and do not lift your lower back off the floor.
5. Repeat the movement to the opposite side, again holding for about 5 seconds.
6. Continue to alternate sides, lowering deeper into each position with each successive repetition (rep).
7. Perform 8 to 10 reps.

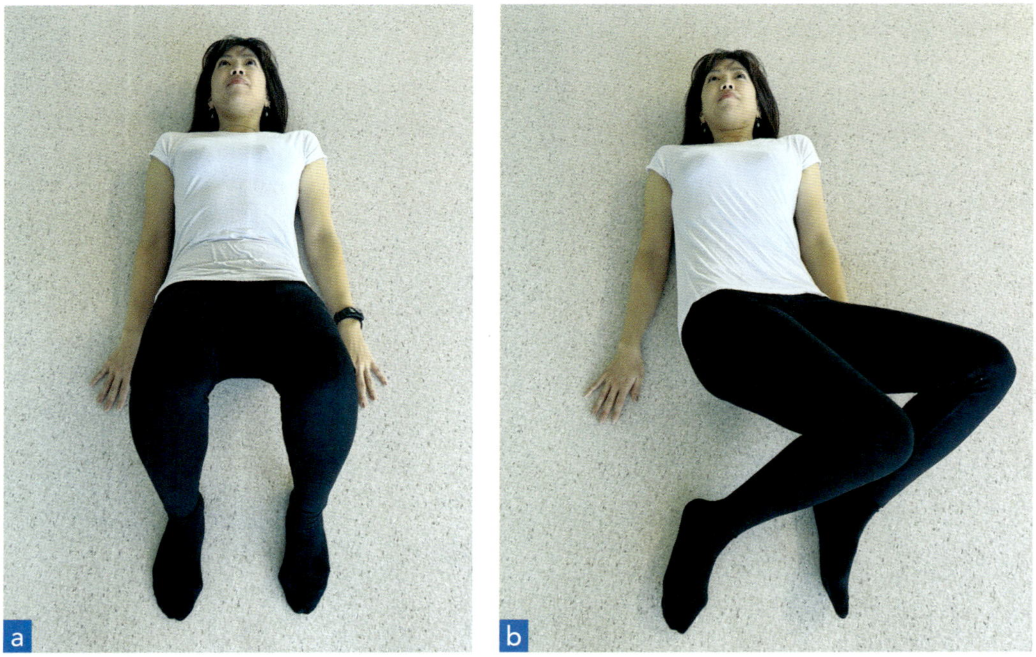

Figure 5.3 Correct positioning for supine hip internal and external rotations. Note that the exercise is done in a controlled fashion to both sides.
Dr. Jeff Russell

The next step for pre-strength training corrective exercise is to strengthen the weak aspects of the musculoskeletal system that are important for overall efficient movement. Most commonly, the **posterior chain system** (muscle groups located at the back of the body) is weaker than the **anterior chain system** (muscle groups located at the front of the body) due to overactivity of the anterior chain during training and dance. The posterior chain is responsible for propelling the body through the frontal, sagittal, and transverse (or horizontal) planes of motion and providing stability for the spine. The structures included in the posterior chain are the calf muscles, hamstring complex, gluteal complex, back and spine stabilizers, upper back and scapular stabilizers, and cervical spine musculature. In addition, the stabilizing system of the **core muscles** should be integrated into all movements of a strengthening program because the core forms the foundation for virtually all movements in dance. Two sample exercises follow.

POSTERIOR CHAIN AND CORE STABILIZING EXERCISE 1: PLANK ALTERNATE ARM/LEG EXTENSION

Benefits of this exercise include improved core connectivity and increased awareness of the anterior and posterior chains.

1. Begin in a plank position (the top of a push-up) with your hands placed on the ground under your shoulders (figure 5.4*a*).
2. Engage the core stabilizers, then push through your right palm into the ground to stabilize your shoulder complex. Raise the left arm, reaching it forward into shoulder forward flexion (figure 5.4*b*).
3. Engage your gluteus maximus, hamstrings, and then your lower back to extend your left hip to lift your right leg, floating it up into a neutral alignment with the body. To avoid overextending your lower back (hyperlordosis) and compromising torso stability, do not extend your leg farther than hip height.
4. Hold the position for 10 to 30 seconds, then return to the starting plank position to complete one rep. Repeat the movement with the opposite arm and leg. Begin with 4 reps. As your strength develops over time, add 2 reps every 1.5 to 2 weeks.

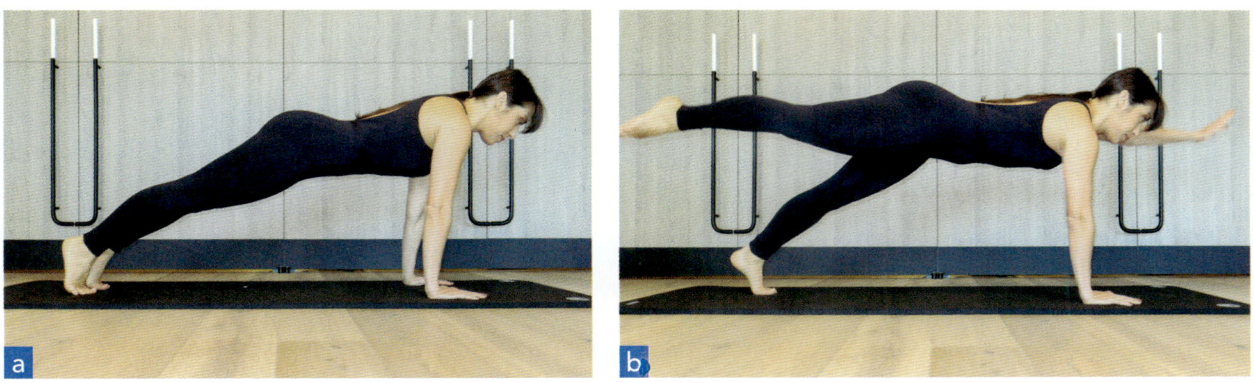

Figure 5.4 Plank progression exercise: *(a)* Starting position. *(b)* Position after properly executing the extremity raises.

Monica Lorenzo

POSTERIOR CHAIN AND CORE STABILIZING EXERCISE 2: OBLIQUE TWISTS (AWAY FROM THE UNSUPPORTED LEG)

1. Begin seated with your legs in front of you, your knees bent to 45 degrees, and your feet dorsiflexed. Place a circular exercise band around both hands; the palms should face each other (figure 5.5*a*).
2. Gently engage your midback, and pull your hands apart to stretch the band.
3. Sense your core stabilizing muscles engaging further after pulling the band. Hold this position.
4. Slightly lean your torso backward, arching it into a C-shaped curve. Then, rotate your torso as one unit toward the right (figure 5.5*b*). Next, rotate to your left.
5. Maintain an open chest position, and do not allow your shoulders to roll forward (figure 5.5*c*).
6. Return to the starting position, and repeat. Perform 2 sets of 10 to 15 rotations to each side.

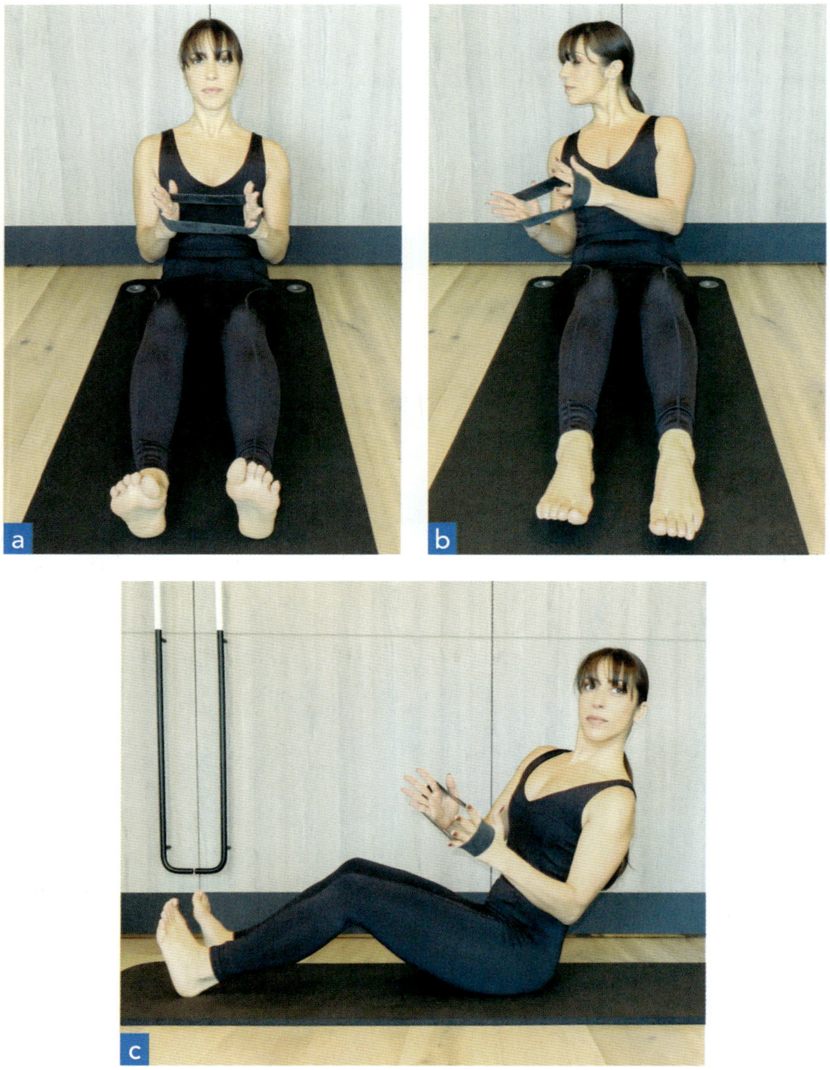

Figure 5.5 Oblique twist exercise: *(a)* Starting position. *(b)* For maximum benefit, positioning is of prime importance. *(c)* During the twist, the chest is open, the shoulders remain back, and the torso maintains its slightly arched position.

Monica Lorenzo

The answer to the personal inventory question about reviewing your current cross-training parameters (discussed earlier) forms the basis for regulating the load of your program. Consider these three important aspects of developing and progressing a program:

1. *Volume*: The amount of work you do in an exercise session
2. *Intensity*: The amount of resistance or physical exertion you undertake, including the duration of a session and repetitions of an exercise
3. *Frequency*: The number of training sessions per day, week, or month

Once you determine the baseline of your capacity for each of these aspects by writing down your current conditioning status and activities, you should build from this baseline. Injury occurs when tissue is exposed to greater volume, intensity, or frequency than it can withstand; this exposure causes the tissue to become overloaded or overworked. Therefore, a gradual increase in all three parameters will produce a safe environment for improvement in your physical capacities.

Recovery is another crucial aspect of strength training. Recovery is not simply a cool-down after exercise. It includes proper nutrition to refuel your body with the nutrients it needs to repair or regenerate tissue. It also includes proper sleep, which contributes to how well you can perform. Sleep deprivation can lead to injury because the musculoskeletal system's regenerative abilities are adversely affected by fatigue. In addition, sleep deprivation negatively affects resiliency and overall performance is negatively affected (Vitale et al., 2019). If your nutrition and sleep are not optimal for recovery, you should reduce the intensity and volume of your training program. Prioritizing improvements in recovery and rest is of paramount importance for reduction of injury risk.

Strength Training Program Guidelines

Answering the questions you asked about your goals for your performance output will help you determine the volume, intensity, and frequency of your program during the allotted time available for a particular training season during the year. An annual training program can be divided into four phases (table 5.1). These phases are based on a dancer's performance or competitive season, and the duration of each season is unique to the dancer's performance schedule. When planning the duration of each phase, keep in mind that it takes about 4 weeks to see appreciable changes in metabolic output and strength (Clark, 2016). At first, strength training load should increase. During performance season, it should be maintained without additional increases as too much resistance could overload the musculature during an already busy period of effort. Using clearly demarcated phases promotes a healthy and sustainable process for you to improve your strength, power, and muscular endurance throughout the year. The goal is to safely load the body over time as a means to mitigate injury.

Specific Strength Training Parameters

Once you have an annual plan in place, you can start creating your weekly program of exercises. Building your exercise program should directly correlate with your strength, endurance, and power goals. Choose exercises that can sustain the balance between the anterior and posterior chains. You can create this balance by alternating muscle groups during the sequence of a program. Incorporate warm-up and cool-down exercises into your program as well.

Finally, determining the level of intensity you should add to your program correlates with how easily you can perform a set of a given exercise. For example, if 12 reps of biceps curls with 10-pound (4.5 kg) dumbbells are easy to accomplish, the recommended progression is to add weight to the resistance so that fewer reps are possible. An adequate weight is one with which 8 to 10 reps in a set is relatively manageable. From there, continue to add reps during your workouts until 12 reps are easy, then increase the weight again.

Frequency of your program should balance on days of lower rehearsal intensity or nondance days. If your rehearsal or class schedule is loaded 5 or 6 days per week, reduce the intensity of the program on heavier dance-intense days. Reducing strength training intensity includes reducing the number of exercises completed in the program as well as reducing resistance. Intensity and volume can increase systematically every week as your resilience and strength improve.

A total body program should alternate segments of the body throughout a week. For example, focus on the upper body on Mondays and Thursdays and the lower body on Tuesdays and Fridays. Another efficient format is to target the total body during

Table 5.1 **Sample Annual Conditioning Program for Dancers**

Phase	Description and duration	Goals
Preseason	Begins at the close of the postseason. The duration of this season can be 1 to 4 months, depending on the duration of the performance season. It may be considered part of the off-season. Dancers use this period with no performance schedule to balance improved strength and conditioning in conjunction with dance training to sustain technique and enhance biomechanical movement.	• Improve total body strengthening and conditioning. • Address corrective exercise protocols. • Gradually increase aerobic training. • Begin power and jump stabilization programs. Do not neglect the core muscles. • Incorporate training for any weaknesses noted during postseason.
Preperformance season	Begins during rehearsal season, or at the initiation of a university or conservatory semester. This phase continues to incorporate strength and conditioning in coordination with a heavier load of dance training. Strength and conditioning loads will directly correlate to duration and load of dance training with care to not overload the tissues.	• Perform 45 to 60 minutes of strengthening and conditioning 4 or 5 days a week in conjunction with 5 to 8 hours of dance training 5 days a week. • Maintain the strength and biomechanical improvements made during preseason. • Improve endurance training. • Acclimate the body to increases in loads. • Implement recovery protocols that address the intensity of training loads.
Performance season	Begins at the start of performance or competitive season. Training loads are moderated. Increasing loads is not a goal; the focus is on training maintenance.	• Engage in 45 to 60 minutes of strengthening and conditioning no more than 3 days a week in conjunction with 4 to 10 performances a week. • Maintain strength and endurance output as well as biomechanical precision in technique. • Follow a strong daily recovery protocol.
Postseason	Begins at the close of performance season. Provides an opportunity for rest, recovery, and preparing for the next preseason cycle.	• Follow a strong recovery protocol. • Address complete injury rehabilitation. • Assess weaknesses noted during performance season, and plan a protocol to manage them.

Adapted from Sands, Wurth, and Hewit (2012).

every session, while alternating agonist and antagonist (muscles on one side of a joint and the other) movements and upper- and lower-body segments every exercise. Table 5.2 presents some ideas for structuring your program.

Format your program on a weekly rotation. Record all of your exercises and movements, including your warm-up, cool-down, and recovery tactics (e.g., myofascial release, foam rolling). Tracking your progress will allow for appropriate and safe increases in intensity and volume of work. The data you gather about your efforts will also provide positive feedback as your capacities improve, which in turn will build your self-efficacy and self-esteem.

Hormone Cycling and Training Programming

When creating a strength training program, one consideration is hormone cycling and its effect on the musculoskeletal system; this factor affects females more than it does males. The female men-

Table 5.2 **Basic Structure of a Strength Training Program**

Program phase	Description	Number of exercises Reps and sets	Sample exercises
Mobility warm-up	Perform dynamic movements that focus on gradually increasing joint range of motion.	• 4-6 exercises • 1-2 sets × 10 reps	• Shoulder controlled articular rotation (CAR) • Hip CAR • Vinyasa (flow) yoga sun salutation
Core connectivity exercises	Begin to activate deliberate core connectivity and balance work that will form a strong foundation of control before you move to more intense movement and strength training exercises.	• 2-3 exercises • 2 sets × 10 reps	• Supine transverse abdominal press • Dead bug • Slow seated torso roll-down to ground • Primal plank • Static plank • Half-ball balance trainer one-legged balance
Low-intensity movement	Strength exercises, including upper- and lower-extremity resistance. Include midlevel weight to your movement to prevent overload in the initial phases. Begin in uniplanar and biplanar movements.	• 2-3 exercises • 2 sets × 10-15 reps	• Biceps curl with mini squat • Lunge with overhead press • Mountain climber
High-intensity movement	Increase intensity of strength exercises. Include multiplanar movements and plyometrics. Increase intensity of movement with heavier weights and increased reps.	• 3-4 exercises • 8-12 reps • 20 sec exercise/1 min rest intervals for plyometrics	• Single-leg deadlift with lateral arm fly • Multiplanar lunge with biceps curl • Suspension training exercises • Box jump • Half-ball balance trainer squat
Core stability cool-down	Begin cool-down with floor work while deeply focusing on core stability. Continue with gentle mobility cool-down exercises and static stretches.	• 3 core exercises • 2 sets × 10 reps • 4-6 stretches and mobility cool-down exercises, 1 set each	• Supine crunch • Prone leg extension • Side plank progression • Mobility and stretching exercises addressing hamstrings, quadriceps, gluteals, torso, shoulders, and neck complex

strual cycle influences the training output of the body and muscular reaction to stress. As a performer, you may not be able to cycle the intensity of your rehearsals or performances; however, you can control your cross-training plan to assist your body in producing strength gains and achieving efficient recovery. You must consider how the rise and fall of hormone levels (primarily estrogen, progesterone, and testosterone) during each phase directly affects the power output and recovery of muscle tissue. Regulating strength and conditioning programs with hormone cycles can provide benefits that include better sleep, faster tissue recovery, less severe menstrual cycle symptoms, improved mood, decreased fatigue, and a heightened sense of overall well-being (Hackney et al., 2019).

The menstrual cycle is composed of four main phases (table 5.3). These phases can be subdivided into seven smaller phases. Fluctuating hormone levels and physiological events across these subphases dictate the best exercises to include in each one. They are described next.

Table 5.3 **Four Main Phases of the Menstrual Cycle**

Phase	Primary event(s)
1: Menstruation	Shedding of the uterine lining
2: Follicular	Development of the follicle Preparation of the egg for release prior to ovulation
3: Ovulation	Release of the egg for potential fertilization in the uterus
4: Luteal	Thickening of the uterine lining to support egg fertilization and maturation

Phase 1A, Days 1 to 5: Menstruation and Early Follicular Phase

During menses and the early follicular phase, progesterone, testosterone, and estrogen levels decrease. A main effect of this drop in hormones can be a reduction in stamina and muscular endurance output. Therefore, restorative exercise is recommended during this phase, especially when creating a training program combined with a rehearsal or performance schedule. Appropriate types of exercise for this phase include walking, short bouts of cycling, vinyasa (flow) yoga, and stretching recovery sessions (slow, controlled movement, including active and passive stretching of the musculoskeletal system).

Phase 2A, Days 6 to 8: Mid-Follicular Phase

During the mid-follicular phase, estrogen begins to rise while progesterone decreases. Growth hormone also elevates during this phase, thus improving synthesis of lean tissue and synthesis of fat into glycogen for energy. Recommended exercise adjustments in this phase include elevation of aerobic exercise and strength training using relatively low resistance, which will help you ramp up your activity from the prior phase. Appropriate types of exercises for this phase include Pilates, power yoga (a blend of vinyasa-style poses that increase heart rate), low-resistance weight training with increased reps, running, and cycling for longer durations than in the early follicular phase.

Phases 2B and 2C, Days 9 to 14: Late Follicular Phase and Ovulation

During the late-follicular phase and ovulation phase, progesterone decreases while testosterone increases. Resting metabolic rate decreases during the late follicular phase, warranting less aerobic training, more HIIT, and more power training to counterbalance the decrease in resting metabolic output. During this phase, you may feel highly energetic. Thus, appropriate types of exercise for this phase include HIIT, anaerobic interval training with running or cycling (short, high-intensity bouts of running and cycling interspersed with low-intensity rest bouts), powerlifting, and strength training using heavier resistance and low reps.

Phase 3A, Days 15 to 20: Early Luteal Phase

During the early luteal phase, estrogen levels remain the same while progesterone levels increase, resulting in an increase in glycogen synthesis within the endometrial cells. The continuation of HIIT and power training are recommended. However, if you begin to notice greater posttraining soreness or early fatigue, you should reduce your overall workout load and continue with anaerobic running or cycling.

Phase 4A, Days 21 to 24: Mid-Luteal Phase

During the mid-luteal phase, progesterone increases while estrogen remains level. This change in balance leads to a continued decrease in power output of the musculoskeletal system. Recovery exercises should be introduced during this time. Make the transition to aerobic training bouts that are longer than those of the prior week. For strength training, reduce the resistance and increase the reps.

Phase 4B, Days 25 to 31: Late Luteal Phase

During the late luteal phase, restorative practices are highly recommended because the musculoskeletal system is under great stress from a decrease in levels of estrogen, progesterone, and testosterone. Examples of appropriate exercises during this phase are yin yoga (slow-paced yoga with asanas, or postures, that are held for longer periods of time than in other styles), walking, and mat-based Pilates with low power output that focuses on core engagement and limb activation.

The Pilates Method

The Pilates Method (named after its creator, Joseph Pilates) is the most widely used form of supplemental training for dancers. It is a means of both injury risk reduction and corrective exercise. Although its widespread popularity increased tremendously from the 2010s to 2020s, dance students and professionals in a variety of dance genres have practiced Pilates since the late 1930s. Legendary choreographer and founder of the New York City Ballet, George Balanchine, recognized the benefits of the Method, and he sent his dancers to Joseph Pilates for strengthening and rehabilitation.

Principal dancer Jacques D'Amboise was directed to Pilates after Balanchine told him his muscles were too big and he had poor posture (Friedman & Eisen, 2005, p. 2). At first reluctant to try the Method, D'Amboise became a devotee, claiming, "The Pilates Method makes me feel exhilarated and absolutely wonderful. The exercises are excellent for strengthening and stretching the entire body, especially the lower abdomen and the back" (p. 2). Celebrated dancer Edward Villella shared how Pilates assisted him in rehabilitation this way: "It was a total toning of the body. What was important to me was just to keep the circulation going when I had to wait to come back to dance" (Kent et al., 1984, p. 163). Other notable dancers of the 20th century who regularly practiced the Pilates Method included choreographer Jerome Robbins; ballerinas Suzanne Farrell, Allegra Kent, Maria Tallchief; and modern dance luminaries Martha Graham, Hanya Holm, Ted Shawn, and Ruth St. Denis.

Numerous studios, gyms, and fitness clubs worldwide offer some kind of Pilates training today. Dance schools, performing arts institutions, professional companies, and universities offer Pilates programs to aid their dancers in strength building, core conditioning, alignment correctives, and—most important—reduction of injury risk. In these programs, highly trained and certified Pilates teachers, physical therapists, and athletic trainers guide dancers on various Pilates apparatus. These ballet companies and universities are some of the many that currently offer Pilates to their dancers: Royal Ballet (London), Boston Ballet, San Francisco Ballet, Houston Ballet, Ballet Austin, University of Utah, University of Alabama, University of Nevada, New York University, and University of California, Irvine.

Marika Molnar, director of physical therapy for the School of American Ballet and New York City Ballet (NYCB), uses Pilates equipment in her practice to rehabilitate and strengthen dancers (Marks, 2017). Ballerinas Tiler Peck of NYCB and Isabela Boylston of American Ballet Theatre (ABT) offered virtual classes from their homes during the COVID-19 pandemic year of 2020 using social media sites. In these classes, they combined Pilates exercises with ballet classes. Peck stated, "These classes are keeping me sane, and giving me something to look forward to" (Lansky, 2020, para. 1).

History of the Pilates Method

Born in Germany in 1880, Joseph Hubertus Pilates was a man of many talents, but he was never a dancer. As a sickly, frail youth, he engaged in a variety of activities to overcome his weaknesses and build his physique. He practiced gymnastics, bodybuilding, swimming, diving, and skiing. He was so successful that he became a model for anatomy charts. In his later years, he found work as a boxer, a circus performer, and a self-defense instructor. Living in England at the outbreak of World War I and imprisoned with other German nationals, he began teaching his fellow inmates about fitness and health. He later claimed that because of his regimen, none of them succumbed to the influenza epidemic of 1918.

In an early relationship to the world of dance, Rudolf von Laban (originator of Labanotation) integrated Pilates' work into his own teaching after meeting him in Germany in the early 1920s. By 1925, after being invited to train the growing German army (and declining the offer), Pilates decided it was time to leave Europe. Emigrating to the United States in 1926, Pilates and his wife, Clara (whom he met on the ship crossing the Atlantic), opened a studio in New York City dedicated to teaching his method of body Contrology (the original name Pilates used to describe his work) (Friedman & Eisen, 2005). In his book *Return to Life Through Contrology* (Pilates & Miller, 1945), Pilates wrote, "Contrology is complete coordination of body, mind and spirit. Contrology develops the body uniformly, corrects wrong postures, restores physical vitality, invigorates the mind and elevates the spirit" (p. 5).

Mind–body fitness or wellness, commonly used to advertise exercise programs and wellness retreats, is not a new idea. Joseph Pilates espoused the relationship of the mind, body, and spirit in his early teachings almost 100 years before this book's publication, writing, "With the body, mind and spirit functioning perfectly as a coordinated whole, what else could reasonably be expected other than an active, alert, disciplined person" (Pilates & Miller, 1945, p. 17)?

These quotes certainly describe the desirable and necessary qualities of a dancer. It is no wonder that the dance community continues to discover the excellent benefits of practicing the Pilates Method as a means of injury reduction.

Pilates Fundamentals

The six fundamentals of the Pilates Method—concentration, control, centering, precision, flowing movement, and breath—are interrelated, and they are crucial to the successful practice of Pilates. These fundamentals are also integral components of a healthy dance technique. Understanding correct breathing and centering is essential for your health and longevity as a dancer; therefore, the following sections focus on these two especially important factors.

Breath

When asked why breath is important, many dancers may answer, "to stay alive!" While this reason is obvious, the multiple benefits of healthy breathing are of paramount importance to your vigorous dance practice. Deep inhalation through the nostrils fills the lungs with fresh oxygen that is carried by the bloodstream to nourish the cells, while exhalation rids the body of carbon dioxide. With the blood flowing throughout the body, your cells are enlivened and waste relating to work and fatigue is carried away. Joseph Pilates taught that the process of complete inhalation and exhalation stimulates muscles into greater activity, and he developed his program with precise breathing patterns for each exercise.

In the teaching of classical ballet, awareness of breath and instructions about how or when to breathe are often not addressed. Traditionally, ballet dancers are expected to demonstrate command of their bodies with little to no apparent effort. They may hold their breath to avoid showing effort and find themselves huffing and puffing between demanding passages; at times, they may be out of breath completely. "Just when dancers need oxygen the most—during a challenging balance or speedy petit allegro—it often seems they instinctively hold their breaths . . . it is an important habit for dance teachers to break" (Thompson, 2020, p. 52).

Proper breathing patterns are important to other genres of dance, too. For example, modern dance practice often uses breath as the initiator of movement, enabling the dancer to perform with a natural fluidity and grace. It is a very positive application of breathing. Additionally, some modern and contemporary choreographers use breath in place of music to cue movement.

Understanding the basic action of the lungs, rib cage, thoracic muscles, and diaphragm (figure 5.6) in the breathing process is fundamental to success in dance. Upon inhalation, the thoracic muscles serve to open the rib cage while the diaphragm drops down, allowing the lungs to fill with oxygen. Ron Fletcher, a Graham dancer and first-generation Pilates teacher, encourages thoracic breathing this way: "Lots of people get into the habit of breathing low in the belly which can lead to distended stomach muscles. Good breathing begins in the chest area, not in the belly" (Fletcher & Ebert, 1978, p. 31). This statement makes sense because the diaphragm sits at the lower margin of the chest region (the **thorax**). Marika Molnar also advocates diaphragmatic breathing, stating in an article in *Dance Teacher* magazine (Thompson, 2020), "This is what happens when you inhale: the diaphragm descends and flattens out, the rib cage expands while the abdominal contents get pushed down and outward, and air rushes into the lungs" (p. 52). It is clear, then, that you must discover proper abdominal awareness and its connection to breath.

Dancers are notoriously faced with stress and tension in an environment of competitiveness and perfectionism. Negativity and emotional upset can trigger poor practice habits that lead to injury. While additional factors must be addressed, mindful and meditative breathing may help alleviate some stressors, thereby assisting in reducing the risk of injuries. Also, taking deep breaths prior to a performance can aid a dancer in calming nerves and reducing perform**ance anxiety** (stage fright).

Breathing Exercise to Support Dance

Given the numerous benefits of mindful breathing as well as the fact that breath can be an inspiration to beautiful movement, this exercise will help you achieve success:

1. Stand tall with your feet and legs parallel and hip-width apart and your arms relaxed at your sides.
2. Take a full breath, inhaling through the nose while feeling the sensation of the lungs expanding in three directions (forward, out to the sides, and across the back).
3. Exhale with slightly pursed lips, slowly and thoroughly emptying the lungs. It helps to imagine the lungs as two balloons or an accordion; they expand to draw the air in, and they compress to force the air out.
4. Continue breathing deeply while concentrating how completely full—then empty—you can make those two balloons, your lungs.

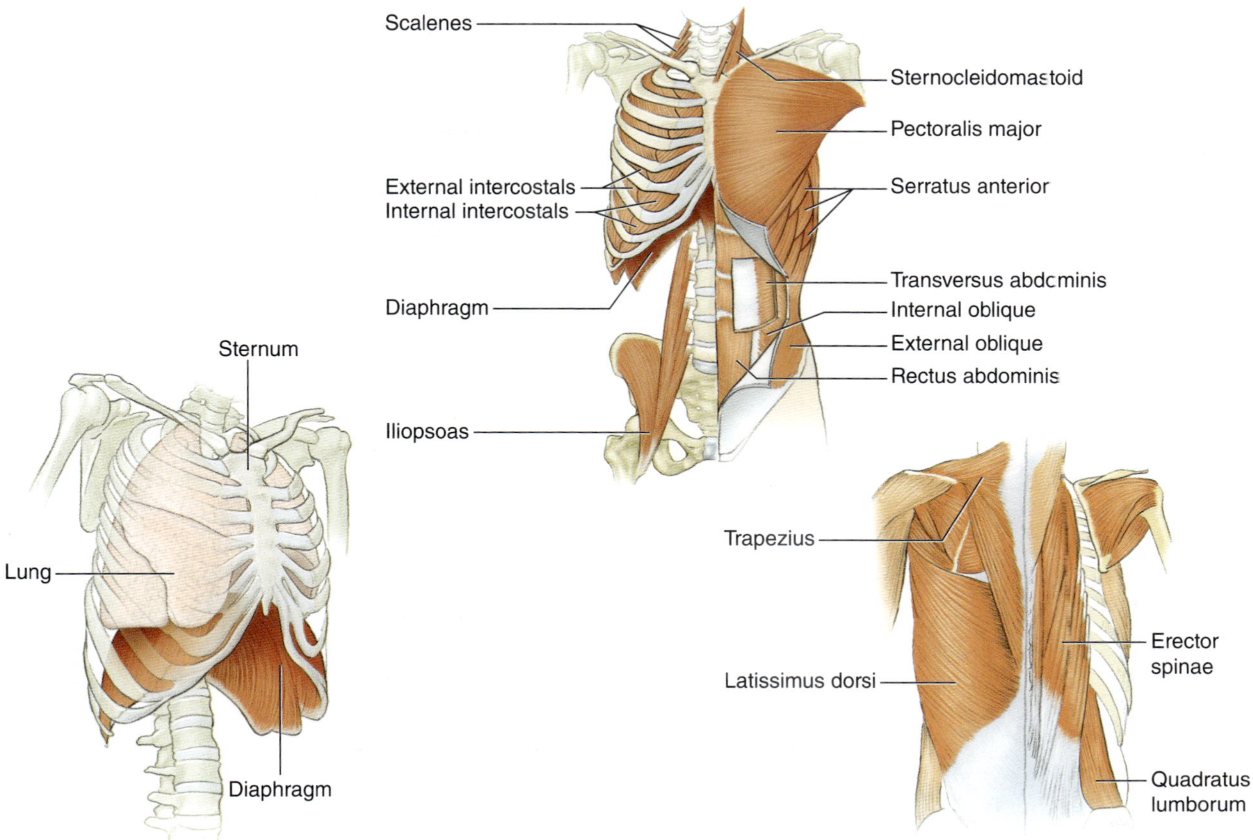

Figure 5.6 The anatomical structures (lungs, bones, and muscles) that allow one to breathe. Note especially the domed shape of the diaphragm muscle, which contracts and moves downward during inhalation and relaxes and moves upward during exhalation.

Make the exercise in the previous sidebar part of your dance practice.

Centering and Abdominal Awareness

In the Pilates Method, the center (figure 5.7) is described as the area of the body that forms a continuous band—front and back—from the bottom of the rib cage to the line across the **iliac crests** (bony borders at the top of the pelvis) (Friedman & Eisen, 2005). Some dance teachers refer to the center simply as the abdominals, the belly, or the tummy. Anatomically, there are several important muscles in this area, such as the rectus abdominis, internal and external obliques, and transversus abdominis. These muscles are described in more detail in chapter 13.

The Centering the Body exercise that follows is excellent for conscious, deep breathing balanced with abdominal support, awareness, and connectivity. A strong center supports the spine and pelvic structure, thus aiding in reducing risk of injury to the dancer.

Being able to both visualize and control the center is an important part of Pilates training. This exercise will assist you in doing so.

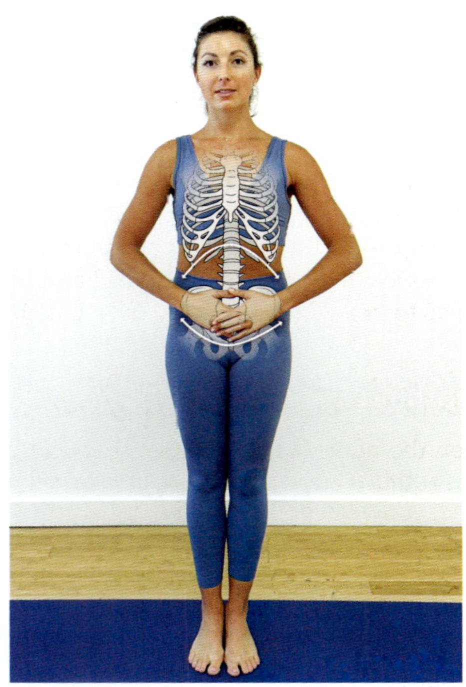

Figure 5.7 The center as it is understood in Pilates practice.

Photo: Diane Diefenderfer; Model: Laura Hanlon

CENTERING THE BODY

1. Stand tall as in the centered posture where you draw your navel to your spine and engage your abdominals to support your spine; your hands are now placed on the lower belly area, below the navel and above the **pubic bone** (figure 5.8).
2. Allow that low belly area to relax and possibly distend.
3. Engage those low abdominal muscles as though you were pulling your navel back toward your spine and your pubic bone toward your **sacrum**. This part of your center is crucial for supporting the low back and maintaining pelvic stability; imagine a tight seat belt extending across this region.
4. Take a deep breath, knowing that the diaphragm will drop, thus causing the belly area to move outward. This movement is normal and necessary for a deep inhalation; however, the lowest area of the belly should not completely relax and hang out. Continue to be aware of abdominal connectivity even while inhaling.
5. Exhale completely, now bringing the navel deeper toward the spine and flattening the lower abdominal area (as if tightening your seat belt).

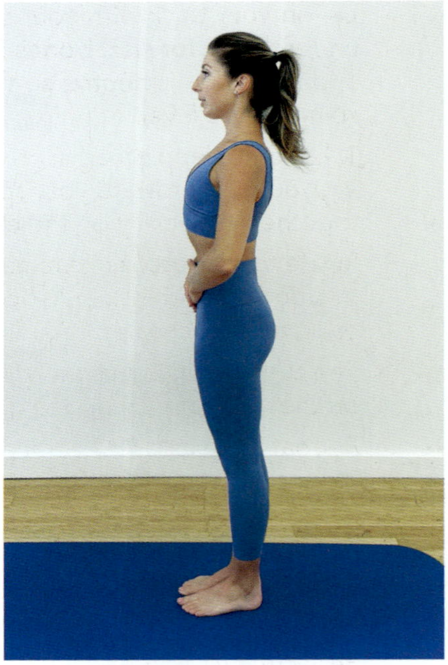

Figure 5.8 Proper positioning for centering the body.
Diane Diefenderfer

It is not uncommon for athletes and dancers (who are performing, artistic athletes) to seek a slim, sleek abdominal area, which is usually considered aesthetically attractive as well as a sign of a strong core. Often, the quest is to achieve the famous six-pack abs, with very noticeable definition of the rectus abdominis muscle in six sections. Performing numerous conventional sit-ups and rapid-fire crunches is a common practice. While it may be considered a sign of superior strength, dancers may benefit more from an understanding of awareness and control using the deeper **transversus abdominis (TA)** muscle. The following exercises will help you explore how the TA can support the low back and pelvis. A Pilates mat or a thick yoga mat would be ideal to support the body during these exercises, which are done in a supine position.

BASIC CURL OR CRUNCH

1. Lie on your back with your arms by your sides, knees bent, and feet parallel on the mat directly under the **sit (or sitz) bones** (in anatomical terms, the ischial tuberosities). Make sure the back is flat and the pelvis is neutral so there is no tucking of the pelvis nor excessive curvature of the lumbar spine (figure 5.9*a*).
2. Take some deep breaths; on each exhalation, try to imprint the lower spine into the mat while drawing your navel toward your spine. The breath and the activation of the low abdominal muscles work together, especially on the exhalation. You should do this movement without tucking the pelvis.
3. Inhale to prepare; while exhaling, begin to lift the head, neck, and upper back into a curl or crunch position. Your chin should hover over the chest (figure 5.9*b*). Move your arms toward your feet, hovering a few inches off the mat. Reach forward with energy, but don't jerk forward.
4. The curl or crunch position is where the bottoms of the **scapulae** (shoulder blades) are slightly resting on the mat—no lower or higher. This movement is not a full sit-up.
5. Repeat the exercise several times. Make sure to inhale to prepare and exhale to crunch while bringing the navel deeply toward the spine, drawing the pubic bone toward the sacrum, and activating the TA. The pelvis should remain in a neutral position; the exercise is performed without tucking or arching the low back.
6. Try to breathe slowly and fully, oxygenating the entire body while discovering the transversus abdominis pressing down toward the spine.
7. Perform 8 to 10 reps.

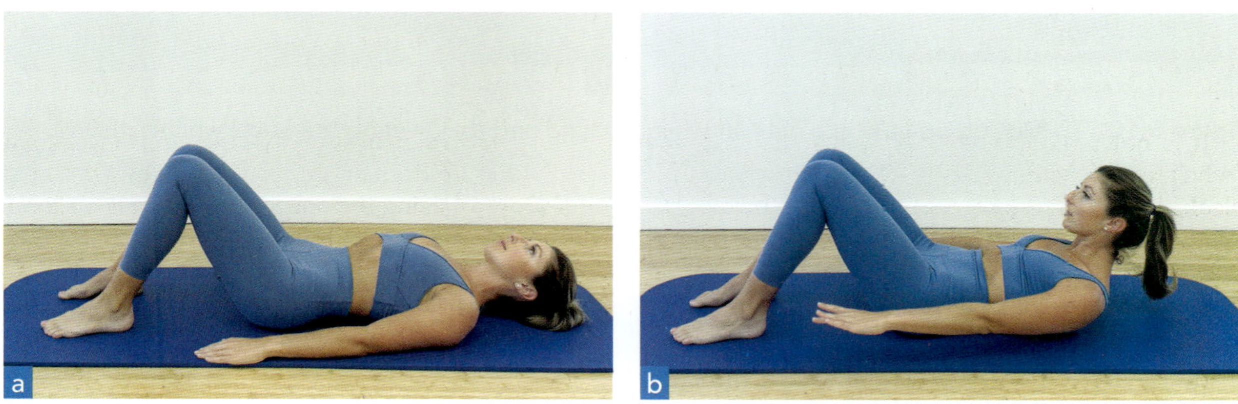

Figure 5.9 Proper *(a)* starting position and *(b)* ending position for a Pilates curl or crunch.
Diane Diefenderfer

HEELS LOWERING

1. Remain on your back with your arms by your sides; keep the spine long, pelvis neutral, and head and neck in proper alignment.
2. With your legs bent and held together, draw your knees into your chest without tucking the pelvis. Keep your feet **dorsiflexed** (flexed), aiming your toes upward toward your knees (figure 5.10*a*).
3. Inhale to prepare; while slowly exhaling, lower your heels toward the mat without arching or tucking the spine (figure 5.10*b*). Do not drop your feet; hover them slightly above the mat. The TA should be working; it is directly responsible for maintaining the neutral pelvis.
4. Return your knees toward your chest. Perform 8 to 10 reps.
5. To make this exercise more challenging, place a tennis ball between your ankles and another one between your knees. Perform the exercise without dropping either ball.

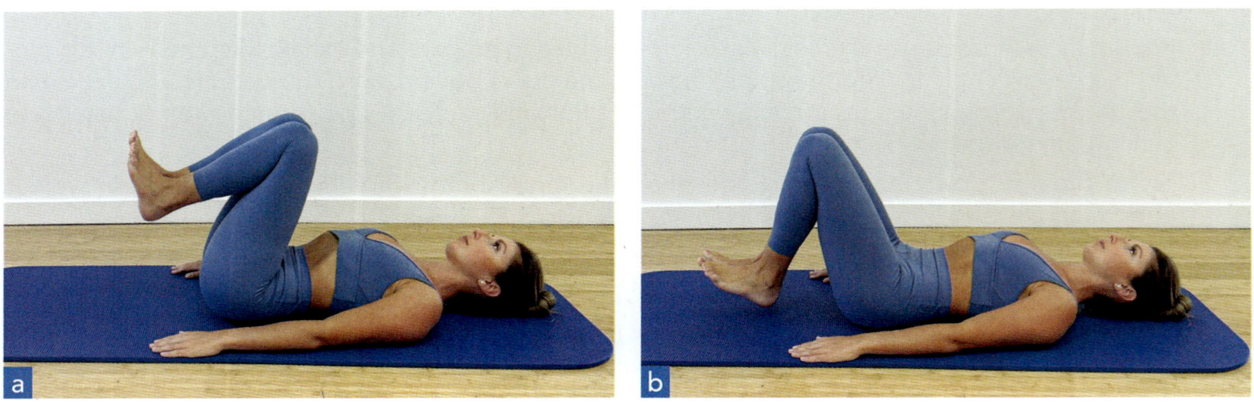

Figure 5.10 *(a)* Moving upward in a heel lift while inhaling and *(b)* lowering the heels while exhaling.
Diane Diefenderfer

Spinal Awareness and Articulation

Dancers are typically known for having beautiful posture and a regal carriage of their bodies, primarily resulting from a strong, flexible spine. Joseph Pilates spoke regularly about the importance of a healthy spine. For example, he once said, "Your posture is as good as your spine is strong, and you are as young as that spine is flexible" (Fletcher & Ebert, 1978, p. 69). Dancers of all genres are required to move their spines in a variety of directions; they bend, arch, twist, rotate, and turn while jumping, landing, balancing, partnering with others, and more. The basic movements of **spinal forward flexion**, **spinal extension**, **spinal hyperextension**, **spinal lateral flexion**, and **spinal rotation** are fundamentals of a strong dance technique. A greater awareness of how the spine moves and supports the body while maintaining abdominal connectivity is essential for reducing injury to the dancer.

Many classical Pilates exercises focus on spinal articulation with support and initiation from the center (abdominals). The roll-up, swan, and pelvic press are three such exercises.

ROLL-UP

This exercise involves spinal flexion from a supine position. The entire sequence is shown in figure 5.11.

1. Lie supine on the mat with your legs fully extended and your arms reaching overhead; the inner thighs are touching, the feet are pointed, the neck remains long, and the abdominals are engaged (figure 5.11*a*).
2. While inhaling, lift your straight arms until they are perpendicular to the floor (figure 5.11*b*).
3. Gently lift your head toward the frame of the arms, bringing the chin toward the chest figure 5.11*c*).
4. While exhaling, continue to roll your spine off the mat, one vertebra at a time, until the body is rounded over the legs (figures 5.11*d* and 5.11*e*); your fingers reach past your toes (figure 5.11*f*). Avoid dropping the torso over your legs; instead, feel the sensation of a thoroughly flexed (rounded) spine and a deeply engaged (contracted) abdominal area. Always think of the cue *navel to spine*.
5. To return, first inhale; then, with a slow exhalation, gradually lower the spine back to the mat, one vertebra at a time (figures 5.11*g* through 5.11*j*). Perform 4 to 5 reps.

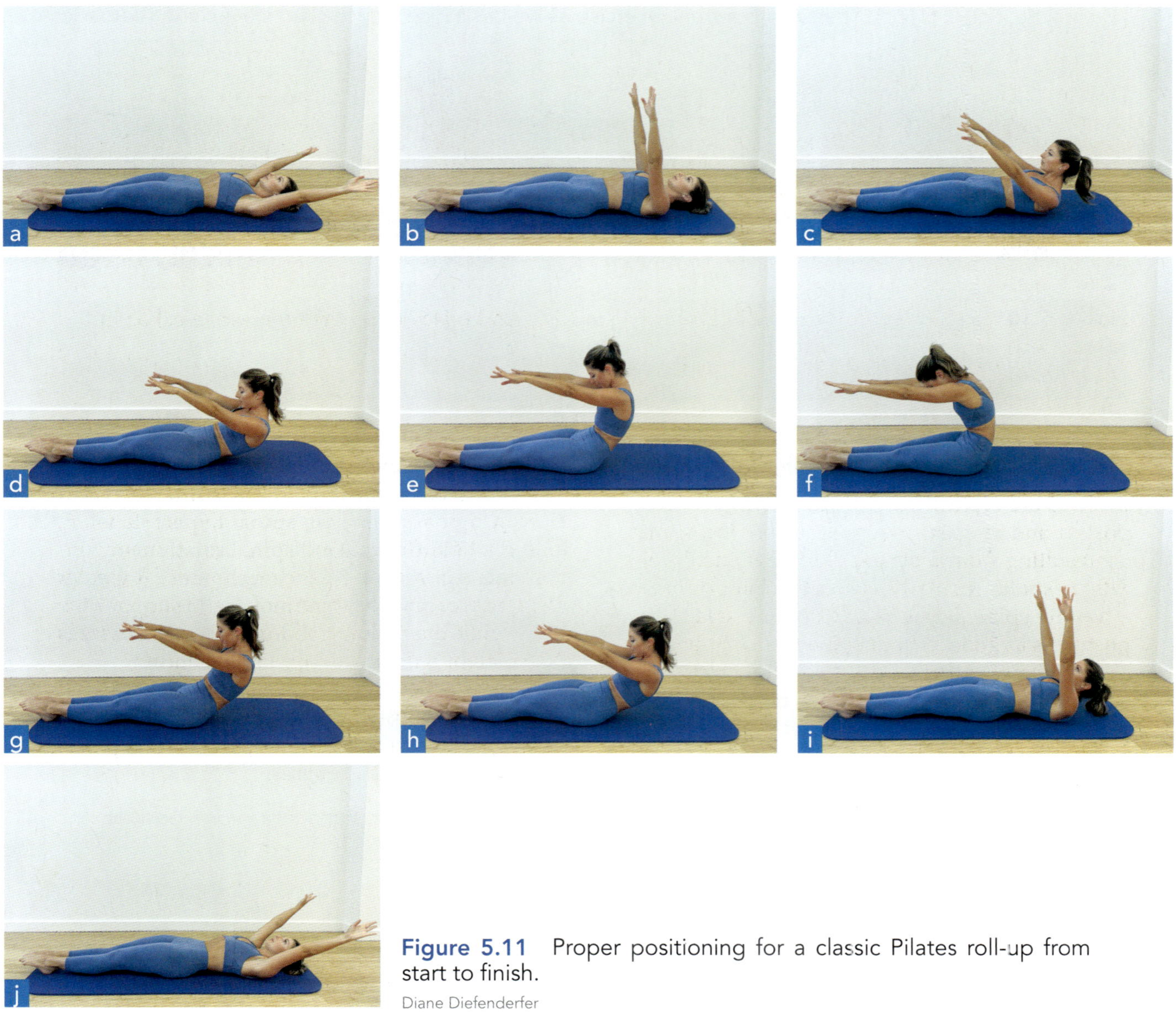

Figure 5.11 Proper positioning for a classic Pilates roll-up from start to finish.

Diane Diefenderfer

SWAN

This exercise involves spinal hyperextension from the **prone** position; the entire sequence is shown in figure 5.12.

1. Lie prone (on the front of the body) with your forehead on the mat and your neck properly aligned; the legs are outstretched and together, and the feet are pointed. Your elbows are bent, and the palms are down (goalpost position) (figure 5.12*a*).
2. Contract your scapular muscles to keep your scapulae depressed. While inhaling, engage your hamstrings, glutes, and abdominals to prepare.
3. While exhaling, lengthen your neck, lifting the head and upper chest carefully off the mat into a slightly arched position (figure 5.12*b*).
4. While inhaling, hold the position with a beautifully lifted sternum and shoulders pressed downward (figure 5.12*c*).
5. While exhaling, return completely to the starting position; be sure to pull the navel toward your spine to protect the back. Perform 4 or 5 reps, going into a deeper or higher arch or hyperextension each time (figure 5.12*d*). The swan is a trunk exercise as well as a nice way to practice arching the back.

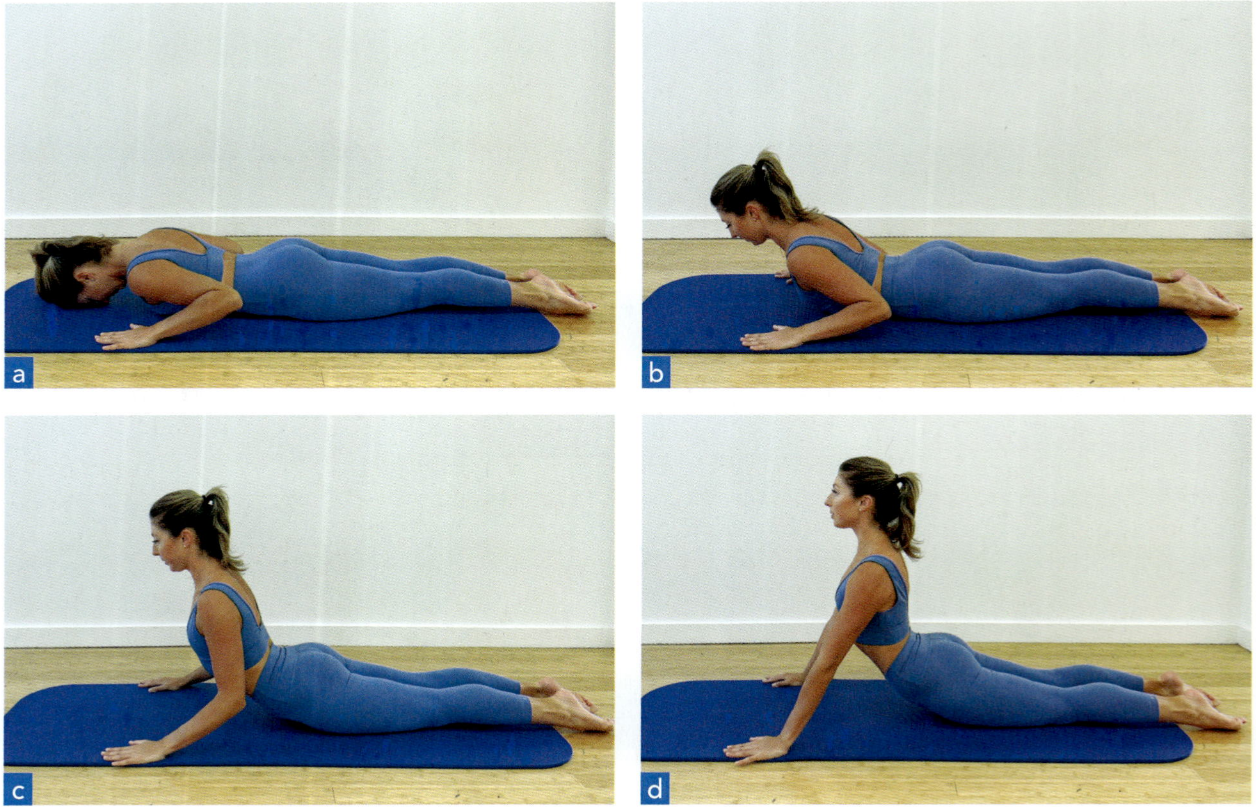

Figure 5.12 Proper positioning for a Pilates swan exercise. The dancer starts in a prone position and moves into spinal hyperextension.
Diane Diefenderfer

PELVIC PRESS

This exercise draws the spine and hips from flexion into extension in the supine position (figure 5.13). It is somewhat similar to a yoga bridge, but the low back does not hyperextend.

1. Lie supine with your knees bent, legs parallel, and feet hip-width apart.
2. Place your arms along your sides. Keeping your head and neck aligned, focus your gaze on the ceiling.
3. Inhale to prepare with a neutral pelvis. While exhaling, deeply contract the abdominals, then engage the TA, **pelvic floor**, glutes, and hamstrings to imprint the spine (figure 5.13*a*), then begin lifting the sacrum off the mat.
4. Continue to lift one vertebra at a time until your back is extended and the torso is supported on the upper shoulder area. The spine should not be hyperextended; imagine drawing a straight diagonal line through the shoulders, ribs, hips, and knees (figure 5.13*b*).
5. While inhaling, hold the position with your legs in proper alignment. Engage your inner thighs to maintain the parallel position of the legs.
6. While exhaling, gradually lower the spine back to the mat, again moving vertebra by vertebra, thinking of making an imprint on the mat as the spine completely returns to the supine position. Perform 4 to 5 reps. For an added challenge, place a block or medium-sized ball between the knees while performing the exercise.

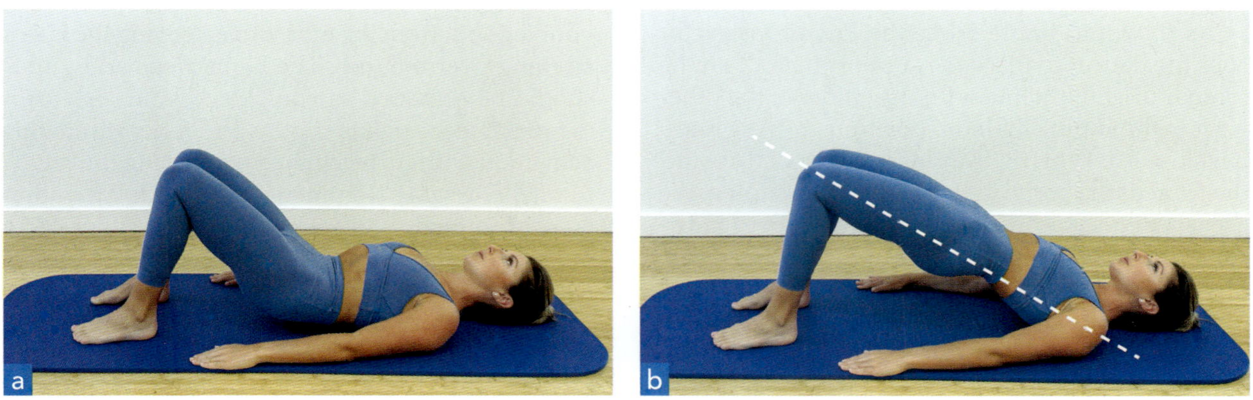

Figure 5.13 Pilates pelvic press: *(a)* After imprinting the spine, begin the exercise with a posterior pelvic tilt. *(b)* The pelvis moves upward, creating a diagonal line connecting the shoulders, ribs, hips, and knees.
Diane Diefenderfer

Alignment of the Foot, Ankle, Knee, and Hip

The majority of Pilates exercises (both on the mat and on various apparatus) are performed with the legs in parallel. Although leg turnout is emphasized mostly in classical ballet, dancers of all genres should be trained in the correct use of external rotation because forcing turnout increases the likelihood of injury. (Chapter 13 includes more specific information about turnout.)

The alignment of your legs must be consistent from the hip to the knee to the ankle to the foot; the cue *knees over toes* in turnout is a frequent correction from a good ballet teacher. However, with the demands of speed, gravity, and working in ever more tightly crossed positions (e.g., fifth position), correct alignment of the hip, knee, and foot is often lost. An excellent means to condition your body against injury is doing footwork exercises on the Pilates Universal Reformer in parallel positions.

As shown in figure 5.14*a*, the Pilates instructor cues the dancer to place the supporting foot on the footbar directly in line with the sit bone; the other leg is in the **supine tabletop position**, moving into a développé devant (figure 5.14*b* leg extended toward the front of the body; in this case, while supine, the leg is extended towards the ceiling). The **quadriceps** should be engaged without locking the knee. The hamstrings and **gluteals** (glutes) should also contract while alignment is maintained from the hip, through the knee, and down to the ankle and toes. To maintain a strong relevé (heel raise) without turning the foot into pronation or supination, the dancer also must engage the inner thigh on the supporting leg. Force on the **metatarsals** in the foot should be centered on the second and third toes. The hips must remain square without any twist or tuck, and the abdominals—as always—should be engaged to maintain the stable and neutral pelvis without tucking.

When moving into a turned-out first position (figure 5.15), dancers must understand the proper use of the **hip external rotators** as well as correct pelvic placement. Unfortunately, in the quest to engage the glutes, dancers often place the pelvis in **posterior tilt** (commonly called tucking under), where the top of the pelvis is tipped backward. To correct this position, maintain a neutral pelvis on the Universal Reformer by engaging the core muscles and drawing in your navel (figure 5.15*a*). Turn your legs out from the hips while keeping the knees tracking over the toes. The hamstrings and glutes should be activated as you extend your legs *without* tucking the pelvis (figure 5.15*b*). Continue this activation with correct placement during the return to plié. The same alignment and muscle activation is incorporated while standing at the ballet barre in first position (as well as in second, third, fourth, and fifth positions).

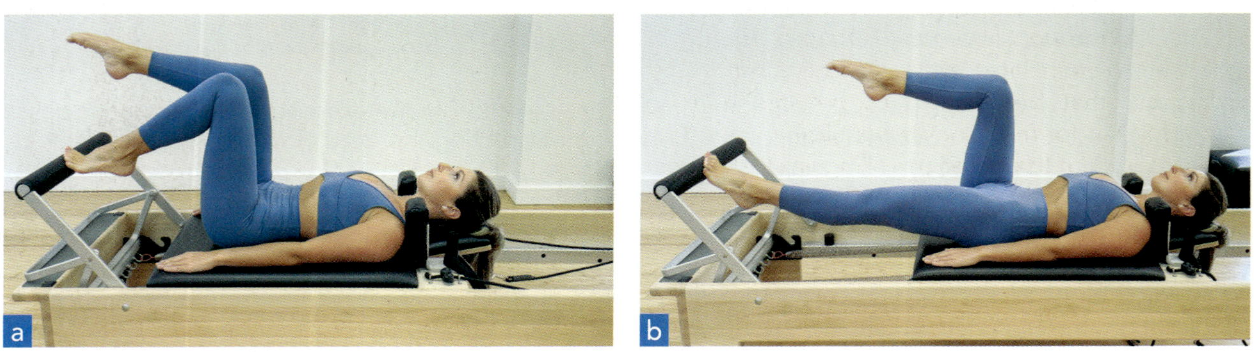

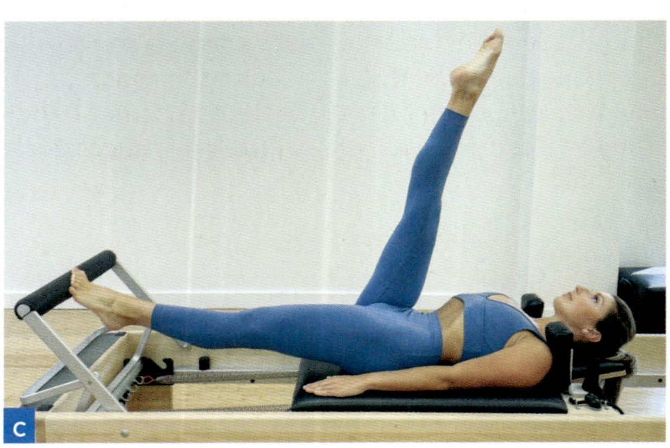

Figure 5.14 Proper positioning for single-leg footwork on the Pilates Universal Reformer.

Diane Diefenderfer

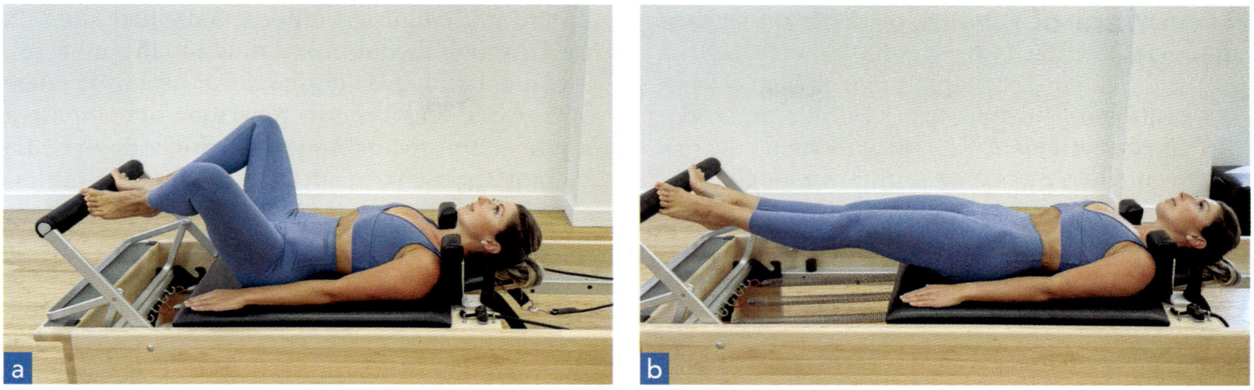

Figure 5.15 Proper use of the Pilates Universal Reformer when in turnout.
Diane Diefenderfer

Case Study: Diane Diefenderfer

I was introduced to the Pilates Method at the Ron Fletcher Studio for Body Contrology in Los Angeles while dancing with the Los Angeles Ballet Company. Fletcher had been a student of and teacher for Joe and Clara Pilates in New York City from the 1940s to 1960s, and his was the only Pilates studio outside of New York at the time. Various intimidating pieces of equipment and sounds of cadenced breathing greeted me as I entered the studio. There were a few clients diligently practicing, and I soon found myself lying on my back on a Reformer. My teacher asked me to breathe deeply as I began doing footwork in parallel positions. My first thoughts were *Why all the breath? Why am I doing pliés in parallel? I am a ballet dancer who works in turnout!*

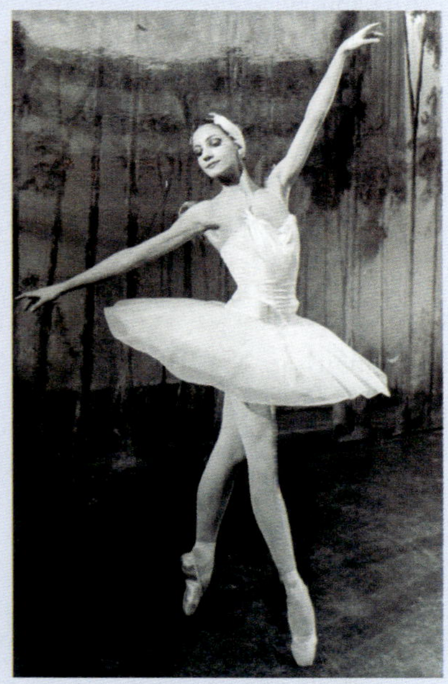

Diane Diefenderfer with the Frankfurt Ballet in *Swan Lake* (ca. 1977).
Diane Diefenderfer

I found the work interesting and challenging; however, it wasn't until a few years later, after surgical repair for a torn medial knee meniscus, that I began to truly appreciate what the Pilates program could mean for me. Conventional physical therapy was certainly necessary, but there was a missing link between the therapy clinic and getting back to company class and ballet performances. I was rather desperate and only too happy to get back on that Reformer and work in parallel. I was able to regain strength in my vastus medialis obliquus (an important part of the anterior thigh muscles) and correct the alignment in both of my long and bowed legs. I was also grateful to discover a keen sense of my deepest abdominal muscles and how so much movement is initiated from the core. Then and there, I became a convert.

I went on to enjoy a long and successful career as a ballet dancer, eventually retiring to teach both ballet and Pilates. More recently as a senior adult, I had a very successful total knee replacement (the knee I hadn't injured years earlier!), and I again credit my Pilates practice with a completely successful rehabilitation.

In its finest demonstration, the Pilates Method is an intelligent movement experience rather than simply another exercise program. When practiced correctly, Pilates enhances your kinesthetic awareness while maintaining a strong, flexible, and properly aligned body with the goal of reducing the risk of injury. When practicing with a combination of positive mental focus, stimulation of breath, and an energetic spirit, dancers are provided with the tools needed for their chosen form of artistic expression.

Myths About Conditioning for Dancers

A number of myths, fables, and partial truths are passed through the ranks of dancers. Teachers pass on what they heard from their teachers, and few people take time to verify whether these unsubstantiated claims are true. The result is that many dancers are hesitant to engage in some advantageous conditioning practices. This section identifies several of these myths to help you reassess the type of conditioning you have been doing or plan to do.

"Strength Training Will Bulk You Up or Mess Up Your Lines"

Strength training has long been a part of traditional training for athletes, including performing athletes (e.g., gymnasts and figure skaters) who are concerned with the aesthetics of their craft. Female dancers tend to be most affected by the myth that strength training will counter the aesthetic requirements of their art. However, they should not be misled into thinking that strength training will create bulky muscles (figure 5.16), lead to unattractive lines, or cause decreased range of motion. This type of muscular development requires an all-in commitment to very specific training regimens. In addition, some weight lifters and bodybuilders use substances (e.g., anabolic steroids) that assist muscle enlargement. If you are a dancer who has this concern, you are encouraged to turn your focus to the benefits of strength training, such as the improved physiology of muscle that reinforces the ability to resist fatigue, the increased bone density that reduces the risk of fractures, the mobilized joint movement that leads to maintaining range of motion, and the enhanced weight control that accompanies the metabolic increases resulting from strength training.

Farmer and Brouner (2021) conducted survey research that suggests variability in how professional dancers, student dancers, and dance teachers view strength training. According to their study (which was conducted in the United Kingdom), both professional dancers and students felt that strength training was more important than did the teachers. However, based on the teachers' answers, teachers did not seem averse to strength training. A wide variety of dance genres were represented in this study, but there was surprising agreement among the dancers, student dancers, and teachers that strength training is beneficial and that it is not an activity more appropriate for males than females or vice versa. Generally, males have more muscle mass than females; therefore, they can exert

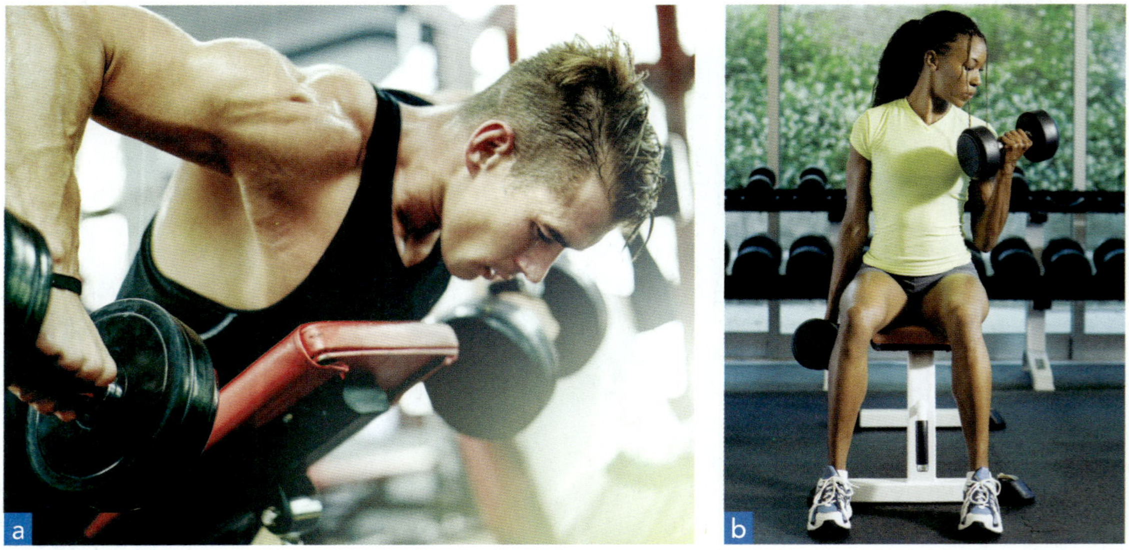

Figure 5.16 Dancers (especially females) need not worry that hypertrophy such as that seen in this male weight lifter *(a)* will occur in them *(b)*.

A: Mikolette/E+/Getty Images; B: Fuse/Corbis RF Stills/Getty Images more force with their muscles. However, when the quantity of muscle fibers producing contractile force is matched between males and females, any differences in strength disappear.

An increase in muscular tension and overload repetitively over time results in strength improvements. Strength development is achieved through a variety of factors that result in muscle hypertrophy, which is the muscle enlargement that many dancers fear. Some strength improvements, especially in the first portion of a strengthening program, are due to better neuromuscular function (the way that the nerves and muscles interact) and not hypertrophy. As noted earlier in this chapter, the type of exercise, circulating hormones, and nutritional intake are some variables that determine how the muscle develops. These variables can be manipulated to best suit any dancer and preserve their desired lines.

Basic differences in anabolic hormone levels in males versus females also contribute to muscle hypertrophy. Testosterone is 20 to 30 times higher in males compared to females (McArdle et al., 2023). Testosterone is known to increase the size and strength of muscle in response to resistance training. In contrast, estrogen (the female sex hormone) has no effect on the size of muscle in response to training (Romero-Moraleda et al., 2019). Strength gains in response to training can be similar in both males and females; however, the size of the muscles will differ, and females typically will not develop overly large muscles. For female dancers who prefer less muscle bulk, this news should be welcome, and it should help them to dismiss the myth that strength training will make them muscle bound.

Why Anabolic Steroids Work but Should Not Be Used

Anabolic steroids seem to be in the news regularly, usually around the time of the Summer Olympic Games but also in connection with elite amateur and professional sports. Olympic athletes, university athletes, professional athletes, and others have been barred from competition because they tested positive for banned substances, of which anabolic steroids are common.

Anabolism is the process of one's metabolism building up tissue. Anabolic steroids do work to increase muscle size—and therefore strength—because their molecules are based on the male hormone testosterone, the sex hormone that gives males several unique characteristics, including muscle enlargement. Females have a relatively small amount of testosterone, which is one reason they do not tend to develop muscle bulk.

Methandrostenolone, nandrolone, tetrahydrogestrinone, and boldenone are some common anabolic steroids. As seen in the molecular models of figure 5.17, the major portion of each anabolic steroid molecule is identical to testosterone. Slight differences give each anabolic steroid its identity. Some of these steroids have bona fide medical uses; others were designed specifically to try to increase sports performance while evading detection by governing authorities. Some are intended for veterinary use only. While using anabolic steroids may increase strength and muscle bulk, they also have substantial negative effects, including the following: cyst formation in the liver; weakened connective tissue; increased aggression; decreased testicular size and impotence in males; and facial hair, chest hair, deepening of the voice, hormonal changes, and clitoral enlargement in females (Kenney et al., 2022). All in all, any training benefits of anabolic steroids are not worth their risks. In addition, their use for nonprescription purposes is unethical and sometimes illegal.

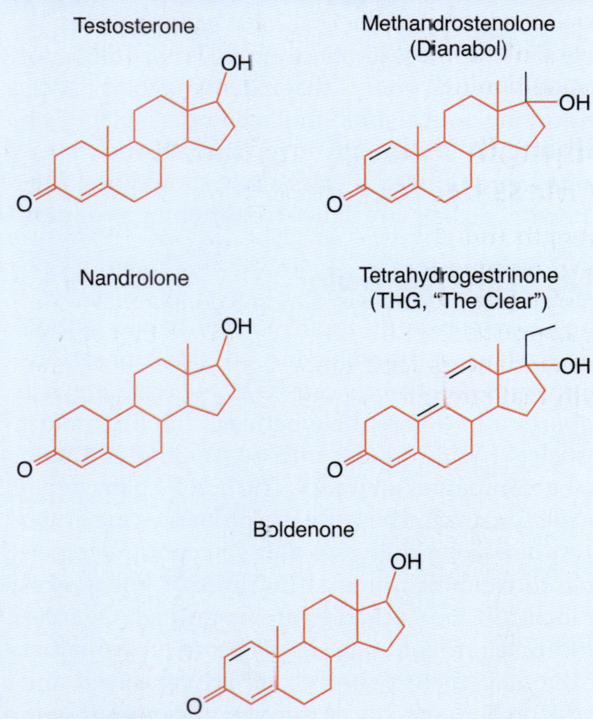

Figure 5.17 The molecular structure of the male sex hormone testosterone compared to the molecular structures of commonly misused and abused anabolic steroids show striking similarities. The identical portions of each molecule are marked in red.

"Dance Technique Training Is Sufficient for Aerobic and Anaerobic Development"

Most forms of dance consist of exercise that is usually short in duration yet high in intensity. The energy system necessary for improving and sustaining this type of exercise is primarily the anaerobic system. Training to improve anaerobic metabolism may be achieved in certain daily dance classes under conditions that include many brief periods of high-intensity effort. In contrast, the aerobic system provides energy as exercise progresses beyond a few minutes and over a sustained period.

In light of this information, dancers who perform continuously—or nearly so—in long pieces of choreography must specifically train their aerobic metabolism to sustain them through an entire performance. This process involves incorporating aerobic training into their overall conditioning program to help boost their aerobic capacity. Plus, as noted in chapter 4, aerobic training has a number of positive health benefits that extend beyond dance. Improving both aerobic and anaerobic metabolism (in addition to strength) over and above what is gained through dance class alone should be a fundamental goal of any dance conditioning program.

"No Pain, No Gain"

Those who choose the motto *No pain, no gain* as their approach to conditioning may be at risk for serious injury, especially injury caused by overtraining. It is important to differentiate between the discomfort associated with regular intense training and pain that accompanies an injury. The body's pain signal must be respected because it is protective in nature.

As a season progresses and you continue repetitive movements, preexisting muscle imbalances or incorrect biomechanics are magnified. Overuse syndromes are common simply based on the nature of the movement patterns that are rehearsed and performed repeatedly. Without sufficient rest, you may fall into an overtraining cycle that becomes evident toward the end stage of your performance schedule (Wyon & Koutedakis, 2013).

Symptoms of overtraining include a decrease in performance, increases in fatigue and irritability, elevated resting pulse, insomnia, continuously sore muscles, and frequent overuse injuries. If you begin experiencing any of these symptoms, you should initiate recovery strategies. Recommended methods to aid recovery include hydration, sleep, proper nutrition, massage or foam rolling, periodic ice treatments, and Epsom salt baths. The role of rest from dance activities cannot be overstated as an important facet of your overall wellness.

"A Double Latte and a Middle Split Is My Warm-Up"

Many dance classes incorporate some type of warm-up as part of the class. Indeed, a typical ballet barre warm-up has all the necessary elements to properly prepare your body to dance. However, in university dance classes, where time is often limited and dancers rush between classes during 10-minute breaks, it may fall to each dancer to perform their warm-up before their teacher begins teaching the class. For early morning classes, for classes during performance seasons, or for other especially busy times such as summer dance intensives, warm-ups (or even certain classes) are often neglected despite their essential role in dancer health and wellness. Thus, a quick stretch and a cup of coffee become the warm-up.

Without a proper warm-up, the body is at increased risk of injury because it has not been primed for the activity it is about to undertake. There are many physiological benefits of completing a warm-up before participating in any physical activity. These benefits include enhanced delivery of oxygen to working muscles, increased body temperature, increased suppleness of the soft tissues that leads to ease of movement, enhanced transmission speed of nerve impulses that improve physical performance, and preparation of the cardiovascular and muscular systems for activity (Asmussen et al., 1978). Dancers empowered with the knowledge of the benefits of an overall warm-up routine should recognize that these benefits are preferred over the risk of getting injured as a result of skipping a proper warm-up.

Conclusions and Practical Relevance

Overall, a healthy dancer is a happy dancer. A healthy lifestyle for a dancer is best viewed cyclically. As the year progresses from a rehearsal schedule to performance schedule, so should your training and recovery cycles. Embracing the ebbs and flows of conditioning and recovery processes will only lead you to tap deeper into your body's needs and abilities.

Initially, take an inventory of your current status in musculoskeletal strength, flexibility and mobility, and the physiological requirements of your specific style of dance. Then, devote the time necessary to equip yourself for dancing at an optimal level. Training goals should be set based on the trajectory necessary to travel from where you are to where you need to be to meet the demands of your class, rehearsal, and performance schedules. Arriving at your destination with a healthy body and the tools to sustain holistic wellness are achievable when you follow appropriate pathways of training and recovery. Recovery and rest are crucial to your effectiveness as you engage in conditioning that will take you to new heights of cardiovascular, strength, power, and muscular endurance output. In short, dancers achieve holistic wellness when they fully embrace their identity as a high-level performance athlete. As Joseph Pilates said, "Physical fitness is the first requisite of happiness" (Pilates & Miller, 1945, p. 3).

Discussion Questions

1. What forms of exercise can train the aerobic energy system, since dance class is not able to do so? How is aerobic exercise different from dance class in the way it conditions your body?
2. While hormonal considerations are important for both males and females, in what ways should female dancers cycle their training in sync with their monthly hormonal cycle?
3. Name three recovery practices that are necessary when bundling a strength and conditioning program.
4. Describe some strategies that dancers can use if they suspect they are having symptoms of overtraining.
5. Breath is a significant fundamental in the practice of the Pilates Method. How might an awareness of breath affect your work as a dancer? How does it affect you in class, rehearsal, performance, and other environments?
6. Reflect on what you have learned about abdominal activation and core control in this chapter. Compare and contrast any types of abdominal workouts or exercises you have previously experienced or currently practice. How might the information in the chapter about abdominal connectivity relate directly to you as a dancer? You may include specific dance movements or choreography.
7. Choose one of the Pilates exercises in the chapter. Following the prompts, practice it correctly for 1 week, then describe your experience. Include challenges, successes, difficulties and whether you feel the movement benefited your dance practice. If it did, continue!

WWW Go to HK*Propel* to access supplemental information and activities connected to chapter content.

6

Flexibility Training for Injury Reduction and Performance

Desiree A. Unsworth, PT, DPT
Merry Lynn Morris, PhD, MFA, LMT
Gary Galbraith, MFA

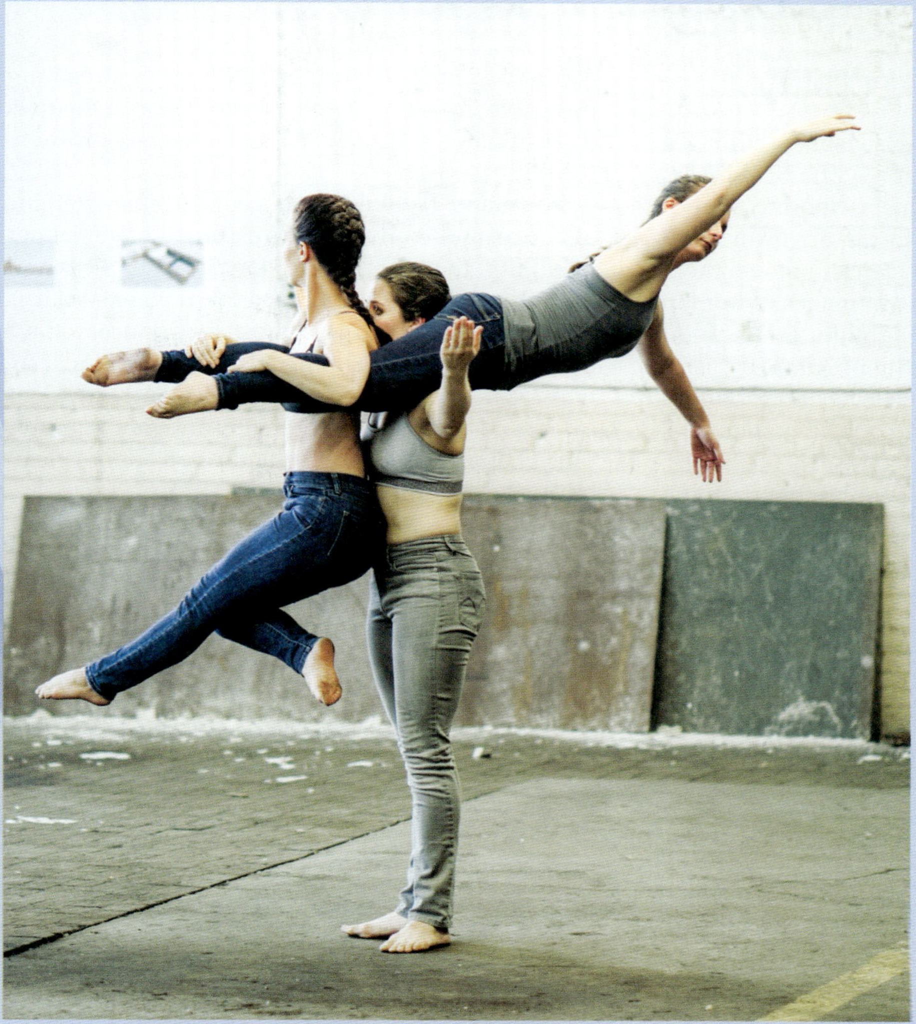

Inlet Dance Theatre, Cleveland, Ohio. *Easter Island Memories*, Choreographed by Bill Wade. Photo: Lauren Stonestreet, www.laurenstonestreetphoto.com; Dancers: Elizabeth Pollert, Emily Stonecipher, Nicole Kapantas.

People often assume that you are flexible because you are a dancer; however, that assumption may or may not be true. Several factors determine an individual's flexibility. In addition, different dance genres require different levels of flexibility, and each genre requires flexibility in different regions of the body. Learning how flexibility works and how it affects dancing will help you manage your flexibility as a component of your whole-dancer health and wellness.

Key Terms

agonist
antagonist
collagen
creep
elastic deformation
elasticity
extensibility
fascia
flexibility
Golgi tendon organs
hypermobility
laxity
mindfulness
motor neuron
muscle spindle
myotatic reflex
plastic deformation
proprioception
reciprocal inhibition
sensory neuron
stretch-shortening cycle
stretch tolerance
thixotropy
viscosity

LEARNING OBJECTIVES

After completing this chapter, you will be able to do the following:

- Describe the various factors that influence flexibility.
- Explain the role of reflexes on flexibility.
- Discuss specific measures that can reduce injury risk for dancers with hypermobility.
- Identify the potential benefits and applications of different types of stretching to support dance activity.
- Design a stretching protocol suitable for your dance specialty.

Introduction to Flexibility

Dance is a powerful moving and visual art. Images abound representing different types of dancers with their bodies arranged in fascinating shapes and actions. Advancements in the art form, pedagogy, training, and dance science and wellness have shaped dancers differently. Images of human bodies in extreme positions highlight the issue of flexibility and significantly influence dancers' aspirations (figure 6.1). While a high level of flexibility is perhaps helpful for completing certain maneuvers, it can also lead to overstressed joints. Nevertheless, social media are full of online sources that promote quick fixes, offer countless examples of stretching protocols (many of which are flawed) and theories of stretching, and advertise devices to promote flexibility.

For many, flexibility is a defining characteristic of dance, and many dancers aspire to have greater flexibility; therefore, understanding what it is and how it works is essential for the dancer. What is flexibility, and what does it mean for a dancer today? Is flexibility really that important for dancers; if so, why? What is involved in flexibility, and how does a dancer address this issue safely and intelligently? This chapter explores these questions about flexibility and other related topics.

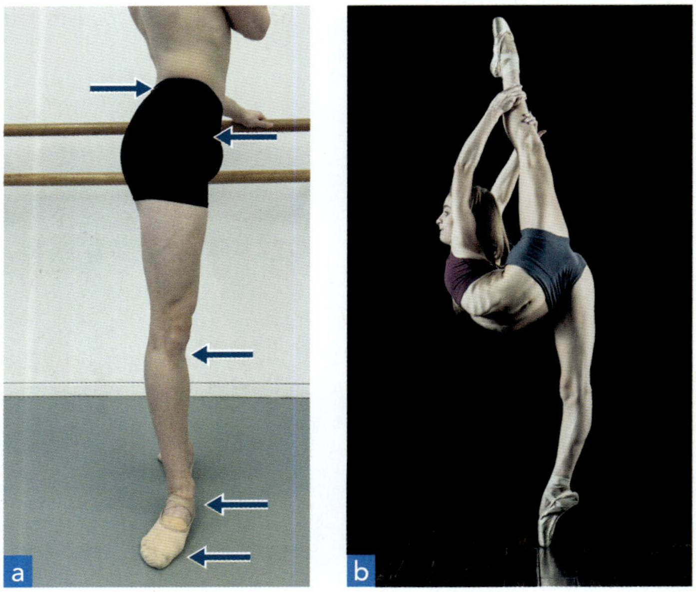

Figure 6.1 Examples of extreme flexibility: *(a)* Turnout well beyond even the usually ideal 180 degrees can create problems in the medial feet, medial ankle, medial knees, anterior hips, and lower back (indicated by the arrows). *(b)* The extent of trunk hyperextension, shoulder mobility, and hip mobility required for a dancer to attain this position is atypical. Forced overstretching in an attempt to achieve this is not recommended.

A: Carina Nasrallah. B: David Hofmann on Unsplash.

Flexibility and Range of Motion

According to the *Oxford English Dictionary*, *flexible* is simply defined as "capable of being bent, admitting of change in figure without breaking" (Oxford University Press, 2023). As simple as this definition may seem, Holt and colleagues (2008) reviewed the complexities of defining flexibility especially with regard to musculoskeletal considerations. Ultimately, they define flexibility as "the disposition of body tissues to allow, without injury, excursions at a joint or a set of joints" (p. 4). In the dance context, people often understand **flexibility** as the distance a body part is able to move, or its range of motion (ROM). However, ROM is the way people see and commonly assess flexibility, but ROM itself is not the same thing as flexibility. Flexibility is more of a qualitative measure, while ROM is a quantitative measure (figure 6.2).

ROM is often seen as how far the limb moves from its standard anatomical position. For example, a ballet dancer who can raise their leg up to shoulder height in a développé à la seconde (leg lifting to the side of the body) could be seen as having a large hip ROM. However, flexibility is just a part of this ability to achieve greater ranges of movement.

Dance and Flexibility

Not all dancers require the same kind of flexibility. The functional demands inherent in the style, form, technique, and culture of a dance form influence the type of flexibility that a dancer needs. For example, classical and contemporary forms differ from folk and ethnic dances and street dance forms. Therefore, the degree and type of flexibility required are unique for each form. In addition, there are so many different types of dancers, and they all have varying flexibility and body types. Simply put, there is no one-size-fits-all approach when it comes to flexibility in dance.

Strength and Flexibility

Discussions of flexibility must also encompass the role of strength. Strength is needed to effectively use ROM and to protect the body throughout the ROM. The distinction between active and passive ROM is important in relation to strength. Passive ROM is the range that can be acquired through the use of other body parts or support from other surfaces or devices; in other words, the target muscles are stretched by forces outside the body. Active ROM is the range that is acquired by contracting applicable muscle groups or when used in conjunction against gravity. For example, a dancer may have worked diligently on their splits to gain greater ROM in the hips and legs, but they may lack the strength to lift the leg upward against gravity or to adequately control the gesture leg, such as in a développé. Strength is also key for the support side of the body because it is where a majority of work actually happens.

In addition, a dancer with greater ROM may have difficulty controlling or protecting a body

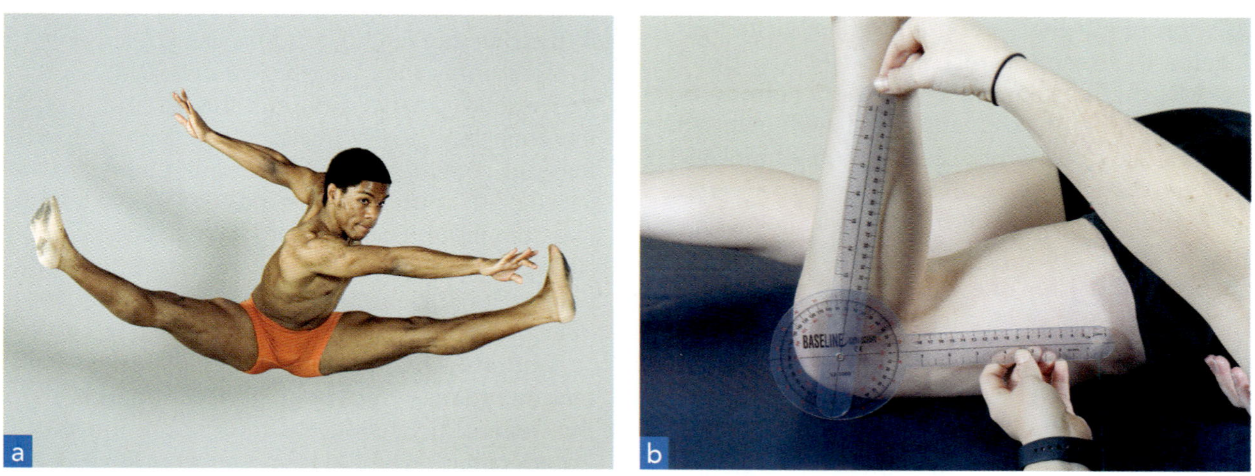

Figure 6.2 Flexibility versus ROM: *(a)* By qualitative observation, the dancer exhibits excellent flexibility in the hips and shoulders, among other joints. *(b)* The dancer's relative flexibility in the knee joint is determined quantitatively by measuring the joint's ROM. This quantitative measurement can then be compared to what is considered typical for the knee.

A: Peter Mueller

part during intense dynamic action or high speed. For example, a dancer without adequate strength performing a Graham technique pitch turn (in which the torso quickly flexes over the standing leg—or *pitches* forward) could incur injury to the hamstrings of the standing leg because of the force of the torso movement on the standing leg during the turn.

Psychology and Stretching

Increasing ROM is not only about mechanically stretching tissues; neurological, cognitive, and psychological factors are also involved. The mind is a part of the process because it helps regulate and assess the injury risk to the body during the stretching process. Given this mind–body connection, remember that the body is your partner and not something to be conquered. Psychological considerations do play an important role in the stretching process.

Effective stretching programs require a mindful approach. As defined in chapter 8, mindfulness is the practice of a nonjudgmental and moment-to-moment awareness toward one's experience (bodily feelings, emotions, thoughts, or activities). It involves actively listening to your body and your thoughts and then responding accordingly. Mindfulness itself is multifaceted, and self-talk may become a component of the process. Your own internal dialogue can hinder your efforts with negative thoughts, but you can also consciously direct your internal dialogue to promote a positive and productive experience. This topic is discussed in more detail in chapter 8.

Appropriate goal setting is an effective tool, and it helps to create a positive mindset for stretching. Measurable changes in muscle length do not happen overnight, so creating goals will help with the process. Goal setting must be done appropriately for each dancer to ensure that the objectives are reasonable; for example, different body types may have different results from stretching, so a reasonable goal for one dancer may not look the same as that for another dancer. Breathing is another important part of the process. Breathing can aid in self-awareness and help induce a restful, receptive state during stretching.

Mental imagery is another effective strategy. Imagery that directly supports the stretching intent is advisable. For example, seeing the relevant anatomy in your mind's eye while stretching may help target the right muscles. Imagery that evokes sensations of release, lengthening, and fluidity may also be useful. For some people, being able to visualize themselves with a greater ROM facilitates confidence and self-affirmation.

Tissues Involved in Flexibility

Various anatomical components contribute to flexibility. Flexibility is influenced by bony joint structure; length and **elasticity** of muscles, ligaments, and tendons; gliding of nerves; elasticity of blood vessels; and all the corresponding interrelated connective tissues, or **fascia**. This section explains how tendons, ligaments, muscular fascia, nerves, and blood vessels are involved in flexibility. All of these parts work in concert during movement.

Tendons

Tendons are composed of dense, fibrous connective tissue that connects muscle to bone. Unlike muscles, tendons are not composed of contractile proteins. A tendon's main role is to connect muscle to bone and transmit the contraction force of the muscle to the bone where the tendon attaches. When a muscle contracts, tension or stretch is placed on the tendon, which in turn applies force to a bone to produce movement around a joint.

The primary component of tendons is **collagen**, which also is plentiful in ligaments and muscle fascia. In addition, the collagen fibers of tendons are almost completely parallel, which gives them excellent strength along their length (figure 6.3). However, because of their high collagen composition and their structure, tendons possess notably less elasticity than muscles. While muscles can stretch up to 50 percent of their resting length, tendons can stretch only up to 4 percent of their length (Simmel, 2014).

There are many different shapes and sizes of tendons; they vary in thickness and length. Specific tendons may also vary in unique characteristics based on their utility in the body. Positional tendons (e.g., tibialis anterior tendon) have a stiffer composition, while energy-storing tendons (e.g., Achilles tendon) have a less stiff matrix that supports power in locomotion (Rumian et al., 2007).

Tendons contain sensory receptors called **Golgi tendon organs**, which help relay information about the degree of tension the muscle-tendon unit is experiencing. When extreme tension force occurs (through muscle contraction or tendon stretch), Golgi tendon organs respond by inhibiting contraction of the muscle, thereby causing muscular relaxation. This topic is discussed further in the section titled Spinal Cord Reflexes.

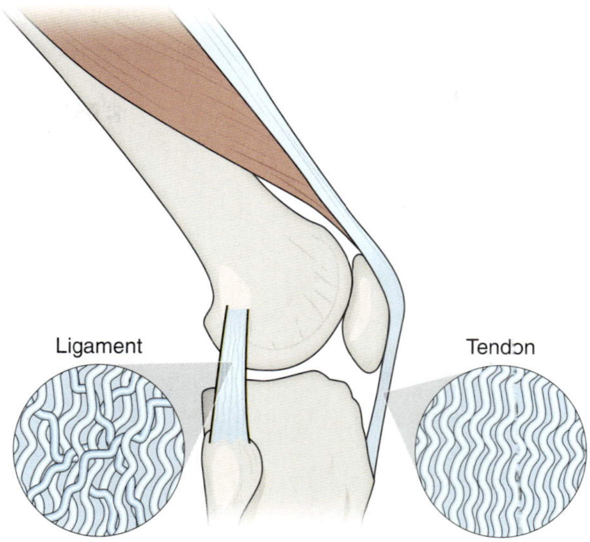

Figure 6.3 Collagen fiber arrangement of tendons and ligaments.

Ligaments

Ligaments consist of bands of fibrous connective tissue, and they usually connect bone to bone. Like tendons, the elasticity of ligaments is low while their strength is high because of the large number of nearly parallel collagen fibers they contain (figure 6.3) (Lis, de Castro, & Nordin, 2012). However, the collagen fibers are not as exclusively parallel as in tendons. While ligaments and tendons have similar composition at the molecular level, the proportion and arrangement of comparable components differ to support their unique roles. Both ligaments and tendons are designed to resist mechanical forces; however, ligaments play an essential role in restricting passive movements of joints and providing stability. Like tendons, they do not have contractile ability.

As in both muscles and tendons, ligaments contain sensory receptors that communicate information about movement to the nervous system. The sensory receptors in ligaments transmit data about joint position, thus permitting accuracy in coordination and balance. When ligaments are stretched too far, they may be permanently deformed and weakened, leading to structural instability of the joint they support. In turn, this instability can negatively impact effective coordination and balance. Generally, overstretching of ligaments (including during injury) can interrupt the proprioceptive signals that allow for accurate positioning of body segments. Thus, it is important that ligaments not be overstretched.

Muscular Fascia

Fascia (from a Latin root meaning "band" or "bandage") may be understood as a thin sheet or wrapping layer of connective tissue that encapsulates every organ, tissue, blood vessel, bone, nerve fiber, and muscle fiber as well as bundles of nerves and muscle fibers, entire nerves and muscles, and groups of muscles. It is a responsive, sensitive tissue monitored by nerves. While definitions vary, *fascia* is best described as a connective system that integrates all parts of the body, creating supportive, three-dimensional, threading relationships throughout. The interconnected fascial tissues enable the sliding and movement of muscles, nerves, and organs alongside one another. Stress may cause the tissues to tighten and become restrictive, creating pain and limited mobility.

The term *muscle fascia* describes the fascial layers around and between muscles. Amid the multiple layers of tissue is a lubricating liquid called hyaluronic acid; this substance facilitates the smooth sliding between fascial layers and enables fluid movement within the tissues. Injury, stress, disease, age, and other factors can cause the fascia to thicken and become sticky or adhesive, leading to rigidity and stiffness (Wilke, 2019). This response may result in restricted mobility and the development of painful, tender lumps or knots in the muscles (see sidebar titled Myofascial Pain Syndrome). Stretching and manual therapy can play a role in improving this condition.

Myofascial Pain Syndrome

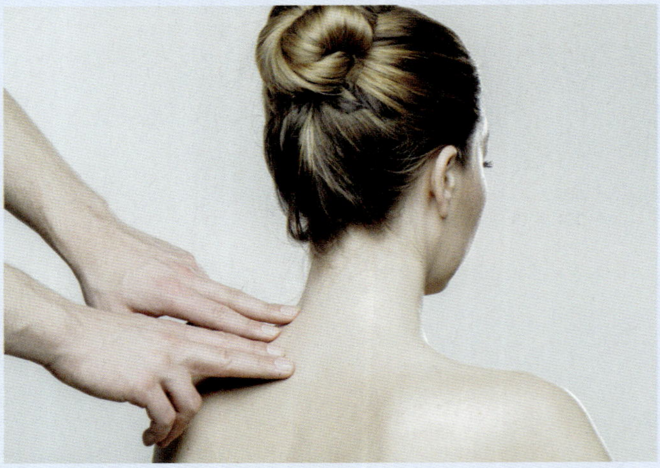

Figure 6.4 The trapezius muscle is an area that is susceptible to myofascial pain syndrome.
Angelo Esslinger via Pixabay

If you place your fingers on your trapezius muscle—the thick muscle that forms the weblike structure on both sides of your neck—and press into the muscle tissue, you are likely to feel some hard lumps, including some that are painful (figure 6.4). These lumps are areas of local hypersensitivity of the muscle called trigger points, and they represent locations of myofascial pain syndrome. These lumps can also elicit pain in other parts of the body (referred pain). The trapezius is one of the muscles most affected by this condition.

The root *my-* means "muscle," and *fasc-* means "fascia." Myofascial pain occurs when part of a muscle tightens into knots or balls of various sizes. It is called *myofascial* because both the muscle and the fascial layers that are woven through the muscle are involved. Often the result of holding an area of the body in one position for an extended period, myofascial pain (especially in the trapezius) is usually exacerbated by stress. Myofascial pain may also occur when a part of the body is injured and the muscles respond by tightening around the injured area. The best treatments for this syndrome are moist heat, gentle stretching, massage, and trigger point pressure, such as with your fingers, a foam roller, an avocado ball, a tennis ball, or another rounded implement. It is not necessarily a serious condition by itself. However, it can be quite annoying, and it may impede your dancing (depending on its location).

Each skeletal muscle is enclosed in a fascial sheath that surrounds the muscle belly and tendon as it connects to the bone. Elasticity of the fascial sheath determines the muscle's capacity for stretch. The fascial sheaths of individual muscles are linked to one another in a chainlike manner. In fact, you can think of the fascia as a network that connects muscles (and other tissues and organs) together all over the body. An understanding of these fascial chains provides insight into how the upper and lower limbs relate to one another functionally as well as how spiral and diagonal relationships manifest from one quadrant of the body to another. Research indicates that attention to the myofascial chains throughout the body can help in injury recovery. For instance, stretching the posterior lower limb muscles—the gastrocnemius and hamstrings—can increase the ROM of the cervical spine in both flexion and extension (Wilke et al., 2017).

Multiple layers of fascial wrappings can be identified in musculature; they include fascia profunda, epimysium, perimysium, and endomysium (figure 6.5*a* through 6.5*c*). All the connective tissue coverings merge to tendons, which attach the muscle to bone. These fascial tissues also help contribute pliability and tone to the muscles (Zugel, 2018). Keep in mind that the body's fascial layers are significantly interwoven, which sometimes creates difficulty in conclusively identifying them.

- *Fascia profunda* (deep fascia) creates a base for the other fascial layers, and it surrounds muscle groups. It is a thick, dense, fibrous tissue with less **extensibility** than other types. Its primary function is to support and protect muscles and soft tissue structures as well as to prevent the spread of infection by providing a barrier. Sensory receptors in the deep fascia allow for monitoring of pain, movement, pressure, vibration, temperature, and chemical status.
- *Epimysium* is made up of dense, irregular connective tissue sheaths that cover a whole muscle, including collagen fibers, as well as fat cells, capillaries, and nerve fibers. The epimysium separates muscles from other nearby tissues and organs.
- *Perimysium* is a connective tissue sheath that binds groups of muscle fibers into bundles or fascicles.
- Finally, *endomysium* is the innermost fine sheath of loose connective tissue that encircles individual muscle fibers.

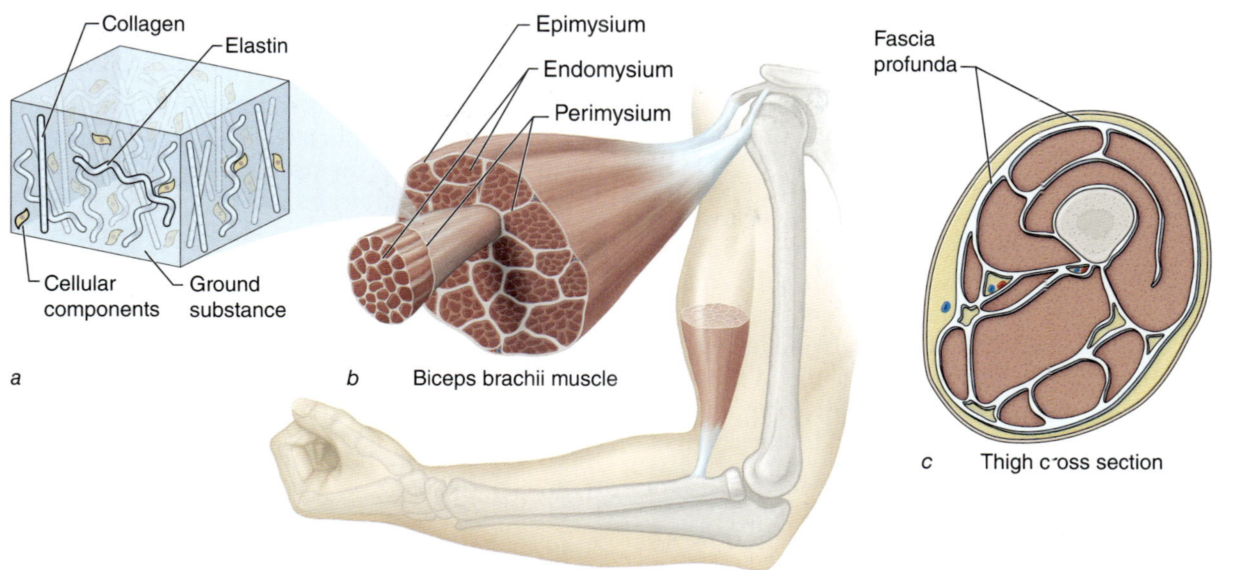

Figure 6.5 *(a)* Fascia is a tissue of high water content that is made up of intersecting and mobile tendrils, as seen under a microscope. *(b)* The three inner layers of muscle fascia—epimysium, perimysium, and endomysium. *(c)* Fascial layers are spread across and through the body, forming an interconnected matrix of support and contours. Fascia profunda is the layer that surrounds all of the muscles of the trunk and extremities while also connecting inward to the other layers.

WWW To visualize and understand these connective tissue layers, see the video in HK*Propel*.

Nerves

Nerves are the pathways by which the brain and body communicate, thus enabling dancers to perform a myriad of physically expressive movements. The nervous system essentially controls the body's movements, determines its level of flexibility, and registers pain. Although the underlying mechanism is yet to be determined, some evidence shows that increasing flexibility may not be due to decreased tissue stiffness but rather involves an analgesic (pain relieving) effect that increases **stretch tolerance** (Shrier & Gossal, 2000). Thus, awareness of pain and respect for your body's boundaries when stretching are paramount in reducing injury risk.

Unlike connective tissue and muscle, nerve cells (neurons) are not made of elastic components; therefore, they do not stretch. Instead, they tolerate tension by gliding within connective tissue and across joints or by slowly adapting to deformation over time. Improving the glide of a nerve around muscles, fascia, and joints may be an important contributor to a dancer's flexibility; however, the research literature examining the effects of neural mobilization on dance injury and performance is presently lacking.

Neural mobilization is a technique that uses manual therapy or exercises to decrease muscular and fascial adhesions surrounding a nerve to promote neural glide. Although the exact underlying mechanism of the effects of neural mobility has yet to be determined, research shows that neural mobilization techniques such as nerve glides, nerve flossing, and nerve tensioners can effectively increase ROM and flexibility in both pathological and healthy populations (Waldhelm et al., 2019).

WWW To explore nerve gliding, see the activity in HK*Propel*.

Blood Vessels

Blood vessels are conduits that carry blood throughout the body. They consist of arteries, arterioles, capillaries, venules, and veins. Because blood vessels are made up of connective tissue, they have the capacity to stretch. Specific blood vessel structure varies depending on its size and function, which also affects blood vessel elasticity. Larger arteries contain elastic connective tissue in their walls, smooth muscle, and an innermost layer of endothelium. This composition allows an artery to recoil between heartbeats to maintain blood pressure and flow. Veins, on the other hand, have little muscle in their walls. Moving blood through them requires assistance by the contraction of skeletal muscles that surround them and a series of one-way valves that close to prevent backflow. Capillaries are made up of a single cell layer of epithelial cells to allow for oxygen and carbon dioxide exchange in the body's organs and tissues. As blood vessels are deformed during a stretch, a cascade of events results in peripheral enlargement of the vessels and increased heart rate, which serve to maximize blood flow.

For dancers, maximizing blood flow is important for efficient nutrient and waste product exchange to support the energy demands of dance, to promote the healing of injured tissues, and to reduce the risk of overstretching. Increased blood flow to tissues being stretched results in increased tissue temperature, which can improve tissue elasticity and ROM. Thus, incorporating a warm-up (e.g., heating pad, warm shower, or dynamic exercise) before stretching may help to increase ROM and reduce risk of injury to the stretched tissue.

Biomechanical Properties of Tissues Impacting Flexibility

As a means to individualize their flexibility training for injury reduction and to enhance performance, dancers should understand the factors impacting tissue extensibility (i.e., stretch capacity). This section examines the biomechanical properties of tissues that influence flexibility, including elastic deformation, plastic deformation, viscoelasticity, and the parallel and series elastic components of muscle.

Elastic Deformation

In flexibility exercises, tissues deform (change their length) differently depending on the amount of tension force applied to them. The greater the stiffness of the tissue, the less extensible it will be because more force is required to deform it. With **elastic deformation**, when the stretching force is removed, the material returns to its original length (as is the case of a gently stretched rubber band that returns to its starting length when released). Elastic deformation does not depend on time; it will return to its original length no matter how long the stretch is held. If tissues were purely elastic, it would not be possible to have permanent gains in flexibility. To achieve permanent ROM gains, plastic (permanent) deformation must occur.

Plastic Deformation

After a tissue has reached its elastic limit, further stress will result in **plastic deformation**. Unlike with elastic deformation, not all of the length change will be recovered when the stretch is removed (as is the case for an overstretched rubber band that, when released, is longer than its starting length. If the tissue has additional tension force applied to it, its breaking point is reached (as is the case for a rubber band that breaks under excess stretch). If your goal is to have a lasting increase in flexibility, you must emphasize plastic deformation over elastic deformation (Clippinger, 2024); at the same time, you need to stay clear of the breaking point in order to reduce injury risk.

Viscoelasticity

All connective tissues exhibit viscoelasticity; in other words, they have properties of both elasticity and viscosity. **Viscosity** can be thought of as a tissue's resistance to deformation under an applied force. It is influenced by speed and duration of the applied stress as well as by temperature. For example, consider what happens to olive oil in a frying pan. When you pour the oil into the pan, it has a syruplike quality; it is viscous. However, once you heat the pan on the stove, the oil becomes loose and runny; its viscosity is now much lower than it was when the oil was cooler. Generally, the faster a stretching force is applied and the cooler the temperature, the higher the viscosity of a substance and the greater its stiffness. Thus, to maximize elongation during stretching, it is beneficial to apply a stretch gradually to warmed tissues over an extended duration.

Creep and Stress Relaxation

Creep is a phenomenon of viscoelastic substances. In the context of a stretch, creep occurs when a constant tension force is applied to a tissue. That tissue will first deform to a certain length, then it will continue to slowly lengthen over time as long as the application of force is maintained.

Stress relaxation is a related term; it is another phenomenon of viscoelastic substances. In the context of a stretch, stress relaxation happens when a tissue is stretched to a certain length and held. Over time, the force required to maintain that tissue length gradually decreases. The force required to maintain the tissue's length is reduced because creep occurs to slightly elongate the tissue.

Thixotropy

The term **thixotropy** comes from the Greek words *thixis* (meaning "stirring" or "shaking") and *trepo* (meaning "turning" or "changing"). It is a property of materials in which the viscosity of a substance decreases under an applied stress (Lakie & Campbell, 2019). An example is a lump of clay that becomes more pliable as you work it with your hands. Muscle and fascia have both been described as having thixotropic properties; in other words, stress (such as movement or pressure) temporarily reduces their stiffness, and conversely, their stiffness increases with time at rest. Thus, to improve tissue extensibility prior to stretching, it can be beneficial to use active movement (e.g., dynamic warm-up) or passive movement (e.g., massage) to temporarily reduce viscosity, which reduces stiffness.

Parallel and Series Elastic Components

A mechanical model consisting of three components explains the properties of muscle contraction as well as tendon and fascia elasticity. The active contractile component (contracting muscle) is discussed in chapter 4. The two passive components are the parallel elastic component (PEC) and the series elastic component (SEC). Keep in mind that in this context, the term *elastic* is a simplification of the viscoelastic properties of tissues for the purpose of understanding a complex system (Herzog, 2019).

Using springs as an idealized representation, PECs lie parallel to the muscle's contractile component while SECs lie in series (in the same line) with the muscle's contractile component (figure 6.6). These elastic components give rise to a muscle's property of elasticity. It has been suggested that the anatomical structures associated with the PEC include fascia, muscle cell membrane, and elastic proteins, while the SEC consists primarily of tendon (Clippinger, 2024).

When stretching a relaxed muscle, deformation occurs across both the PEC and SEC. In contrast, when a muscle is actively contracted, it can offload stress from the PEC while deforming the SEC. Such is the case during the **stretch-shortening cycle** (eccentric contraction of a muscle immediately followed by concentric contraction of that same muscle, such as in the quadriceps muscles when executing a jump), which contributes to greater force production than can be produced by a muscle's active contractile component alone. The SEC essentially acts like a spring that stores potential energy; it is released to become kinetic energy that is added to the kinetic energy supplied by the muscle contraction. The stretch-shortening cycle is the basis for plyometric exercises as well as most explosive, powerful movements in sports, dance, and other activities.

Spinal Cord Reflexes

Spinal cord reflexes are automatic responses to stimuli that do not necessarily involve the brain. These neural pathways form a framework for more complicated motor activity that is controlled by the brain, specifically, the motor cortex (Kandel et al., 2013). Having a fundamental framework of reflexes frees a dancer's motor cortex to plan complex sequences of movements. For example,

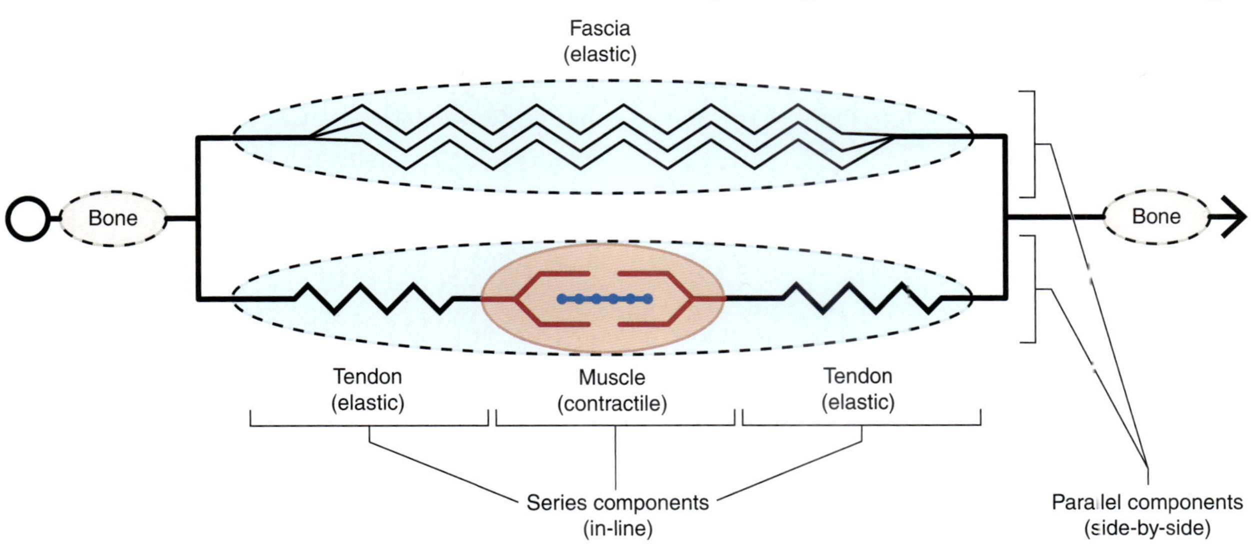

Figure 6.6 The contractile, series elastic, and parallel elastic components in a typical muscle-tendon complex.

the motor cortex may send a command to maintain one's posture, then rely on the myotatic reflex (see next section) through a negative feedback loop that makes adjustments to the posture as necessary.

Myotatic Reflex

The **myotatic reflex** (also called the stretch reflex) is a spinal cord reflex activated by rapid stretching of a muscle that causes a contraction of the stretching muscle to resist the muscle's lengthening (Knierim, 2020). This reflex involves a two-neuron pathway (figure 6.7*ab*). For example, when a pitcher of water is unexpectedly placed on a restaurant server's empty tray, sensory receptors called **muscle spindles** in the biceps brachii muscle of the upper arm sense a change of length in the muscle and send a signal via a **sensory neuron** to the spinal cord. There, the sensory neuron connects to a **motor neuron** that takes its signal to the biceps. This signal causes the biceps to contract so that the pitcher of water is supported and does not spill. Rapid stretching, which can be characteristic of ballistic stretching or bouncing into a stretch, may elicit the myotatic reflex and result in painful muscle spasms rather than allowing a muscle to relax (Fox, 2011).

The sensitivity of the stretch reflex is regulated by a system called the gamma efferent pathway. In this pathway, gamma motor neurons innervate muscle spindles, keeping them taut and thereby maintaining the spindles' sensitivity to changes in the muscle length. The net effect of this system is control of muscle tone and **proprioception**. Generally speaking, low muscle tone (hypotonia) contributes to increased flexibility, while high muscle tone (hypertonia) contributes to decreased flexibility.

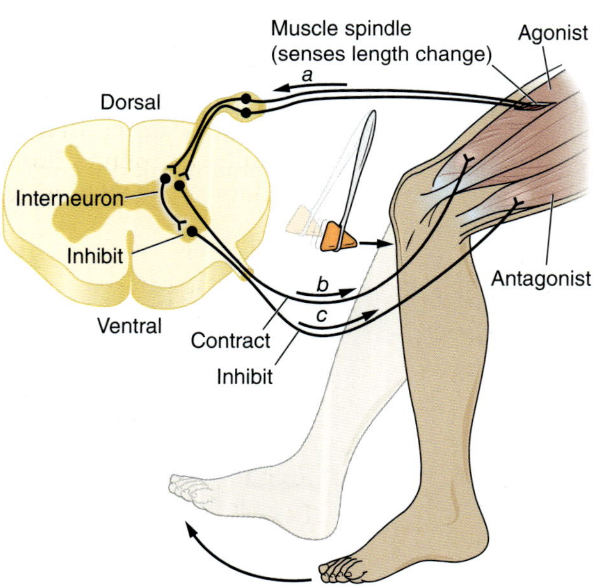

Figure 6.7 The myotatic (stretch) reflex arc showing the (*a*) sensory (afferent, or incoming) nerve input from the muscle spindle to the spinal cord and the (*b*) responding motor (efferent, or outgoing) nerve signals that cause the stretched muscle (agonist) to contract and the antagonist to relax (reciprocal inhibition).

Reciprocal Inhibition

Reciprocal inhibition occurs when muscles on one side of the joint relax to accommodate contraction on the other side of the joint, which is an integral part of the myotatic reflex. In the previous example of the waiter's tray, when the biceps brachii is suddenly stretched and the stretch reflex is activated, the opposing muscle group (the triceps brachii) must be inhibited so it does not counteract the contraction of the biceps. This inhibition occurs through a three-neuron pathway. The muscle spindles (a PEC) sense a change of length in the stretched biceps muscle and send a signal via a sensory neuron to an inhibitory interneuron in the spinal cord, which innervates a motor neuron that sends its signal to the triceps muscle. This efferent inhibitory action is also seen in figure 6.7*c*. Because the interneuron is inhibitory, it prevents the opposing motor neuron from firing, thereby reducing the contraction of the triceps. Without reciprocal inhibition, both the biceps and triceps in the example might contract simultaneously and work against each other. This organizational feature simplifies the control of voluntary movements; the central nervous system does not have to send separate commands to the opposing muscles. Reciprocal inhibition has been proposed as one of the theoretical physiological mechanisms behind proprioceptive neuromuscular facilitation (PNF) (Hindle et al., 2012) (discussed later in the chapter).

Inverse Myotatic Reflex

The inverse myotatic reflex (also called the inverse stretch reflex, autogenic inhibition, or Golgi tendon reflex) is a spinal cord reflex activated when tension is applied to a muscle-tendon unit. It causes the tensioned muscle to stop contracting. In other words, its action is inverse to (opposite) that of the myotatic reflex.

This reflex involves a three-neuron pathway. The sensory receptors involved in this reflex are located in the muscle-tendon unit; they are called Golgi tendon organs. Because the Golgi tendon organs are part of a SEC, they sense changes in muscle tension through muscle contraction or tendon stretch. They send a signal via a sensory neuron to the spinal cord, where it synapses with an inhibitory interneuron that then synapses with a motor neuron that carries its inhibitory signal to the muscle, thus keeping that muscle from contracting. In this way it is a protective reflex, creating what is known as autogenic (self-generated) inhibition. For example, if a heavy barbell exceeds the lifting capacity of the biceps brachii muscle, the excessive tension in the muscle-tendon unit may trigger the inverse myotatic reflex to inhibit the biceps, causing it to relax and the weight to fall to the ground. Autogenic inhibition also has been postulated as one of the physiological mechanisms behind proprioceptive neuromuscular facilitation (PNF) (Hindle et al., 2012).

Golgi tendon organs were first thought to have only a protective function, namely, keeping muscles from being injured by excessive amounts of tension (as in the previous example). However, research indicates that Golgi tendon organ receptors are not only activated at high tension levels, they also fire at low tension levels as in a static stretch when the stretched muscle relaxes after being held for a short period (15 to 60 seconds). Additionally, the Golgi tendon organ receptors provide the nervous system with precise information about the state of a muscle's contraction. This communication allows for very specific, fine-tuned movements (Kandel et al., 2013). Such complexity stems from the fact that the inhibitory interneuron also receives input from the cerebral cortex, muscle spindles, cutaneous (skin) receptors, and joint receptors. One theory is that this varied input allows the amount of work of a muscle's motor units to be spread out more evenly. If some muscle fibers are bearing more of the load than others, their Golgi tendon organs will be more active, which will inhibit the contraction of those fibers. As a result, less active muscle fibers will increase their contractions to "pick up the slack, thereby sharing the workload more efficiently" (Knierim, 2020, para. 8).

Hypermobility

In some forms of dance, abnormally large joint ranges of motion may be seen as advantageous, resulting in self-selection for that form of dance. Some research suggests as many as 44 percent of dance students are hypermobile (Day et al., 2011). **Hypermobility** can be defined as a larger than average ROM in a joint or joints (Blackmon & Faulkner, 2019). Hypermobility is best understood as a characteristic existing along a spectrum that may or may not be associated with symptoms and that depends on various factors, including genetics, age, sex, weight, and training. However, hypermobility, which can be inherited or acquired through training, can predispose a dancer to greater risk of pain and injury due to delayed tissue healing, decreased joint proprioception, and excessive joint **laxity** (Knight et al., 2012).

WWW To screen for joint hypermobility, see the activity in HK*Propel*.

Hypermobility in Pregnancy and Postpartum

Should a dancer become pregnant, increased levels of the hormone relaxin are associated with increased joint laxity. This increased flexibility is desirable to prepare the birth canal for delivery of the baby, but it can also contribute to increased stress to the dancer's ligaments and tendons (Manejias, 2020). Hormonal changes associated with raised estrogen levels mid-menstruation may also contribute to joint laxity in females (McCormack et al., 2004). Pregnant dancers should be cautioned against large jumps and overstretching, especially of the adductor muscles that attach at the pubic symphysis at the front of the pelvis; stretching these muscles during pregnancy may cause the pubic symphysis to separate. Supportive shoe wear is also recommended to reduce overstretching the ligaments of the foot and ankle due to naturally increasing body weight during pregnancy (Manejias, 2020). Musculoskeletal changes occur postpartum, as well, and adequate rest and gradual return to activity are needed to reduce risk of injury. Consulting a pelvic floor physical therapist can be helpful (Blackmon & Kirollos, 2020).

Hypermobility Implications for Dancers

While joint hypermobility can contribute to a dancer's flexibility—which might be aesthetically desirable in some dance forms—it also increases the potential for injury. Although joint hypermobility certainly is not a reason to abandon dance, greater care is required in a dancer's technical training to prevent excessive joint stress and reduce injury risk. Stability, strength, balance, and proprioception should be emphasized over flexibility, which already comes more naturally to dancers with hypermobile joints (Knight et al., 2012).

For example, using a compression sleeve or kinesiology tape over the back of a hyperextended knee might improve sensory input from joint proprioceptors and allow the dancer to decrease knee hyperextension. An external wrap, bandage, or tape also can act as an extra layer of connective tissue to provide further stability. Additionally, training at a slower pace may be necessary to ensure adequate strength gains and optimal movement patterns for hypermobile dancers who fatigue more quickly and heal more slowly. Adequate nutrition, rest, and recovery are essential, and seeking medical care from providers familiar with joint hypermobility will be beneficial.

WWW Go to HK*Propel* for more information about hypermobility, including hypermobility syndromes.

Types of Stretching

There are several types of stretching, and a few of them are discussed in this section. For any stretching effort to be effective, efficient, and safe, it must be done correctly. Anatomical knowledge, including basic understanding of muscles and connective tissues, is beneficial. A key part of this knowledge is knowing each muscle involved, how to target that muscle, and what part of the muscle is being stretched by a specific exercise. With any stretch, working the muscle toward its lengthened end range is important. Therefore, the two ends of the muscle (the origin and the insertion) must be moved away from each other.

For example, the origin of the three hamstring muscles is the ischial tuberosity of the pelvis (sit bone). The insertions (distal attachments) are below the knee on the tibia and fibula. Importantly, the hamstrings cross two joints—the hip and the knee; thus, these muscles are responsible for both hip extension and knee flexion. To acquire the best stretch, then, the opposite actions are required—hip flexion and knee extension.

Static Stretching

The two kinds of static stretching are passive and active. Passive static stretching requires the muscle to be extended to its maximum range and held for a short period using body weight, a partner, or an apparatus to achieve and hold that position. Take the muscle into the far end of its length, and gently push it a little farther to feel its tension (but not pain). A short hold period (15 to 60 seconds) will help the tissues to slowly adapt and increase their length without serious injury.

Active static stretching requires that the target muscle or group of muscles (considered the **antagonist** muscle) be placed in a stretched position by contraction of the **agonist** muscle or group. Thus, the force of the agonist is what stretches the antagonist on the other side of the joint. For example, contracting the lateral flexors of the cervical spine (agonist) would elicit a stretch in the lateral flexors on the opposite side of the neck (antagonist). A straight leg raise while supine on the floor would require contracting the hip flexors/quadriceps (agonist) while the hip extensors/hamstrings (antagonist) would be stretched. Static active stretches are harder to maintain than passive stretches, but they do promote mobility and strength through a joint's ROM.

Ballistic and Dynamic Stretching

Ballistic stretching entails using forceful bouncing movements of the body or limb to take the targeted muscle beyond its normal range. An example of a ballistic stretch would be a dancer trying to force their split by bouncing into and lengthening the muscle beyond its typical range. Although for some people it is a familiar or favorite type of stretching, a disadvantage is that ballistic stretching elicits the stretch reflex. Thus, it may not be the safest or most effective form of stretching to increase ROM.

Dynamic stretching is similar because it is a movement-based stretch, but it differs in that body segments are not pushed beyond their normal range and the movement does not involve bouncing. Dynamic stretching involves taking the targeted muscles through a full ROM; with each repetition there may be a small increase in range, but the goal is not to push significantly beyond the maximum range. This type of stretch is best to help with increasing your dynamic ROM, and it is an effective preparticipation warm-up activity. Often dynamic stretching activities are controlled or low-intensity versions of those that are part of sports or dance.

Proprioceptive Neuromuscular Facilitation (PNF) Stretching

PNF is a technique or sequence of actions used to create a stretch. It makes use of multiple approaches. Although it can be done alone, it is most effective when executed with a partner. At the heart of the PNF stretch is an isometric muscle contraction followed by a release or relaxation, which is done in specified sequences.

A basic sequence is contract–relax PNF stretching. In this form, the targeted muscle engages in an isometric contraction, which is held for a short period, then the muscle relaxes into a static (passive) stretch. A partner can help hold the body in position while in the isometric portion of the maneuver and then add assistance during the passive static stretch segment (figure 6.8).

Another sequence is contract–relax–contract PNF stretching. It is almost the same as the previous example, but the passive static stretch is replaced by an active static stretch when the dancer doing the exercise contracts the antagonist muscles to assist the stretch. For example, in the hamstring stretch performed in figure 6.8, the dancer would contract the hip flexors to assist the movement of the leg toward the torso, thus adding additional force to the stretch.

Stretching for Warm-Up and Cool-Down

Stretching is an important part of a preparticipation activity (warm-up). When addressing stretching before classes, rehearsals, or performances, consider the following guidelines.

In general, stretching before an activity should focus on increasing heart rate and body temperature while reacquiring dynamic or functional flexibility. Sitting on the floor with the legs in second position emphasizes static stretching, and it does not promote a rise in body temperature; therefore, it is not an adequate way to prepare for activity. Static stretching requires warm body tissues to elicit an effect; your cooler tissues prior to dancing are not conducive to increasing their length via static stretches. Dynamic stretching raises your body temperature and promotes blood flow so that ROM can increase to the extent required for dancing.

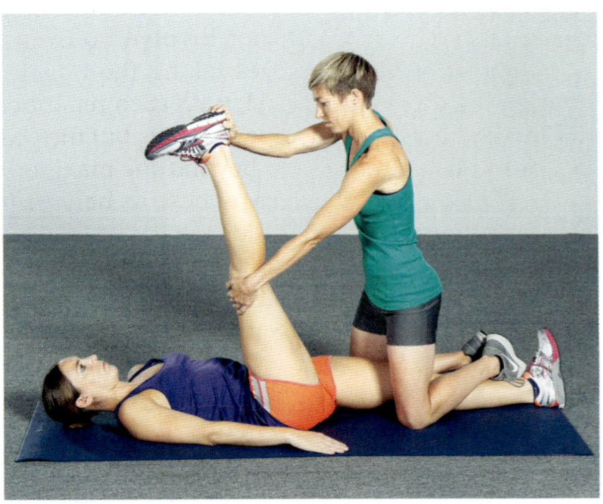

Figure 6.8 A partner assisting during contract–relax PNF stretching. The assistant provides resistance to isometric contraction of the hamstrings of the person who is stretching. After the isometric contraction is released, the assistant gently pushes the leg toward the person's torso, thus stretching the hamstrings.

When stretching before any kind of activity with the intention of increasing tissue length, it is important to be careful. Conflicting research results exist with regard to the impact of static stretching on strength and power output, but the general consensus is that long-duration static stretching may negatively affect high-performance activities such as dance, at least acutely (Kozai & Surgenor, 2017; Lima et al., 2019). Stretches designed to lengthen muscle and fascia should be done after activity during the cool-down period. At that time, the body is already warm with ample blood flow to allow effective elongation of muscles, fascia, and other tissues. Also, the muscles will have enough time to recover after stretching before any kind of power or strength output is required of them again.

Another important consideration—regardless of when you stretch in relation to activity—is balanced stretching. Even though a joint on one side of the body may have greater ROM than the same joint on the other side, a stretching program should work both sides evenly. Also, muscles on either side of a joint should be balanced. For example, any attention given to hamstring flexibility should also be directed at the quadriceps and hip flexors. Finally, appropriate strengthening is also important for optimum support of the joints. Chapter 5 will help you construct an appropriate strengthening program.

Risks of Stretching

Performing a stretch for a long duration (more than 60 seconds), overstretching joints (extremist stretching), and warm-ups that rely solely on sustained static stretching in preparation for dance activity are unhelpful applications of stretching that may decrease peak performance and increase injury risk. A review of the research literature on stretching reveals a consensus for these issues. Lima and colleagues (2016) showed that both static and ballistic stretching decreased hamstring strength immediately after stretching. They recommended that these particular types of stretching not be performed prior to activities requiring strength application. Less clearly understood is whether or in what ways flexibility is associated with a reduction in injury risk or, conversely, whether or how it increases injury risk.

Flexibility and Injury Risk

While stretching can increase ROM at joints (due to increased tissue length), there is conflicting scientific evidence indicating that stretching or flexibility prevents injury or reduces injury risk (specifically static, PNF, and ballistic stretching). You are encouraged to explore the research literature yourself using the tools described in chapter 3 so you can assess the strengths and weaknesses in the various research methodologies and rationales (e.g., Lauersen et al., 2014; Small et al., 2008; Holt et al., 2008; Woods et al., 2007; Wyon, 2010).

Stretching protocols are regularly applied in clinical practice for rehabilitation during injury recovery, and they possess a variety of potential benefits. Research demonstrates that acute stretching can increase blood flow, resulting in improved endothelial (blood vessel cell lining) function, reduced arterial blood vessel stiffness, and lower blood pressure (Kruse & Scheuermann, 2017; Shinno et al., 2017; Hotta et al., 2018).

Stretching can also decrease muscle pain and alleviate muscle tension. Intentional stretching where positions are held for a sustained period (e.g., static) is broadly used within most dance and other athletic practices, often in both warm-up and cool-down phases. In ballet technique classes, some form of static or active static stretching is frequently employed during barre work before working in the center. Keep in mind that most dance technique classes inherently involve dynamic stretching within the design of exercises or combinations (e.g., ballet—cambrés (bending of the torso forward, side, back, or in a circular motion); jazz—isolations; modern—spinal roll-down; Graham—turns around the back).

To the extent that stretching increases joint ROM, it is reasonable to assume a benefit for physical preparation in dance, where specific joints need adequate ROM according to the dance style or form practiced. As introduced earlier in the chapter many different types of stretching exist; therefore, stretches should be strategically chosen for maximum benefit based on each dancer, the dance style or form, and the associated goals.

Extremist Stretching

Hypermobility of joints (whether genetic or induced by extreme stretching regimens) can compromise the integrity of joints, potentially creating instability and joint degeneration (Simmel, 2014). Practices in which the arch of the foot is forced into extreme plantar flexion by placing a weight or structure on top of the foot should be avoided. Similarly, practices in which turnout (external rotation) of the legs at the hip joint is forced to or beyond 180 degrees places strain along the kinetic chain from the lower back to the feet. Ankle and knee injuries and weaknesses can result from this type of forced turnout. As mentioned previously, forcing joints into extreme stretched positions repetitively can compromise the integrity of the joint structure, creating ligament laxity and joint instability, reduced proprioception, and decreased muscular power. For long-term health and a sustainable career, dancers should build optimum strength and stability, taking considerable care to moderate the degree of stretching of joints.

Methods for Flexibility Training

The core temperature of the body should be raised before any type of sustained stretching occurs. When you stretch, push only to the point where you feel muscle tension and a mild sense of pull or elongation. If you experience sharp or stabbing pains or spasms, you may be damaging your tissues. Overstretching can create strains or sprains. Aches, soreness, bruising, swelling, and muscle spasms indicate overstretching.

Four stretch parameters have been identified as potentially influencing the increase or decrease of flexibility of a joint: intensity, duration, frequency, and stretch position (Apostolopoulos et al., 2015). *Intensity* relates to the magnitude of the force being applied, *duration* is how long the stretch is held, *frequency* is how often the stretch is performed, and *stretch position* is how the body is positioned during the stretch.

Stretch duration recommendations range from 15 to 60 seconds, and the intensity of a static stretch is estimated at 8 out of 10 (with 10 being the highest intensity). This recommendation is just under the level where the muscle begins to twitch. The twitching usually indicates that the autogenic inhibition reflex is protecting the muscle from tissue damage. At this level, you should not feel pain when stretching, although you may feel moderate discomfort (Wyon, 2010).

The American College of Sports Medicine (ACSM) advises stretching regularly with an intensity of stretching to the point of feeling tightness or slight discomfort (Liguori & ACSM, 2020). While they are general, these guidelines may be applied to a dance-specific environment. The duration should be two to four repetitions (reps) of 15 to 60 seconds each. Efforts to change long-term length of muscle-tendon-fascia units (rather than a focus on maintaining active ROM with dynamic stretching) should be carefully evaluated. Adequate time for tissues to heal requires a frequency that includes rest periods between stretching sessions; therefore, two or three stretching sessions per week may be best.

An alternative to the more moderate- or high-intensity stretching discussed above is low-intensity stretching. Termed *microstretching*, this strategy encourages the application of a stretch at approximately 30 to 40 percent of maximal perceived force for a 60-second duration (or an intensity of 3 out of 10, with 10 being the most intense). The rationale is that this type of low-intensity stretch performed regularly (even daily) enables fuller relaxation of the muscle without stimulating the stretch reflex or creating undue trauma such as might be experienced in high-intensity stretching. In this type of stretch, you should not feel pain or discomfort (Apostolopoulos, 2010).

Stretch position is not a well-researched topic. However, it is important to consider how your positioning affects muscle line of pull as well as to what extent your position is conducive to maximal relaxation of the joint and muscle being targeted. For instance, consider that a hamstring stretch would be more effectively achieved in a supine position versus a standing position; when standing, the hamstrings are less relaxed because they are devoted to maintaining balance. Likewise, to stretch the hip flexors, you might experiment with lying on your back on an elevated surface (e.g., a table) and pulling one knee to your chest; the other leg extends off the end of table and relaxes, allowing gravity to assist stretch of the hip flexors in the extended leg (figure 6.9). This method is preferable to performing a lunge-type stretch in which the hip flexors must contract to help maintain balance. In general, consider whether you can relax your full body and mind during a stretch. If the stretch position chosen is quite difficult or awkward to hold, relaxation may be difficult and inhibit the effectiveness of the stretch, especially when more lengthening or plasticity of the tissue is desirable.

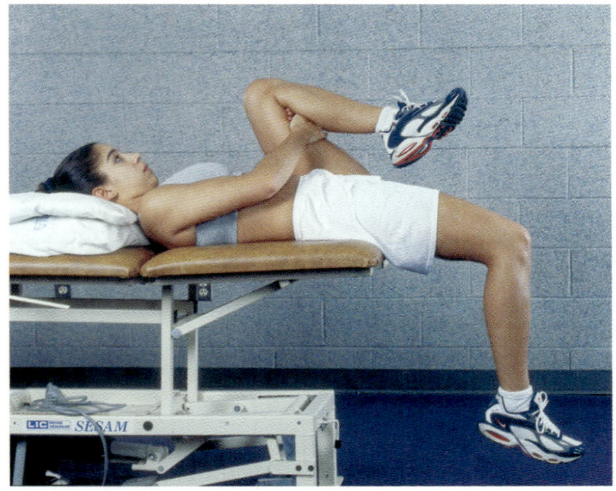

Figure 6.9 A hip flexor stretch in the limb hanging off the table. This position allows the hip flexors to fully relax.

A simple method to evaluate possibly overlooked areas that need stretching is to analyze which joint positions are frequently held or used in a partial range in your dance practice and which joints move through a full ROM during your activity. For example, in a ballet technique class, most of the class is spent with hip joints outwardly (externally) rotated; the external rotators of the hip are essentially in perpetual contraction. Therefore, it is likely that the hip external rotators will need to be stretched while the inward (internal) rotators will need strengthening. Similarly, when the arms are held in second position with the elbows lifted, the shoulder joints' abductors and rotators are in a constant isometric contraction. In other words, the abductors and internal and external rotators of the shoulder joints all must be stretched (as well as strengthened through their full range). In short, muscles that experience repetitive use in an isolated range during your regular dance practice should receive flexibility training through their full excursion.

An effective stretch positions a joint in a way that allows a muscle or muscle group to be elongated. For example, stretching the external rotators of the hip requires that the hip be positioned in internal rotation. If you want to target the lateral hamstring (biceps femoris) rather than the medial hamstrings in a stretch, you should assume a position that isolates the lateral hamstring. The biceps femoris externally rotates, extends, and abducts the hip while also flexing the knee; therefore, a position or action of internal rotation, flexion, and adduction of the hip with the knee extended would stretch the biceps femoris. On the other hand, the medial hamstrings (semitendinosus and semimembranosus) internally rotate, extend, and adduct the hip, while also flexing the knee; therefore, a position or action of external rotation, flexion, and abduction of the hip with the knee extended would stretch the medial hamstrings. Note that when a muscle acts on two joints, such as the hamstrings that cross the hip and knee joints, a maximal stretch will be accomplished only when you take into account the positions of both joints in relation to the muscle's line of pull (e.g., extending the knee while the hip is flexed). Be mindful that not all muscles and associated fascial tissues have the same type of sensory responsiveness or composition; therefore, you may need to perform some stretches longer than others for maximal benefit. Moreover, this responsiveness can also vary between individuals.

In addition to paying attention to how you use your joints and muscles in your dance experiences, be intentional about noticing the ways you hold your body in your nondance activities throughout the day. Notice your postures and positions; what ranges of motion are missing from your daily habitual activities? Constant computer work and phone use, including texting, can create muscular imbalances throughout the spine. Carrying a purse, backpack, or dance bag on one shoulder consistently can also create postural deviances and core muscle imbalances. Sleeping positions, sitting postures, and standing postures can all contribute to your overall biomechanical patterns and challenge your dance practice.

In closing, be aware of times when it is not advisable to stretch. Circumstances that preclude stretching include significant soft tissue injury, joint instability, reduced or impaired joint receptor and pain sensations (including reduced pain from analgesic medication), certain types of fractures, presence of surgical supportive devices such as plates and screws, genetic conditions causing excess soft tissue laxity, mornings right after waking up, painful conditions triggered by stretching, and other conditions noted as contraindications by a health professional (Holt et al., 2008).

Warm-Up Practices

During the warm-up phase, when you are preparing your body for dance activity, dynamic stretching and light stretching (with holds under 15 sec) are recommended. Static stretching (with holds more than 15 sec) is not advised due to the potential negative impact to force, power, and strength (Kozai & Surgenor, 2017). When blood flow increases and the core temperature of the body has been raised, tissues become more pliable. Your specific movement choices for a warm-up should be relevant to the activity you intend to do. If you are warming up for a specific type of choreography with significant upper-body weight-bearing demands, your warm-up would be different than if you were preparing for a traditional ballet or tap class or preparing to perform Indian classical dance, such as bharata natyam. In general, any warm-up should include segments of gentle pulse raising, joint mobilization, and muscle lengthening (dynamic stretching) as well as mental preparation (Kozai & Surgenor, 2017).

Pulse raising involves movements to increase heart rate, such as prances, light jogging, burpees, jumping jacks, or cycling. These movements should be done until the heart rate increases (1-5 min). During this period, focus on large, full-body movements, and gently mobilize all the joints of the body. You may include arm circles, hip circles, ankle circles, and spinal motions (flexion, extension, lateral flexion in both directions, rotation in both directions). For the muscle-lengthening phase of a warm-up, the focus should be on dynamic stretching. Joints should be taken through their full ROM in a continuous, gradual manner from full flexion to full extension. Dynamic stretching helps maintain an elevated core body temperature while enabling dynamic flexibility and stimulating the contracting muscles.

Incorporate proprioceptive exercises into your warm-up, such as balancing on one leg while circling the other leg around in a controlled manner (moving the gesture leg front, side, back; and vice versa), or try using a balance board. Also, try standing on one leg and closing your eyes. Shift your weight from one leg to the other with your eyes closed to challenge your proprioceptive receptors. You can also try it while taking the torso off its vertical axis (right or left lateral flexion) and through weight shifts with the upper body.

Incorporating a tactile warm-up at the beginning of your general warm-up is a complementary method to help stimulate blood flow and body connectivity. Try tapping lightly on the muscles you want to warm up, squeeze or press them, then slide a hand across them (e.g., imagine spreading oil or lotion; start at the upper chest and slide one hand down the opposite upper arm, forearm, and hand). Tapping can have a stimulating effect; while pressing, squeezing, and sliding may be more calming. The warmth and pressure of your hands aid in manually warming up the tissues. If some places in your body feel disconnected, a tactile warm-up may help the body feel more integrated by facilitating neural awareness through touch.

Be careful not to overstretch muscles involved in joint and postural stability as it may contribute to joint instability (Wyon, 2010). Dancers with joint hypermobility and existing joint instability should be particularly careful in their warm-up and in all of their stretching choices.

Postactivity Practices

In general, sustained, static stretching is appropriate after a dance class. Immediately following vigorous activity, the proprioception system may not be as acutely attuned to sensing your body's limitations as it is before activity; therefore, waiting until the body readjusts closer to its baseline may help you avoid exceeding these individual limitations. This area of research is controversial (Wyon, 2010); evidence is inconclusive, therefore more research is necessary.

You might consider initially doing fast stretching, where joints are taken through their full ROM but held for only 5 or 6 seconds at their endpoints (Wyon, 2010). Pay attention to what parts of your body feel most tense or restricted, and consider targeting those areas. If you did a repetitive motion during class or rehearsal that required the muscles of a joint to engage in excessive holding or isometric contraction within a restricted range (e.g., sustained relevé, continual hip turnout, or an overhead lift), be sure to address the opposite actions of that joint, moving the joint through its full dynamic range with gentle lengthening.

External Tools to Enhance Flexibility

Other methods for stretching the muscles and connective tissues involve using external tools such as balls, foam rollers, heat, vibration, and touch or manual pressure (Behara & Jacobson, 2017; Fagnani et al., 2006; Osawa & Oguma, 2013; Sands et al., 2006; Škarabot et al., 2015; Weerapong et al., 2005; Monteiro et al., 2018; Capobianco et al., 2019). Research indicates that heat applications can be effective in assisting the extensibility of muscles (Petrofsky et al., 2013). Heat tends to increase tissue elasticity through a relaxation effect on collagen fibers, vasodilation, pain relief, reduction of muscle tone and spasticity, increased cellular metabolism, decreased joint stiffness, and promotion of hyperemia (a transient increase in blood flow) (Eby & Alfano, 2012). For optimal benefit, 10- to 15-minute heat applications are recommended.

Manual massage (by a massage therapist or other professional, or self-administered) can also serve to create pliability in the tissues (recall the concept of thixotropy from earlier in the chapter). Foam rollers and balls are external massage tools that have similar effects due to the pressure the instruments apply on the muscle tissues. Vibration may likewise cause a relaxation effect in the muscles and facilitate muscle lengthening. Dancers may want to incorporate these tools in conjunction with their stretching regimen.

Conclusions and Practical Relevance

This chapter addressed flexibility. In dance, it is called the quality of suppleness in movement through effective joint range of motion (ROM). Flexibility goals should be tailored to dancers' specific individual needs and the dance form they practice. Anatomical components influencing flexibility include bony structure, tendons, ligaments, muscle fascia, nerves, and blood vessels. Proprioceptive and reflex mechanisms within tissues regulate and impact flexibility neurologically. Other influential factors include age, sex, genetic disposition, and pregnancy.

Different types of stretching used to support flexibility include static (active and passive), ballistic, dynamic, and proprioceptive neuromuscular facilitation (PNF); all have varying benefits and goals. In your stretch protocols, you should consider intensity, frequency, duration, and position as well as the vital role of mindfulness. Tools that may support stretching goals include foam rollers, balls, heat, vibration, and touch or manual pressure. Extreme stretching is not advised for long-term career sustainability, and overstretching can disrupt proprioceptive integrity of joints, thus increasing injury risk. Generally, dynamic stretching is helpful prior to dance activity, and more sustained stretching is appropriate after a dance session. You should seek a balance of stability and mobility by incorporating effective stretching with strengthening techniques to support your long-term health and reduce injury risk.

Discussion Questions

1. Using your understanding of the biomechanical properties of tissues, explain why a dancer might feel more flexible after repeated stretching and why that same dancer might feel stiff again after a rest period.
2. In preparation for dance activity (warm-up phase), what type of stretching is most advisable? Why? Using the ideas presented in the chapter, design a short warm-up for yourself.
3. In your own words, distinguish between each type of stretching introduced in the chapter. Try each of these types on your own or with a partner, and compare your experiences.
4. Explain how overstretching can be detrimental for a dancer. Incorporate the anatomical information presented in the chapter.
5. What role does muscle fascia play in stretch capacity? What factors can increase and decrease the stiffness of fascia? How can an understanding of myofascial chains inform your movement practice and/or approach to stretching?
6. Experiment with an external tool, such as a foam roller, ball, heating source, or manual pressure, to address an area of tightness in your body. Describe your experience, and reflect on the qualitative differences before and after using the tool.

WWW Go to HK*Propel* to access supplemental information and activities connected to chapter content.

7

Nutrition, Hydration, Rest, and Recovery

Ann F. Brown, PhD, CISSN, FIADMS
Meghan A. Brown, PhD, FHEA, SENR
Jasmine D. Challis, RD, MRes

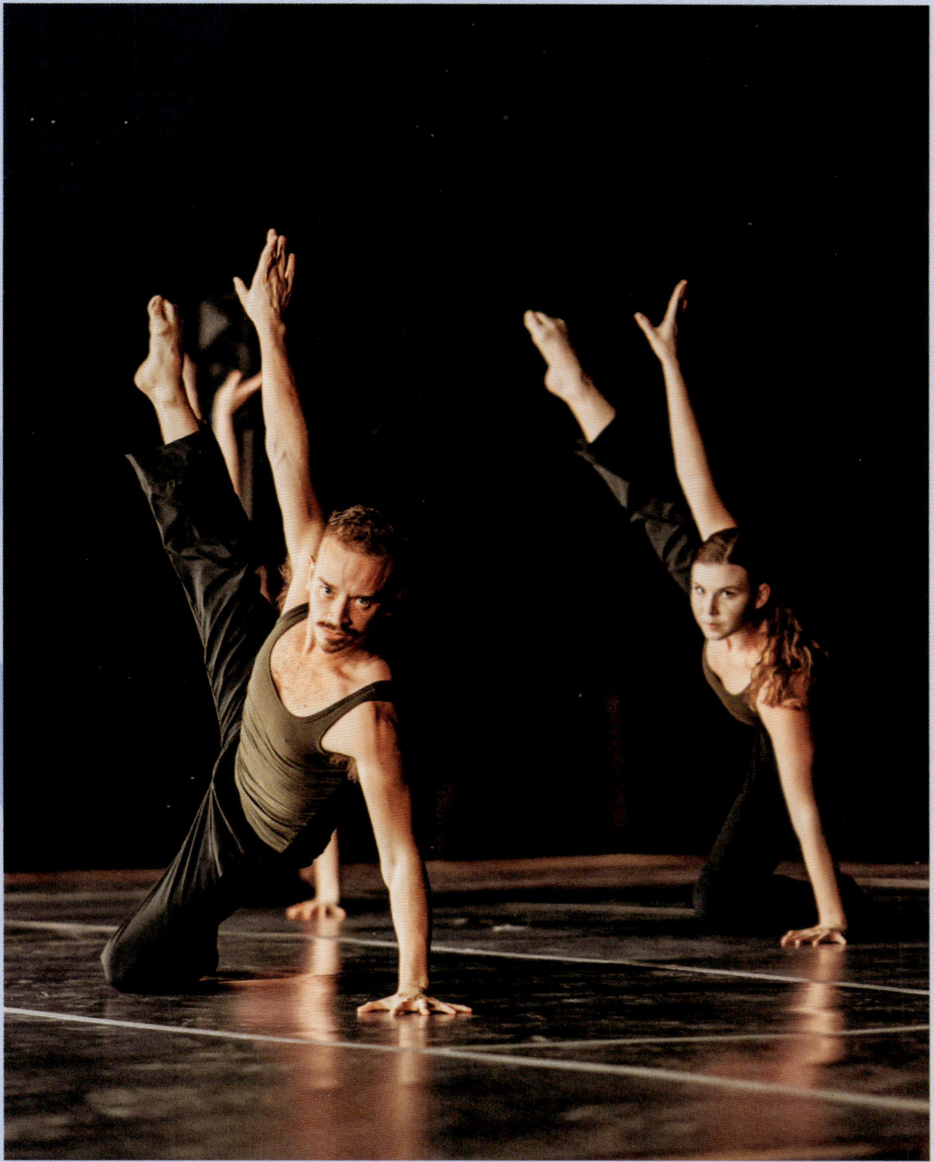

Ad Deum Dance Company, Houston, Texas. *No More Monsters,* choreographed by Steve Rooks. Courtesy Randall Flinn, Artistic Director. Dancers: Dylan Allen, Rachel Chouinard.

Few topics are as broad ranging and impactful on health—but so poorly understood—as nutrition and hydration. If you are like most people, you need help navigating the myriad of nutritional information and resources that are available. With some guidance, you can obtain the information necessary to be an excellent dancer who runs on fuel that enhances—rather than inhibits—your performance, rest, and recovery.

Key Terms

antioxidant
basal metabolic rate
carbohydrate
energy availability
fat
fat-free mass
fiber
glycemic index (GI)
hypertonic
hypotonic
isotonic
macronutrients
micronutrients
net protein balance
phytonutrients
polyphenol
postprandial
protein
relative energy deficiency in sport (REDs)
resting metabolic rate
tryptophan

LEARNING OBJECTIVES

After completing this chapter, you will be able to do the following:

- Describe the role of each macronutrient and selected micronutrients to dancer well-being and injury risk reduction.
- Discuss differences in nutrient requirements based on the goals of a dancer, timing during the day, and timing during a dancer's "season."
- Adjust fluid intake to avoid injuries linked to dehydration.
- Outline health conditions and lifestyle choices that influence nutrition requirements.
- Explain the current nutrition recommendations associated with injury risk reduction.
- Discuss the role of sleep, rest, and recovery in supporting dancers' well-being.

Sound evidence shows that diet and nutritional status can influence sport and exercise injury risk and recovery (Close et al., 2019). However, nutrition advice related to injury is often neglected in dance populations. This fact is surprising and concerning given the prevalence of injury (Ramkumar et al., 2016) and suboptimal nutrition intakes (Challis et al., 2020) in dancers. When dancers understand nutrition recommendations, they are better able to improve their nutritional choices. This chapter addresses the gap in information and guidance for dancers, encouraging optimal strategies relating to nutrition, hydration, rest, and recovery to minimize injury risk and support recovery.

Relationship of Proper Nutrition to Whole-Person Wellness

Dancers are artistic athletes; to perform at their best, they need the nutrients (fuel) to support dance training, performance, and recovery. While the human body is designed to cope as well as possible with less-than-optimal food or fluid, when the amounts, types, and timing of the nutrients obtained from the food and fluid you consume are not enough for the workload undertaken, your risk of injury increases and your recovery process is delayed (Academy of Nutrition and Dietetics et al., 2016).

Dancers are at risk of food insecurity. The term *food insecurity* has been defined by the Food and Agriculture Organization of the United Nations (FAO) as "the state of being without reliable access to a sufficient quantity of affordable, nutritious food" (FAO et al., 2022). Dancers who are not able to access adequate food will not be able to train and perform at their best. Dancers who are unable to afford adequate food are advised to explore all possible options for support. Where genuine financial hardship exists, many educational establishments offer funds and food banks, and they also may be able to offer suggestions for other potential remedies. For professionals experiencing food insecurity, seeking advice from support organizations is an initial step toward finding ways to meet nutritional needs.

The foods you consume provide energy, nutrients, and substances to sustain metabolism and activity, create and maintain muscle strength and stamina for dance, and enable the body to repair itself and to mount the best possible defense against disease. The immune system mounts this defense when infections arise, whether they stem from bacteria, viruses, or other causes (e.g., yeast or molds).

A diet consisting of few types of foods is less likely to be adequate for the dancer's wellness than a varied diet. Moreover, a diet that relies on highly processed foods is less likely to be nutrient rich than a diet that includes minimally processed foods. For example, a chicken or tofu and mixed vegetable stir-fry served with brown rice provides a better range of essential nutrients than a meal consisting of a chicken burger with a lettuce garnish served with fries. A varied diet that is rich in plant-based foods and contains sufficient nutrients to meet all nutritional requirements, adequate hydration, and enough rest to allow the body to recover from the impact of dance training and performance will give you the best chance of minimizing both illness and risk of injury. Although getting suboptimal nutrition and rest increases your risk of impaired wellness, evidence suggests that dancers do not meet their nutritional requirements (Challis et al., 2020).

Nutrigenomics and Individualized Nutrition

The term *nutrigenomics* is defined as the relationship between nutrients, diet, and gene expression (Chadwick, 2004). It is a fast-moving field exploring how genes respond to the influence of nutrition. For example, a person may be genetically more prone to insulin resistance, which can impact energy levels and concentration. However, their food choices can minimize their risk of insulin resistance and its consequences.

Individualized nutrition plans recognize that while people are broadly similar, differences such as variations in your genes mean that you will benefit from adopting advice to take account of your individual requirements. For instance, because iron absorption has a genetic component, you may be at higher or lower risk of iron deficiency than your peers (Camaschella, 2019). Genetic nutrition tests are currently not accurate enough to give individual diet advice, so you should approach them with caution and consult with a dietitian who will take genetics and other factors into account when advising you.

Food and Society

Human beings are social animals; therefore, prolonged isolation compromises your well-being. Food is your fuel, but it also has a social role. Thus, meals eaten with others not only provide nutrition but also allow time for essential rest. Dancers are familiar with the concept of combining rest times with taking in fluid and food; however, when schedules are less hectic, breaks are not just for nutrition and hydration. Every dancer has different preferences for food, whether in minor ways (e.g., taste for seasoning) or major ways (e.g., being vegetarian or vegan, having a food allergy). These areas are explored later in this chapter.

Given that food has both a physiological and an emotional effect on people, perhaps it is not surprising that so many people (often those with no nutrition training at all) are passionate—but variably accurate—about the information they disseminate through social media. You should always check the source of any information you obtain on social media. (See chapter 3 for tips on how to approach resources to gain information you desire.) Globally, there are many reputable dietitians and nutritionists who promote evidence-based dance nutrition strategies and advice—in person and via social media or other virtual means—and who also are experienced in working with dancers.

Macronutrients

Macronutrients are needed in large amounts (measured in grams) to supply energy daily; the main macronutrients are **carbohydrate**, **protein**, and **fat**. Energy from food is measured in kilocalories (kcal, which is commonly called a calorie in reference to food) or kilojoules (kJ). Alcohol is a macronutrient, but it is unhelpful as a source of energy for dancers. Carbohydrate and protein both provide approximately 4 kcal of energy per gram, alcohol provides approximately 7 kcal of energy per gram, and fat provides approximately 9 kcal per gram. To dance with minimal risk of injury or illness, energy intake must match energy output. Clear evidence from work on **relative energy deficiency in sport (REDs)** (Mountjoy et al., 2023) shows that not meeting nutritional requirements has a significant number of health consequences. Overconsuming macronutrients is only helpful for the underweight dancer needing to restore body fat and muscle to healthy levels. Figure 7.1 provides an overview of the components of energy balance, and table 7.1 shows how to estimate energy requirements by estimating total daily energy expenditure (TDEE). Prediction equations for resting metabolic rate (RMR), arguably the most convenient way to estimate basal metabolic rate (BMR) (Jagim, 2018), use information about an individual to predict BMR (e.g., age, stature, and body mass). Table 7.1 provides information about one such equation.

Carbohydrates

Carbohydrate is a compound of carbon, hydrogen, and oxygen; the three main types of carbohydrate are sugars, starches, and fiber. They can be metabolized aerobically (with oxygen) and anaerobically (without oxygen), which means they can be used to produce energy when exercise intensity is high. Carbohydrate recommendations are based on body weight and exercise intensity; they will vary day to day according to your workload, but will be included in every meal.

Glycogen is the human storage form of carbohydrate; it is stored in the liver and muscles. These stores are limited, so low-carbohydrate diets are not advocated for the dancer. Details about the optimal amounts of carbohydrate for dancers are provided in the section "Nutritional Considerations for Dance"; these amounts vary by duration and intensity of workload. In general, most dancers need between 200 and 500 grams of carbohydrate per day.

Fiber is the term for the parts of food not digested in the small intestine. Some of it will pass through

Table 7.1 **Estimating Total Daily Energy Expenditure (TDEE) to Estimate Energy Requirements**

Component of TDEE	Description	Sample estimation of TDEE (energy requirements)
Basal metabolic rate (BMR) ~60% of TDEE	Aside from laboratory or equipment-based methods (e.g., direct or indirect calorimetry [the analysis of heat production and gas exchange] and heart rate monitoring), BMR is most commonly estimated using prediction equations such as the Harris-Benedict equation (Harris & Benedict, 1918).*	This case study involves a female dancer who is 25 years old. She weighs 132 lbs (60 kg), and she is 5.6 ft (170 cm) tall. She has a typical rehearsal day that includes a few hours of activity. Her predicted BMR using the Harris-Benedict equation would be • BMR = (9.5634 × weight in kg) + (1.8496 × height in cm) − (4.6756 × age in years) + 655.0955 • BMR = (9.5634 × 60) + (1.8496 × 170) − (4.6756 × 25) + 655.0955 • BMR = 573.804 + 314.432 − 116.89 + 655.0955 • BMR = 1,426 kcal To account for physical activity, BMR is typically multiplied by an appropriate PAL. Her estimated TDEE would be TDEE = BMR × PAL TDEE = 1,426 kcal × 1.75 TDEE = 2,496 kcal Therefore, her energy requirement is ~2,500 kcal on this day.
Physical activity (exercise and nonexercise) ~30% of TDEE	Aside from laboratory and equipment-based methods, arbitrary physical activity levels (PALs) can be assigned to express a person's daily activity in this way: 1.2 = very inactive, sedentary, or immobile 1.5 = nondance or rest day 1.75 = training or rehearsal day 2.0 = performance day	
Thermic effect of food/dietary-induced thermogenesis ~10% of TDEE	Thermic effect is the energy for food digestion, absorption, and metabolism; it depends on diet composition because it varies for different macronutrients. It typically equates to approximately 10% of ingested energy.	

*Some valid critiques and limitations exist with using prediction equations, and they should only be used to estimate BMR.

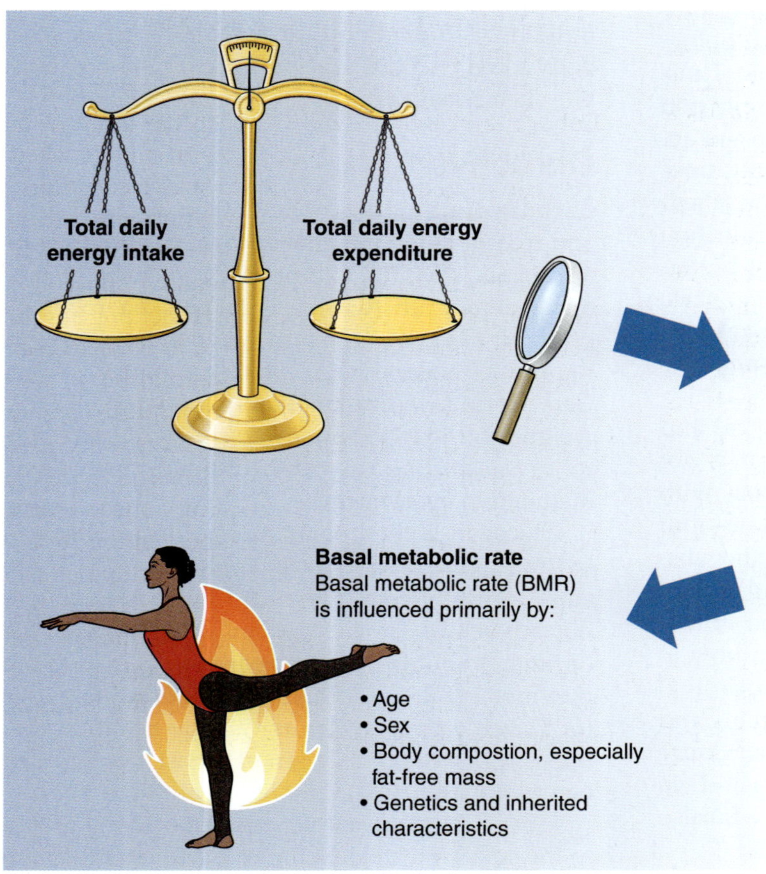

Figure 7.1 Overview of the components of energy balance.

the large intestine undigested, while some will be used by bacteria to produce fatty acids that, in turn, are used by your body. Fiber is a mixture of substances such as pectin, beta glucan, resistant starch, and cellulose. These substances have many different effects, including preventing constipation, helping to regulate blood sugar levels and cholesterol levels in blood, and supporting the gut microbiome (the microorganisms in the digestive system). There are different ways of measuring fiber content, and different countries recommend different amounts for nutritional health. Dancers should include at least five portions daily of fruits and vegetables and a range of grains and pulses (beans and lentils) in amounts that meet their carbohydrate requirements. Doing so will almost certainly provide adequate fiber, too.

Fats

Fat is also composed of carbon, hydrogen, and oxygen, but the oxygen content of fat is lower than that of carbohydrates. Fat is metabolized aerobically during activity of relatively low intensity. Fat is energy dense, yielding over twice the energy of carbohydrates, and fat stores are considerably larger than those of carbohydrate in all dancers. Fat is very important for many body functions. Fat in the body acts as an insulator from cold and damage, and it serves as an energy reserve. Average daily fat intake must be enough to meet your body's needs. Roughly 1 gram per kilogram of body weight per day is a useful guide. Depending on their structure, fats are described as unsaturated (usually plant based) or saturated (found in animal products and often also in manufactured products such as cakes, biscuits, and cookies). Dancers are advised to opt for unsaturated fat as the major proportion of their intake.

Essential fatty acids are unsaturated fats that you must eat because your body is not able to synthesize them itself. The two types of essential fatty acids are omega-3 and omega-6. Adequate amounts of the omega-6 group are found in plant-based oils, so you are likely to meet your requirement provided your diet does not overly restrict fat. Omega-3 fats, on the other hand, are found in oily fish, sea algae (algal oil), linseeds, pumpkin seeds, walnuts, rapeseed oil, and soybeans, or in dietary supplements.

High-fat foods include oils, butter, margarine, nut butter, hard cheese, cream, pastry, cake, most cookies (British biscuits), and many fried foods—especially deep-fried foods, such as French fries (British chips), potato chips (British crisps), and fried chicken. Fat is slower to digest than carbohydrate and protein. Therefore, although small amounts are both necessary and useful to help appetite regulation, high-fat meals eaten before dancing are likely to limit performance while the body tries to balance the demands of dance and digestion.

Proteins

Protein is composed of carbon, hydrogen, and oxygen, with the addition of nitrogen and sulfur to form amino acids that are linked together via peptide bonds. There are 21 amino acids, 9 of which are described as essential (including the three branched-chain amino acids, or BCAAs); that is, you must consume them in your diet for many purposes, including promotion of sound sleep. Protein recommendations are discussed later in the chapter.

Micronutrients

Micronutrients include more than 30 vitamins and minerals. Although they are all important to the human body, the ones of particular interest for dancers are listed and described in table 7.2.

Hydration, Sweat Loss, and Fluid Needs

Euhydration is the state in which the amount of water in the body is optimal; it is commonly called being hydrated. The body loses water constantly through breathing, skin perspiration, and urine production. Dehydration, the state in which body fluid levels are suboptimal, has negative short- and long-term side effects. Your body functions best at a core temperature of around 96.8 to 98.6 degrees Fahrenheit (36-37 °C). Many essential body processes do not work as well at temperatures above and below this range; at temperature extremes, dance is not possible.

All physical activities—including dance—result in heat production. Sweating is the main route for heat loss during physical activity in humans; the evaporation of sweat reduces the body's temperature. Although sweat rates vary, approximate average values are 800 to 1,200 milliliters (mL) (27-41 fl oz) per hour for males and 400 to 600 mL (14-20 fl oz) per hour for females (Baker, 2017).

Table 7.2 **Micronutrients Relevant to Injury Risk Reduction: Functions and Food Sources**

Micronutrient	Functions relevant to dancer injury risk reduction	Good food sources
Iron	Normal red blood cell production	Well absorbed from red meat, liver, kidney, dark chicken meat, and oily fish Less well absorbed from eggs, grains, pulses, nuts and seeds, fruits, and vegetables (although including foods rich in vitamin C can help absorption) Supplement (advised for vegetarian and vegan dancers—particularly those who menstruate—to reduce risk of iron deficiency)
Calcium	Bone health Normal muscle function	Higher amounts in most dairy products, fortified milk substitutes, sardines, sesame seeds, salmon, and herring Useful amounts in beans, some vegetables, grains, and some nuts
Selenium	Normal immune function Mood regulation	Brazil nuts, seafood, fish, eggs, lentils, and offal (e.g., liver, kidney) Grains and other nuts and seeds (fair sources)
Zinc	Normal immune function Wound healing	Meat, seafood, green vegetables, and seeds
Iodine	Normal metabolism	Dairy foods and white fish Fortified salt (where available) Supplement (advised for vegans)
Vitamin A: retinol Vitamin A: carotenoids	Normal wound healing Helps prevent cell damage (**antioxidants**)	Dairy foods, egg yolk, liver, some fatty fish Orange and green vegetables and fruits
B vitamin group	Energy release from food Healthy nervous system Normal blood cell formation	Grains, protein-rich foods, some vegetables B_{12} (present only in foods of animal origin): milk, cheese, yogurt, and B_{12}-fortified foods; aim for 2.4-4 micrograms (mcg) per day
Vitamin C	Normal immune function Normal wound healing	Many fruits and vegetables; 5 to 7 portions of a variety of vegetables, fruit, and salad per day (400-550 g)
Vitamin D	Healthy bones Normal immune function Normal muscle function (Deficiency linked to inflammation and cancer risk)	Sunlight: check local/national weather guidelines for timing; 10-15 mcg or 400-600 international units (IU) of vitamin D_3 supplement daily (more in places with less sunlight, but usually no more than 20 mcg or 800 IU daily*
Vitamin E	Prevents cell damage (antioxidant)	Oils, nuts, seeds, whole grains

*Spiro & Buttriss, 2014

Rehydration

To cover the essential water requirements of the adult body, female dancers typically need at least 1,500 mL (50 fl oz) of fluid per day, and male dancers typically need about 2,500 mL (85 fl oz) per day. Additional fluid is required to replace sweat losses; research recommends 1.25 to 1.5 mL for every 1 mL lost (Academy of Nutrition and Dietetics et al., 2016). The benefits of fluids other than water are discussed later in this chapter. Aim to start any exercise—including dance—in a state of euhydration.

It is helpful to know you can tolerate longer periods—up to an hour during training—without taking fluids; however, during training, the main priority should be staying hydrated to reduce injury risk (Jones et al., 2008). Some foods—particularly vegetables, salads, and fruit—have a very high water content, so those who include large amounts of these foods in their diets may find their need for fluid is slightly less than it would be otherwise. Your body will use fluid most effectively if

1. you have done a suitable warm-up; it diverts blood from the kidneys and thus it reduces urine formation.
2. you take in fluid regularly when exercising for more than an hour (e.g., 150-300 mL [5-10 fl oz] about every 20 minutes).
3. you continue to drink fluids regularly to restore euhydration after exercise.

From a practical perspective, being aware of the volume and color of urine you produce is a good guide to hydration. Thirst can be a reliable guide to fluid requirement, but it is often not sensitive enough in physically active individuals with moderate to high sweat rates, especially for those dancers who find it hard to judge thirst. Lower urine volumes and darker color suggest dehydration. The method of measuring weight change (in dry clothing) from pre- to postexercise can help identify inadequate hydration. A rule of thumb is for every kilogram (2.2 lb) of body weight lost, replace it with 1.5 liters (50 fl oz) of fluid. Replacing this fluid is essential for recovery and for maintaining performance.

Sports Drinks

Sports drinks traditionally aim to be **isotonic** (having a composition similar to body fluids), in which typically it has a carbohydrate content between 4 and 8 grams per 100 mL (3.4 fl oz) plus electrolytes. Electrolytes are important minerals involved in the body's fluid regulation and are often lost in sweat. Sodium, potassium, and chloride are found in virtually all sports drinks; however, some drinks may also contain calcium, phosphate, or magnesium. These liquids are designed to be absorbed readily, replace losses, and provide a small amount of energy for ongoing activity. See the Homemade Sports Drinks sidebar.

Many additional options are labeled as sports drinks; some of them supply only electrolytes, or perhaps they include a very small amount of carbohydrate. These types of drinks are **hypotonic**, which means they are less concentrated than body fluids. Water is hypotonic, and it is adequate for low-intensity dance classes. While research suggests that isotonic drinks can improve sports performance compared with plain water (Coso et al., 2008), evidence on hypotonic drinks is more limited. You should try different drinks, keep notes on their

Homemade Sports Drinks

Generally, sports drinks tend to be isotonic (they have a mixture of electrolytes with a concentration similar to that found in your body), and they aim to replace fluid and electrolytes lost in sweat (including sodium, which is found in salt) as well as some carbohydrate (4-8 g per 100 mL [3.4 fl oz] of liquid). While there are many sports drinks on the market, they are easy to make at home. Following are a few sample recipes for you to try. Note that the lower amount of salt is adequate in most situations; however, use the higher amount of salt if you are dancing or training in conditions where you sweat heavily. Shake each of these drinks well after combining the ingredients.

1. Mix 400 to 600 mL (14-20 fl oz) of your preferred fruit juice with enough water to make 1000 mL (34 fl oz) of liquid. Add 0.5 - 1 level teaspoon (tsp) of salt.
2. Mix 1000 mL (34 fl oz) of water with 50 g (4 tbsp) of glucose and 0.5-1 level tsp of salt.
3. Mix 750 mL (25 fl oz) of coconut water with 250 mL (8 fl oz) of pineapple juice and 0.5-1 level tsp of salt.
4. Mix 900 mL (30 fl oz) water, the juice of two lemons, and 2 tbsp of honey. For a flavor twist, you can add sliced ginger to the water for an hour and then remove it before adding the other ingredients.

Hypertonic beverages have concentrations of dissolved components that are higher than what is found in your body. These concentrations are useful to consider for recovery. During recovery, the aim is to rehydrate as well as to provide both carbohydrate and protein for restoring glycogen stores and to start the repair of the muscle fibers damaged during intense exercise, including dance.

A great example of a hypertonic drink is a 500 mL (17 fl oz) glass of milk with 1 to 2 percent fat content. Soy milk is the most comparable plant-based source. This also includes milk with any flavoring that contains some carbohydrate, such as chocolate milk. Syrups, powders, and fruits (including berries) can be added to create milkshakes or smoothies with additional nutrients.

palatability and any unpleasant gut side effects, and opt for the one (or more) that works best for you. Always check the list of ingredients; you may prefer to avoid some of the additives, which can include artificial colorings, flavorings, sweeteners, and—in the United States—high-fructose corn syrup (HFCS). HFCS can raise blood glucose levels very rapidly. For dancers working intensively, this rise will likely not cause any problems because carbohydrate use is rapid. However, caution is advised under other circumstances. You should always have some water with you both as a drink and as a mouth rinse (to minimize adverse dental effects) after consuming carbohydrate-containing drinks.

For rapid hydration, avoid **hypertonic** drinks. These drinks usually have a sugar content of over 8 grams of carbohydrate per 100 mL (3.4 fl oz). They include fruit juices, smoothies, most fizzy drinks (sodas), and milk-based drinks. Cordials and other concentrated drink syrups should be diluted to a suitable level. Moreover, sports drinks can be diluted with water, too, as some border on hypertonicity.

Translating Nutrients Into Food: Reading Food Labels

Looking at ingredients and nutrition labeling can be helpful; however, knowing what you are looking for will make the process more useful. Food labels in the United States and United Kingdom list ingredients in a specified way, with the most plentiful ingredient first and the remaining ingredients in descending order by weight contained in the food. Knowing this information is useful, but the proportions are not always listed; therefore, you should choose foods where the first few ingredients best meet your requirements.

In general, the fewer ingredients a product contains, the less processed it is. It is important to remember that while some additives (e.g., artificial flavoring and coloring) do not provide any nutritional benefits, others (e.g., preservatives) help keep food safe. While you should focus on less processed foods as the basis for your diet, you need to make individual, day-to-day choices about how best to meet your nutritional needs. For example, you might include balanced, ready-to-eat meals that simply need re-heating. When you encounter a busy schedule, this option is far better than consuming cereal, toast, instant noodles, or worst of all, nothing.

Nutrition labels offer the amounts of specific nutrients; macronutrient information is compulsory in many countries, and micronutrient and other important information vary by country. Certain government websites provide information on labeling requirements. For more guidance, see the sidebar Learn to Use Nutrition Labels to Your Advantage.

Food allergens are identified on food labels in many countries, but which allergens are noted varies by country. While 8 major allergens are highlighted in the United States, the UK and Europe list 14, and Australia and New Zealand acknowledge 10. If you have food allergies and you are touring internationally, plan ahead for each country you will visit so that you can eat safely.

Grocery Shopping Challenges

If you have a generous food budget, you can choose to eat organic foods or foods free of genetically modified organisms (GMOs). If, on the other hand, you have a limited budget, then be reassured that you can still eat healthily. In fact, the data suggesting that organic foods offer significantly better nutrition are quite limited, and organic foods usually come at a much higher price. Your priority, then, is to obtain the nutrients you need within the constraints of your budget.

An ongoing debate centers on the benefits and disadvantages of GMO foods. In terms of nutrition, they seem to be as good as their conventional counterparts; however, their long-term effects need further research. Overall, focus primarily on meeting your nutritional requirements to give yourself the best chance of achieving your dance goals.

Beware of using coupons and offers in supermarkets unless they fit with your plans. Avoid shopping when you are hungry, which may lead to impulse buying. Major food retailers spend much effort and money on store layouts that increase purchasing; thus, go shopping with a plan and a shopping list. Planning and flexibility will allow you to take advantage of genuinely useful offers. Remember that you should buy only what you will eat. There are both financial and environmental reasons to avoid wasting food.

Basic Nutrition Recommendations for Highly Physically Active Individuals

All athletes—including dancers, who are performance athletes—have increased nutrient demands compared to less physically active individuals. Increased demands are inclusive of all macronutrients; however, these demands differ depending on the goal

Learn to Use Nutrition Labels to Your Advantage

Nutrition labels on food products offer a wealth of information. Here, you will find out how to dissect what is in a selected food product. Figure 7.2 presents a label from a frozen lasagna. The label's first component shows you how many servings are in the package or container. This number is crucial because the rest of the label provides details on the indicated serving.

Now notice the other three sections on the label: calories, nutrients, and percent of daily value (%DV). There are four servings in the package. When examining the label, you can easily see that one portion of the frozen lasagna contains 280 kilocalories. Therefore, if you ate half of the lasagna, you consumed 560 kilocalories. Another important detail is that two servings of this lasagna, by themselves, would not be sufficient to meet your daily nutritional needs. In fact, they would supply less than one-third—and perhaps as little as one-fourth (or even less)—of your needs. Additionally, you can see that by consuming two servings of the frozen lasagna, you would consume 68 grams (g) of carbohydrate (8 g fiber) and 30 g of protein to support recovery from a long day of classes and rehearsals. The sodium content in two servings (1,700 mg) would replenish sodium lost throughout the day from sweat.

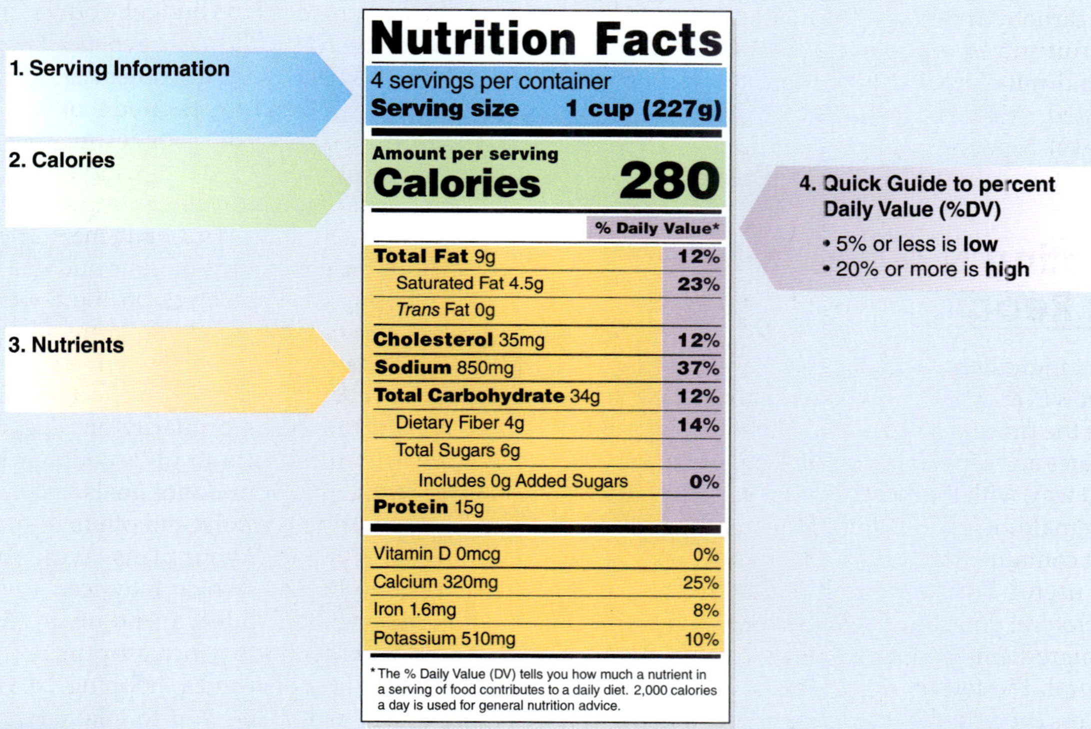

Figure 7.2 When you visit your grocery store or prepare your meals, use nutrition labels like this one to guide your decision making.

Reprinted from U.S. Food & Drug Administration. Available: https://www.fda.gov/food/new-nutrition-facts-label/how-understand-and-use-nutrition-facts-label.

of the athlete or performer. Therefore, the following sections explain nutrition recommendations based on three broad categories: strength, endurance, and dance. Dance is separated into its own category because both strength and endurance are components of most dance forms. Thomas et al. (2016) offers these overall ranges for athlete macronutrient consumption:

- Carbohydrate: 6-10 grams per kilogram of body weight per day (45%-65% of total energy intake)
- Protein: 1.2-2.0 grams per kilogram of body weight per day (10%-35% of total energy intake)
- Fat: 1.0 gram per kilogram of body weight per day (20%-35% of total energy intake)

Table 7.3 provides detailed information on food items that are commonly suggested for a training or performance meal plan, including the approximate amounts of macronutrients they provide.

Table 7.3 **Approximate Amounts of Macronutrients Provided by Typical Foods in a Training or Performance Meal Plan**

Food and amount	Protein (g)	Carbohydrate (g)	Fat (g)	Additional information
Bowl of oatmeal or porridge made with 3/4 cup oats and 1-1/2 cups milk, or 3/4 cup muesli with 1-1/2 cups milk and fruit	10+	40-50	3-5	Oats have a low **glycemic index (GI)**; oatmeal is good for a long morning. Adjust portion size to requirements (upward from 40 g oats); add nuts or seeds.
2 slices whole-grain bread, 80 g	8	30	1	White bread is similar, but it is lower in micronutrients and fiber.
2 eggs, boiled	16	negligible	11	Eggs have high-quality protein; they are inexpensive and a good source of micronutrients.
Brown rice, 1/2 cup (70 g) before cooking	8	77	2	Brown rice is richer in vitamins, minerals, and fiber than white rice.
Tofu, firm or extra firm, 100 g	12	2	7	Tofu has less protein per 100g compared to meat/fish: use a bigger portion than 100g if possible.
Mixed vegetables, 80 g (1 portion)	3	5	<1	Vegetables vary in content; variety gives the best range of nutrients. Salad provides fewer carbohydrates and protein, but is useful for micronutrients.
Banana, medium	1	20	negligible	A banana is a source of carbohydrates and micronutrients, including potassium.
Low-fat plain yogurt, 125 g	6	10	1	Check the nutritional value of non-dairy alternatives.
Cereal bar, ~45 g	4	20-30	8	Small bars are ~50% of these values; check ingredients for more grains, fruits, nuts, and less sugar.
Medium baked potato: ~200 g	5	45	<1	A baked potato is great as a basis for easy meals.
Cooked salmon steak, 100 g cooked weight	25	0	16	It is an excellent source of omega-3 fatty acids.
Cooked lentils, 3 tbsp	3	7	<1	Large portions are needed to meet protein needs, or mix with other sources.
Glass of 2% milk, 200 mL	7	9	3	Milk is a good source of calcium; if using plant-based alternatives, check the nutrition label.
Mixed nuts, 21 g	6	3	12	Nuts also contain a variety of micronutrients; the fat is largely unsaturated.

Nutrition Considerations for Strength

Participants in sports demanding strength and explosive power often engage in a resistance training program to supplement their sport-specific training regimen. Resistance training induces muscle damage; muscles then go through a process of repair and growth. Muscle growth requires additional protein in the diet—primarily essential amino acids—to facilitate protein synthesis. Athletes and performers engaged in regular resistance training may have the ability to use consumed protein sources more efficiently than those not participating in resistance training. Therefore, they may require less dietary protein than those athletes not participating in resistance training (Academy of Nutrition and Dietetics et al., 2016). Strength athletes should consume approximately twice that recommended for the general public, which amounts to 1.6 to 2.0 grams per kilogram of body weight per day (Academy of Nutrition and Dietetics et al., 2016; Phillips, 2004).

Resistance training also significantly reduces muscle glycogen (stored carbohydrate) and results in impaired performance if carbohydrate is not adequately consumed. For the strength athlete, carbohydrate timing is of primary importance to ensure the carbohydrate is available at the most optimal time during performance. Resistance training is often periodized; thus, the carbohydrate recommendation may change depending on the phase of training. The range in which strength athletes should consume carbohydrate is 4 to 7 grams per kilogram of body weight per day.

Nutrition Considerations for Endurance

Although the goals of an endurance athlete or other endurance-focused performer do not include muscle growth to the same extent as someone wanting to develop strength, protein requirements are nonetheless elevated to aid in repair of muscle damage. Endurance athletes and dancers should consume at least 1.4 grams per kilogram of body weight per day; more specifically, they should spread out their protein consumption throughout the day (every 3-5 hours) to ensure proper absorption.

Special considerations for endurance athletes depend greatly on intensity of exercise per week. For example, according to Vitale and Getzin (2019), if someone runs 1 hour per day at a moderate intensity, they should consume 5 to 7 grams of carbohydrate per kilogram of body weight per day; however, if they run 4 to 5 hours per day at a moderate to high intensity, their recommended carbohydrate intake should be 8 to 12 grams of carbohydrate per kilogram of body weight per day. Longer-lasting activities rely heavily on carbohydrate to sustain the activity. Without sufficient carbohydrate, one runs the risk of depleting carbohydrate stores. Due to the length of some endurance events, athletes should not only prepare well in advance to load the muscle with stored carbohydrate, but they also may need to consider fueling during the event to avoid performance detriments.

Nutrition Considerations for Dance

Recommendations specifically for dance are primarily based on recommendations for other athletic groups such as those mentioned previously. These recommendations have been adapted from the position statement on nutrition for athletes from the American College of Sports Medicine, American Dietetic Association, and Dietitians of Canada (Rodriguez et al., 2009). Protein recommendations for dance range from 1.2 to 2.0 grams per kilogram of body weight per day; however, more recent research indicates that protein needs may be higher (~2.3 g per kg of body weight per day) to optimize body composition (Brown et al., 2020).

When dance classes and training are relatively low in intensity, the carbohydrate recommendation is approximately 5 grams per kilogram of body weight per day (Sousa et al., 2013), a quantity lower than the general recommendations for athletes. This is a relatively low level of carbohydrate that should only be followed for low-intensity training. Intensity differs between dance styles, and it depends on the phase within a season. Carbohydrate intake should be monitored carefully to ensure adequate consumption.

For moderate-intensity bouts (e.g., performances), carbohydrate should be increased to recommendations similar to those for strength and endurance athletes as explained previously. A specific carbohydrate recommendation exists for speedy recovery from activity such as continuous or high-intensity dance classes or performances; it is around 1 to 1.2 grams per kilogram of body weight per hour for up to two hours post exercise. This amount should be part of one's daily total intake and not in addition to total energy intake.

Nutrient timing is critical for any athlete, but it is especially important for dancers in light of their extensive time dedicated to classes, rehearsals, and performances. The body must have enough fuel prior to exercise as well as fuel to support optimal

Table 7.4 **Approximate Seasonal Macronutrient Recommendations for Dancers***

	Preseason (rehearse and train)	In-season (performances)	Postseason (rest and recover)
Carbohydrate	5-7	5-12	4+
Fat	0.8-1.3	1.0-1.5	1.0-1.2
Protein	1.2-2.5	1.4-2.0	1.5-2.3

*Expressed in grams per kilogram of body weight per day. Dancers should be mindful to meet total energy requirements alongside these approximate macronutrient recommendations.

recovery after exercise. Periodization of nutrition is the planned use of nutrition to enhance exercise adaptations. It allows for the diet to ebb and flow with changes in the dance seasons (Jeukendrup, 2017). To properly fuel the body, the dancer needs to first consider their training schedule and what season they are in (e.g., preseason, in-season, postseason). Table 7.4 shows recommendations for macronutrient intake during the three seasonal phases (Ambegaonkar & Brown, 2021).

Considerations for Dietary Practices

As highlighted previously, nutritional requirements are variable from person to person and from day to day. Moreover, specific considerations exist for those who have additional dietary requirements because of a health condition, lifestyle choice, or cultural or religious reason. Indeed, many health conditions result in an individual having specific dietary requirements. Examples include clinical conditions such as phenylketonuria (PKU, in which the amino acid phenylalanine cannot be broken down in the body), diabetes (in which blood sugar levels are not well controlled without intervention), and celiac disease (an autoimmune disorder in which gluten ingestion damages the digestive tract). It is important to note that all dancers can meet nutritional requirements when attention is given to these additional considerations.

Food Allergies and Intolerances

Some individuals experience adverse reactions following the ingestion of specific foods. Many foods or food additives (including peanuts, fish, milk, celery, soy, and dyes) are responsible for food reactions. A food allergy results when the body's immunological mechanisms are involved in creating a reaction to ingesting the food or additive. In this instance, one's body uses an immune response to treat the ingested item as a foreign invader. The magnitude of such allergies varies; in some cases of severe allergies, it may include death. A food intolerance, on the other hand, is a nonallergic or non-immune-mediated (but still undesirable) reaction to food, such as that which occurs after drinking cow's milk in the case of lactose intolerance.

Symptoms that follow food reactions vary substantially (figure 7.3). Mild symptoms may include itching, nausea, vomiting, bloating, and constipation; more severe symptoms may include swelling under the skin, hives (raised itchy rash patches), and anaphylaxis (occurs when a body is under allergic attack). The more severe results are generally associated with allergic reactions. Dietary management of food allergies, intolerances, and sensitivities differs. Therefore, dancers who experience symptoms of a food reaction should confer with their physician and a registered and accredited dietitian, nutritionist, or other health professional; the professional should be qualified to diagnose and manage suspected conditions using appropriate testing, treatments, and dietary guidance.

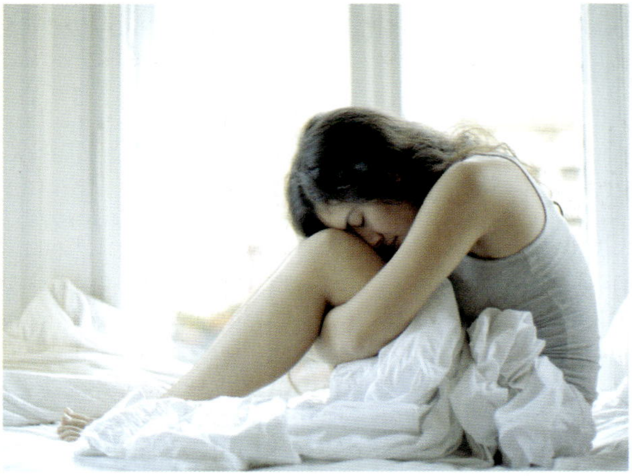

Figure 7.3 Symptoms of a food reaction can vary significantly, but they often include nausea and gastrointestinal discomfort.

Andrea Piacquadio on Pexels

Tips for Avoiding Fad Diets

There are thousands of fad diets; as the term *fad* suggests, they can come and go as fashions and fancies change. Being aware of several red flags will help you spot fad diets. Common warning signals include the following:

- *Diets or supplements that promise quick fixes with minimal effort.* They typically promote rapid changes to performance; body weight, shape, or composition; health; or energy. Only if your diet is very poor and you correct important deficiencies are you likely to see significant changes to any of these measures in a short time. In general, a true fix is not quick, and something that is quick is not a true fix.
- *Diets that ask you to remove entire food groups from your nutritional intake without a clinical need for such a restriction.* Any diet that limits your range of foods makes it harder to get the energy and nutrients you need. The more variety you have in your diet, the greater your chance of achieving nutrient recommendations. If you limit food groups unnecessarily, you could miss out on some great nutrient sources.
- *Diets that limit the times when you can eat.* While these plans may offer some benefits to specific groups of people, they are usually unsuitable for active individuals such as dancers, particularly if their activity takes place over several hours each day. Limiting your food intake to certain times can prevent you from receiving proper fuel to sustain you through training or performance; moreover, it can keep your body from adequately refueling, recovering, and rehydrating after training or performance.
- *Diets that ask you to invest in expensive supplements.* It is good practice to follow a *food first* approach for your dietary needs; in other words, first obtain your nutrition from good food choices. Supplements may have a place in your diet, but you should consider the need and the risks of using them. Do you have a specific deficiency for which you need supplementation? Has sufficient research shown the supplements to improve health or dance-specific performance? Learn the likely effects of a supplement; if you see good evidence to use one, determine the best value option. Always prioritize your spending on the whole foods your body needs.
- *Diets in which meals are replaced with shakes or other products.* This approach is problematic for many reasons. Of particular importance is that these meal substitutes are likely to be much more expensive than the recommended whole-food dietary approach. Meal replacements may provide a known quantity of nutrients, but humans benefit from enjoyable food that is available across the whole food matrix. For example, some plant nutrients are best obtained from eating a wide range of whole fruits and vegetables; they cannot be adequately replaced by other sources. Moreover, seeking so-called convenience in food intake is not necessarily a good practice; stopping to eat a well-balanced meal includes benefits to health that extend beyond nutritional value.

Gluten-Free Diet (GFD)

Gluten is a protein that is present in wheat, barley, and rye grains. It can cause significant physical problems for those whose bodies cannot properly process it. One example is celiac disease, a clinical and lifelong autoimmune disease caused by a reaction to gluten that decreases the ability of the small intestine to absorb nutrients from food (figure 7.4). It affects approximately 1 percent of the global population, and genetics appears to play a role in an individual's susceptibility to it (Singh et al., 2018). Celiac disease has no cure, but treatment and management by following a gluten-free diet (GFD) resolves the associated symptoms. Although oats contain a protein that is similar to gluten, most people on a GFD can consume them. However, because oats are often processed and handled in the same environment as other grains, they can become contaminated with gluten. The same is true for any other type of food produced in an environment

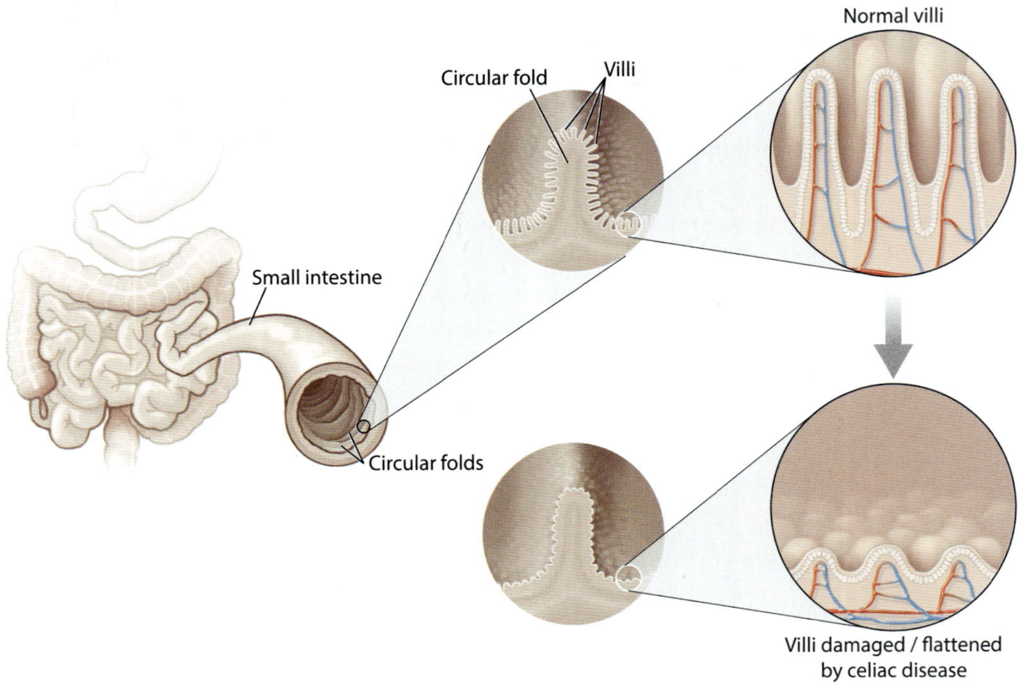

Figure 7.4 For people who have celiac disease, the normal fingerlike projections (villi) inside the walls of the small intestine are flattened. Because the villi assist nutrient absorption by increasing the surface area of the intestinal walls, the flatter, damaged villi are severely limited in their ability to provide this function.

(including restaurants) with gluten-containing food sources. For this reason, people adhering to a GFD are advised to check that foods are certified and labeled "gluten free" (GF).

The popularity of a GFD has increased in people without celiac disease across both the general population and athletic groups due to beliefs that this diet is healthful, augments weight loss, reduces gastrointestinal stress, and may have ergogenic (performance-enhancing) benefits (Lis et al., 2015). While some indications are that a GFD might be useful for those with health challenges, including wheat allergy, nonceliac gluten sensitivity, and irritable bowel syndrome (IBS), overall, the evidence for benefits to adhering to a GFD outside of celiac disease is limited (Lerner et al., 2019). Indeed, research has demonstrated that following a GFD without medical reason increases the risk of energy and nutrient deficiencies as well as compromised gut health (Bulka et al., 2017; Niland & Cash, 2018). As a result, given several characteristics of gluten-containing foods that are important to overall health (e.g., they are typically high in fiber, carbohydrates, and micronutrients), individuals without gluten-related issues are not advised to adopt a GFD.

Plant-Based Diet

A plant-based diet consists mostly or entirely of plants (e.g., vegetables, fruits, grains, legumes, seeds, and nuts); there are many different types that limit animal-based products to different extents. The popularity of these diets—particularly vegetarian and vegan diets—has increased dramatically globally (especially in the United States and in Europe) in the years since the turn of the Millenium. Research suggests that the prevalence of vegetarianism, veganism, or actively avoiding red meat is between 28 percent and 60 percent in dancers (Brown, 2018). This figure is concurrent with a fast-growing consumer market and media interest in plant-based foods and other meat alternatives. While there is evidence that plant-based diets are associated with a reduced risk of several chronic diseases and that they may be more environmentally sustainable (Craig et al., 2021), currently little evidence exists for their use in supporting athletic performance, particularly for exercise recovery.

A plant-based diet may increase the risk of energy and micronutrient deficiencies (e.g., vitamin B_{12}, iron, and zinc). Additionally, compared to animal-based proteins, plant-based proteins are typically lower in quality when considering their amino acid profile (specifically of the nine essential amino acids that the body cannot produce itself), digestibility, bioavailability, and **postprandial** protein synthesis. All these considerations are important in injury and postexercise recovery contexts. Therefore, dancers who choose to follow a plant-based diet should carefully consider their total energy, protein, and micronutrient intakes to ensure that their body's requirements are met.

Body Composition in Dance

The term *body composition* describes the physical components that contribute to a person's mass. In many cases, health professionals use body weight and body mass index (BMI) to assess health. (BMI is your body weight in kilograms divided by the square of your height in meters.) However, body weight and BMI fail to consider the body's proportional composition and patterning. Body composition provides detailed information about what the body is composed of and what contributes to body weight.

Because of the great variability in dance styles and training, the optimal body composition for a dancer depends on the demands of their chosen style and training regimen. Not all dance styles have the same physical or aesthetic demands; therefore, dancers do not have one body type recommendation that should be considered optimal. Rather, body composition is a more detailed picture of health compared to body weight and BMI, and it is critical to understand the parameters of your healthy body composition to optimize performance and reduce risk for injury.

Relative Energy Deficiency in Sport (REDs)

To maintain healthy body composition as a dancer, you must consume adequate energy (food calories). If energy consumed does not meet the needs required for dance training and performance, normal body functions can be impaired. This reduced function caused by inadequate calorie consumption is known as **relative energy deficiency in sport (REDs)** (Mountjoy et al., 2014). REDs can lead to decreased metabolic rate; disrupted menstrual function; and compromised bone health, immunity, and protein synthesis in both men and women. Although REDs can affect many body systems, maintenance of bone and muscle health is of primary importance for dancers to reduce the risk of injury. A number of studies have reported that dance populations have low **energy availability** and are at risk of REDs (Brown et al., 2017; Keay et al., 2020).

Proper caloric consumption is required to maintain the hormone function in the body that directly impacts the health of bones (Mountjoy et al., 2014). Low bone mineral density can lead to serious skeletal injury, and it has lifelong impacts through the aging process. It is also well known that inadequate calorie consumption can dramatically slow muscle repair and synthesis of muscle tissue. To ensure that you properly recover and can prepare for the next day of training, calorie demands must continuously be met to avoid the detrimental effects of REDs.

Maintenance of Lean Mass

Dance often places a strong emphasis on leanness and body weight as opposed to body composition. Approximate body composition normative values are shown in figure 7.5; they comprise fat mass and fat-free (lean) mass. Body image stressors can lead to a heightened focus on weight loss, but muscle (part of lean mass) is usually (if unintentionally) included in this weight reduction. This loss of muscle mass leads to decreased physical function and overall performance. In a physical activity focused on leanness (as is the tendency in dance), it is of utmost importance to focus on maintaining lean mass. Lean mass not only provides the basis for all human movement, it also contributes to metabolic rate, hormone regulation, and fitness status. Research shows that increasing protein intake can help to reduce lean mass loss during periods of high activity and low-calorie consumption in athletes (Mettler et al., 2010). Protein intake is an important consideration, especially while trying to consume enough calories for the demands of dance.

Implications of Low-Fat Mass

Body fat often gets a bad rap among lean athletes, but it is necessary for normal physiological functioning and overall health. Body fat is categorized as either essential or storage, where essential fat consists of fat located around or in the heart, lungs, liver, spleen, kidneys, intestines, muscles, and central nervous system. The minimal essential fat threshold for adult females is higher (12% body fat) than for adult males (3% body fat) because of sex-specific differences (McArdle et al., 2015). However, if an athlete or dancer were to approach these low body fat values, normal menstrual function would be adversely affected, and other medical complications could occur. Many female weight-sensitive athletes have a high chance of delayed, irregular, or absent menstrual cycles due to extremely low body fat. This response can lead to bone loss over time and increased risk for musculoskeletal injuries (McArdle et al., 2015). Overall, body fat must be sufficient to

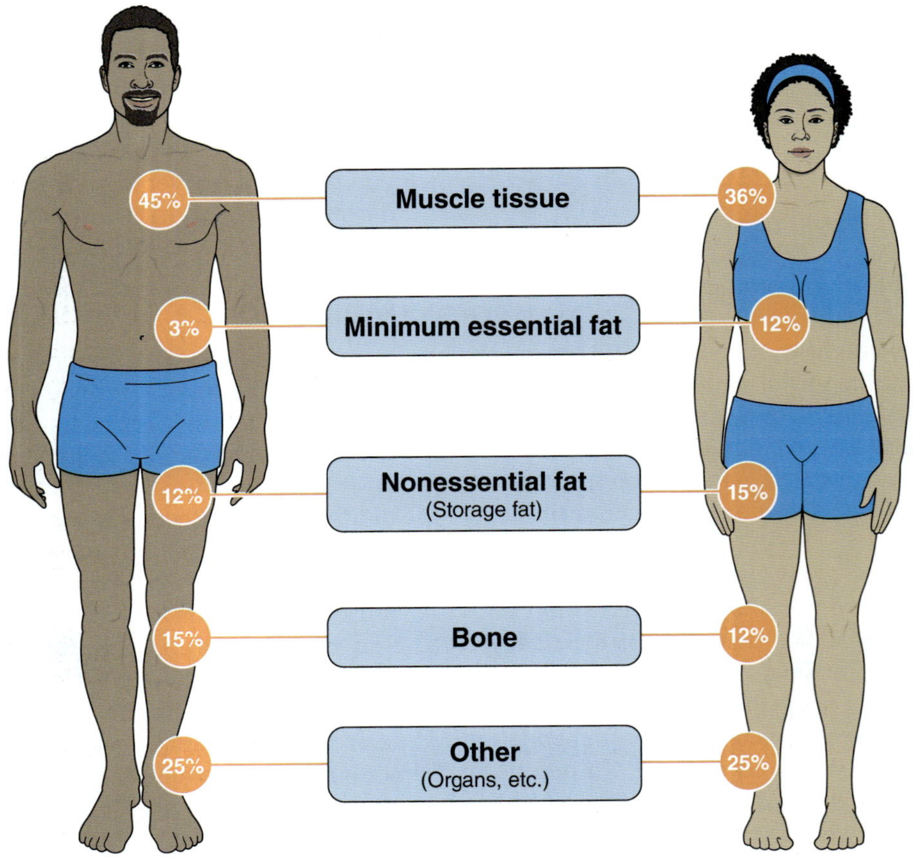

Figure 7.5 The components of body composition for males and females. Important points include the necessity of essential fat for protection of body organs, insulation, and a variety of physiological functions. Some aspects of body composition are genetically influenced, and some are modifiable by physical training and dietary practices.

support menstrual function in females to protect against negative health effects and serious injury.

Nutritional Strategies for Injury Prevention, Recovery, and Rehabilitation

The causes of injury are multifaceted. While common contributing factors such as accidents, unsafe environments, excessive workloads, and fatigue are well reported, few people acknowledge the role of the diet and dancers' nutritional status in influencing injury risk. Similarly, recommendations for optimal recovery and rehabilitation from dance-related injuries do not always recognize the role of nutrition. While specific requirements are largely governed by the severity and type of injury (e.g., bone vs. muscle vs. tendon or ligament) and the stage of the injury process (e.g., healing, recovery, immobilization, rehabilitation, or return to activity), some general nutrition recommendations exist for supporting injury and rehabilitation; they are shown in figure 7.6. Dancers should seek advice from a registered and accredited dietitian or nutritionist to establish their individual requirements.

Energy

As mentioned in the discussion of body composition, dancers are at risk of low energy availability and REDs. These conditions can increase the likelihood of impaired bone and muscle health or result in reduced lean body mass, thus leading to impaired strength and performance and increasing susceptibility to bone- and muscle-related injury (Carbone et al., 2012). Initial research with ballet dancers has demonstrated that very lean dancers are more prone to injury and may take longer to recover (Benson et al., 1989). Similarly, a study by Frusztajer and colleagues (1990) found that most ballet dancers with stress fractures were at less than 75 percent of their ideal body weight; they had a greater incidence of eating disorders and lower fat intake and they had a higher intake of low-energy foods.

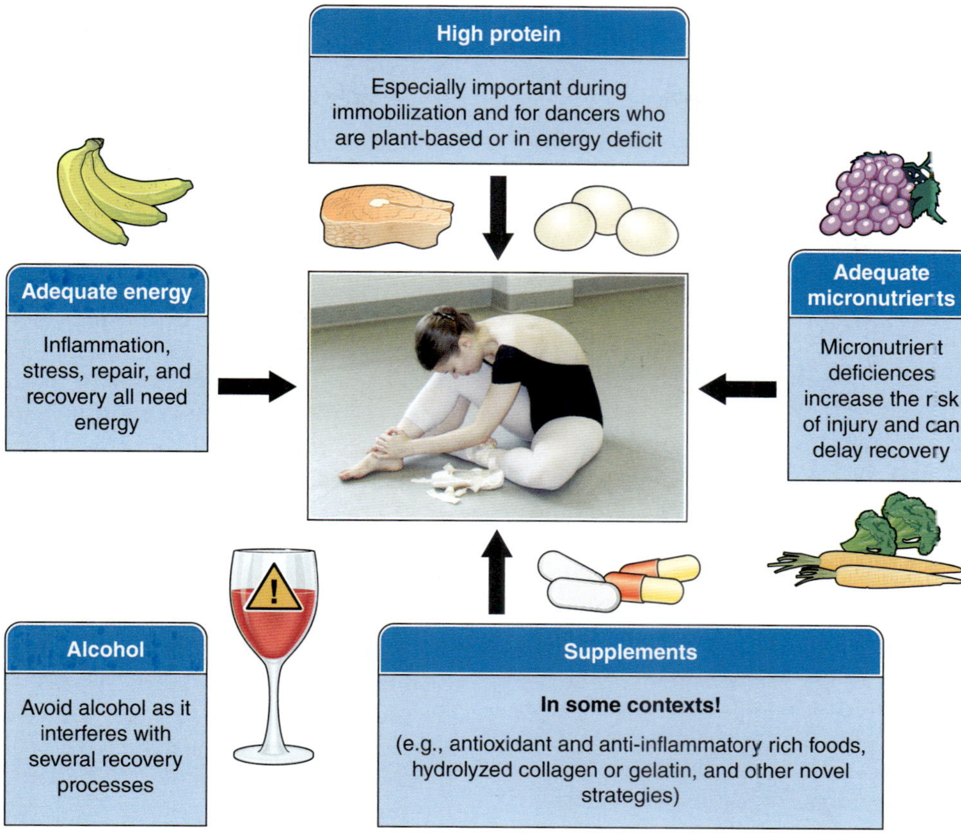

Figure 7.6 Overview of nutritional recommendations to support injury prevention, recovery, and rehabilitation.
Photo: Dr. Jeff Russell

In addition, it is important to note that the inflammatory and stress responses, the repair of damaged muscle (due to the increased protein turnover), and processes associated with rehabilitation from injury combine to increase energy expenditure by 15 to 50 percent (Frankenfield, 2006). Therefore, while a reduction in total energy intake may be appropriate to avoid significant changes in body composition during periods of reduced activity due to injury, it should be managed and monitored as carefully as possible. Dancers should maintain an adequate energy availability of 45 kilocalories per kilogram of **fat-free mass** per day after accounting for exercise energy expenditure to support their general health and also to help reduce injury risk (particularly of bone-related injury) and support recovery processes. One way to assess energy availability is to first assess exercise energy expenditure and body composition to determine fat-free mass. Various body composition analysis techniques, including bioelectrical impedance analysis, air displacement plethysmography, and dual-energy X-ray absorptiometry can be used to assess body composition.

Protein

Protein has an enormous number of roles in the body, including as a key constituent of muscle, bone, and collagen (the main structural protein of tendons and ligaments). Therefore, adequate protein intake is important for minimizing risk of injury in dancers. Given that protein turnover increases following injury (and even a few days of immobilization or inactivity tends to reduce muscle protein synthesis, muscles' sensitivity to the anabolic effects of amino acids and lean body mass), it is not surprising that protein requirements are increased during periods of injury and rehabilitation. At the very least, protein consumption should not be reduced when overall energy intake is reduced.

To prevent muscle loss and to facilitate recovery, relatively high protein intakes of approximately 2.0 to 2.5 grams per kilogram of body weight per day are recommended (Tipton, 2015). A high protein intake is particularly important during periods of immobilization as well as for dancers following a plant-based diet or who are in energy deficiency. Protein intake should be spread out (~20-40 g per meal every 3-5 hr) to encourage a positive **net protein balance** throughout the day. Moreover, dancers are encouraged to include high-quality proteins, such as milk (e.g., whey) or soy protein, with more complete amino acid profiles than those found in low-quality proteins. The essential amino acid leucine is especially important; it is thought to be the most potent stimulator of muscle protein synthesis. Dancers who supplemented their diets with whey protein—of which approximately 14% is leucine (van Vliet et al., 2015)—observed accelerated recovery following acute exercise-induced muscle damage (Brown et al., 2018).

Micronutrients

Many **micronutrients** have essential roles in wound healing (vitamins A, B, and C) and muscle repair (B-complex vitamins and vitamin C) as well as maintenance of bone (calcium, vitamin D, magnesium, and phosphorus) and collagen (vitamins A and C). Interestingly, little evidence exists to suggest that increasing micronutrient intake beyond typical recommendations improves or accelerates recovery from injury. Therefore, extra supplementation is not necessary when no evidence of deficiency exists.

Instead, an adequate supply of micronutrients will help reduce the risk of injury and support recovery from injury. Nevertheless, given that the research that has consistently demonstrated vitamin D insufficiency in dance populations (Vella & Cameron-Smith, 2010; Wolman et al., 2013; Wyon et al., 2018), dancers will likely benefit from supplementation with vitamin D_3 (the form of vitamin D most available in stores), particularly during winter months when sun exposure is limited. A study reported lower traumatic injury occurrence in adolescent dancers who supplemented with vitamin D compared to dancers who did not undergo supplementation (Wyon et al., 2018). Some micronutrients also possess **antioxidant** properties that may confer additional benefits in recovery contexts, at least during acute stages of injury.

Alcohol

Injury rates in athletes who do not consume alcoholic beverages appear to be significantly lower compared to those who do (O'Brien & Lyons, 2000). Importantly, alcohol ingestion should be avoided during recovery and periods of illness and injury because it has been found to interfere with several recovery processes (Vella & Cameron-Smith, 2010; Lakićević, 2019), particularly when alcohol volume is beyond a modest intake. Effects of alcohol ingestion related to body recovery include impairments in muscle protein synthesis, glycogen resynthesis, rehydration, wound healing, cognitive function, performance, and sleep quality.

Additional Supplements

While nutritional strategies for the prevention and treatment of injuries should consider adequate energy, protein, and micronutrient intakes as described previously, some dietary supplements show promising results. Some of the research evidence is equivocal, but many nutrients purport to help injury recovery. The most well-researched are summarized next.

Antioxidant and Anti-Inflammatory Products

The body's inflammatory response is initiated following an injury. Depending on the type and severity of the injury, this response can last several days. The process is thought to be associated with several symptoms, including muscle swelling and soreness. In addition, the production of oxidants (including free radicals, which are unstable forms of atoms) increases during exercise itself and in response to acute inflammation and injury. Oxidants tend to break down the body by damaging cells, while antioxidants tend to counteract this oxidation process.

The body's antioxidant enzymes promote biochemical reactions that help neutralize free radicals. If oxidant formation exceeds antioxidant capacity, oxidative stress can result, causing excessive damage to proteins, lipids (fatty molecules), and even DNA (which carries genetic information). Antioxidant capacity can be increased and the inflammatory response dampened by ingestion of foods and drinks rich in antioxidants and anti-inflammatory compounds (table 7.5). Including them in your diet may be beneficial to your postdance and postexercise recovery. A few nutrients with antioxidant properties have been investigated, mainly in acute recovery contexts. These nutrients include antioxidant micronutrients (e.g., vitamins A, C, and E), plant-derived **polyphenol**-rich foods (e.g., berries and cherries), and omega-3 fatty acids. One study reported some evidence of accelerated recovery from acute muscle-damaging exercise in dancers who supplemented with tart cherry juice (Brown et al., 2019).

While some negative symptoms associated with oxidative stress and inflammation may interfere with training and performance (particularly when only short periods of recovery are allowed in schedules), free radicals and the inflammatory process are a natural part of your body's functioning; they play an important role in wound healing and physiological adaptation to exercise (Owens et al., 2019). Therefore, the goal is not to eliminate them; rather, it is to moderate them effectively when considering supplementation with antioxidant and anti-inflammatory foods and drinks.

Collagen

Collagen is the main protein found in connective tissues, including tendons and ligaments. Therefore, interest in nutritional strategies to increase collagen production has grown as a means of potentially reducing injury rates in athletes. Novel nutritional strategies that have been explored include supplementation with gelatin (which contains amino acids similar to those in collagen) and hydrolyzed collagen (collagen that is broken down into small molecular pieces). Some support exists for their use in managing injuries in athletes (Dressler et al., 2018; Shaw et al., 2017).

Rest as a Necessary Component of Dance

Minimal research has been performed on rest and sleep requirements for the dancer, so this section follows recommendations and information appropriate to the broader athletic population. Normal sleep patterning is broken into two categories: non–rapid eye movement sleep (non-REM sleep) and REM sleep. Non-REM sleep includes three separate stages ranging from light to deep sleep, while REM sleep is its own individual sleep stage. The duration of all four stages of sleep changes throughout life. Walsh and colleagues (2021) report that from adolescence to young adulthood (15-30 years old), light sleep (stages 1 and 2) is approximately 57 to 65 percent, deep sleep (stage 3) is 16 to 22 percent, and REM sleep (stage 4) is 21 to 23 percent of a sleep span of 7 to 10 hours. In addition, they confirm that with reduced sleep stages and inadequate rest, athletes are at risk for impaired cognition, disrupted tissue repair and growth processes, and a lowered immune response.

Importance of Rest and Sleep

Sleep duration and quality are both important factors to consider for an athlete trying to optimize performance and maintain health. Research suggests that sleep requirements are higher in athletic groups to ensure adequate recovery as well as metabolic and muscular adaptations between training bouts. A research review (Gupta et al., 2017) found that poor sleep quality is most prevalent in female aesthetic athletes (the most similar to dancers, although dancers have not been studied). Moreover, Schaal and colleagues (2011) found more sleep disturbances in aesthetic athletes than any other category of athlete.

Table 7.5 **Foods Generally Associated With High Levels of Antioxidant Properties**

Antioxidant compound	Contained in these foods (among others)
Vitamin C	Broccoli, Brussels sprouts, cantaloupe, cauliflower, grapefruit, leafy greens (turnip, mustard, beet, collard), honeydew, kale, kiwi, lemon, orange, papaya, snow peas, strawberries, sweet potato, tomatoes, bell peppers
Vitamin E	Almonds, avocados, Swiss chard, leafy greens (beet, mustard, turnip), peanuts, red peppers, spinach, sunflower seeds
Carotenoids	Apricots, asparagus, beets, broccoli, cantaloupe, carrots, bell peppers, kale, mangoes, turnip and collard greens, oranges, peaches, pink grapefruit, pumpkin, winter squash, spinach, sweet potato, tangerines, tomatoes, watermelon
Selenium	Brazil nuts, fish, shellfish, beef, poultry, barley, brown rice
Zinc	Beef, poultry, oysters, shrimp, sesame seeds, pumpkin seeds, chickpeas, lentils, cashews, fortified cereals
Phenolic compounds • Quercetin • Catechins • Resveratrol • Coumaric acid • Anthocyanins	 • Apples, onions • Tea, cocoa, berries • Grapes, peanuts, berries • Spices, berries • Blueberries, strawberries

Data from Harvard University T.H. Chan School of Public Health (2023).

Although many athletic cultures idealize the ability to function on little sleep, it is an avoidable problem that unnecessarily compromises performance. Training schedules may be inappropriately planned (e.g., excessive classes and rehearsals for dancers) to not allow proper rest and sleep (Watson, 2017). Rest and sleep must be prioritized to allow the body to fully recover and prepare for the next training bout or performance.

Sleep Requirements for Optimal Sport Performance

Unique factors must be considered prior to understanding sleep recommendations for athletes. Compared to the typical population, athletes (especially dancers) perform and practice (rehearse) late into the evening, have high training loads, may travel and sleep in unfamiliar places, and may train early in the morning. An expert consensus statement synthesizes sleep recommendations for athletes (Walsh et al., 2021). Following are the five key educational items presented in that statement.

1. Nighttime sleep quantity targets are 7 to 9 hours for adults, 8 to 10 hours for teenagers, and possibly more than 10 hours for athletes.
2. Daytime naps may supplement nighttime sleep when schedule changes are not possible.
3. Good sleep hygiene improves sleep quality (discussed next).
4. Consider chronotypes (so-called larks and night owls) for sleeping and training; avoid training too early in the morning or too late at night.
5. Resist preoccupation with sleep monitors and sleep information that may increase anxiety around sleep.

Sleep Hygiene Habits

Sleep hygiene includes both having a bedtime routine and a bedroom that promote uninterrupted sleep. Enabling good sleep hygiene can improve sleep quality, ultimately aiding exercise recovery. Positive sleep hygiene habits include going to bed and waking up at the same time every day; preparing yourself for bed (reading, shower or bath, etc.); avoiding screen time (phones, tablets, computers, televisions) in bed; avoiding caffeine after noon; avoiding alcohol and nicotine; sleeping in a quiet, dark, cool bedroom; consuming foods rich in melatonin or taking a melatonin supplement (2-10 mg) before bedtime; and using aids such as a sleeping mask and earplugs to block sensory stimulation that may interrupt sleep.

Conclusions and Practical Relevance

Nutrition plays an important role in the health and well-being of dancers. Each dancer's situation should be assessed so that nutritional strategies are

Nutritional Practices That Support Sleep

Diet and sleep have been linked due to the physiological processes involved in sleep regulation. The body primarily relies on neurotransmitters such as serotonin and melatonin to regulate the sleep cycle, and these neurotransmitters can be influenced by nutrition. What you eat can affect your sleep quality and duration; therefore, you should consider nutrition and sleep together to enhance performance, optimize recovery, and reduce risk of injury.

A research review identified three common nutritional findings that elicited improvements in sleep (Binks et al., 2020). These suggestions for sleep-promoting foods are outlined here:

1. A high-glycemic-index (GI) carbohydrate meal can shorten the time to fall asleep (Afaghi et al., 2007).
2. Foods with **tryptophan** (animal meats, tofu, beans, nuts, seeds) are important; a diet low in tryptophan impairs sleep because tryptophan is a molecule the body uses to produce serotonin (Bravo et al., 2013).
3. Foods with melatonin (animal products, grapes, tomatoes, pistachios) and **phytonutrients** (tart cherries, kiwi) are reported to improve sleep duration and quality (Howatson et al., 2012).

tailored to their individual requirements. Broadly, in order to minimize your risk of injury and optimize recovery from injury, it is essential that you maintain appropriate dietary intake and avoid nutrient deficiencies. Dancers must consume adequate quantities of energy, protein, and micronutrients, and they must ensure that their sleep is not compromised.

There is little evidence connecting the role of diet and nutrition *directly* in injury contexts for athletes and dancers; much remains to be learned. Thus, it is important to appreciate that the field of performance nutrition and how it relates to injury prevention, recovery, and rehabilitation is growing, which explains why it cannot be fully explored in this chapter. Additional related topics for consideration include the specific nutrition requirements that are best when undergoing surgery or recovering from traumatic brain injury, as well as the emerging evidence in more novel applications of nutrition supplements in recovery and injury contexts (e.g., use of cannabidiol [CBD] products, milk-based beverages, pro- and prebiotics, creatine, and beta-hydroxy-beta-methylbutyric acid [HMB]). Interested readers are directed to additional literature to supplement this chapter (e.g., Close et al., 2019; Smith-Ryan et al., 2020). Finally, dancers will benefit immensely from access to qualified nutritionists or dietitians who can help support their goals without compromising health or performance.

Discussion Questions

1. Have you previously considered nutrition to be important in your dance training and performance context? Elaborate on nutritional areas you could improve in your daily life to optimize your performance and reduce your risk for injury.
2. Have you previously changed your dietary intake in response to injury and, if so, in what ways? In light of this chapter, describe dietary adjustments you would make should you become injured.
3. How can you manipulate and optimize your nutritional intake during recovery after strenuous rehearsals and performances? What are some lessons you can adopt from what is known about athletes' recovery nutrition practices?
4. While rest and sleep often are not considered a part of nutrition, clearly they are highly related to both nutrition and physical performance. What rest and sleep practices do you feel would help your dancing if you adopted them? Identify any roadblocks standing in your way of doing so and then develop a plan to improve this area of your life.

WWW Go to HK*Propel* to access supplemental information and activities connected to chapter content.

Psychological Wellness and Mental Health

Jo-Anne La Flèche, MPsy, MA
Bonnie Robson, MD, FRCPC
Kathleen McGuire Gaines, BA

8

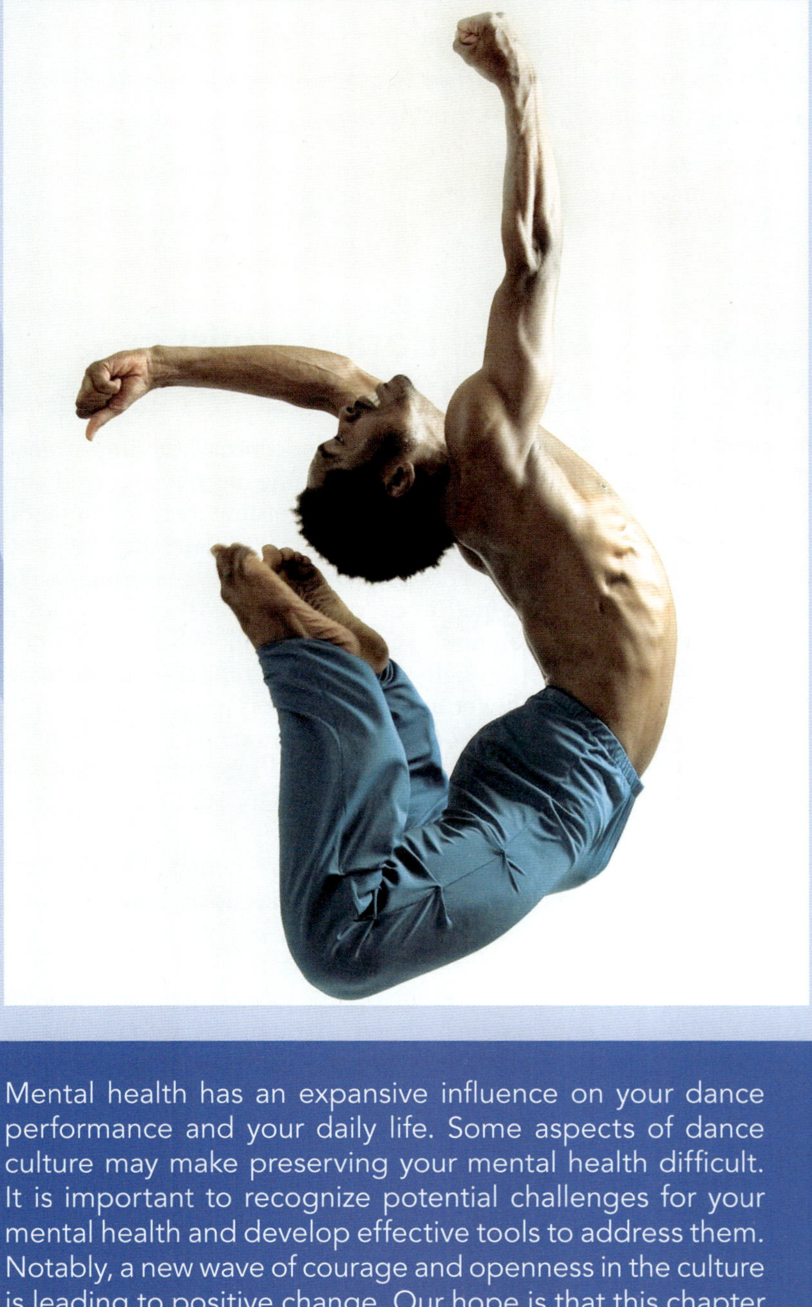

Photo: Anita Buzzy Prentiss; Dancer: Simon Phillips

Mental health has an expansive influence on your dance performance and your daily life. Some aspects of dance culture may make preserving your mental health difficult. It is important to recognize potential challenges for your mental health and develop effective tools to address them. Notably, a new wave of courage and openness in the culture is leading to positive change. Our hope is that this chapter will help you to be part of the solution.

- anorexia nervosa
- anxiety
- avoidant/restrictive food intake disorder (ARFID)
- body exploitation
- body image
- bulimia nervosa
- burnout
- depression
- disordered eating
- distress
- eating disorder
- eustress
- gender disparity
- mental imagery
- mindfulness
- perfectionistic concerns
- personal identity
- post-traumatic stress disorder (PTSD)
- power-based culture
- psychosocial factors
- self-compassion
- self-directed abuse
- self-esteem
- self-fulfilling prophecies
- self-talk
- stoicism
- stress
- virtuosity

LEARNING OBJECTIVES

After completing this chapter, you will be able to do the following:

- Discuss how the body–mind connection and mental health relate to success in dance.
- Outline common aesthetic and performance ideals for dancers of all genders.
- Identify and describe common negative challenges that can hinder dancers' mental health, including strong perfectionistic concerns, destructive self-talk, negative body image, low self-esteem, and traumatic experiences.
- Explain the negative effects of unconstructive life habits on dancer wellness.
- Differentiate between disordered eating and eating disorders, and examine how these habits affect dancer wellness.
- Outline the main mental health issues and symptoms that dancers may experience.
- Summarize the difficulties dancers experience in trying to voice their needs and discomforts, including how power structures and maltreatment can affect their perspective.
- Incorporate self-care and other practices into a daily safe dance routine.

Martha Graham once said, "Dance is the hidden language of the soul" ("Martha Graham Reflects on Her Art", 1985, H1) These profound words highlight the intimate links interconnecting body sensations; states of mind; and feelings, past experiences, values, beliefs, and hopes for the future. As a dancer, your expressed movement is the language by which you communicate your lived experience.

You devote a significant amount of time and energy learning technical and artistic skills for the mastery of your art. However, attending to your physical needs is not enough to ensure artistic growth or reduce the risk of injury. Dance practice can be very challenging mentally and emotionally because it involves tremendous commitment, perseverance, and engagement of your whole being—body, mind, and soul. You must cultivate whole-person wellness (discussed in chapter 1) in order to achieve your full potential while decreasing your risk of getting injured.

This concept of wellness includes your mental health. Since your physical wellness is directly tied to your mental health, this chapter addresses common mental health challenges that dancers face and the ripple effects on injury risk. Mental health skills and resources are provided to heighten dance injury management and prevention.

Mental Health Statistics and Injury

Since the turn of the 21st century, the importance of mental health has become more recognized and accepted. While stigma regarding mental illness still exists in popular culture, star athletes such as gymnast Simone Biles and tennis player Naomi Osaka have helped to normalize these discussions for a new generation by going public with their mental health struggles. Within dance, the conversation has been slower to follow, but it is moving in the right direction. For example, famous ballerina Kathryn Morgan shocked the dance world by leaving her soloist position at Miami City Ballet in protest of body shaming.

Research and treatment of mental illness among dancers is an emerging and quickly growing field. Even 5 years before the writing of this book, statistics on dancers' mental health were scarce; today, more information on this topic is available. In general, research shows that dancers are more likely to struggle with mental health challenges than the general population. Most dancers report feeling that mental health is neither valued nor supported within dance culture. Data consistently suggest that the primary mental health concerns for dancers are anxiety, low self-esteem, perfectionism, and disordered eating.

Such findings have been confirmed in an unpublished study by the mental health advocacy group for dancers, Minding the Gap (www.WeAreMindingTheGap.com). They surveyed U.S. collegiate dancers in November 2020 at the height of the COVID-19 pandemic (Araújo et al., 2021); they found that 48 percent of dancers exhibited high levels of anxiety and 44 percent showed low self-esteem. Both of these numbers indicate poor mental health. In addition, 55 percent of the dancers reported anxiety regarding their physical appearance. In each measure, dancers' scores were less favorable than the normative data of the general population of the same age. Moreover, ballet dancers presented poorer overall mental health than their dance counterparts in jazz and modern dance.

In the Netherlands, 44.6 percent of contemporary dance students reported mental health issues during a single academic year, and almost 30 percent of them experienced substantial mental health impairment affecting their dance performance and whole-person wellness. General anxiety, stress related to external factors, and constant fatigue were the most prevalent problems experienced by the participants (van Winden et al., 2020a).

Mental Health Statistics

In the United States, almost half of adults (46.4 %) will be challenged with a mental illness during their lifetime (National Alliance on Mental Illness, 2021). These prevalence rates are consistent in other countries as well; the rate is 50 percent in Canada (Canadian Mental Health Association, 2022) and 44 percent in Australia (Australian Institute of Health and Welfare, 2022). Among all forms of mental ailments, anxiety is the most common, with a prevalence of 18.1 percent of the U.S. population (National Alliance on Mental Illness, 2021).

In the United Kingdom, one male adult out of every eight, and one woman out of five (average 17% of the population) face mental illness each year (McManus et al., 2016). In the United States, adults aged 18 to 25 years old are at greatest risk; prevalence rates are 29.4 percent for any mental illness and 8.6 percent for severe mental illness (National Alliance on Mental Illness, 2021).

Aesthetic and Performance Ideals

Since the 1960s Western society has been obsessed with images of body perfection, thinness, and apparent eternal beauty for all genders. The body is viewed as an object, a commercial by-product that is part of a billion-dollar industry promoted by publicity, fashion models, magazines, television, and the movie industry. The dance world reinforces exaggerated and unreasonable expectations of what constitutes the so-called *right body*. These social ideals and the view of the body as a machine for performance are found in ballet as well as many other concert dance genres (Oliver, 2005, 2008; Pickard, 2012).

Classical ballet stemmed from European monarchy, and it became codified in the middle of the 17th century. This elite art form has always pursued poetic ideals of perfection, body lightness, and elevation—**virtuosity** executed with apparent ease—to create the illusion of supernatural grace and beauty. These aesthetic values were magnified in many ballets blancs (literally "white ballets," in which the dancers wore white dresses or tutus) during the Romantic era of the 19th century (Lee, 1999).

In the Romantic era and until the 1960s, ballerinas were generally portrayed as sensuous, supernatural beings with round body shapes (figure 8.1). Male dancers had to be strong and muscular to lift their female partners with ease and grace. In the 1960s, along with Twiggy and other fashion models, the prepubescent, waiflike, long-limbed and lightly-clothed ballerina of George "Mr. B" Balanchine's New York City Ballet set a new trend. Images of the Balanchine ballerina were identical to body types found in women's magazines and dance books for children (Ritenburg, 2010).

Mr. B set standards of stellar virtuosity, aerial grace, and tremendous speed for his dancers (Lee, 1999). These aesthetic and performance paradigms became the absolute and universal landmark in major professional dance companies around the world. This implicit body ideal is seen in most dance genres; since Balanchine's death in 1983, the ballet aesthetic has continued to get thinner, and it has evolved beyond the choreographer's ideal into an assumption of what he might have loved (Kelly, 2012; Pickard, 2012). Women are now expected to be slender, muscular, *and* graceful. Such a standard may lead to insufficient food intake, which dance research has shown is linked to injury and lack of peak performance (van Winden et al., 2020b).

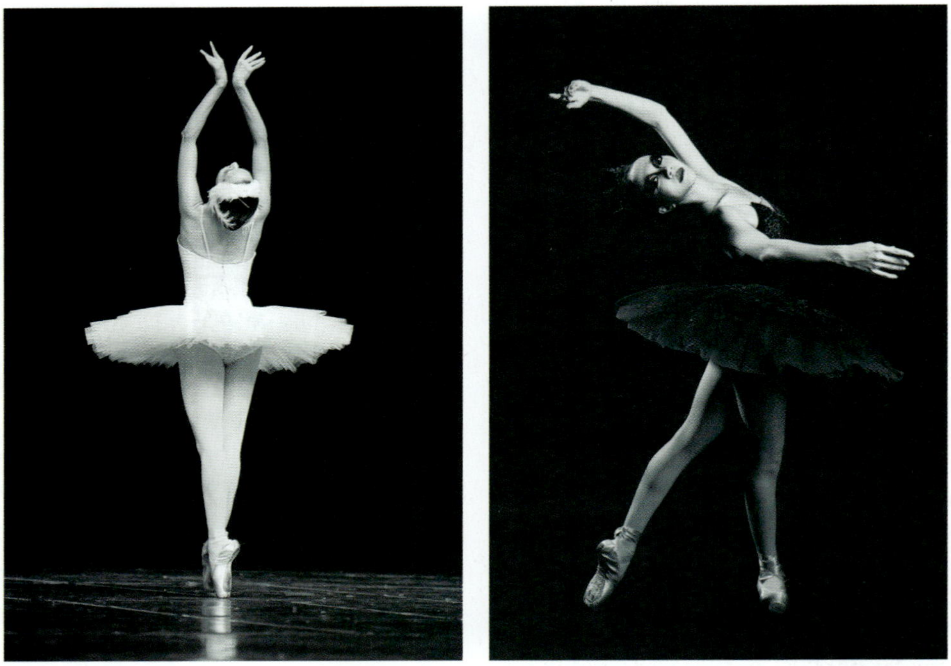

Figure 8.1 As ballet evolved over the years, ballet dancers were expected to be of slender form with the ephemeral appearance of floating across a stage.

Left—Gang Hao on Unsplash; Right—Knight Duong on Unsplash

Psychological Issues in Dance Practice

In your dancing, aesthetic and performance ideals may strongly influence your expectations and create added pressure that puts a toll on your stress level along with the great challenges of daily training. The following text addresses psychological issues involved in dance practice.

Perfectionistic Concerns

Throughout intensive training in pursuit of aesthetic and performance ideals, dancers often develop high levels of **perfectionistic concerns** that are manifested by excessive worries about making mistakes, a fear of failure, and a rigid quest for the absence of flaws. They may be reinforced by a parent's or a teacher's own perfectionism. Striving for perfectionistic excellence can motivate you to engage intensely in your art, set high standards, and maintain focus. In contrast, strong perfectionistic concerns may have maladaptive consequences, such as obsessive thinking, hypercritical self-talk, invalidating comparisons with others and with ideal models, and a general dissatisfaction with yourself and your dancing (figure 8.2). Perfectionistic strivings and perfectionistic concerns may interact in a more or less adaptive way, depending on their degree of intensity (high or low). For example, you might set high goals for yourself while accepting that making mistakes is inevitable in dance performance (Kveton-Bohnert, 2017; Nordin-Bates, 2020, 2023).

Research shows that perfectionistic tendencies are common in classical ballet and contemporary dance for dancers and teachers alike, and they are likely to negatively affect performance, intrinsic motivation, creativity, and general well-being (Nordin-Bates, 2020). Eventually, dancers with strong perfectionistic concerns may experience low self-esteem, anxiety, or depression. They are also at greater risk of disordered eating or developing an eating disorder (Nordin-Bates, 2020, 2023; Smith-Theodore, 2021; Taylor & Estanol, 2015).

The 2019 International Olympic Committee (IOC) Consensus Statement indicated that limited coping resources and perfectionism are significant mental risk factors for sport injuries (Reardon et al., 2019). Dance research has not yet established a direct causal link between perfectionism and the occurrence of injury. However, this relationship may not be explicit because perfectionism has an indirect effect on stress, and stress is linked to injury. If you have perfectionist tendencies, you may

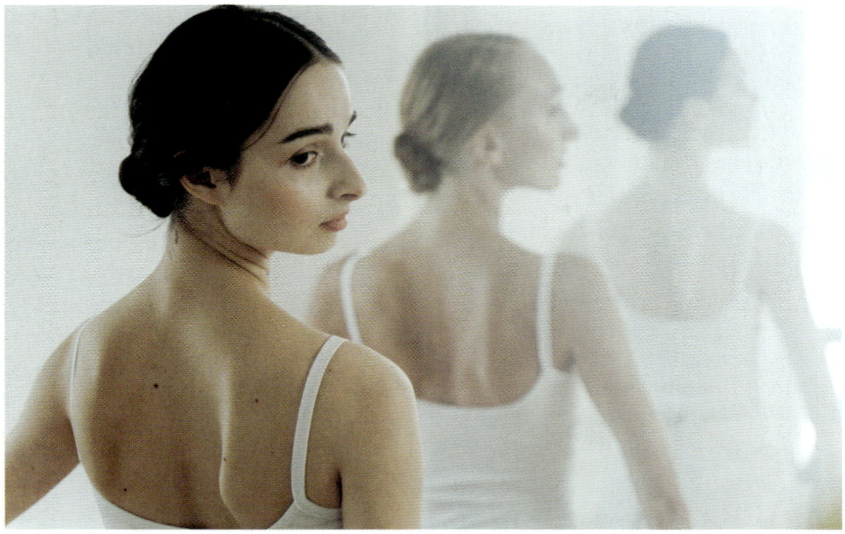

Figure 8.2 Comparing oneself to other dancers can lead to self-criticism, and it is l kely to accentuate perceived flaws.
Cottonbro on Pexels

experience greater performance anxiety and lower self-confidence than other dancers, which can lead to negative stress responses, thus heightening the probability of injury (van Winden et al., 2020b).

Self-Talk

Maladaptive perfectionism is linked to destructive self-talk. **Self-talk** is defined as statements or verbalizations regarding oneself. These statements may be explicit and audible to an outside observer, or they may be covert inner dialogue. They can be positive and motivating in the face of challenges, or they can be negative, stressful, and self-defeating (Hardy, 2006). If you harbor rigid demands to perform well, your inner critics may become cynical tyrants regardless of objective accomplishments. This toxic attitude perpetuates negative thoughts, emotions, and **self-fulfilling prophecies** (e.g., predicting failure).

It can be easy to confuse your thoughts with reality. Therefore, you should pay close attention to the quality of your inner dialogue; it affects how you perceive and react to daily events as well as on how you view your body (body image) and your worth (self-esteem).

Identifying Perfectionistic Thinking

The language of perfectionistic dancers is often downplayed or taken for granted because it is easily confused with the quest for performance excellence. Nonetheless, this language does reveal the tremendous pressures that needlessly burden dancers. You may recognize yourself or one of your colleagues in the following examples (Smith-Theodore, 2021). Such destructive self-talk must be confronted with positive self-talk. Accountability with a trusted peer, teacher, or mental health professional will also be helpful.

- *I know I am the worst dancer in the class because it takes me a lot longer to pick up the choreography.*
- *I hate the way I did the combination across the floor. Everyone was staring at me, and I was horrible.*
- *If I don't push myself harder, I will never be perfect.*
- *My turnout is worse than anyone in the class. That is why the teacher never looks at me when I'm at the barre.*

Body Image

Body image is defined in various ways in psychology, dance, and sport literature. Body image comprises two inseparable elements: the lived body (inner) and the perceived body (outer). The lived body relates to physical sensations from inside, including proprioception. The perceived body concerns your perceptions and attitudes toward your physical appearance that are forged by past experiences, self-judgments, and beliefs about how your body is judged by others. Body image begins

Common Types of Negative Self-Talk in Dancers

Scholars have identified several kinds of negative self-talk that are typical in dancers (Kveton-Bohnert, 2017; Smith-Theodore, 2021).

- *Filtering*—Focusing only on the negative events despite your victories.
- *Personalizing*—Falsely viewing every negative event as related to yourself.
- *Catastrophizing*—Believing a situation is far worse than it actually is.
- *Polarizing*—Thinking thoughts that are either all bad or all good.
- *Superstition*—Thinking or behaviors that are based on irrational beliefs and a view of yourself as being driven by outside forces (positive or negative).

to develop from early childhood and evolves positively or negatively throughout adolescence and adult life; it depends on life experiences (Nasio, 2007; Papalia & Martorell, 2021).

By making unhealthy comparisons to other bodies, you may view your physical appearance as being intrinsic to your personal value. This perspective can put your body image ahead of your daily progress and improvements; furthermore, it increases risk of body dissatisfaction, disordered eating, and eating disorders. Mirrored studios; negative comments on appearance, weight, and physical abilities; and toxic comparisons to images of a so-called ideal can heighten the risk of challenges to your body image (Alexia & Dimitropoulou, 2011; Oliver, 2008; Pickard, 2012; Pollatou et al., 2010; Price & Pettijohn, 2006; Radell et al., 2017, 2020).

Because dance is an aesthetic art form, dancers are particularly vulnerable to negative comments about their bodies, and they depend heavily on teachers' and mentors' positive feedback to build self-confidence and succeed (Pickard, 2012) (figure 8.3). For example, when combined with other risk factors such as anxiety or poor self-esteem, one hurtful remark about weight or appearance can seriously damage a dancer's body image and even trigger disordered eating (Garcia-Dantas et al., 2018; Green, 2001; Hobden, 2009; Taylor & Estanol, 2015).

Because these cultural and social factors may hinder body image, you should be mindful of their possible negative impact on how you feel about your body. Given that your dancing body is both the medium and the creator of your art (and it is always on display and evaluated by others in the studio or onstage), body image is at the very core of your daily practice. Consequently, you may feel insecure and more critical about your body. However, to stay psychologically well, you must cultivate positive perceptions, attitudes, and actions toward your body-instrument and lower any self-defeating comparisons with unrealistic standards or with your peers (Mainwaring & Aujla, 2017). As the next section demonstrates, how you feel about your physical appearance and abilities is also intimately linked to your self-esteem.

Self-Esteem

Self-esteem has been researched extensively in the field of humanistic and positive psychology, and it has been defined in various ways. This chapter uses this definition: Self-esteem is a balanced relationship between feelings of personal self-competence to face life's challenges and a sense of self-worth and personal dignity, such that you act according to your human values. Self-esteem is continually changing, and it may fluctuate depending on your present context and the phase of your life cycle.

One's opinion about oneself typically grows during childhood through nurturing relationships with authority figures and those close to the child. In the teenage years, with the onset of puberty and many challenges to be faced, self-esteem often becomes more fragile, and it is largely influenced by the acceptance of peers as well as personal and social success. Body esteem (the perception of one's beauty) weighs heavily on the person's general self-esteem throughout life but even more so during childhood and adolescence (Mruk, 2013). From the life stage you are in now, self-esteem will evolve for the span of your lifetime. Feelings of personal competence and self-worth also may vary within your life. For example, you may feel quite confident about your personality traits and your intellectual, academic, or creative abilities, but you may also feel insecure about your looks or dancing prowess.

When compared to the general population, the self-esteem of high-level dancers is considerably more ingrained in body image and ideals of perfection. This finding is not surprising given that dance is a physical art form; you can't simply detach yourself from your body-instrument. With time, your dance becomes intertwined with your sense of personal identity and self-esteem; eventually, you *become* your dance. On good days, the closer you reach your performance and aesthetic ideals,

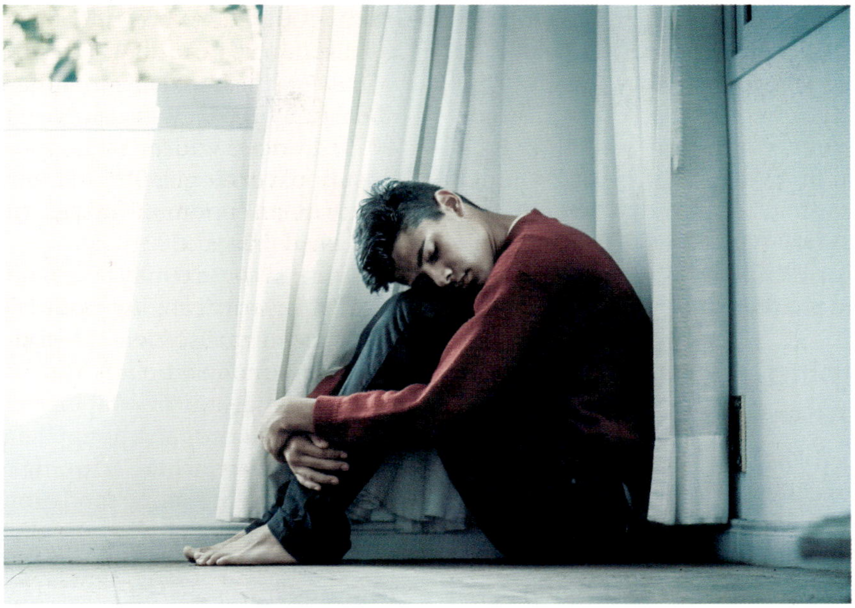

Figure 8.3 Negative comments from others—especially teachers—can be destructive to one's body image and overall self-esteem, initiating a cycle of mental health challenges.
Fernando on Unsplash

the better you feel about your appearance and self-worth. Dancing can make you feel vibrant and elated! Unfortunately, the same rule applies when you do not feel on par with your expectations or when you face a setback (Oliver, 2008).

Research suggests that dancers' body esteem and self-esteem vary depending on social context, such as being in class or onstage versus being at a social gathering. Ballerinas score lower on self-esteem assessments than their contemporary counterparts, which may be due to strict ballet ideals and perfectionism, which reinforce feelings of inferiority (van Zelst et al., 2004).

No matter the objective success and dance genre, most artists tend to feel dissatisfied with their dance performances. They compare themselves negatively to dance idols and dancers they admire and compete with, most often through the lens of perfectionism and negative self-talk (Alexias & Dimitropoulou, 2011; Jackson, 2005; Mainwaring & Krasnow, 2010; Pickard, 2012). The late Balanchine ballerina Irma Sandrey once said, "No ballerina is ever totally satisfied with herself. You *always* want to do better, to do more" (La Flèche, 2014).

As a general principle for success, the potential for negative views of yourself must be actively challenged. Regardless of your emotional highs and lows, and your feats or setbacks, embrace your unique richness as a person. Remind yourself that you are so much more than your dance—no matter how passionate you feel about your art. This is a fundamental aspect of the spiritual dimension of whole-person wellness (presented in chapter 1).

Unconstructive Life Habits

The rigorous schedules and high expectations (from yourself and others) of dance can lead you into the trap of neglecting basic needs or using poor coping strategies. These strategies may become unconstructive life habits, which can eventually impair your global wellness and promote injury. The following sections discuss these habits.

Insufficient Sleep and Rest

Some dancers consider rest and recovery as more or less a waste of time compared to the thrill and excitement of developing their artistic skills. In this case, it may be tempting to forsake sleep hours to accomplish all the tasks you want to get done in your day. However, you should keep in mind that most adult dancers need 8 to 9 hours of sleep. Adolescents must sleep an average of 9 to 10 hours per night to meet energy demands of puberty and growth spurts during training years (Papalia & Martorell, 2021). These figures may vary depending on your personal needs and the intensity of performance challenges you face at any given time, but it is true that sleep and rest are crucial.

Insufficient sleep or overtraining occasionally may not have a serious impact on your health, so it may be tempting to minimize these. Eventually, however, your body will settle its accounts. Chronic fatigue impairs your motor and learning skills while putting you at great risk of getting injured or developing symptoms of burnout, anxiety, and depression (Batson & Wilson, 2017; Krasnow & Wilmerding, 2015). Additional insights into rest and recovery appear in chapter 7.

Smoking, Vaping, Alcohol Abuse, and Drug Abuse

Dancers may be seen smoking outside dance schools and performance venues as they seek to unwind, relax, and control their weight. However, whatever the perceived advantages of smoking and vaping are, these activities are discouraged. They reduce physical endurance, aerobic fitness, bone health, tissue healing, and recovery from injury (Quin et al., 2015; Sterne & Patsalidou, 2017).

As a rule, dancers should avoid consuming alcohol and drug substances the evening before and on the day of dance practice. If they consume them at other times, they should do so moderately and occasionally, and always within health guidelines. Using alcohol or drugs of any kind (e.g., marijuana, prescription, or over-the-counter drugs such as laxatives) may be tempting at some point in order to alleviate excessive stress, to conform to thin body ideals, or just to fit in with a peer group. However, it is known that in addition to the commonly known negative physical effects that include potential dangers of being under the influence of alcohol and drugs, regular intake of these substances alters your energy level, mood, and general coping abilities (Taylor & Estanol, 2015).

Disordered Eating and Eating Disorders

The tragic 1997 death of Boston Ballet dancer Heidi Guenther from eating disorder complications caused a major shift in the way companies and schools address dancers' weight. Almost overnight, nutritionists and mental health professionals were brought into studios. Dancer weigh-ins remained under the assertion that they would help identify dancers with eating disorders.

Despite this shift, dancers are still three times more likely to have an eating disorder than the general population (Arcelus et al., 2014). The pressure to attain the standard of a so-called perfect, lean and mean body in the hope of achieving success puts female dancers and some male dancers at high risk of developing imbalanced eating behaviors (Oliver, 2008; Kelly, 2012; Quin et al., 2015; Taylor & Estanol, 2015). Dancers with an eating-related problem may not appear underweight, and they generally do not reveal their condition for fear of being judged or punished (Saigal, 2021).

Eating disorders may be classified along a continuum of severity ranging from disordered eating to clinical eating disorders. **Disordered eating** refers to behaviors and beliefs that prevent you from consuming the nutritional ingredients required for your energy needs and optimal dance performance. Behaviors may include skipping meals, taking only light meals, eliminating food groups, chewing gum instead of eating, fasting, and dieting. On the other hand, an **eating disorder** is a clinically diagnosed eating disturbance that has damaging effects on your global wellness; this condition is most often associated with body image concerns and distortions (Quin et al., 2015; Sterne & Patsalidou, 2017; Taylor & Estanol, 2015).

Most adolescents experiment with disordered eating at some point. In the dance world, 73 percent of female dancers consider that being of low body weight improves their chances of being cast in significant dance roles. In fact, 44 percent of females and 33 percent of males report having been advised to lose weight at some point in their dance career (Keah et al., 2020). However, the physical and psychological harm caused by disordered eating is largely underestimated. Following are common forms of disordered eating and eating disorders observed in dancers.

Dieting

Despite the documented inefficiency of weight-loss programs, dieting is very common in Western society. It is often linked to low self-esteem, low mood, and body dissatisfaction. Dieting moralizes your food choices, increases concerns with food, and reinforces black-and-white thinking about food—and yourself—as either good or bad. In the general population, a third of normal dieting becomes pathological dieting; of those cases, 20 to 25 percent develop a full eating disorder or syndrome.

Dancers who eat in a disordered way to stay thin are at tremendous risk of developing an eating disorder, especially if they have received a negative comment about their physicality (Saigal, 2021). Consider this example: A female dancer who battled against anorexia for the past year finally came to terms with her new hourglass body shape. Then, a few weeks prior to showtime, her rehearsal director said, "You dance the role of Giselle so graciously. You would look so much better if you lost 10 pounds." This single comment may be all that is needed to reactivate the dancer's eating disorder.

Orthorexia

Orthorexia relates to obsessive concerns and rigid behaviors regarding healthy nutrition, perfect food standards, and food preparation. This subclinical eating disorder has not yet been officially classified in the *Diagnostic and Statistical Manual of Mental Disorders, Fifth Edition* (commonly known as the *DSM-5*) (American Psychiatric Association, 2022), but it has gained increasing attention in recent years both from dance scholars and health professionals. Most often, the excessive concern for food correctness (e.g., eating food containing no salt, no sugar, no additives) goes unnoticed, being mistaken for trendy healthy food values. However, the desire to eat well crosses the fine line toward obsession when it creates emotional **distress**. In this case, people with orthorexia will most likely lose weight and isolate themselves socially (Cena et al., 2018). Since athletes and dancers concerned about good nutrition are at risk of developing orthorexia, you are encouraged to be mindful of warning signals when something good becomes too much or takes a substantial amount of your attention.

Avoidant/Restrictive Food Intake Disorder (ARFID)

Avoidant/restrictive food intake disorder (ARFID) is defined as avoidance or restriction of certain foods (for reasons other than religious practices) that prevents you from meeting nutritional or energy needs. A person with ARFID may experience a lack of interest toward eating, a sudden disgust toward the sensory quality of certain foods (e.g., its appearance or smell), or a fear of a digestive ailment. ARFID symptoms include significant weight loss, dependence on nutritional supplements, and impaired social relations. Exclusion of food groups by choice are reported by 50 percent of female dancers and 33 percent of male dancers (Keah et al., 2020; Taylor & Estanol, 2015).

Anorexia Nervosa

Dancers eating in a disordered way may eventually develop an eating disorder, the most common of which is **anorexia nervosa**. This malady is marked by voluntary restrictions of food intake—which may reduce body weight below 85 percent of average body mass index (BMI)—denial of hunger, intense fears of gaining weight, and distorted body image. Other common physical symptoms are loss of muscle mass, paleness, very dry skin, brittle nails and hair, amenorrhea, delayed growth, immune problems, frequent injuries, stress fractures, and osteoporosis.

Dancers with symptoms of anorexia also experience loss of energy, depressive and anxiety states, and extreme need for control. People with this disorder are typically described as high achievers, perfectionists, and people pleasers. In addition, the rigid mindsets and reactions (e.g., all-or-nothing thinking) that are characteristic of those with anorexia are reinforced by food deprivation. People with anorexia tend to battle with feelings of toxic guilt and shame while trying to be perfect; these feelings come from low self-esteem (Steiger & Thaler, 2016). While they restrict their own intake of food, people experiencing anorexia often develop a strong interest in cooking for others.

Bulimia Nervosa

Dancers with **bulimia nervosa** alternate between frequent and compulsive binging within 2 hours of their last meal, and compensatory behaviors (e.g., overtraining, laxatives) with or without purging. Dancers with bulimia often exhibit an obsessive need for self-control and a strong concern about food, body weight, and physical appearance. At the same time, they tend to be impulsive and have mood swings as well as substance abuse issues. In general, approximately 1 percent of female teenagers and women will encounter anorexia, while 2 to 4 percent of them will be challenged with bulimia during their lives (Hobden, 2009; Steiger & Thaler, 2016).

Factors Involved in Eating Disorders

A literature review reveals a lifetime prevalence of overall eating disorders of 12 percent for female dancers (16.4% for ballet dancers), 2.0 percent for anorexia (4% for ballet dancers), 4.4 percent for bulimia (2% for ballet dancers), and 9.5 percent for eating disorders not otherwise specified (EDNOS) (14.9% for ballet dancers). Compared to the general population, dancers have a three times higher risk of experiencing eating disorders, particularly anorexia nervosa and EDNOS; however, their risk of experiencing bulimia nervosa is no higher (Arcelus et al., 2014).

Multiple factors interact in triggering eating disorders. Genetic predispositions, such as anxiety, may heighten your sensitivity to stress. **Psychosocial factors**, such as a culture of thinness, adverse childhood experiences (ACE), family problems, dependency issues, or current stressful events increase your risk of developing an eating disorder. The probability increases 10 times if you are female and have an immediate female relative with an eating disorder (Taylor & Estanol, 2015; Steiger & Thaler, 2016). Like anorexia, bulimia threatens dancers' health, especially in cases of frequent purging. Most concerning is the fact that eating disorders may lead to death if left untreated (Taylor & Estanol, 2015). Chapter 7 provides more information about disordered eating and eating disorders from a nutritional perspective.

If you suspect you have disordered eating or eating disorder symptoms, or if you recognize them in a fellow dancer, you are strongly encouraged to seek professional help quickly. Since eating disorders reinforce rigid thinking; denial; and feelings of guilt, fear, and shame, acknowledging the problem and seeking appropriate help may be very challenging. However, waiting longer increases the health consequences, and it likely increases complexity and difficulty of treatment. A number of international mental health resources are available in appendix A.

Common Mental Health Challenges

Modern values of hyper-performance, efficiency, and fast daily living have led to an explosion of stress-related health problems. While stress is an unavoidable fact of life, dancers must cope with the added challenges of intense training and performance demands so that they can dance freely and safely. Growing research indicates how unconstructive attitudes and behaviors, high levels of emotional pain and distress, and poor coping skills in dance and in daily life interact at the onset and for the duration of dance injuries (Mainwaring & Finney, 2017; van Winden et al., 2020b).

Stress and Burnout

Stress is an instinctive bodily response to a perceived threat to your well-being in the face of a challenging situation. Stress responses are warning signals regarding physical, psychological, or interpersonal issues you must address in order to restore life balance. Some types of stress are considered a positive action force rather than a problem to control. Optimal amounts of these types of stress, called **eustress**, energize and may even heighten dancers' performance. As stress factors multiply or become chronic, mental *dis*tress (the opposite of *eu*stress) sets in, and it may eventually lead to **burnout** (Mainwaring & Aujla, 2017; Quin et al., 2005; Taylor & Estanol, 2015). Once you identify the causes of your distress, you will be in a better position to either take appropriate self-care measures or find solutions to deal with stressors over which you have no control.

WWW Go to HK*Propel* for a list of distress and anxiety symptoms in the Common Mental Health Challenges resource.

Anxiety

While stress is an instinctive and global bodily response, **anxiety** is an emotional and mental reaction to an anticipated future event or situation that does not exist yet or is unlikely to exist. Anxiety disorders affect an average of 40 million people in the United States per year (ADAA, 2021), and they cover a wide range of types and degrees of intensity. Anxiety manifests itself in one's body, mind, social interactions, and behaviors.

Anxiety disorders have nothing to do with a dancer's ill-will or attention-seeking, but usually result from a mixture of biological and psychological factors. For example, your family may be genetically inclined to react anxiously to unexpected or challenging events. Chemical changes in the brain may alter your ability to self-regulate stress efficiently and, therefore, produce physical responses typical of anxiety states (e.g., fight/flight/freeze). This explains why some dancers are born with anxious personality traits that affect the way they perceive and react to daily events, while others only feel anxious when faced with a challenge.

Psychological factors of anxiety include how you learned to think about certain situations or cues, the fears you associate with events (e.g., forgetting choreography), and finally, the amount of control you believe you have over situations. Adverse Childhood Experiences (ACE) can also have an impact on how you currently react to events and deal with anxiety. Lastly, anxiety symptoms can be induced by medication and other substances such as caffeine, alcohol, and drug use, as well as in certain medical conditions (e.g., infections).

Given the high levels of stress dancers usually contend with in daily practice, it is useful to distinguish between various types of anxiety disorders and learn how to cope with more serious signs of anxiety. Below are two common forms of anxiety experienced by dancers.

Adjustment disorders are not classified in the *DSM-5* under anxiety disorders, but are characterized by anxiety symptoms stemming from an acute stressor. Common events in the dance world such as an injury, the loss of a contract, a poor performance, relationship issues, or even a joyous event (e.g., obtaining a principal role in a show) may trigger an adjustment disorder with anxiety symptoms.

Performance-only anxiety disorder, commonly known as *stage fright*, is a form of social anxiety and is based on the subjective fear of not being on par with artistic challenges and events. Prior to performing, you may suddenly get very tense, have butterflies in your stomach, or feel the urge to urinate. According to scholars, a certain degree of pre-performance nervousness—or jitters—provides an optimal level of arousal that enhances artistic excellence. Normally, these reactions subside during or after the artistic event (Mainwaring & Aujla, 2017).

Regardless of talent or experience, performing artists commonly report having problems dealing with performance anxiety at some point. Anxious performers may often feel torn between their desire to share their artistry with the audience and irrational fears of proving inadequate and being humiliated or rejected.

If you have perfectionistic tendencies, are hyper-competitive with peers, seek social recognition, or are overly focused on end-results, you are prone to experiencing performance-only anxiety symptoms. They can include catastrophic and negative thinking, intense fears (e.g., fear of forgetting, being criticized, or disapproved), distractibility, feeling irritable or emotionally unstable, and feeling out of control (Kenny, 2011). You also may sabotage your chances of success with self-defeating behaviors (e.g., arriving late, procrastinating). High levels of performance anxiety are liable to back-fire and trigger debilitating levels of stress that could hinder your ability to dance and heighten your injury risk.

If you experience anxiety almost daily for six months or more, have a very sudden onset with physical symptoms (similar to symptoms of heart problems), or anxiety impacts your ability to leave your home or spend time with people, you may need professional counseling or medication to help you cope with your circumstances. Moreover, a dancer exhibiting anxiety disorder symptoms often suffers from depression and vice versa. According to the Anxiety & Depression Association of America (2021), nearly one-half of those diagnosed with depression also are diagnosed with an anxiety disorder.

Depression

Dancers often go through difficult episodes of sadness or physical or emotional fatigue, due to high performance demands. However, normal depressed states (e.g., being moody after a bad day or a disappointing outcome) are usually temporary and should not be confused with mood disorders or grieving after a painful loss.

Clinical **depression** is a fairly common mood disorder. According to the Anxiety and Depression Association of America (ADAA) (2021), in 2017, 6.7 percent of all adults in the United States had experienced at least one major depressive episode in the past year. Depressive illness is identified with the following ailments (figure 8.4): low mood most of the day; lowered interest in activities you usually enjoy; significant changes in weight, appetite, or sleeping habits; feeling agitated or without energy; impaired concentration and decision-making abilities; feelings of worthlessness or toxic guilt; and thoughts about death or suicide, with or without a plan (American Psychiatric Association, 2022).

No matter how resilient you are, you may experience depressive symptoms at some point in your career due to a wide number of reasons, including poor self-esteem and body dissatisfaction, financial hardship, social isolation or relationship turmoil, social inequity and discrimination of minority groups, and traumatic interpersonal experiences. In addition, difficult career transitions or severe injury can prevent you from dancing for a long period or even end your career. These events can challenge your sense of self and purpose in life, which are deeply ingrained in dance (McGuire, 2016).

As with anxiety, depressive disorders may vary in duration and severity. The following disorders are seen most commonly in dancers:

› *Adjustment disorder with a depressed mood* elicits symptoms of depression that are triggered within 3 months of the occurrence of a stressor, which usually involves a major change in your life (positive or negative). Even if your distress is out

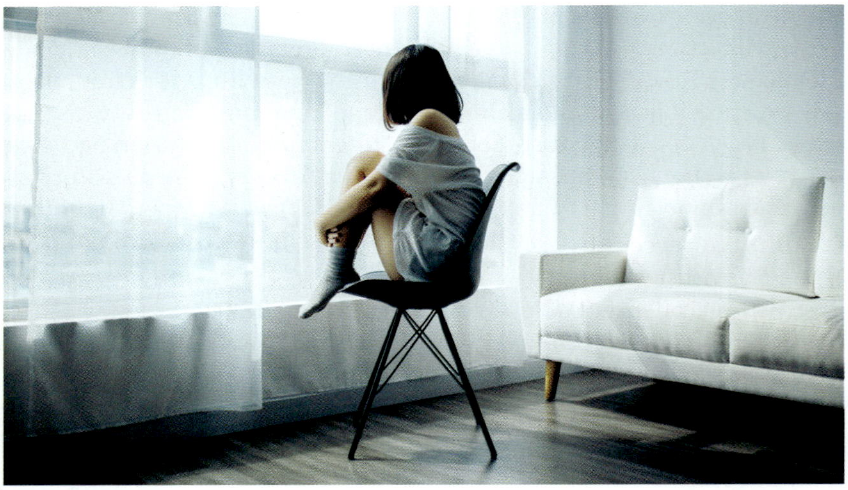

Figure 8.4 Isolating oneself, lowered mood, and disinterest in one's usual activities are three signs that may indicate depression.
Anthony Tran on Unsplash

of proportion with the situation and impairs your daily functioning, symptoms will likely resolve within 6 months as you adapt to your new reality or the stressor subsides. Short-term support is usually effective in facilitating your recovery.

› *Premenstrual dysphoric disorder* (PMDD) involves significant physical and psychological symptoms during specific phases of a female dancer's menstrual cycle. These symptoms may include mood swings, irritability, and low self-esteem. Premenstrual dysphoric disorder is distinct from (and more serious than) premenstrual syndrome (PMS).

› *Postperformance depression* is a nonclinical form of depression that is very common among dancers following a significant show or series of shows, a disappointing performance, or receiving negative feedback. This body–mind letdown process manifests itself as a general decrease in energy level; feelings of sadness, listlessness, and irritability; harsh self-criticism; ruminating on flaws following performances; and, at times, a loss of purpose related to one's art.

WWW Go to the HK*Propel* resource Common Mental Health Challenges for more on this topic.

Contrary to more serious depressive disorders, this adjustment process is necessary for physical and psychological recovery from the stress of high-intensity performing. When the curtain falls on a final performance in a run, you may also have to deal with a brief mourning period related to the joys, thrills, and sense of personal identity connected with your project (La Flèche, 2018; Taylor & Estanol, 2015).

Generally, you should consider seeking help if you are experiencing depression symptoms for a sustained period of 2 weeks or longer, or if you have dramatic swings ranging from manic joy to depressive states. Individual and group psychotherapy sessions may be useful for dancers coping with depression.

A Culture of Silence and Pain

Before considering self-care and injury risk reduction measures, this section reflects on the tremendous and covert impact of stoicism and power-based relationships on dancers' global wellness. Silencing discomfort and pain can eventually cause great damage to dancers' mental and physical health. Identifying such negative behaviors and replacing them with proper self-care will help dancers achieve their full potential.

Stoicism and the Stigma of Vulnerability

Western concert dance has always valued aesthetic and performance perfection, risk-taking, and **stoicism** (showing indifference to pain or hardship) to obtain artistic excellence. Despite massive research-based evidence that promotes dancers' self-care, implicit pressures to succeed at all costs remain culturally accepted. The tough competitiveness of the dance world may lead to body neglect or misuse. Pain and injury are often falsely considered as part and parcel of dance, indeed as signs of technical improvement or even as types of war trophies. Many dancers learn from an early age to repress bodily feelings (e.g., hunger, thirst, fatigue) to achieve their goals (Alexias & Dimitropoulou, 2011; Pickard, 2012).

Because of the culture of accepting pain and risk-taking, the ability to withstand hardship and cruelty is linked to artistic excellence (Lakes, 2005; McEwen & Young, 2011; Papaefstathiou et al., 2013; Rip et al., 2006). Warning signs of physical or psychological imbalance may be ignored or downplayed because of obsessive passion. After all, *the show must go on!* Dancers report having danced injured or returned to training too soon following an injury out of fear of losing a role or a contract. Unattended needs lead to growing exertional pain and injuries that may hamper or even terminate dance practice (Akehurst & Oliver, 2014; Fortin et al., 2009; Rip et al., 2006).

Power Structures and Toxic Competition

Most professional dancers enter recreational dance school in childhood and graduate in their early twenties. Students quickly learn and assimilate the rules, values, and traditions of the institution and dance genre (e.g., attire, hairdo, class routines). These values and practices become deeply ingrained into their ways of thinking, feeling, and reacting. For you as a dancer, **personal identity** is fused with your dancing body as you actively engage in your artistic project (Pickard, 2013). Because you *become* your dance, you look up to successful dance teachers with high regard; you see them as gateways to fulfilling your dreams.

On the other hand, dance is a **power-based culture** that stems from a long heritage of authoritarian pedagogy. Teachers and directors are most often viewed as gurus, and they have enormous influence on dancers' careers. Due to high social status, the teachers' and directors' attitudes and behaviors are rarely discussed, while dancers are expected to be docile and speedy learners who mold their body-machines to accommodate their mentors' requirements. Power plays out in dance classes and rehearsals regardless of teachers' goodwill (e.g., their intention may be to help). Since painful experiences are normalized in the dance culture, you may have trouble recognizing doubtful or abusive teaching practices and seeking help. Emotional and physical harm often result from well-intentioned, shame-based dance instruction (Forcier, 2017; Green, 2001; Kelly, 2012; Lakes, 2005; Moola & Krahn, 2018).

Regardless of their dance genres, most professional companies and preprofessional schools are based on hierarchy and fierce competition. Young dancers are highly vulnerable to unfair treatment and **body exploitation** by powerful principal dancers or authority figures; they feel they must pay this price as they actively seek to move up in the pecking order. For this reason, a code of silence prevails in the dance community in regard to all forms of maltreatment, including sexual offenses (Green, 2001; Forcier, 2017; Lakes, 2005; Moola & Krahn, 2018; Pickard, 2012; Wingenroth, 2018). As in sports, maltreatment and abuse in dance stem from power structures and practices in a culture that has failed to recognize and prevent such problems; this jeopardizes dancers' physical and psychological integrity (Mountjoy et al., 2016; Papaefstathiou et al., 2013).

Gender disparity between dancers contributes to power struggles. In dance, females outnumber males by far; therefore, if you are a female dancer, the competition in your field is higher. In other words, you must work harder to obtain a teacher's or director's approval as well as to eventually gain dance favors such as desirable roles. You may fear displeasing an authority figure, losing artistic status, or losing already scarce dance contracts. Many female artists silence their personal needs and discomforts or rely on male partners to voice the group's needs (Fortin et al., 2009).

On the other hand, as part of the privileged few, male dancers have special status throughout their career, holding power in most professional dance schools and companies. Training or academic requirements may be more easily tailored to accommodate male dancers' desires or limitations to ensure their continued participation in dance. Men who transition out of their performance career often continue to occupy leadership positions in a largely female world. Statistics from the Dance Data Project (2021) show that during the 2019 to 2020 season, only 28 percent of artistic directors of the top U.S. professional dance companies were women, and they were paid a third less than their male counterparts. In addition, 72 percent of the total works presented during the 2019 to 2020 season were created by men.

Traumatic Experiences in Dance

Statistics indicate that 60 percent of men and 50 percent of women in the United States have a history of at least one trauma in their lives. Moreover, 7 to

Examples of Psychological Abuse in Dance

1. A female dancer with a balanced silhouette recalls her ballet teacher constantly calling her the nickname "Tubby." For years following that experience, she battled with anorexia.
2. A lead dancer giving a technique class, believing that one of his male pupils was not lean enough, asked the pupil to hold his extended leg in the air as punishment for eating too much. The lead dancer told the student, "You fed it [the leg], now hold it!"

8 percent of the U.S. population experiences symptoms of **post-traumatic stress disorder (PTSD)**, including depression, flashbacks, nightmares, and panic episodes (U.S. Department of Veterans Affairs, 2020; Stop Street Harassment, 2018). According to Thompson and Jaque (2016), in the United States PTSD prevalence rates climb to 25 percent for dancers and 13 percent for athletes. Clinical symptoms in both populations correlate highly with experiences of intentionally perpetrated sexual or nonsexual trauma. Experiences of dancer maltreatment were first reported in the late 1970s, but abusive practices have been tolerated for many years prior. Dancers who have lived through traumatic events have been governed by a code of silence. In general, these events fall into the four main categories described next.

Self-Directed Abuse

Excess body objectification and stoicism eventually lead to the absence of self and one's misuse of their body—if it seems to serve the dancer's interests and goals (e.g., to become thinner). A lack of body and emotional awareness disrupts one's ability to self-regulate basic needs such as hunger and thirst and one's ability to respect personal limits (Alexias & Dimitropoulou, 2011; Fortin et al., 2009; Jackson, 2005; La Flèche, 2019; La Flèche, 2020; Pickard, 2012; Ritenburg, 2010). **Self-directed abuse** also relates to the neglect and normalization of discomfort, pain, and injury, which lead to physical or emotional distress. For instance, you may not distinguish routine performance pain from injury pain, especially if you feel fearful of the possible consequences of that pain (Fortin et al., 2009; Moola & Krahn, 2018).

Psychological Abuse

Sport science research shows that sexual, physical, and psychological abuse are highly correlated (Parent & Fortier, 2018); this correlation may apply to dancers, too. With the explosion of social media platforms, cyberbullying (which is a form of abuse) has become frequent and highly problematic for young, vulnerable dancers who are sensitive to social judgment. Intentionally aggressive verbal and nonverbal behaviors perpetrated by mentors or peers are very harmful. For athletes, rejection and deliberate denial of attention or training are particularly devastating (Kveton-Bohnert, 2017; Papaefstathiou et al., 2013; Stirling & Kerr, 2013). Unfortunately, various forms of inequity and discrimination plague the dance world (as in wider society), and they add to the negative psychological load. For instance, a substantial racial imbalance is observed in dance, especially in ballet. Black female dancers are underrepresented in predominantly white American ballet companies. While dance companies such as the Alvin Ailey American Dance Theater and the Dance Theatre of Harlem are notable exceptions, they certainly do not represent a trend of racial inclusion among dance organizations.

Physical Abuse

Harmful training practices go unnoticed due to dancer stoicism and silencing (Kveton-Bohnert, 2017). In sports, neglect is considered another form of physical abuse (Mountjoy et al., 2016). This abusive practice may also occur in dance. For instance, preprofessional dancers have reported to the authors feeling uncomfortable about asking a choreographer for a break after hours of rehearsing. They feared being perceived as unmotivated and losing dance roles.

Sexual Abuse

Since 2018, an increased number of cases of sexual misconduct from fellow dancers and dance community members occupying positions of power have been disclosed. Sport research shows that sexually abusive coaches use different tactics with female victims than with male victims. Females are likely to be subjected to intimate behaviors and manipulative strategies, such as being pressured to pose nude or in sexually provocative positions. Male victims may experience more aggressive and intrusive behaviors, such as being shown pornography or pushed into

Examples of Physical Abuse in Dance

1. During private classes, a professional ballet dancer reported feeling uneasy due to her teacher repeatedly squeezing the back of her neck for so-called alignment purposes. The teacher persisted in this action despite the dancer's pleas for him to stop. When she confronted him about it, the teacher stopped coaching her.
2. Numerous dancers have reported being pressured to dance while injured or before fully recovering from an injury. Their refusal to dance under those circumstances was covertly considered a lack of commitment.

sex under the influence of alcohol (Brackenridge et al., 2008).

A key factor found in most sexual abuse is a process of grooming a target victim by a perpetrator. Elliott (2017) proposed a self-regulation model of sexual grooming that comprises two phases: (1) the *potentiality phase* of strengthening the relationship, providing rewards, breaking down inhibitions, and creating security; and (2) the *disclosure phase*, during which the target victim is desensitized and gradually and purposefully introduced to information and actions that lead to the abuse. This type of methodology is the perpetrator's attempt to achieve their goal with a minimum of resistance and without detection by authorities. Sadly, research shows that dancer maltreatment is likely to be ignored because when considered separately, each episode may seem negligible in that moment. However, the accumulation of abusive situations may become traumatic over time, and it may affect dancers' overall wellness (Moola & Krahn, 2018).

Winds of Change

Since the advent of the *Me Too* movement in 2017, the abusive landscape is slowly changing. Allegations of misconduct perpetrated within prestigious U.S. and European dance companies have multiplied. Dancers—along with dance scholars, teachers, and administrators—have begun to address this delicate but important topic. This chapter attempts to do the same.

According to Angyal (2021), dancers are now more willing to voice their experiences of interpersonal maltreatment in public dance literature. These articles have brought increasing awareness and discussion in the dance space. Growing attention is now being given to the specific needs of marginalized communities and to developing new initiatives that include mental health skills training. Nonetheless, great effort is still needed to eradicate abuse, violence, and discrimination in an effort to make the dance space a safe and happy place for all stakeholders.

Given the systemic risk factors of abuse and maltreatment, sport studies advocate for a multipronged approach to ensure personal safety and prevent further trauma (Mountjoy et al., 2016). This approach involves engaging all members of the dance community—including institutions, administrators, teachers, parents, and dancers—to identify the first warning signals and act quickly. Everyone must gain knowledge and openly discuss abuse and violence, their causes, and the silencing of those who experience them. The first step in this approach is becoming aware of your own abusive attitudes or behaviors as well as those of others, no matter how small or insignificant they may seem.

Open communication and valuing other people's views and feelings are essential. You are encouraged to cultivate embodied self-awareness, learn more about your rights and responsibilities, express personal needs and discomforts, identify and disclose abuse (as a victim or a witness), and reflect on personal traps (e.g., an excessive desire to please others). Self-care and empowerment measures are described in the next section.

Mental Health Tools and Self-Care Measures

Self-care is a crucial part of maintaining your mental health. It falls on your shoulders to participate in and achieve self-care as a means of reducing your likelihood of being adversely affected by mental concerns. Self-care measures help you cultivate psychological wellness, self-discipline, and resilience. You are encouraged to experiment with and adapt the tools offered in this section according to what works best for you.

Balanced Life Habits

With heavy schedules and long hours, maintaining personal equilibrium can be very demanding for dancers, regardless of social context (recreational, preprofessional, or professional dance). All too often, you may end your dance day feeling exhausted and left with very little spare time for yourself. Nonetheless, you should devote some personal time to rest and recover physically and psychologically. This time is necessary to help you recharge your body's energy systems, restore tissue damage caused by high-level dance activity, and prepare to perform efficiently the next day. By doing so, you will also lower your risk of injury by refreshing your fatigued state.

At least 1 hour before sleeping, create a relaxation ritual based on your favorite activities. Take a walk, enjoy a warm bath, listen to soft music, read a book, or draw. To better engage in restful sleep just before bedtime, try deep breathing while imagining yourself in a safe and happy space. As a general principle, it is best to ignore the urge to use your phone or computer, or to watch television, as these keep your brain stimulated and make it harder to fall asleep. In addition, sleep quality has been associated with both alcohol and cannabis use, such that individuals—especially young adults—who use more alcohol and cannabis report poorer sleep (Troxel et al., 2022).

Dancers are increasingly aware of the importance of well-balanced eating to attain their performance goals and reduce injury risk. Despite a tight schedule, you should never sacrifice sufficient food intake and hydration. Taking time off from dancing to snack or share a good meal with others is also a great way to relax and experience pleasure. As with rest and sleep, occasionally skipping meals may not be overly detrimental, but doing so consistently over time could lead to malnutrition which opens the door to body imbalance and injury (e.g., osteoporosis, stress fractures), not to mention depression and anxiety.

To stay balanced and motivated, you must also learn to do, think, and talk about topics other than dance—no matter how passionate you are about dancing. Taking part in a variety of activities (especially some you have never done before) and staying in touch with family and nondancer friends will help maintain a safe emotional distance between you and your art, and it can prevent you from falling into obsessive passion that can lead to losing your sense of self. By developing other skills and interests, you also refuel your energy and nourish your joy for dance.

Breathing, Relaxation, and Mindfulness

Efficient breathing is essential for dancers' energy intake and body self-regulation during and outside of dance practice. Many dancers become so wrapped up in their practice that their breathing is disrupted; they get very tired or tense. These occurrences may reduce performance and heighten injury risk. Taking time to relax and breathe deeply in a mindful way (figure 8.5) raises moment-to-moment somatic awareness, and it enables you to address your needs and limits accordingly.

If you are tired, intense breathing (e.g., repeated, hard exhaling) increases your drive and focus. On the other hand, deep, slow breathing reduces your heart rate and stress level while also alleviating body tension and negative thoughts. Slower breathing also improves dance flow and recovery between sessions (Karin et al., 2017; Mainwaring & Aujla, 2017; Taylor & Estanol, 2015). In light of this information, while you breathe mindfully, try slowing down your pace in daily activities to restore energy as you go.

Many deep breathing and relaxation exercises are available online; examples include inhaling slowly from your abdomen for 5 counts and exhaling for 6 counts. In addition, progressive muscular relaxation (PMR) training may be helpful. Although research on its application is generally confined to using it as an adjunct treatment for medical conditions, it has proven to be effective in reducing stress in a variety of situations (Aalami et al., 2016; Dehdari et al., 2009; Zhao et al., 2012). PMR involves tensing, holding, and releasing each group of muscles repeatedly. In summary, you may want to try various types of exercises before settling on the ones that best suit you.

Self-Compassion

Self-compassion refers to unconditional kindness and comfort toward self and others. Every person is fallible, and every person is faced with challenging experiences. Becoming aware and accepting of your own experiences in a clear manner—without condemning or finding excuses—arises from **mindfulness**. Self-acceptance and kindness lower stress, make you more available to dance, and nourish your sense of connectedness and collaboration with other artists. These tools also help you balance

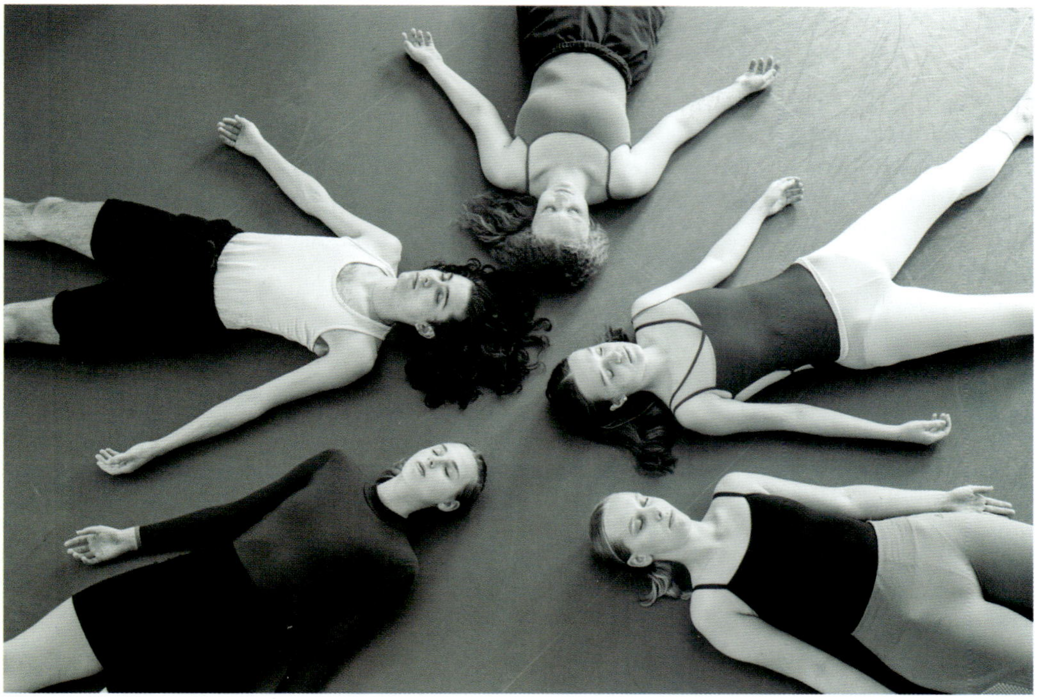

Figure 8.5 Pausing for rest, relaxation, purposeful breathing, and collecting oneself pays great dividends in the midst of a busy dancer's life.

your goals and expectations realistically as well as accept victories and mistakes as they occur. These honest acknowledgments allow you to appreciate your efforts and learning experiences along the way (Mainwaring & Aujla, 2017; Neff & Knox, 2017).

To build self-compassion, begin by practicing mindful activities such as deep breathing, relaxation, and **mental imagery**. Pinpoint harsh self-judgments, and replace them with compassionate and constructive thoughts (see the next section). Following a relaxation session, you actively engage in self-kindness. For example, imagine in vivid detail a safe place—a place where you encounter your perfect nurturer or your best friend. What would that person say to you about your flaws or setbacks?

Positive Self-Talk

Negative thoughts are usually taken for granted or considered a fixed reality. Learning to pay close attention to what you say to yourself and challenge unconstructive perceptions or reactions is vital to your psychological wellness. Try lowering expectations, and replace unhelpful or rigid thinking (described earlier) with positive self-talk. Rather than requiring yourself to be flawless, try pursuing excellence (being and doing *your* best). Talk yourself through setting clear and realistic goals, recall your past successes to build self-confidence, accept mistakes as part of learning, and focus on dancing with joy. Let dance be enjoyable!

Self-Awareness and Spiritual Wellness

Psychological wellness is closely linked to building self-awareness (discovering who you are beyond your immediate thoughts, sensations, feelings, or behaviors). Reflecting without judgment on your beliefs, values, strengths, boundaries, and ultimate goals helps you learn from past experiences and guides future actions. It also helps you relate to others in a more authentic and satisfying way. Common reflective questions might include *Why do I dance? With whom do I wish to work and why? What really matters to me? What changes could I make to be happier and pursue my goals more effectively?*

Self-awareness is a never-ending process; you evolve and change throughout your life. It requires you to take time alone to reflect on how you are feeling and where you are going. Meditative activities can be helpful, including journaling, walks in nature, and so-called *nondoing* activities such as

Managing Negative Self-Talk

Being able to counteract the negative parts of conversations you have with yourself—those lies in your mind that drag you down—requires proactive steps. Here are some examples:

- Instead of dwelling on negative events, celebrate small victories and count your blessings daily. Many people find it nourishing to be grateful for what they have.
- To fight off personalizing, view a problem as if it were someone else's. How would you recommend they handle it?
- To avoid blowing disappointing situations out of proportion, look at the big picture and place them in a larger time frame. Proper perspective will be your friend.
- Instead of black-and-white (all good or all bad) thinking, see yourself as a growing artist. Seek ways to improve and be creative.
- Add the word *yet* to soften self-criticism (e.g., "I can't complete this turn *yet*.") (Kveton-Bohnert, 2017; Mainwaring & Aujla, 2017).
- Acknowledge negative thinking, and add a challenge statement that includes a time frame to raise your performance endurance (DeWolfe et al., 2021). Instead of thinking *I am so tired, I won't make it through this rehearsal*, reframe your thinking to *I am really tired, but if I taper the intensity of my dancing for the next 30 minutes, I can safely finish the rehearsal.*

admiring the clouds and people watching (Kabat-Zinn, 2016).

Spiritual wellness is attached to your purpose for being on Earth, your life meaning, and your belief system. Mindful and self-reflective practices may lead to your quest for spiritual wellness—a desire to connect to something greater than yourself and your role on planet Earth (e.g., the universe, nature, or a religious practice)—and the need to act on your values and beliefs both within and outside of dance. Finding meaning and fulfillment in what you are doing or experiencing—no matter how vague or how small it may seem at the time—provides an extra layer of satisfaction and joy in good times and emotional support to get through adversity.

Planning Your Workload and Setting Goals

Learning to plan your daily talks and to set goals are great assets for managing your time and energy efficiently while also mitigating avoidable stress. Goal setting helps you focus more clearly on what you must do and when to do it. Short-term goals offer a sense of direction, while long-term goals serve as benchmarks for your gains. Both are needed to nurture healthy motivation.

In any given day, group your tasks in order of priority. Generally, begin with tasks that are both urgent and important, followed by those tasks that are important but less urgent. Next, either do the tasks that are urgent but less important, or—better yet—get someone to help you, or delegate all these tasks. Finally, try not to put much effort into tasks that are neither urgent nor important. One widely employed tool to assist you with this process is the Eisenhower matrix (Victorino, 2020), a planning template named after the 34th president of the United States, Dwight D. Eisenhower, who popularized its concept (figure 8.6). It provides a way to track your effectiveness at accomplishing your work. Do not neglect to reward yourself when you complete important projects!

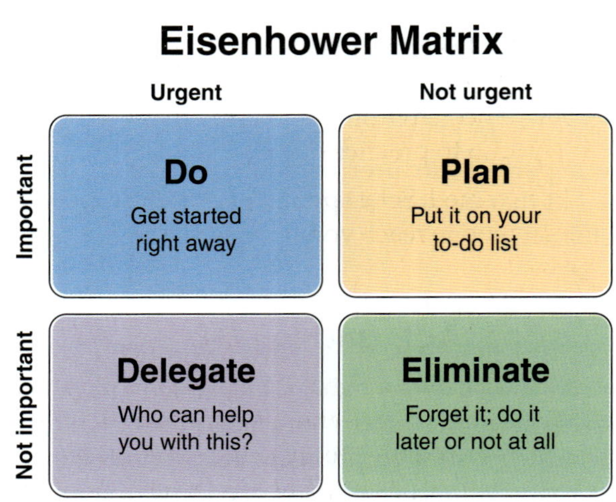

Figure 8.6 An example of an Eisenhower matrix that is used for planning how to accomplish tasks and responsibilities. It is usually used daily.

Go to HKPropel to download a blank Eisenhower matrix.

Here is another technique for completing your tasks by priority: It starts similarly to the Eisenhower method. Prepare a list of what you want to accomplish. Then begin by doing what is urgent, followed by what is important. Toward the end of your day or your week, work on those items that are less important. Within each block of work, proceed from the tasks you find the most difficult or least pleasurable to those that are easier or more fun. Overall, this process helps you reduce counterproductive behaviors such as procrastination and scattered attention while boosting feelings of self-empowerment, satisfaction, and self-esteem.

In preparing your goals, the SMART planning acronym is a widely recommended and useful approach for dancers who deal with loaded schedules (Mainwaring & Aujla, 2017; Quin et al., 2015). The letters of SMART correspond to characteristics you should build into each goal (specific, measurable, action-oriented, realistic, and time-framed). For example, imagine you want to learn to perform a double pirouette. Here are some possible SMART goals:

Specific: Define exactly what you want to achieve (e.g., a double pirouette).

Measurable: Set observable standards to track your progress (e.g., turning with proper alignment).

Action-oriented: Identify the actions needed to achieve your goals (e.g., practice daily for 10 minutes).

Realistic: Determine achievable goals, taking into account your physical and artistic abilities and your dance environment (e.g., having access to the studio to practice daily).

Time-framed: Set a specific period during which you intend to reach your goal (e.g., the day, week, year).

Choose, Act, and Let Go

Once you clarify your goals, you must make choices and act on them. Some choices may be difficult—or even heartbreaking—because they involve leaving behind someone or something you really care about. For example, moving away from family and friends to attend a preprofessional dance school is quite challenging, as is moving from your hometown to attend college several hours or more away. You cannot always have exactly what you want, but your life circumstances will be easier if you commit positively to your choices, move forward with confidence, count your blessings, and be grateful; at the same time, you can develop creative ways to remember and transform what you left behind and maintain appropriate connections so that you do not lose touch completely.

Taking action and letting go are also necessary for situations or events over which you have no control. For instance, you do your best to prepare for an audition, execute what is required as well as possible, and appreciate the learning experience, but you have no say about its outcome. Once you finish the audition, the decision is in other people's hands. You may devote time and energy to help a friend, but you cannot control how your help will be received or what actions your friend will take afterward. In such situations, you will benefit from focusing on giving your best and not concentrating too heavily on the results.

Mental Imagery

Imagery is the mental representation of objects, ideas, or situations that are stored in your memory bank or in your imagination; it forms the basic language of dance. Images are different from dreams because when you form an image, you are fully aware. Effective mental imagery, or visualization, incorporates all the senses (visual, auditory, tactile, kinetic, and olfactory). Performers and viewers both experience dance through a series of physical and mental images that affect the body's physiological and emotional states. Dancers' body mechanics are also affected by imagery. The psychological skill of creating mental images can be very effective during training and onstage. Widely used by high-level performers, this practice involves either concrete images to review dance roles or sequences, or metaphorical images to change body states and develop artistry. Mental practice has the same effect on the neuromuscular system as physical exertion. Moreover, the effect is stronger if there is a short delay between mental practice and actual work. Rehearsing mentally improves technical artistic performance and learning efficiency; it reduces distractions, it reinforces memory, and it highlights memory blanks and causes of error. Imaging successful phrases and dance scenarios may be incorporated in preperformance routines. By helping you feel better equipped mentally, imagery boosts motivation and self-confidence, which reduces performance anxiety before a production (Karin et al., 2017; Taylor & Estanol, 2016).

Furthermore, mental practice may contribute to alleviating physical strain and maintaining balanced rest and recovery during intense training and rehearsal. It prevents dancer burnout and accidents by helping you stay better attuned to your body signals, needs, and proper alignment while also identifying any triggers that may cause needless tension and anxiety. Imagery may even contribute to speeding up recovery following an injury; it allows you to stay connected with dance practice and work on your goals while you take the time to fully rest and recover before resuming regular activities (Karin et al., 2017; Taylor & Estanol, 2015).

Strong Social Network

Over time, the intensity of daily high-level dance practice forces some dancers to become estranged from family and loved ones. You may gradually stop confiding in your parents, caregivers, or others about your challenging emotions and situations to prevent them from being worried or feeling disappointed in you. This disconnection from those you care about—and who care about you—may lead you to eventually lose touch with your body and self-awareness as well as with your ability to regulate your personal needs. To maintain psychological wellness, you need to build a strong social network. You are encouraged to stay connected with trusted people (either virtually or in person) to discuss challenges you encounter, keep things in perspective, and get adequate support when needed. Keep in mind that others need you to be a strong social support for them, too (figure 8.7). In addition, you should explore current dance research and publicly available dance literature so that you can stay up-to-date with current knowledge and be able to exchange viewpoints with fellow dancers. (Chapter 3 explains how to engage with scientific literature.)

Help-Seeking Behaviors

If you feel overwhelmed by challenges or unexpected losses despite your best effort at self-care measures, you may consider seeking help from an experienced dance mentor or a mental health practitioner in your community (e.g., physician, psychologist, mental coach). These professionals can help you clarify the elements of your distress and guide you to the appropriate resource for assistance.

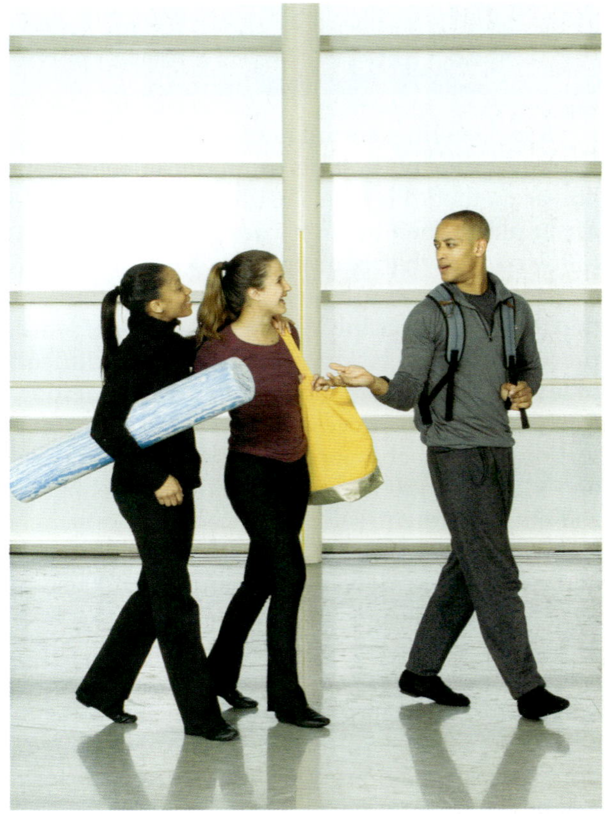

Figure 8.7 Find opportunities to encourage others in the same way that you want to be encouraged.

Any dancer with a history of depression or anxiety disorders should develop a prevention plan to deal efficiently with predictable sources of stress (e.g., dance productions, touring, academic loads). Keep a list of contact information for helpful services, consult your physician to discuss possible medications or other beneficial health measures, and schedule psychotherapy sessions during your tough times. The saying *It's okay to not be okay* is true, but it is important to seek help when necessary.

Helping Someone in Crisis

If a distressed dancer confides in you about their feelings, engage active listening procedures. In other words, listen intently without judging, trying to appease the person, or finding a quick solution. Most often, talking things over with someone who holds a compassionate ear helps people gain clarity on what they are experiencing. However, if an individual you encounter is in a mental health crisis, then in addition to active listening, you should discuss practical self-care and help-seeking measures with them (figure 8.8).

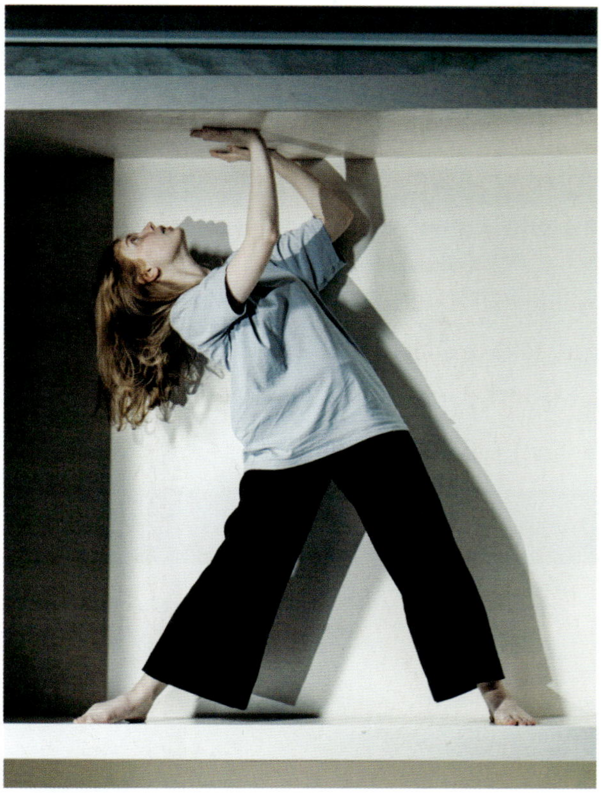

Figure 8.8 Someone experiencing a mental health crisis may feel trapped. Learn the appropriate methods of guiding them toward the care they need.

Mart Production on Pexels

If you fear for the person's life or physical integrity, discuss your feelings openly and encourage them to consult a health care professional. Never promise confidentiality if the person's life is in danger or if they are in a crisis. In the United States, immediately call 988 (emergency number for mental health challenges) or 911 (if 988 is not available in your area). Other countries have their own numbers for summoning emergency care. Do your best to support and guide the person in distress toward helpful resources. Do not take on the role of a mental health professional unless you are licensed to do so. It may be difficult to watch the circumstances unfold, so summon professional assistance. Ultimately, the outcome is up to the person unless they are an imminent danger to themselves or others.

If you want to equip yourself for helping people with mental health challenges, consider earning a certification in mental health first aid. The certification course is offered in the United States (www.mentalhealthfirstaid.org/) and in many other countries (https://mhfainternational.org/). It is intended to help you be an effective first responder when you come across someone who is experiencing a mental health crisis.

Conclusions and Practical Relevance

Many factors contribute to overall wellness. These factors have a deep impact on the instance of injury and length of recovery, and they also affect virtually every other part of dancers' well-being. If you want to be successful and healthy as a dancer, caring for your mental health is just as important as caring for your physical health. Foundational aspects of dance training—including perfectionism, criticism of a dancer's body, and lowered self-esteem resulting from these standards in dance—may poorly impact your mental health as well as lead to physical injury if they are not attended to properly.

While the correlation between mental and physical health is accepted in the wider medical community, dance culture has been slow to follow; fortunately, this is beginning to change. Dancers may find themselves in both training and professional spaces where best practices to support mental health are not in place. Thus, it is important that you understand the most common mental health challenges dancers face, recognize the early signs of distress, and identify resources available to you. Participating in unconstructive life habits is detrimental to your well-being, so incorporate the tools provided in this chapter as you move forward in dance and any other field in which you find yourself.

The dance community has a shared responsibility to confront its culture of silence, to embrace its vulnerability, and to celebrate the whole dancer—that human being who is dancing. As people in this community achieve greater ranks or positions of power, they must find ways to make dance a more supportive and inclusive environment so that the art form can thrive while producing happy, fulfilled people within it. You, dear dancer, are the future. You have the opportunity more than anyone else to increase the winds of change through own your self-care, empathy, and actions every single day that you enter a studio or step onto a stage.

In closing, please go to appendix A which provides a wealth of resources to help you find mental health support for yourself or others.

Discussion Questions

1. When you consider dance aesthetics, what do you think of the current efforts of inclusion and diversity to change the traditional ideals of the female and male dancing bodies?
2. In what ways may poor body image predispose dancers to develop eating disorders?
3. In order to prevent burnout, what distress symptoms should you watch for in your daily dance practice?
4. What obstacles can you identify that may contribute to the culture of silence in dance?
5. What steps or actions would you suggest a dancer take to alleviate toxic perfectionism?
6. What unconstructive life habits could you change to take better care of your global wellness? What practical tools could you use?

WWW Go to HK*Propel* to access supplemental information and activities connected to chapter content.

9

First Aid and Emergency Planning for the Studio and Stage

Kevin M. Brown, MEd, ATC
Melody Hrubes, MD
Laura Santos, MS, LAT, ATC

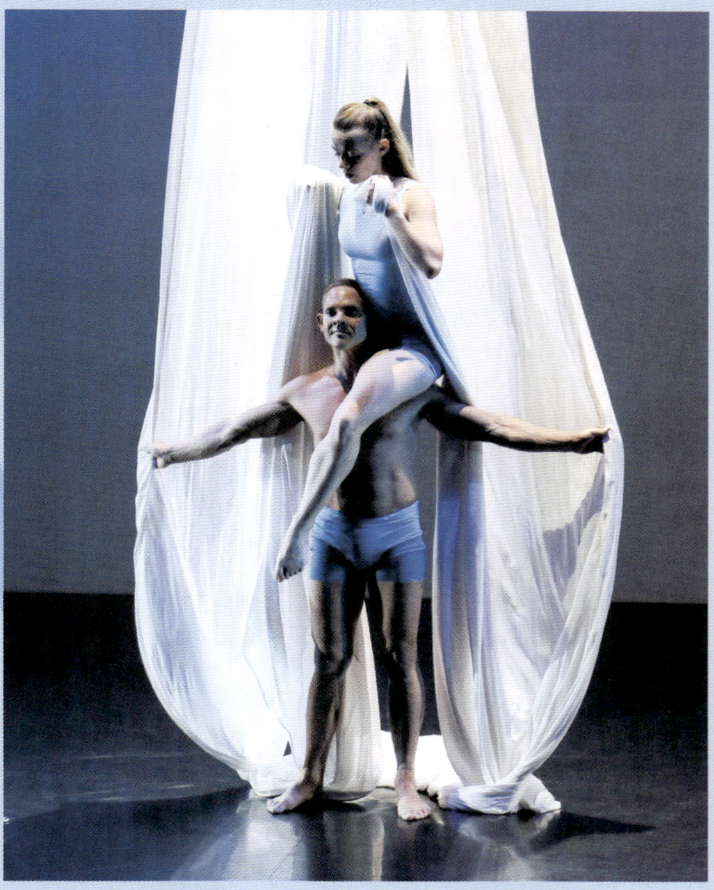

Case Western Reserve University Department of Dance, Cleveland, Ohio. Katherine Averill and Richard Oaxaca in Karen Potter's "Into the Wind". Photo: Brad Petot

When injury strikes a dancer—indeed, it is likely to strike at some point—it will usually occur when a health care professional is not in the immediate vicinity. Therefore, dancers and dance teachers must know the basics of how to handle such a situation, including one that is an emergency. Well-devised advance plans combined with calm, rational management during an injury event are the keys to success and to ensuring that the person who is injured has the optimal opportunity for appropriate care and successful restoration to dancing.

Key Terms

- emergency action plan (EAP)
- first aid
- first responder
- immediate responder
- personal protective equipment (PPE)
- standard precautions

LEARNING OBJECTIVES

After completing this chapter, you will be able to do the following:

- Discuss the components of an emergency action plan (EAP) for a specific dance setting.
- Assess potential emergency risk.
- Determine the severity of an injury or emergency.
- Choose an appropriate response to perceived first aid or emergency situations.
- Identify typical components of a first aid kit.

A university dance program is an amalgam of students, faculty, accompanists, and other department staff. Once a program goes into production or performance, the number of people involved increases to include theater staff, technicians, and many others. As discussed in previous chapters, dance injuries are going to occur at some point and the concern is whether you are prepared for them. Increased exposures in classes, rehearsals, and performances lead to an increase in the potential for a serious injury or emergency that may require help from outside the dance program. This chapter discusses the why and how of emergency preparation for the student in a university dance program.

Role of Health and Safety in Dance Training and Performance

No, dance injuries are not fully preventable. As with injuries in general, it's *when*—not *if*—an emergency will occur in the university dance setting. As mentioned in chapter 1, while reducing potential for injury is the ultimate goal, it is not always possible. This is true for all involved, including students, teachers, technicians, musicians, and health care workers. Therefore, preparation becomes paramount to establishing an environment that feels optimized for students to work on their skills and deepen their knowledge. Planning for unexpected situations allows those involved to be prepared for any circumstance and feel confident when emergencies occur. Students must feel safe in order to fully engage in the work required for the rigors of learning in a university context. In addition, awareness of the injury risk in dance training and performance deepens student and faculty respect for themselves and others. Proper application of first aid and the knowledge of appropriate actions in emergency situations can help limit the severity of an injury, prevent additional injury, and reduce disruptions to training, both for the injured person and their peers.

Responsibility for Health and Safety

In the university setting, the responsibility for health and safety in dance training and performance is a shared one that should involve students. Health care professionals and faculty members are ideally situated to manage urgent or emergent incidents due to their experience with a variety of situations and their consistent availability during the school year. However, students should understand and take responsibility for their own safety as well as the safety of others.

When students learn emergency preparedness and management, they gain awareness of their own health risks in class and performance, and they realize that they have a stake in helping others when adverse circumstances arise. Knowing the potential risks to your own body may inform certain choices regarding risk assessment and mitigation strategies. Classes such as ballet en pointe and partnered lifting, or repetitive stress such as tap dancing, present specific physical challenges; additional challenges include the length and structure of such classes and rehearsals as well as unfamiliarity with new choreographers.

Awareness of the importance of your own health and safety can inform your decisions for how to structure your semesters in your university to prepare for your desired career. This awareness can also lead to the knowledge required to advocate for yourself when you think your health and safety are at risk, such as when you are fatigued or encounter risk due to environmental factors (table 9.1). Educating students on habits that promote health and safety reinforces self-responsibility. Students should arrive to class, rehearsals, and performances rested and alert and with an adequate level of fitness for what is expected during that time. Ultimate responsibility for the care of your own dancer's instrument—your body—belongs to you.

A university is an excellent environment to build this foundation in young dancers because it is an optimal time for them to learn it; given the transient nature of the profession (once students graduate, they may often change companies, cities, and teachers throughout their careers), the opportunity may not present itself again. Improving self-awareness, learning to monitor symptoms, and knowing how to advocate for themselves are truly their continuity of care because dancers themselves may be their only constant between contracts and locations.

In a group setting (figure 9.1), promoting safety is a shared responsibility among all involved. Faculty training is valuable in reducing injury risk (and therefore injuries). For example, one strategy could involve shortening rehearsal duration early in the semester when dancer aerobic conditioning might not be ideal. Resources vary, as does the level of preparedness, between universities. Medical services may not be consistently available, increasing the importance that everyone knows the basics of how to help in an urgent or emergent situation. Early intervention and coordination of care may be essential (depending on the type of emergency), so training in early recognition along with appropriate action may improve the outcome after an injury, and it may even save a life (Mitchell et al., 2008). **Immediate responders** are the first helpers on the scene. Depending on the situation, their main roles are to (1) initiate the emergency medical response and (2) provide care until a higher level of care becomes available.

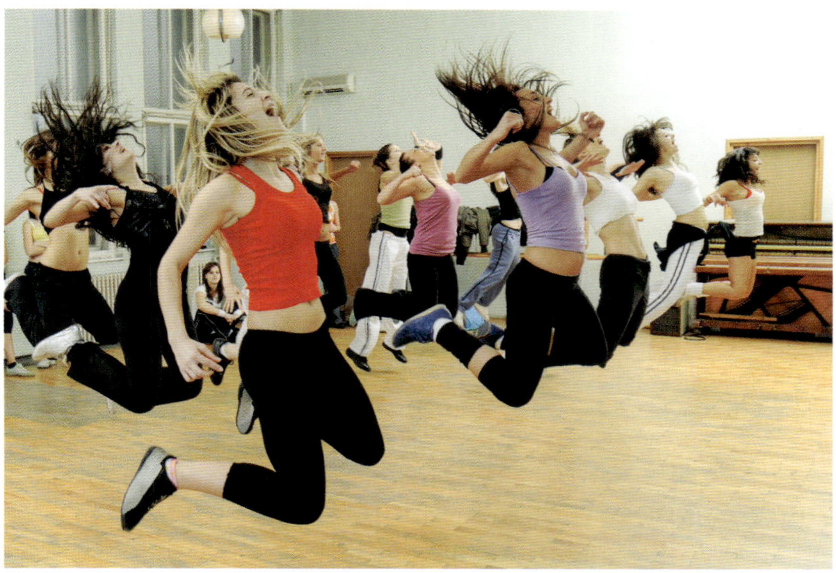

Figure 9.1 Dance often occurs in close quarters, thus increasing the likelihood of collisions that could lead to serious injuries. All members of the group share responsibility for everyone's well-being.

Dragan Trifunovic/fotolia.com

Table 9.1 Environmental Risk Factors That Can Affect the Risk of Dance Injuries

Stage floor	Weather/ambient conditions	Spacing	Visibility	Costume/equipment
Sprung (or not) Raked Steel Outdoor (grass, cement, multiple terrains)	Temperature/heat Humidity Rain or wet surfaces Lightning	Between performers Edge of stage Wall Set pieces	Strobe lighting Low lighting Intense lighting/ spotlights	Corsets Footwear Head pieces Props

Immediate responders may or may not have formal medical training, but they do serve a role that Ashkenazi and Hunt (2019) call "valuable and unique . . . in reducing mortality, morbidity, and suffering from emergency events" (p. 1). **First responders**, on the other hand, are professionals such as police officers, firefighters, emergency medical technicians, and paramedics (titles vary internationally) (figure 9.2). Be aware of local and national laws that may exist relating to emergency circumstances. Good Samaritan laws protect individuals from criminal prosecution should they unintentionally cause harm in the course of providing assistance to an urgently ill or injured person. Some Good Samaritan laws also include a duty to assist, holding capable individuals liable if they do not aid a person in need. Research the laws in your area to understand your rights and responsibilities.

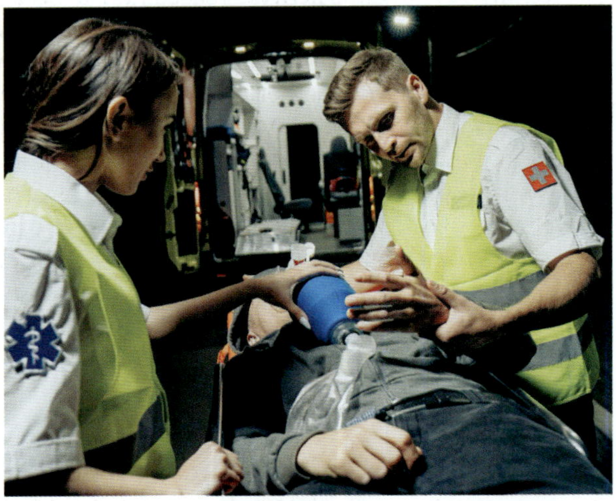

Figure 9.2 First responders are trained professionals who take over care from immediate responders at the scene of an emergency.

Mikhail Nilov on Pexels

How to Manage Emergencies as an Immediate Responder

An essential early step in any emergency response is to determine the level of care needed. Summoning appropriate help is the next step, and the third is to apply lifesaving measures within the scope of your training. Certification in first aid, cardiopulmonary resuscitation (CPR) or basic life support (BLS), and mental health first aid are important preparatory measures for both dancers and dance teachers. Training resources are listed later in this chapter.

Signs of a Health-Related Emergency

As an immediate responder, you should observe the scene to gather as much information as you can about the situation. Quickly interview affected persons and bystanders. Observe how many people appear to be ill or injured, and note their current level of injury. Look for indications of a life- or limb-threatening injury. If you note any of the signs of a health-related emergency found in table 9.2, contact emergency medical services immediately to summon first responders to the scene. If you are unsure about the severity of an illness or injury, err on the side of caution; contact emergency medical services.

Table 9.2 **Common Signs of a Health-Related Emergency**

Sign	Details to watch for
Loss of consciousness	Completely lax body Unresponsiveness to attempts to arouse
Trouble breathing	Shortness of breath, wheezing, gasping, shallow or rapid breathing that may be accompanied by skin color changes (bluish, grayish)
Severe bleeding	Rapid loss of blood
Altered consciousness	Confusion, garbled speech, disorientation to time and place
Severe deformity	Bone broken and/or protruding through the skin Joint/limb at odd angle(s)
Severe neck or back pain following trauma	Fall from greater than standing height Collision

Safety Considerations

In responding to an emergency, take care to avoid potential harm to yourself and others. When forming your initial impression of the circumstances, consider whether the scene is safe for you to enter into or remain in. Check for hazards such as slippery floors, sharp or falling objects, live electricity, or fire. If the scene is too unsafe for you to enter into or to stay in, move to a safe place and call for help. If necessary and possible, bring any ill or injured people with you.

Standard Precautions

There is a principle in health care that when providing care, one should assume that both the caregiver and the patient may be carrying and be capable of transmitting harmful pathogens. Health care professionals use physical barriers and take other measures to limit or prevent infection. This combination of risk mitigation approaches is called **standard precautions** (Centers for Disease Control and Prevention, 2019). People who are not health care professionals should also employ these tools when possible to lessen the risk of infection when providing care to others.

Personal protective equipment (PPE) is one of the most important features of standard precautions (figure 9.3). Gloves, face masks, eye shields, and gowns provide physical barriers to keep blood, saliva, respiratory droplets, and other bodily fluids away from entry points such as broken skin, the eyes, the nose, and the mouth. Other components of standard precautions include handwashing before and after providing care; managing supplies to avoid contamination between patients; following cough etiquette; and following protocols to clean and disinfect surfaces, instruments, and equipment (World Health Organization, 2007). Even in an urgent scenario, taking the time to use PPE and incorporate appropriate controls is important for the health and safety of everyone involved.

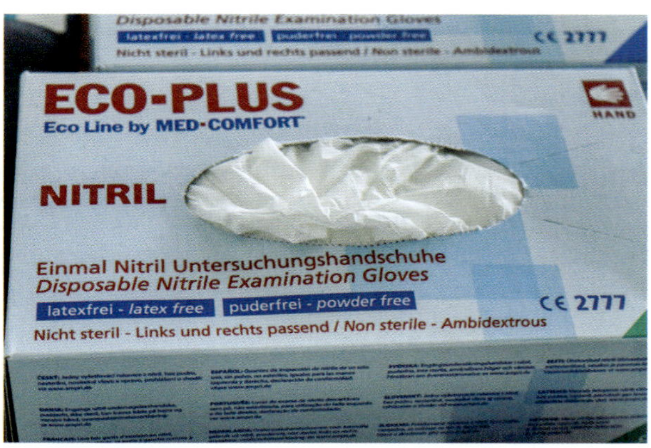

Figure 9.3 Gloves are the first pieces of PPE that should be available to immediate responders. Depending on the circumstances, a mask, eyewear, and a disposable gown may be added. PPE gloves should be made of hypoallergenic material (e.g., nitrile) rather than latex.

Alexander Fox via Pixabay

First Aid Knowledge for the University Dancer

Fortunately, catastrophic injuries are rare occurrences in dance (Vassallo et al., 2017). Injuries that are serious but nonemergent are more likely to occur in the studio and onstage. When these accidents happen, immediate responders providing timely care on-site can limit further harm and serve as a bridge to same- or next-day professional medical attention. **First aid** is the early care provided for an acute injury or illness. For injury, the type of care required depends on the type of injury that occurs. This type of care is the focus of the following section. Some forms of care beyond first aid are presented in other chapters about specific body regions.

Wounds

Barefoot dancing, partnering, and floor work may expose dancers to injuries that disrupt the skin, creating open wounds. The four major types of open wounds are as follows:

- *Lacerations* are cuts. They can be shallow or deep. They are often the result of contact with sharp objects, such as pieces of broken glass or protruding pieces of metal.
- *Abrasions* are injuries to the superficial layers of skin. A floor burn is a common type of abrasion in contemporary dance, breaking, and other dance styles that include slides and falls. An open blister can be considered an abrasion because it likely started from continual friction on an area of the body.
- *Puncture wounds* occur when an object with relatively small surface area (and often pointed) is driven into the skin and perhaps into deeper tissues. Stepping on a nail is a classic mode of sustaining a puncture wound. In some puncture wounds, all or part of the penetrating object remains in the body.

› *Avulsions* are tearing away of the skin and other tissues. An avulsion occurs as a companion to shearing (sideways) force application.

First aid for wounds requires initial compression to stop active bleeding. Apply pressure to the area with a gloved hand and a piece of clean, absorbent material (paper towel, gauze, or clean article of clothing, if nothing else is available). Continue applying pressure until the bleeding slows or stops.

Among its variety of functions, skin acts as a barrier to potentially infectious pathogens. It is important to clean and cover wounds in a timely manner; doing so can prevent infections and scarring. Use a combination of soap and running water to clean simple wounds. If a sink is not available, bottled water or a saline rinse (found in some first aid kits) are acceptable alternatives (Singletary et al., 2020). Once the area is rinsed, pat it dry, and apply a clean bandage.

Certain wounds require urgent (within hours) medical intervention for the best outcomes. They include the following:

› Wounds that are very deep or will not stop bleeding require appropriate investigation and bleeding control measures (e.g., suturing). Excessive loss of blood is a medical emergency.
› Lacerations to the palm of the hand or web spaces between the fingers can affect hand function, and they may require plastic surgery intervention.
› Facial wounds may require plastic surgery intervention.
› Puncture wounds may need imaging such as an ultrasound or X-ray to completely visualize the puncturing object and prophylactic (preventive) antibiotics to protect against infection.
› Wounds resulting from contact with rusty or visibly soiled objects may indicate the need for a tetanus vaccination or booster to prevent serious infection throughout the body.

Monitor every wound over several days for signs of infection (e.g., local heat, drainage, discoloration, swelling), and seek professional care if any of those signs appear.

Traumatic Musculoskeletal Injuries

Musculoskeletal injuries involve damage to the muscles, bones, joints, or associated tissues. Acute musculoskeletal injuries occur suddenly and are often the result of accidents like slips, falls, collisions, or awkward movements.

Dislocations

A joint dislocation is an injury in which a bone that is part of a joint slips or is forced out of normal alignment. The shoulder and patella (kneecap) are common places where dislocation may occur in dancers. Ankle, toe, wrist, and finger joints also may become dislocated. Do not ask the injured person to return the joint to a normal position—nor try to force it yourself—because it may cause further damage to the joint or its surrounding tissues.

Fractures

Fractures are bone injuries; *fracture* and *break* mean the same thing when talking about bone. In the dance setting, their occurrence is secondary to high-energy incidents (e.g., slips, trips, odd jump landings, and falls). Even seasoned medical professionals often need diagnostic imaging to confirm the presence of a fracture, so in the initial response when providing first aid, it is best to assume that a bone could be fractured.

Sprains and Strains

Sprains are injuries to ligaments (tissues that connect bone to bone). They can be mild, moderate, or severe; severe sprains can result in joint instability, and they may also involve fractures. Strains, on the other hand, are stretching or tearing of muscles or tendons (tissues that connect muscle to bone). They can be mild, moderate, or severe. Complete tears can be accompanied by immediate disability and perhaps mild deformity.

Managing Traumatic Musculoskeletal Injuries

The initial management of serious traumatic musculoskeletal injuries involves minimizing movement of the affected area to prevent further stress or injury. Provide crutches (if available) to limit or eliminate weight bearing for lower-extremity injuries. A sling for the elbow or shoulder can be helpful for relieving pressure in upper-extremity injuries, or the dancer might feel more comfortable simply supporting the affected arm against their trunk with their opposite limb. Fingers or toes can be buddy taped (using tape to secure the injured digit to its neighbor) for increased stability and comfort. Someone who sustains a dislocation, fracture, or severe sprain should be transported to a medical facility with the affected area immobilized as much as possible. If there is any obvious threat to circulation or a loss of sensation in the injured limb, or if the injured area cannot be stabilized sufficiently for transport, summon emergency medical services. Moreover, do not attempt to move an individual complaining of neck or back pain after a fall or collision; keep them still and calm until first responders arrive.

Head Injuries

In dance, a blow to the head might come during a collision with another dancer, a flying object, a prop, or the ground. Such injuries also are common backstage where the lighting is subdued and props and technical equipment are present. Concussions and related injuries to the brain are addressed in chapter 14. Two facial injuries that may result from a blow to the head are nosebleeds and dental injury.

Nosebleeds

Bleeding from the nose that occurs secondary to a trauma (i.e., a fall or a blow to the head) should be evaluated medically to rule out rare but serious injury (Weir, 1997). For initial management at the scene, control bleeding by having the injured individual lean forward slightly and pinch the nostrils together, applying pressure to the lower 1/3 of the nose (Jamshaid et al., 2023). Instruct them to breathe through their mouth and hold the pressure for 5 to 15 minutes until bleeding stops. Inserting a cotton nose plug or piece of a tampon can help absorb a large amount of blood. If bleeding continues beyond 20 minutes, is severe, or if the individual is having trouble breathing, summon emergency medical services.

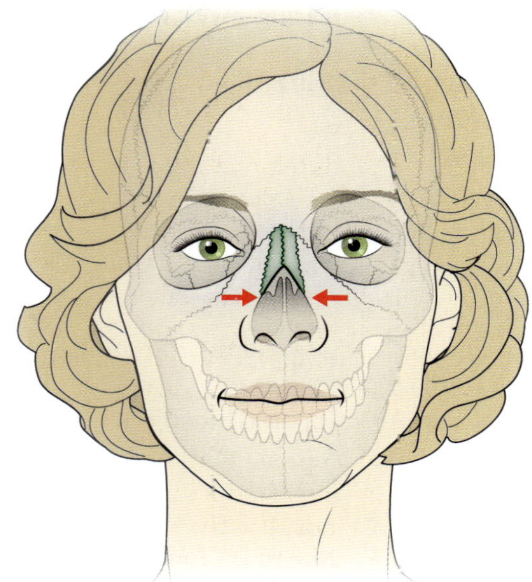

Figure 9.4 Managing a nosebleed includes application of pressure to the lower 1/3 of the nose by pinching the nostrils together.

Dental Injury

If a tooth is knocked loose in the studio, backstage, or onstage, pick it up by the crown (the part that shows in the mouth), not the root. International Association of Dental Traumatology guidelines for the management of traumatic dental injuries call for rinsing of a visibly dirty tooth with milk, saline, or saliva (Fouad et al., 2020). If possible, replace the tooth in the open socket, have the individual bite down gently on a clean cloth or piece of gauze to hold the tooth in place, and refer them to a dentist immediately. If the tooth cannot be replaced on site, place it in a solution designed for temporary tooth storage. If no such product is available, place the tooth in milk, saline, or saliva. The sooner the tooth can be stabilized in its socket, the better; therefore, urgent dental care is advised (Fouad et al., 2020). Follow the same procedure for a broken tooth without the reimplantation step. More information about managing dental injuries is available at www.iadt-dentaltrauma.org.

Whenever providing first aid care for these head injuries, remember to employ standard precautions. In the case of a wound or a nosebleed, you can offer an absorbent material to the affected dancer to apply pressure themselves while you put on gloves. Use other PPE as needed, and wash your hands when you are finished providing care.

Emergency Action Planning

Emergencies require quick and correct action, availability of the appropriate supplies, communication, and teamwork. Emergencies can involve medical, traumatic, or environmental situations that occur to an individual or a group. Figure 9.5 identifies potential emergency scenarios for which an **emergency action plan (EAP)** is needed.

Whereas injuries (whether minor, major, or emergent) are an inevitability in dance, it is important to have procedural plans should the need for advanced medical care arise. An EAP is a living document that outlines steps that will be undertaken during an emergency. The saying *Failing to plan is planning*

MEDICAL EMERGENCY

- Respiratory distress (asthma, allergy, anxiety, suffocation)
- Seizure
- Diabetic coma
- Cardiac event
- Anaphylaxis
- Drug overdose
- Compound fracture (bone protruding through the skin)
- Significant/unstoppable bleeding

Head injury

- Falling set piece
- Fallen dancer/dropped by partner
- Collision with another dancer
- Noncontact injury (e.g., whiplash)

General medical concerns

- Respiratory illness (dancer being sent home)
- Gastrointestinal illness
- Fainting/passing out
- Mental health crisis

Urgent/emergent acute injury

- Suspected spinal injury (neck or back)
- Dislocation (e.g., patella [kneecap], shoulder, etc.)
- Fracture
  - Closed
  - Displaced
- Severe sprain
- Muscle tear/tendon rupture

Blood

- Wounds
- Cuts
- Nosebleeds

Emergency of nonmedical cause

- Violence
- Active shooter
- Violent student
- Bomb threat/suspicious package
- Civil unrest
- Fire
- Explosion (nonviolent, e.g., gas main)
- Weather/acts of God
  - Earthquake
  - Severe weather/tornado/flooding

Figure 9.5 Possible circumstances requiring an EAP in dance facilities.

to fail has been attributed to many different well-known historical figures, but the sentiment remains the same. A comprehensive emergency action plan is a vital component to any university dance program as well as to any location where people are physically active. As Hernandez and Strickland (2005) acknowledge, it is incumbent on dance programs to reduce risk and provide a safe environment. As a dance student, you have an obligation to assist your fellow dancers in reducing their chance of injury as well as to help them should they become seriously injured. Additionally, if you transition to being a dance teacher, this obligation grows into a duty to keep your students safe from harm.

Emergency action planning is not only a moral and ethical standard, but a legal standard in the United States, as well. In the wrongful death legal case *Kleinknecht v. Gettysburg College* (1993), the court ultimately found in favor of the parents of an athlete who had suffered cardiac arrest on the lacrosse field. In the final ruling, it was found that the college had a duty to care for the player as well as a duty to take reasonable precautions against the risk of reasonably foreseeable life-threatening injuries. In this case, there was no EAP in place, there was significant delay in providing the athlete care because no on-site medical care was available, coaches on-site were not trained in CPR, and locked gates caused a delay in accessing the athlete. An EAP could have precluded all of these unfortunate contributors to a poor outcome. Thus, it is essential to have a comprehensive EAP to not only protect dancers and other physically active individuals should an emergency occur but also to help mitigate any liability on the university or location where an activity is taking place.

Elements of an EAP

The ultimate goal of any EAP is to make it as easy as possible to contact assistance and to get that assistance to the location of the emergency in the easiest and fastest way possible. These components must be included in a complete emergency action plan:

- Listing of personnel and their roles
- Methods of emergency communication
- Emergency equipment availability and location
- Transportation options
- Venue information and directions to access the scene

Figure 9.6 shows an example of an EAP that includes all of these components. This type of plan should be posted in the venue to which it applies; copies should be kept in the department office and with all key department leaders.

WWW Go to HK*Propel* for a blank emergency action plan template based on figure 9.6.

Personnel and Roles

The first step in constructing an EAP is to define the roles of those involved. Consider who may be at the location when an injury or other emergency occurs; it could include dance faculty, choreographers, other dance department staff, additional building staff, and the dancers. It is important that those involved know their roles should an injury or other emergency occur, be comfortable with those roles, and be willing to perform them if called upon to do so. Additionally, it is ideal that multiple people be assigned to each role to account for the potential of one being the injured party or not being present at the time of the emergency.

At a minimum, people serving as immediate responders should be designated for the following roles:

- *Scene safety*—Responsible for assessing immediate safety of the scene and providing care to the injured party. This person should be the individual with the highest degree of training in emergency and medical management.
- *Summoning help*—Responsible for calling for help. This call may be to EMS, campus police, or other appropriate parties. This person should be calm under pressure and communicate well.
- *Retrieving equipment*—Responsible for retrieving equipment from its storage location and bringing it to the emergency scene. Equipment may include an automated external defibrillator (AED), splints, ice, or anything else the immediate responders may need.
- *EMS arrival*—Responsible for coordinating EMS arrival and ensuring EMS can reach the emergency scene as quickly as possible. This role may involve drafting others into service to help direct personnel if the scene is not directly accessible (e.g., a location being on a different floor from the building access or behind a locked door).

Each of these roles is identified in the following exploration of the other EAP components.

Emergency Communication

The call for emergency help by the immediate responder assigned to this role is the most critical step in activating the EAP. You must know who to call and how to reach them. Each university, theater, and studio space will have its own idiosyncrasies. You may be able to call 911 (or your local emergency number) directly, or you may be required to contact campus security or another intermediate agency. In a situation that is nonemergent but still serious, you may be asked to contact campus health services or a medical provider within the dance department such as an athletic trainer. It is essential that this information be included in your EAP and discussed with everyone who may be responsible for making an emergency call.

Along with knowing *who* to call, it is also important to know *how* to call. EAPs should include location of the nearest landline telephone, especially in areas where cellular phone service may be limited. Wording for specific statements that provide key pieces of information can be included in the EAP to reduce the risk of mistakes when people are under the pressure of an actual emergency.

SAMPLE UNIVERSITY DEPARTMENT OF DANCE

EMERGENCY ACTION PLAN
Rehearsal Studio #2

EMERGENCY PERSONNEL:

- **Class:** Dance faculty, accompanist, other Dance Department staff as needed on site
- **Rehearsal:** Artistic staff, choreographer, other Dance Department staff as required by daily schedule on site

EMERGENCY COMMUNICATION:

- Cellular telephone on site with Dance faculty and artistic staff
- Land line telephone available at Dance Department front desk (*must dial "9" for outside line)*

EMERGENCY EQUIPMENT:

- First aid supplies available under sound system during class and rehearsals
- AED available in hallway between Studio #1 and Studio #2 (exit Studio #2 and turn left)

EMERGENCY PROCEDURES:

1. Check dancer for signs of emergency and information needed for EMS.
2. Call 911 and provide the following information:
   a. Name, location, and phone number of the caller
   b. Nature of emergency
   c. Condition of dancer(s) involved
   d. Any treatment that has been provided
   e. Directions to the emergency scene
      SAMPLE UNIVERSITY DANCE DEPARTMENT STUDIO #2
      JOHN JONES FINE ARTS BUILDING ROOM 202
      1234 SOUTH MAIN STREET
      ANYWHERE, USA 98765
      "Come to the main entrance (Door #1). Someone will be there to meet you."
   f. Other requested information
3. Call department head and Dance Department front desk to notify of emergency.
4. Meet the ambulance and direct to the appropriate site.
   a. Someone should be outside to meet the ambulance and direct to elevator
   b. Someone should be at elevator holding doors to allow immediate access and send to second floor
   c. Someone should be at elevator on second floor to direct down the hall to the right to Studio #2
5. Control the scene.
   a. Move other dancers away and limit access to the scene.
   b. Keep everyone calm.
6. Once scene is safe and care is established, contact remaining emergency contacts.

EMERGENCY PHONE NUMBERS:

Name	Position	Phone
Jane Smith	Dance Department Chair	(123) 555-1212
Bob Johnson	Dance Department Athletic Trainer	(123) 555-8989
Susan Walker	Dean, College of Fine Arts	(123) 555-4554
Dance Department Front Desk		(123) 444-3434
Campus Security		(123) 444-9191

Figure 9.6 Sample emergency action plan (EAP).

When calling for emergency help, the caller should provide these pieces of information:

- Name, location, and phone number of the caller (in case of a disconnection)
- Nature of the emergency
- Condition of the dancer involved
- Treatment currently being provided
- Directions to the scene and how to access the injured dancer

It is important to stay on the phone until all information that is requested has been provided. Let the emergency dispatcher hang up first.

Emergency Equipment

Information about available equipment and its location should be part of an EAP. It is imperative that whoever assumes the role to retrieve the necessary equipment during an emergency be able to locate and access that equipment in a timely fashion. It is equally important to ensure the equipment is accessible whenever the facility is in use. For example, an AED behind a locked door after hours will not help a patient who is experiencing cardiac arrest. Additional discussion of emergency equipment occurs later in this chapter.

Venue Information and Scene Access

The final piece of an EAP is facilitating first responders' arrival where the emergency has occurred. The immediate responder who coordinates this process assists first responders in navigating as quickly as possible any barriers that impede access. The EAP and instructions given during the emergency call should include the address of the facility as well as any room information or additional directions. However, the immediate responder identified for this coordination role must ensure proper access to the area is available and that emergency responders are directed along the most expedient route. Consider stairs, locked doors, locked gates, and other barriers to access, such as doors requiring a key card or biometric data for entrance and elevators. As discussed in the Personnel and Roles section, in order to ensure success, enough people should be assigned to this operation to direct responders and to eliminate any obstacles they may encounter.

It is important to customize your EAPs for a variety of possible situations and locations. Separate areas of the same building may have different access points or accessibility for emergency personnel. Additionally, some areas within a theater or other performance venue may provide a more complex challenge; examples include potential emergencies on the rail, on a catwalk, in a lighting grid, in a trap room, or in an orchestra pit.

Who Else to Contact

Once an emergency is under control and help has arrived, undoubtedly other individuals will need to be notified. You must keep in mind applicable privacy laws at the local or national level as well as the preference of the dancer. People on this list could include the following:

- On-site medical providers for the dance department (if they are not already present)
- Campus police or security
- Campus health service
- Dance department leadership, including the department chair, other faculty, and the dean
- Parents, roommates, or significant other of the injured dancer
- University maintenance staff, such as environmental services or physical plant workers needed for clean-up and similar functions

Communication and Rehearsal

The EAP should be periodically reviewed—and adjusted as necessary—by the department's athletic trainer or health care consultants as well as the dance faculty. No matter how well an EAP is written, if it is not executed as written, it has the potential to fail. Potter and Martin (2009) suggest scheduling frequent rehearsals of your EAP with all parties who have the potential to be involved. This rehearsal should include not only those specifically identified in the EAP, such as faculty, accompanists, and dance department staff, but also those who may be tangentially involved, such as production staff, theater staff, and dancers themselves. Like rehearsal for a performance, rehearsal of an emergency action plan ensures that the choreography of potentially saving a life goes as planned.

Posting the EAP

The best way for everyone involved to know the EAP should an emergency occur is for the EAP to be posted in conspicuous places throughout the facility. Andersen and colleagues (2002) suggest posting it near each accessible telephone. However, should the facility not have a telephone in each area an emergency could occur, a designated place can be identified to allow anyone involved to locate the specific plan for that facility. For example, this area could be near the sound system or above the light switches for the room. Additionally, having a copy near a call board or daily schedule is also a good practice.

Nonmedical Emergencies

In addition to various medical emergencies that can occur, it also is prudent to plan for nonmedical emergencies; they also happen with little warning. Such events could include weather emergencies such as severe thunderstorms with damaging winds or tornadoes, and earthquakes. Also consider strategies for events that require other emergency responses that are not medically related, including violent students, active shooters, and bomb threats. Finally, plans should be in place for events such as civil unrest or other potentially destructive events, such as a gas main explosion.

Emergency Equipment

When injuries occur—be they small or large—having the proper supplies and equipment available may be the difference between a positive and negative (or more difficult) outcome. This section discusses some common emergency equipment that is helpful in the university dance setting.

First Aid Kit

A well-stocked first aid kit is often the key to successful injury management. The kit should contain supplies for wound care, tape for joint support in the case of sprains, medications for common ailments, and emergency supplies for more serious injuries (e.g., splints). Additionally, the kit should include items of PPE, including gloves, eye protection, gowns, and masks, to protect those who provide care in instances when a dancer is bleeding or becomes ill. Figure 9.7 contains a list of essential and recommended items for a well-stocked first aid kit. The contents of such a kit must be reviewed often to both replenish items whose stock is low and replace items that have passed their expiration date.

Blood Control and Biohazard Spill Kits

Whether maintained as part of the first aid kit or as a separate kit, it is vital to have items available to control bleeding should a major wound occur as well as biohazard clean-up kits for emergencies when blood, vomit, urine, feces, or other bodily fluids are present. These kits are available from first aid supply vendors. They include items such as tourniquets for bleeding control and absorbent powders to help with fluid clean-up. Training in bleeding control is discussed later in the chapter.

While evaluating your options for blood control and clean-up, it would also be prudent to evaluate and discuss your procedures with the appropriate departments within your university. Facilities, maintenance, physical plant, and campus risk management and safety staff often have policies requiring they be contacted for removal of more than a minor amount of biohazardous material. Moreover, cleaning supplies that are used, such as cloths, wipes, and gloves, must be disposed of in biohazard receptacles.

Automated External Defibrillator (AED)

Perhaps the most essential emergency item that should be on hand is an automated external defibrillator (AED). Pelto and Drezner (2020) recommend that an AED be accessible at all venues where sports or physical activity are taking place and that it be close enough to have an interval of less than 3 minutes between collapse and first shock. Someone with knowledge and training in the use of an AED should be present any time physical activity occurs; that suggestion is a practical reason for encouraging CPR or BLS training of dance department faculty and staff.

Having an on-site AED is only the first step in the chain of survival for a cardiac arrest patient. The AED also must be accessible at all times; it must have a charged battery, as well as pads that are in good condition and not expired. It is essential that the AED remain at a consistent location when not in use. Any deviation from this placement must be communicated to everyone who may need to locate it in the event of a cardiac emergency.

Ice and Other Cold Therapy

Ice is frequently used as a source of immediate pain relief following injury. As injuries in dance are inevitable, a small ice machine is a good investment for a dance department or studio. Care should be taken to ensure proper maintenance of the machine to produce the best results. The ice produced by machines falls into three major categories: cubes, pellets or nuggets, and crushed. Pellet or nugget ice tends to be most popular for injuries because it conforms to

First Aid +

Medications and Topical Ointments	**First Aid**
Albuterol inhaler*	**Ace (elastic) bandages in assorted sizes (2", 4", 6" wide)**
Aloe or similar soothing topical cream	**Rubbing alcohol (isopropyl)**
Antacid	_Alcohol wipes_
Anti-diarrheal medication	**Bandaids (various sizes and appropriate skin tones)**
Antihistamine (like Benadryl)	_Cotton swabs, balls, Q-tips_
Anti-inflammatory medication (Ibuprofen, Naproxen)	_Dermabond / super glue_
Baby aspirin	**Gauze pads**
Calamine lotion	**Hydrogen peroxide to clean wounds**
Cold sore ointment	_Kerlix gauze, 4" and 6"_
Cough drops	**Nitrile gloves**
Decongestant tablets and nasal spray	_Non-adhering dressings (Telfa)_
Epi-Pen*	_Nose plugs (cotton rods or tampon pieces)_
Eyedrops (lubricating, artificial tears)	_Occlusive dressing_
Eyewash and eye cups	_Roller gauze_
Glucagon*	_Steri-strips_
Hydrocortisone cream	_Wound care debridement kit_
Indigestion medication	
Mineral oil (for tape removal)	**Infection Control**
Naloxone*	_Antiseptic wipes_
Pain medication (Tylenol)	**Face shield/goggles**
Saline solution	**Hand sanitizer**
Sugar or glucose solution (candy)	_N-95 mask_
Topical anti-Inflammatory gel (Arnica, Voltaren gel)	**Paper gown**
Triple antibiotic ointment	_Spill clean-up kit_
	Face masks
*May require prescription and/or written standing orders. Please consult your local regulations.	
Taping and Padding	**General Medical/General Needs**
Adhesive and non-adhesive felt	**BP cuff and stethoscope**
Adhesive and non-adhesive foam (1/8" and 1/4")	_Energy bars and powdered electrolyte replacement drinks_
Adhesive stretch tape	_Heating pad_
Adhesive tape (white, cloth)	_Matches or lighter_
Duct tape	**Nail clippers (finger and toenail)**
Elastikon/Elastoplast tape	**Penlight / flashlight**
Kinesiology tape	**Plastic bags (for ice)**
Leukotape (McConnell) and Cover-Roll stretch tape	_Pulse oximeter_
Moleskin	_Reflex hammer_
Orthoplast	_Safety pins_
Pre-wrap	_Scalpel_
Second Skin (1" squares and 3" circles)	**Scissors**
Self-adherent tape (Powerflex, Coban)	**Tampons**
Tuf-Skin, QDA, or other spray tape adhesive	**Thermometer**
	Tongue depressors (disposable wood)
Emergency Supplies	_Towels_
Air stirrup brace for ankle sprain	_Tweezers / needle_
Automated external defibrillator (AED)	
CPR mouthpiece / face mask	**Site/Venue-Specific**
Crutches	_Insect repellent_
Knee immobilizer	_Space blanket_
Sling	_Sunscreen_
Splints–finger, leg, and arm or **universal (SAM) splint**	
Tooth saver	**Essential items**
	Recommended items

Figure 9.7 A list of essential and recommended items for a well-stocked first aid kit.

body parts better than cubes but does not melt as quickly as crushed ice. A supply of zip-top plastic bags or produce-style grocery bags in the first aid kit are excellent resources for applying an ice pack.

Options for cold therapy beyond ice include reusable gel cold packs and chemical instant cold packs. Reusable gel cold packs are popular because they are pliable, thus allowing them to conform to body parts. They also stay cold longer than ice bags, and they do not melt. Instant cold packs work through a chemical reaction that occurs when a pouch inside the cold pack is broken by squeezing it. The squeezing action mixes the compounds in the pack to create the cold. Special care is required with both of these options. There must be a barrier—a damp cloth is a good choice—between the skin and the cold pack, because these items maintain a low temperature that may cause frostbite in the skin areas they contact. A dry cloth is less desirable for this purpose because it will not allow as efficient a tissue cooling effect as a damp cloth.

Emergency Medications

Several medications may be useful to have available should an emergency occur. Be certain to consult local laws prior to obtaining these medications; many require a prescription from a physician and training in their use. They must be maintained under strict security, and under no circumstances should such medications be administered to anyone other than the individual for whom they are intended. These medications could include the following:

- Albuterol inhaler for asthma and breathing emergencies
- Epinephrine auto-injector for allergic reactions
- Glucagon for diabetic emergencies
- Naloxone (e.g., Narcan, Kloxxado, Zimhi) for opioid overdose (figure 9.8)

Recommended Training for Dancers and Teachers

Once you have accepted the responsibility to become involved in the safety of your fellow dancers and students, there are several certification courses you can take to help develop and refine the skills needed to play an active role in your EAP. These trainings and several others may be available through your university, local organizations, or online education as well as the nonprofit commu-

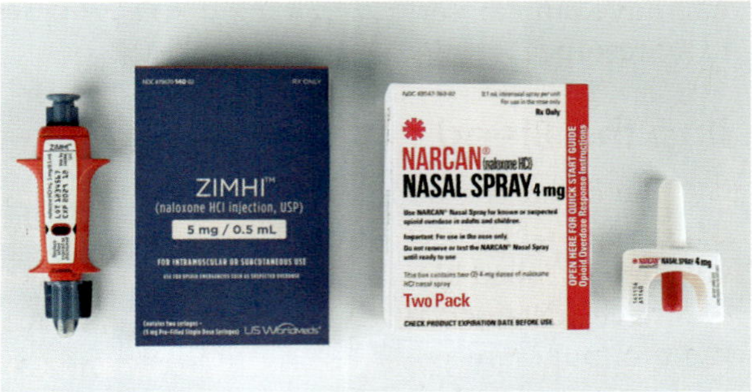

Figure 9.8 Two types of naloxone products to counteract opioid overdose—the injectable Zimhi (left) and the nasal spray Narcan. Either of these medications must be administered by an immediate responder as soon as signs of an overdose are recognized.

Pharmacy Images on Unsplash

nity organization ICSAVE (Integrated Community Solutions, 2023). See the sidebar for contact details of key organizations.

First Aid and Cardiopulmonary Resuscitation (CPR)

Cardiopulmonary resuscitation (CPR), basic life support (BLS), and first aid training include the essential basics of emergency care. You will learn how to give rescue breathing, treat someone you suspect is having cardiac arrest or another heart problem, and apply an AED. You will also learn how to care for a dancer who sustains a significant injury, including splinting and treatment for shock. These courses will prepare you to help a dancer until more highly trained help arrives.

Mental Health Emergency Training

Mental health first aid training teaches you about the signs of mental illness and substance use disorders as well as how to identify, understand, and respond to them. Question, Persuade, Refer (QPR) training focuses on suicide prevention for those who may recognize the signs that a dancer may be considering suicide. Note that both courses are basic training for emergencies. Just as taking a first aid and CPR class does not make you a doctor, taking mental health emergency training does not make you a mental health expert. Once again, the purpose of all of this recommended training is to equip you to address the needs of someone in distress until qualified first responders arrive. Another important point in the United States is knowing the mental health crisis line number *988*; this can be contacted either by phone or text message. Other countries may have similar services. Appendix A provides many resources related to mental health.

Stop the Bleed Training

Stop the Bleed is a national organization devoted to training that focuses on treatment for those who have uncontrolled bleeding. It can include dancers who have sustained injuries such as a compound fracture, puncture wounds, or other injuries that produce significant bleeding.

Emergency Planning and Response in the Context of Whole-Person Wellness

Hettler's six dimensions of wellness model (presented in chapter 1) represents interconnected facets of holistic well-being. Consider how emergency planning and response play a role in each of the six dimensions.

Occupational

Deepening one's skill set through the acquisition and cultivation of emergency response training is an investment in occupational competence and value. Some dance companies involve their dancers in emergency response, so having background knowledge and skills as an immediate responder may make a dancer more attractive to prospective employers. Safety training is often a requirement for professional positions such as dance captain, coach, or teacher. In more immediate terms, this chapter may lead you to recognize that workplace safety and emergency preparedness are part of your current responsibilities as a dancer in training. Advocating for a safe training environment for yourself and others will be important throughout your schooling and future career.

Physical

Many dancers dedicate considerable time and attention to training their bodies. An unexpected incident could—in an instant—set back their hard work or jeopardize their ability to participate in their chosen art. Emergency planning and first aid prioritize quick and effective response to life- and limb-threatening illnesses and injuries for the purpose of preserving life and function of the physical body. While the risk of catastrophic injury may be low, time-loss and temporarily debilitating injuries are more common among dancers at various levels of training. The National Wellness Institute (n.d.) states, "The physical dimension of wellness entails personal responsibility and care for minor illnesses and also knowing when professional medical attention is needed" (p. 1). Embracing emergency preparedness and first aid training can be strategic for you as a dancer, as can developing an understanding of the medical and wellness resources available in your area.

Social

Emergencies can happen anytime and anywhere, so immediate response training and first aid knowledge may be useful outside the dance setting to help family, friends, or others in the community when the unexpected occurs. Emergency action planning relies on a team approach in mitigating risks and responding to emergencies. Keeping emergency response skills current and being willing to act when the need arises demonstrate care for others and an awareness that all have a role to play in keeping each other safe. Equally important is knowing the scope of your role and when to bring in more qualified responders and medical professionals.

National Organizations Providing Emergency Response Training Certifications (USA)

Cardiopulmonary Resuscitation, Basic Life Support, Heartsaver

American Heart Association: www.heart.org

American Red Cross: www.redcross.org

First Aid

American Red Cross: www.redcross.org

Stop the Bleed: www.stopthebleed.org

Immediate Responder Training Resources

Integrated Community Solutions: https://icsave.org (also serves as a clearinghouse to provide training from several other emergency care organizations)

Mental Health First Aid: www.mentalhealthfirstaid.org (https://mhfainternational.org is the website for non-USA readers; it connects to accredited providers in other countries, including Canada, Australia, New Zealand, Hong Kong, India, Japan, Malaysia, and several European countries.)

Intellectual

As noted by Hernandez and Strickland (2005), safety standards are foundational to dance education. Absorbing choreography and executing technique may be especially difficult when a student is distracted by safety hazards; ask any student who has taken class in a sweltering studio or performed on a stage with a slick spot. At the very least, the training environment must be safe for students to learn effectively.

Beyond the basics of dance education, incorporation of first aid training into curricula introduces another mode of learning and expands overall knowledge of dance students. Emergency response planning and implementation encourage adaptive learning as students apply a framework of action to a virtual scenario or a real-life event. Finally, the recommendation to maintain current knowledge and to regularly refresh skills encourages lifelong learning.

Spiritual

The spiritual dimension of wellness encompasses the development of one's worldview and understanding of their purpose in life (National Wellness Institute, n.d.). Many people endorse a moral responsibility to help others in need, but they do not feel equipped to provide that help in a meaningful way. Obtaining training in first aid and other immediate responder procedures and acknowledging oneself as capable of helping (within a defined scope of care) promote self-efficacy, confidence, and realization of purpose.

Emotional

The mere thought of an emergent situation may produce feelings of anxiety and fear. Although emergencies can be frightening, the actions of immediate responders can positively affect their outcomes (Oliver et al., 2017). Rationale for first aid training and emergency response planning includes the understanding that having the knowledge and tools to respond in an emergency empowers people to act and can decrease fear of the unknown.

Conclusions and Practical Relevance

Injuries are inevitable in the university dance world. While most of these injuries will be relatively minor and self-treatable using techniques found throughout this book, some injuries may be serious and require outside assistance. This chapter described several potential emergency situations as well as the importance of being prepared for those emergencies, including being an immediate responder. Although everyone hopes that emergencies do not occur, familiarity with the components of an emergency action plan (EAP) and how dancers, dance teachers, and others can take part in it will help ensure that these situations are handled well when they do arise. You now have several recommendations for formal training you can undertake to learn how to help others when emergencies occur. Preparing for emergencies is the right thing to do, and it may be a legal duty in some areas. Do not plan to fail by failing to plan.

Discussion Questions

1. Describe a situation in which you participated because you had formal emergency response training, or describe a situation in which you could have participated if you had received such training beforehand.
2. Identify three potential barriers to emergency personnel access in your setting that should be addressed in your emergency action plan (EAP). For example, at which points is a university ID required to access your classroom or building? Alternatively, what special location instructions are needed for first responders to arrive as quickly as possible?
3. Which five components of a first aid kit do you consider the most essential? Why?
4. Discuss how you would remove an immobile performer from a challenging or unsafe physical environment. What circumstances and possibilities would you have to take into consideration?
5. Create a sample EAP for your performance space.

WWW Go to HK*Propel* to access supplemental information and activities connected to chapter content.

10

General Principles of Caring for Injuries

Selina Shah, MD, FACP, FAMSSM
Jacqui Greene Haas, MA, ATC Ret.
Debra A. Crookshanks, BSc, PT

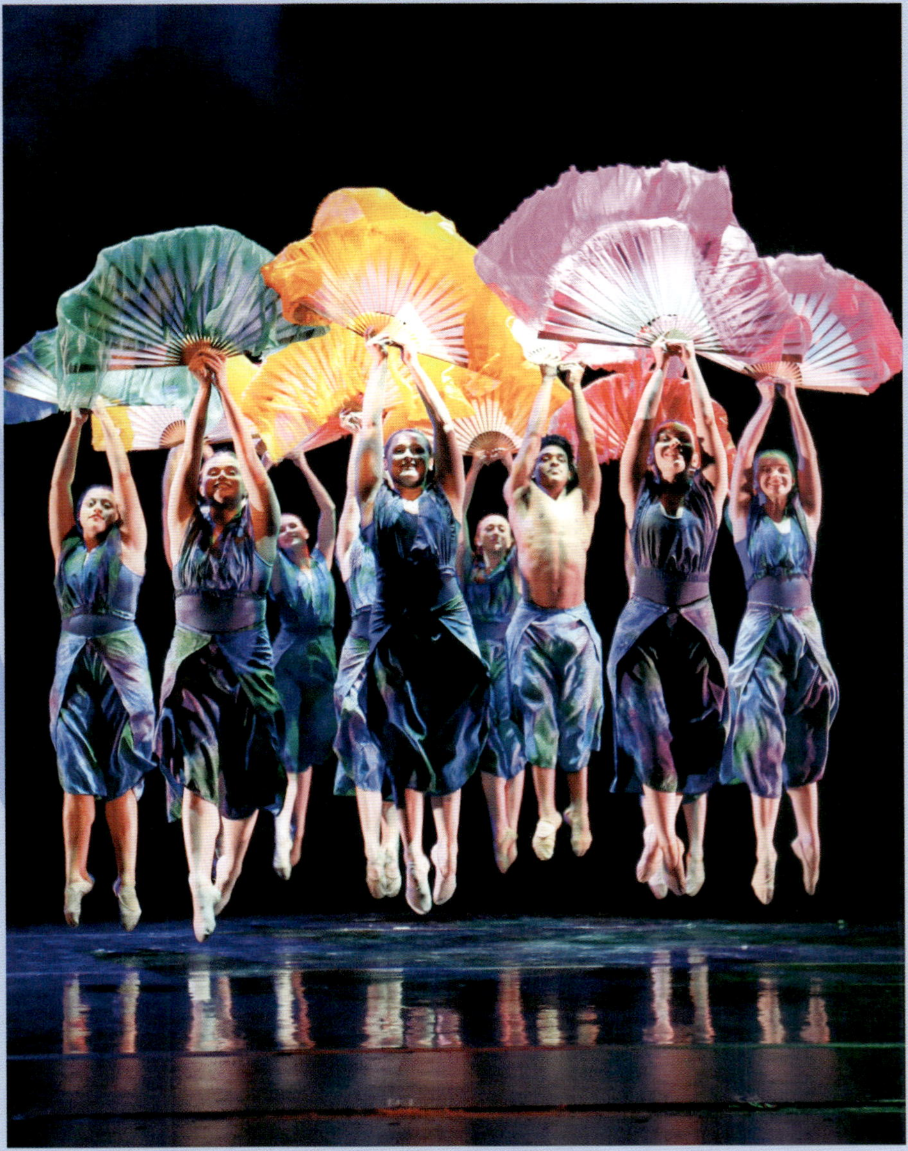

Shenandoah Conservatory, Winchester, Virginia. *Heart Blossom*, choreographed by Ting-Yu Chen. Photo: Jeff Taylor

Key Terms

- acute injury
- chronic injury
- contusion
- cryotherapy
- edema
- fracture
- healing environment
- hematoma
- injury
- integrated health care
- ligament
- rehabilitation phases
- relative rest
- sprain
- strain
- synovial sheath
- tendinopathy
- tendinosis
- tendon
- tenosynovitis

Injuries happen in dance; therefore, you must learn how to best manage them. Sometimes you may need the care of a health care professional, but you also have access to ways to help yourself when confronted with pain and other factors that limit your dancing. When these limitations occur, giving them prompt and proper attention is the way to long-term success.

LEARNING OBJECTIVES

After completing this chapter, you will be able to do the following:

- Identify different types of soft tissue.
- Describe different types of injuries.
- Explain the immediate management of injuries.
- Discuss common types of medical imaging that can be used to assess injuries.
- Create an environment best suited for healing that emphasizes a holistic approach to injury recovery.
- Integrate core elements of treatment and rehabilitation into personal injury care.
- Relate how an integrated health care team should work in caring for dance injuries.

Understanding the basics of injuries will help you understand what is happening in your body when you experience an injury. This knowledge will assist you in communicating with your health care team to facilitate your recovery and return to the studio in a healthy manner. The goal of this chapter is to guide you in learning injury basics, including the categories and types of injuries as well as how best to care for them.

Types of Injuries

Injuries can be classified into these two main categories: acute injuries and chronic injuries. **Acute injuries** (also known as traumatic injuries) occur during a sudden, traumatic event. Because they occur in a single memorable moment, it is relatively easy to describe specific details about how they happened, such as the date, the time, the dance move that caused the injury, and the circumstances that led to the injury during that move. For example, an injury may result from landing a jump incorrectly and rolling onto the outer edge of the foot, thus causing a fall during rehearsal for an upcoming performance.

On the other hand, **chronic injuries** (also known as overuse injuries) occur from repetitive use. They are accompanied by a gradual onset of pain, swelling, or both, which can interfere with the ability to dance fully without discomfort. For example, over the last few weeks, a dancer may have noticed pain in the back of the ankle that is worsening. Initially, the pain may have only accompanied relevés, but now the dancer notes pain with jumps and pliés, too.

Another way to characterize injuries is by type. The most common categories include contusions, sprains, strains, fractures, and tendinopathies (painful conditions occurring in tendons). Contusions, sprains, strains, and traumatic fractures are acute injuries, whereas stress fractures and tendinopathies are chronic.

Contusions

Contusions (bruises) are caused by the impact of a force on the body. They range from minor to severe depending on the level of that force. Minor bruises involve some tenderness, swelling, and darkening of the skin from mild capillary bleeding. A more severe blow can lead to the development of a **hematoma**, a collection of blood that pools under the skin (figure 10.1) due to bleeding from larger blood vessels into the muscles and surrounding tissues following a hard impact. Contusions usually heal over time; compression and icing may help this process proceed more efficiently.

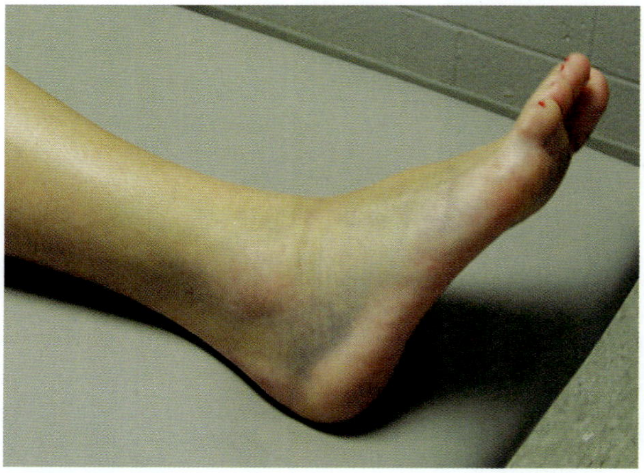

Figure 10.1 Bruising often accompanies a contusion or other injury where blood escapes from blood vessels and becomes apparent as discoloration under the skin.
Dr. Jeff Russell

Sprains

Sprains involve damage to the ligaments. **Ligaments** are soft tissue structures that help hold the joints together by connecting bone to bone. Their primary structure is made of collagen—the most common protein in the body—whose molecules look like long, tubular, mostly parallel strands. Ligaments contain some collagen fibers that are not parallel to the rest of their fibers, thus giving them strength in several directions (figure 10.2). Ligaments can handle a certain amount of force that stretches, pulls, and compresses them while they help hold joints together during movement. Sprains are acute injuries that occur when a ligament is overstretched or twisted in a direction it is not used to handling. Sprains are categorized as grade I, II, or III. Grade I involves a simple overstretch to the ligament, grade II involves partial tearing of the fibers of the ligament, and grade III involves complete tearing of the ligament (figure 10.3).

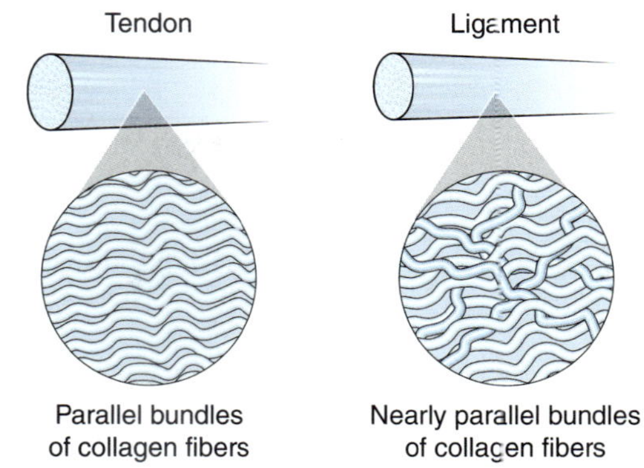

Figure 10.2 The collagen fibers of tendons and ligaments contribute to their strength. In tendons, the fibers are generally parallel. In ligaments, most of the fibers are parallel; the ones that are not parallel provide strength to the tissue in directions other than those parallel to it. This variation is necessary for the function of ligaments to support joints.

Strains

Strains are acute injuries to either tendon or muscle. **Tendons** are usually bands or cordlike structures that connect muscle to bone; however, they can also be flat and broad. They are made primarily of collagen fibers that in a normal tendon—unlike in ligaments—are almost all lined up parallel to each other. They transmit the force of a muscle's contraction through the tendon to a bone to create movement in a joint. In addition, as force is applied to either a tendon or a ligament, the usually rippled parallel collagen fibers straighten out (figure 10.4); if that force is too great, they are injured. As with sprains, strains are classified as grade I, II, or III. Grade I involves stretching of the fibers, grade II involves partial tearing of the fibers, and grade III involves complete tearing of the fibers; this scheme is similar to the grading of ligament injuries shown in figure 10.3.

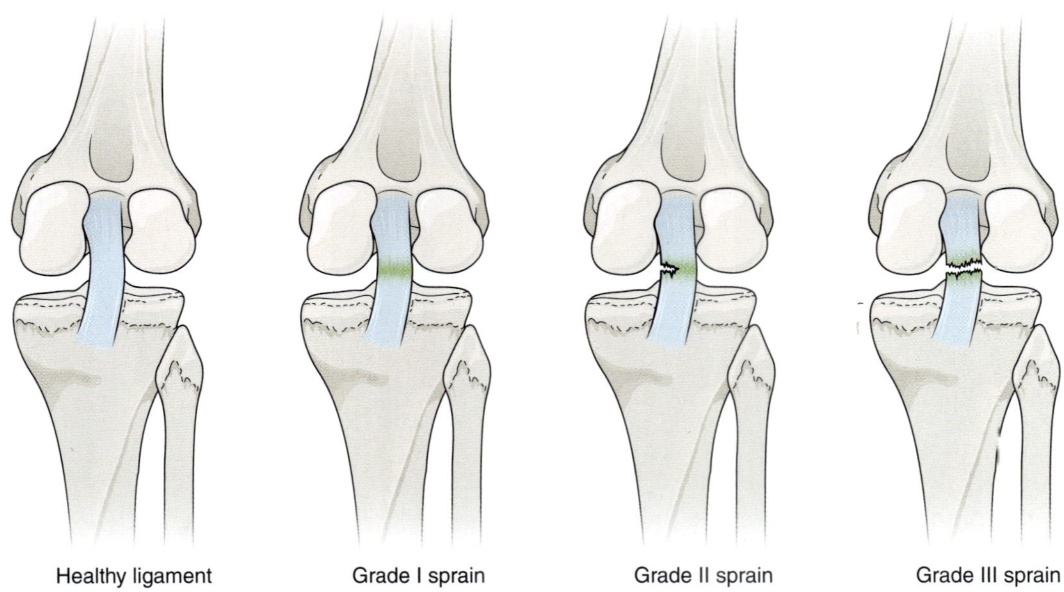

Figure 10.3 The amount of tissue damage determines categorizing sprains as grade I, II, or III. This scheme is also used for muscle and tendon tissue.

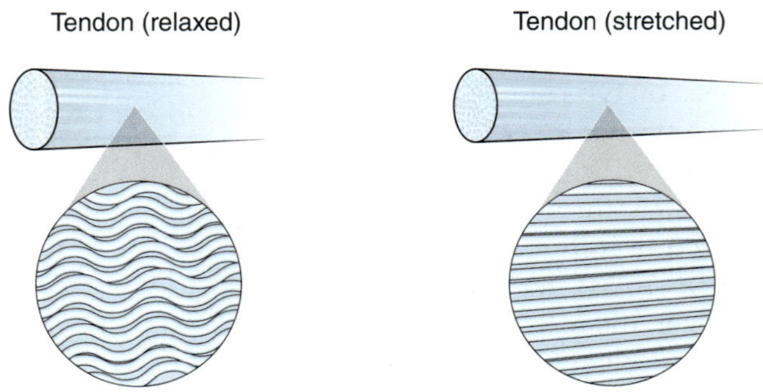

Figure 10.4 When a muscle is relaxed, the collagen fibers of the tendon connecting it to a bone appear wavy. However, once the muscle contracts or is stretched, the force of the contraction or the stretch lengthens the tendon and elongates its collagen fibers, thus removing much of the wavy pattern.

Fractures

Fractures are disruptions of bone. When most people think of an acute fracture, usually they think of a break in the bone. This type of fracture is often seen on radiographs (X-rays). However, some acute fractures, called occult fractures, are not visible on X-rays. If a physician suspects a fracture after obtaining an X-ray where a fracture does not appear, a magnetic resonance imaging (MRI) or computed tomography (CT) scan is ordered to provide further evidence that confirms or rules out the fracture.

The bones of children who are still growing are more supple than the bones of adults, so rather than break, youngsters' bones tend to bend. This type of injury is called a torus—or buckle—fracture; they are still considered fractures even without an apparent break. However, if a crack in the bone is seen on an X-ray, the injury may be called a greenstick fracture because of its similarity to what happens when one tries to break a branch on a live (green) tree. The branch will bend—and may crack—but it won't break all the way through. Figures 10.5*a* through 10.5*c* show different types of fractures. The fractures in figures 10.5*a* and 10.5*b* are seen in children, while the one in figure 10.5*c* is typically seen in adults.

Stress Fractures

Stress fractures are categorized as overuse injuries. When repeated forces are placed on a bone (e.g., from jump landings), it endures stress. If a bone cannot keep up with the constant repair necessary to handle this stress, it starts to develop a stress injury, which eventually results in a stress fracture. This injury is much like bending a paper clip back and forth. At first, the clip's metal bends; however,

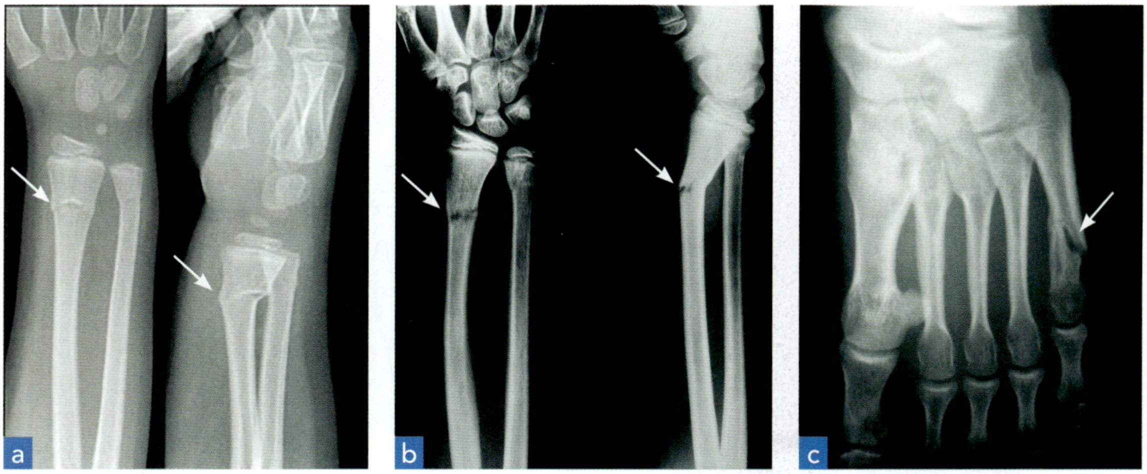

Figure 10.5 Comparison of different types of fractures. *(a)* Torus fracture. *(b)* Greenstick fracture. *(c)* Simple fracture of the shaft of the 5th metatarsal of the foot, an injury known as a dancer's fracture.

after many bends back and forth, the metal weakens, begins to crack, and eventually breaks through. Stress fractures are often not seen on typical X-rays; they usually require an MRI or a special X-ray technique called a bone scan to confirm.

For example, consider figures 10.6*a* through 10.6*c*, which depict a tibial stress fracture in three types of imaging. In the X-ray (figure 10.6*a*), the stress fracture is not apparent. However, the MRI (figure 10.6*b*) shows the stress fracture clearly. Notice the textured area of the bone inside the yellow box (which indicates swelling). A bone scan is an imaging technique that uses a low-level radioactive substance injected into the body followed by an X-ray. In places where increased bone metabolism occurs (e.g., the location of a stress fracture), the substance becomes concentrated, thus showing a so-called hot spot on the image. The bone scan in figure 10.6*c* allows comparison between the right and left tibias. The black concentration seen inside the blue boxes indicates the stress fracture location.

Tendinopathy and Tendinosis

Tendinopathy refers to an overuse injury to a tendon; it is the preferred term—rather than tendinitis—for most such injuries. *Tendinitis* implies inflammation of a tendon, and most tendon injuries are not inflammatory in nature. They often occur in the portion of a tendon that attaches to a bone or in the main body of the tendon. In either case, the tendinopathy creates pain and sometimes causes swelling in these localized areas.

Tendinopathies—especially those that are neglected when dancers dance through pain—can be related to another injury known as tendinosis. **Tendinosis** is a condition involving a complex series of events at the cellular level that results in degeneration of the tendon. This degeneration creates disruption of the normal collagen fibers in tendons. In general, tendons have poor blood supply, so the tendinosis persists rather than resolves. Over time, if the collagen degenerates enough, the tendon may

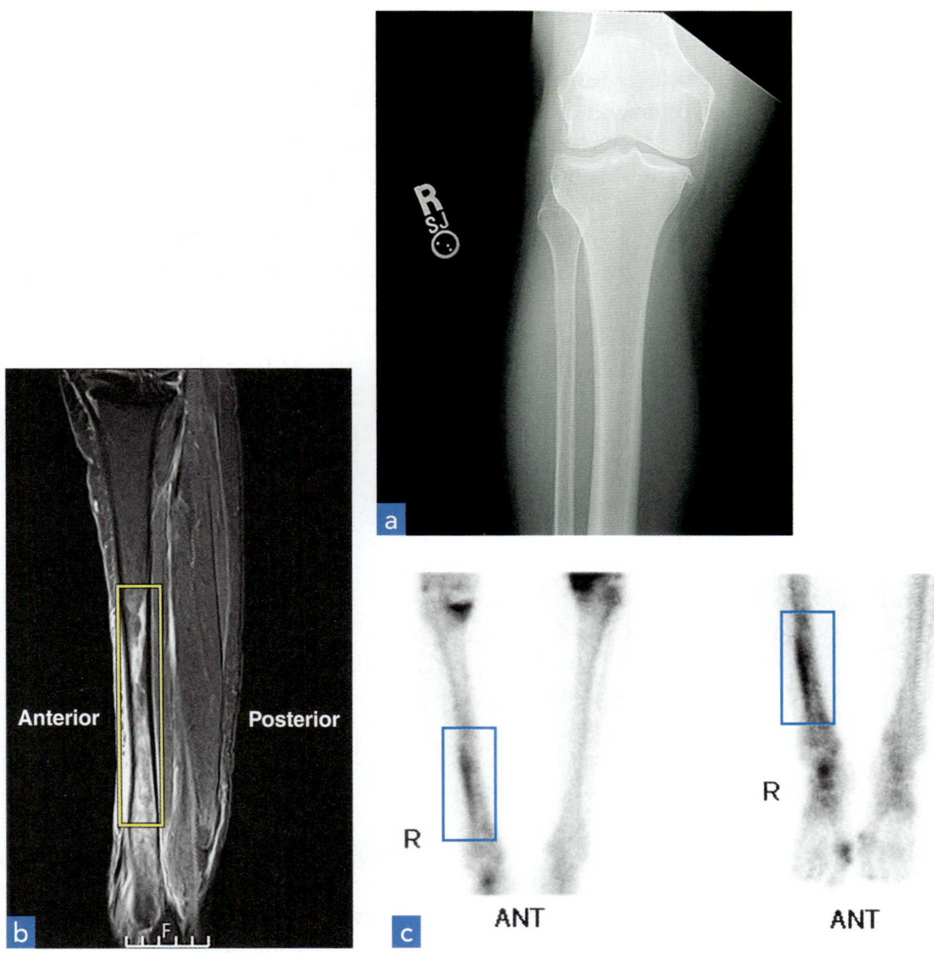

Figure 10.6 A stress fracture of the tibia shown in three types of imaging: *(a)* Plain X-ray; *(b)* MRI; and *(c)* bone scan.

Dr. Selina Shah

become weakened to the point of a strain and—at its worst—a complete rupture. This course of events significantly complicates the injury.

Much research still is needed to understand exactly what leads to tendinosis. It may be a complicated interplay between inflammatory and degenerative processes. Often, the initial stages of tendinosis do not create symptoms, but they do make a tendon more susceptible to injury. A strain may occur more easily in a tendon with active tendinosis compared to a normal, healthy tendon. Such strains may be difficult to heal because of the underlying tendinosis in the tendon and the lack of adequate blood supply that is needed to help promote healing.

Some tendons are housed in a **synovial sheath** of connective tissue. A specialized connective tissue called the synovium (or synovial sheath) makes fluid to provide lubrication for the tendons. Synovial sheaths are like tunnels that allow tendons to slide back and forth, especially in areas with a tight space for a tendon to operate. When the space between the tendon and sheath becomes inflamed from repeated friction of the tendon moving back and forth or from a strain that causes the tendon to swell in its sheath, an injury called **tenosynovitis** results. You can see what this word means when you break down its parts in this way: *ten-* = "tendon;" *synov-* = "synovial sheath;" and *-itis* = "inflammation."

Left untreated—such as when a dancer ignores the pain and tries to keep dancing—this injury can become quite severe to the point where the tendon begins to stick inside the synovial sheath. This advanced inflammation is called adhesive tenosynovitis, which can lead to a condition known as triggering of the tendon. Triggering is the sensation when a swollen part of a tendon feels as though it pops as it moves through the tight space in the inflamed synovial sheath. A common example of this condition in dancers is in the flexor hallucis longus tendon, the tendon that flexes the great toe downward. When the tendon is thickened and activated to flex the great toe, it has to push through the tunnel in this tightened space and can lead to a palpable pop—a trigger.

Physiological Stages of Healing

Healing an injury involves three main phases: inflammation, proliferation, and remodeling. Each of these dynamic stages is complex, and they all work together to repair damaged tissue (figure 10.7*a-e*). Rushing through any of the physiological changes that occur during the healing process can slow down recovery or cause chronic discomfort and an inability to regain full function of the injured area.

The acute inflammatory process starts immediately upon injury; cells congregate to the damaged site to start the healing process of removing damaged tissue, thus ridding the area of any contamination if there is an open wound and limiting further damage. Once the inflammatory process is underway (at approximately day 3), the proliferative phase begins; this phase can last for a few weeks. During this phase, cells are brought to the area to construct collagen that replaces the injured tissues. Pain and swelling improve, thus allowing for a return to simple activities depending on injury severity. At this point, the collagen is in the early stages of organization and is not strong enough to be stressed. It is important to not rush through this

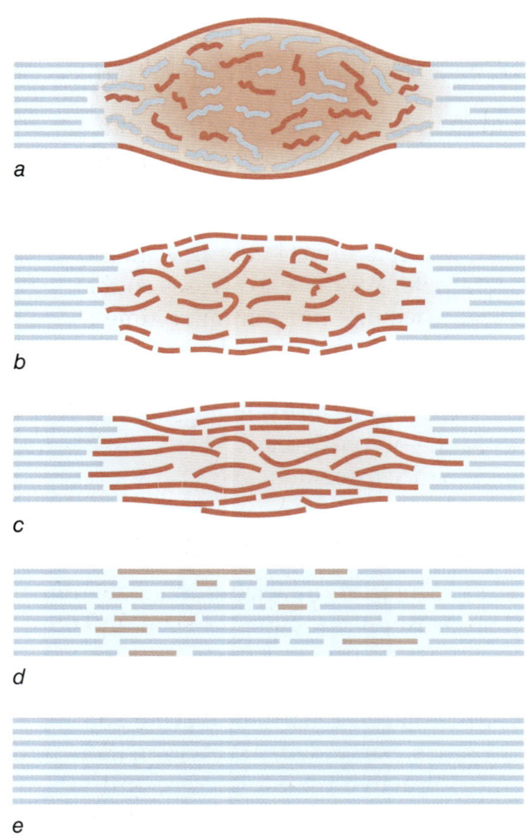

Figure 10.7 The phases of tissue healing. *(a)* Inflammation phase, with damaged tissue and blood vessels resulting in edema. *(b)* Proliferation phase, in which reparative cells start to regenerate. *(c-e)* Steps of the remodeling phase showing reorganization of collagen fibers until tissue is fully remodeled.

phase to get back to dance; follow your health care provider's advice in terms of what you can and cannot do in dance and other activities.

The final phase of healing—the remodeling phase—begins at about week 3; this phase can last for up to 12 months (or even longer) depending on the severity of injury. During this phase, collagen fibers are organized into their normal configuration, and development of tensile strength capable of handling stress loads occurs. It is important to follow your health care provider's guidance on proper exercises for strength, joint range of motion, and flexibility during the remodeling phase while the damaged tissues become stronger. A progressive and challenging exercise program stimulates growth in the injured tissue, and it improves function. The goal is to rebuild the damaged tissue to allow a safe return to rehearsals and performances. Rushing any of the physiological stages of healing can cause chronic inflammation or chronic instability, either of which can hamper performance.

Care of Soft Tissue Injuries

The human body is designed to optimize healing for return to normal function. It is important to understand how healing occurs; therefore, this section expands the discussion of the healing phases. Dancers must know how to work within the parameters of these processes so that they can maximize healing and minimize time away from dance while recuperating. Trying to short-circuit proper care—or ignoring it altogether—may lead to increased injury severity, increased time loss from dance, and—in particularly severe cases—the end of one's dance career.

The Inflammatory Process

Soft tissue injuries cause an immediate inflammatory response in the injured tissue. Inflammation is an important process; the body uses it to fight foreign invaders such as bacteria and viruses, to remove damaged cells, and to bring about healing of its tissues. Some signs of inflammation are pain, swelling, reactive muscle spasm, and limitations in functional movements. The goals of the early inflammatory response are to protect damaged tissue from further injury, prepare the injured site for repair, and stimulate the recruitment and activation of repairing cells. The inflammatory phase usually persists for 48 to 72 hours after injury; however, its duration varies between individuals. In addition, it can be influenced by the type of tissue damaged, the severity of the damage, and how an injury is initially cared for (Brukner & Khan, 2018).

While inflammation is an essential process that initiates tissue regeneration and repair, excessive bleeding and swelling (**edema**) can delay recovery and may cause secondary damage to nearby tissues by reducing their blood flow. Therefore, the goal of acute injury management is to prevent excessive bleeding and edema, reduce pain, provide an ideal environment for tissue repair, and promote a faster return to function (Brukner & Khan, 2018).

During the body's important inflammatory phase of the healing process, it is tempting to use anti-inflammatory medications to reduce pain and swelling as a means of returning to dance sooner. However, the use of these medications is controversial because evidence suggests that they might not be more effective than acetaminophen (e.g., Tylenol) or paracetamol (e.g., Panadol) and they may impair the healing process (Lyrtzis et al., 2011; Stovitz & Johnson, 2003). That is, a medication that is anti-inflammatory opposes the important work of the inflammatory process. As research continues to uncover mechanisms involved in inflammation and how medications operate, avoiding these medications may be better in the long run in order to give the body's natural efforts a better chance to heal the injury. In addition, anti-inflammatory drugs can cause distress in the gastrointestinal system.

Dancers may want to weigh the risks against the benefits of using anti-inflammatory medications by discussing them with their physician. Anti-inflammatory medications include aspirin or aspirin-containing products as well as other nonsteroidal anti-inflammatory drugs (NSAIDs) such as ibuprofen (e.g., brand names Motrin, Advil, and Nurofen) and naproxen sodium (e.g., brand names Aleve and Naprosyn). Medication specifically for pain relief such as acetaminophen and paracetamol (e.g., brand names Tylenol, Panadol) do not contain anti-inflammatory compounds. Overall, it is best to seek the advice of your qualified medical professional regarding how to manage your pain.

Acute (Early) Care of Soft Tissue Injuries

The acute period of an injury extends from immediately after the injury to approximately 48 hours postinjury. Early management of injuries historically centered on the ICE (Ice, Compression, Elevation) method or the RICE (Rest, Ice, Compression, Elevation) method (Mirkin & Hoffman, 1978). Recommended injury care further evolved to become PRICE (Protection, Rest, Ice, Compression, Elevation) and—more recently—POLICE (Protection, Optimal Loading, Ice, Compression, Elevation) (Bleakley et al., 2012). The strategies to guide management using POLICE are shown in table 10.1. Ice, compression, and elevation (ICE) remain part of the basic principles of early injury management. In addition, it is important that an injured dancer do no HARM (by not using Heat, avoiding Alcohol intake, avoiding Return to activity prematurely, and not using Massage) during the initial 3 days after an injury occurs because any of those actions may increase recovery time (see sidebar Do No HARM).

Table 10.1 **Steps Involved in Acute Soft Tissue Injury Management: POLICE**

P	Protection	Protection after injury provides a stress shield to vulnerable tissues by unloading or preventing joint movement for a period. It allows injured tissue time to heal, and it limits the possibility of further injury. Examples include taping, braces, and a walking boot. Rest should be of limited duration, followed by progressive mechanical loading to restore strength and function. This process is best done under the guidance of a qualified health care professional.
O L	Optimal Loading	Optimal loading replaces rest with a balanced and incremental rehabilitation program during which early activity encourages early recovery.
I	Ice	The most common form of cold treatment, **cryotherapy** is the application of ice or cold packs to the injured area to limit injury-induced tissue damage by reducing tissue temperature at the site of injury. Ice lowers the metabolic rate of cells in the injured area, thus lowering the cells' demand for oxygen. Oxygen is more difficult for blood circulation to deliver to the cells because of damaged blood cells in the area. The state of not having enough oxygen is called hypoxia. Aims: • Reduce swelling and edema through vasoconstriction of local blood vessels. • Reduce pain associated with tissue damage via slowing of sensory nerve impulses. • Reduce painful muscle spasm via slowing of motor nerve conduction velocity (Herrera et al., 2010). • Reduce secondary hypoxic injury by lowering the metabolic demand of injured tissues (Brukner & Khan, 2018). Recommended treatment: Short, intermittent applications (Bleakley et al., 2006), with 5-10 minutes on, 20 minutes off, 5-10 minutes on. Repeat this sequence once or twice daily for the first 24-48 hours. The duration depends on the depth of injured tissues and the size of the injured area (e.g., ankle ligament [superficial, smaller] versus hamstring muscle [deep, larger]).
C	Compression	Compression is used following acute soft tissue injury to increase pressure in the veins and lymphatic vessels to counteract edema (swelling) (Brukner & Khan, 2018). Standard protocols recommend a pressure of 15-35 mmHg. Elastic bandaging is the most common technique with which to apply compression; it should start just below the injury site with each layer of the elastic wrap overlapping the preceding layer by one-half its width. Finish wrapping about 4 inches (10 cm) above the upper injury margin. A standard elastic bandage is a versatile and effective solution; select a width that will provide good coverage for the size of the injured area.
E	Elevation	Elevating an injured extremity above the level of the heart results in a decrease of the fluid pressure inside the limb, and it subsequently reduces the accumulation of fluid contained around the cells of the tissues at the site of the injury (Brukner & Khan, 2018). It aims to promote drainage of the swelling via the lymphatic vessels as well as to assist the veins in removing additional excess fluid.

Adapted from C.M. Bleakley, P. Glasgow, and D.C. MacAuley, "PRICE needs updating, should we call the POLICE?" *British Journal of Sports Medicine* 46, no. 4 (2012): 220-221. https://doi.org/10.1136/bjsports-2011-090297.

Do No HARM

In the first 72 hours following injury, these HARMful factors should be avoided:

Heat, Alcohol intake, Return to activity prematurely, Massage

H—heat. Heat may increase the bleeding at the injured site by enlarging the blood vessels. Avoid hot baths, showers, saunas, heat packs, and heat rubs.

A—alcohol intake. Drinking alcohol may mask pain and the severity of the injury, thus increasing the risk of reinjury. Additionally, alcohol has been shown to have negative consequences on a number of factors related to tissue healing (Jung, 2011).

R—return to activity prematurely (dancing, running, etc.). Trying to return to activity too early may cause further damage at the injury site.

M—massage or vigorous soft tissue therapy. Vigorous massage should be avoided in the first 24 to 48 hours because it may cause further bleeding and swelling at the injury site (Brukner & Khan, 2018).

Subacute Care of Soft Tissue Injuries

The subacute period of an injury occurs from about 48 hours postinjury to 1 or 2 weeks postinjury. In 2020, Dubois and Esculier proposed that the previously coined acronyms focused on acute management while they ignored subacute and longer-term stages of tissue healing. They suggested a new acronym be implemented; it is called PEACE (Protection, Elevation, Avoid anti-inflammatories, Compression, Education) & LOVE (Load, Optimism, Vascularization, Exercise). The steps involved in this contemporary PEACE & LOVE approach (table 10.2) encompass the rehabilitation continuum from immediate care (PEACE) to subsequent management (LOVE). An advantage of this approach is its aim to educate patients as well as address psychosocial factors to enhance recovery.

The path to treating any dance-related injury, from immediate acute care through subacute and longer-term stages, is well supported by research.

Three Clinical Pearls About Cryotherapy (Cold Treatment)

1. In addition to its use in the initial stage of an injury, cryotherapy is advantageous during late-stage rehabilitation to reduce the sensation of pain, thus enabling a window of opportunity for supervised exercise rehabilitation (Mitchell & Thain, 2011).
2. Cryotherapy is not indicated in the management of exercise-induced muscle soreness, previously referred to as delayed-onset muscle soreness (DOMS) (Wang et al., 2021; Malanga et al., 2015).
3. Cryotherapy should not be used prior to activities requiring advanced motor control or proprioception. A reduction in motor and sensory nerve conduction velocity (a side effect of cryotherapy) reduces dynamic stability (Macedo et al., 2014), and it may place the dancer at risk of reinjury or further injury (Alexander et al., 2018).

Become familiar with these processes of managing injuries so that if you experience a dance injury, you can facilitate your efficient and effective return to dancing, reduce your risk of reinjury, and prolong your career.

Rehabilitation Measures

Rehabilitation of dance injuries restores range of motion, strength, flexibility, and function for a successful return to dance. Some physical benefits of rehabilitation include addressing pain and pain management, swelling, movement dysfunction, coordination, and balance skills. The psychological benefits include building self-esteem, confidence, and motivation to combat the stressors associated with injury. For the best outcomes, rehabilitation measures should include effective communication between health care providers and dancers, quality assessment and diagnosis, effective progression of the plan of care, functional assessments, dance-specific interventions, dance modification, and return to dance guidelines. Success depends on full participation from the dancer and the health care team. Every patient is unique, as is every injury, so the plan of rehabilitation care must be individualized.

Table 10.2 **The PEACE & LOVE Method of Caring for a Dance Injury**

P	Protection	Avoid activities and movements that increase pain and bleeding during the first few days after injury.
E	Elevation	Elevate the injured limb higher than the heart as often as possible to promote fluid flow out of the injured tissues.
A	Avoid anti-inflammatories	Avoid anti-inflammatories; they inhibit the inflammatory process required for tissue healing.
C	Compression	Compress with an elastic bandage or other compression device to reduce swelling.
E	Education	Educate the patient about the benefits of an active approach to recovery; avoid unnecessary passive treatments and medical investigations.
&		
L	Load	Load an injured area by letting pain guide the gradual return to normal activities; optimal loading promotes repair, remodeling, and tissue tolerance.
O	Optimism	Optimism in one's approach conditions the brain for optimal recovery through confidence and positivity.
V	Vascularization	Vascularization (the restoration of blood flow) is done by choosing pain-free, aerobic activities to increase blood flow and oxygen delivery to repairing tissues.
E	Exercise	Exercise for rehabilitation restores mobility, strength, and proprioception, and it leads to an active approach to recovery.

Adapted from B. Dubois and J.F. Esculier, "Soft-Tissue Injuries Simply need PEACE and LOVE," *British Journal of Sports Medicine* 54, no. 2 (2020): 72-73. https://doi.org/10.1136/bjsports-2019-101253.

Communication

Developing a quality relationship with the health care team will help build communication skills and promote education for both parties. The physician can diagnose and evaluate injuries, order and review imaging, discuss potential procedures, and refer the injured dancer to other health care providers to create an integrated approach to recovery. Health care team members may not know dance, but they still can help with injury evaluation and management; in such cases, communication is key. Explaining training demands and dance movements, plus demonstrating how the injury occurred and identifying any aggravating factors, can help the health care provider optimally manage the injury. In this way, health care practitioners and dancers can learn from each other and work together toward optimizing the integrated approach to injury management. More information about how to work with a variety of health care providers is presented in chapter 15.

Relative Rest

Unfortunately, many dancers report that visits to health care providers result in a prescription to stop dancing. While complete rest may be required to protect the dancer during certain injuries, the command *Stop dancing*—given without any understanding of how abrasive those words sound to dancers—is met with disdain. Thus, another important factor in provider–dancer communication is the goal of defining **relative rest**. Generally speaking, relative rest involves avoiding certain movements while continuing with others under the guidance of the physician, athletic trainer or physical therapist, and dance instructor(s). Such modifications may include decreasing the intensity and frequency of dance activities and avoiding certain movements during rehabilitation to prevent overload of healing tissue.

Many dancers compare their passion for dancing to an addiction, and the thought of not dancing is extremely difficult. Dancers should try to work with their provider to establish an agreeable and safe way for the dancer to participate in a modified portion of training. If full rest is needed due to a more severe injury, the provider may be able to prescribe rehabilitative alternatives (Russell, 2013) such as teaching class, performing floor barre (non-weight bearing floor exercises that relate directly to basic ballet training), or incorporating motor learning with mental practice (Sabo, 2013).

Pain Perception

Communication regarding perception of pain can be difficult. Many dancers have difficulties distinguishing the difference between performance pain and injury pain. They continue to dance with the pain, which results in the risk of further injury. Both performance pain and injury pain involve a physical sensation and a psychological response. Performance pain is more acute and can be voluntarily reproduced, whereas injury pain is typically involuntary and threatens performance (Anderson, 2008). Education and communication from the health care team can help a dancer differentiate between the two pain experiences to reduce the risk of chronic injury.

Clinical Assessment

As previously discussed, injuries can be chronic or acute, and the clinical evaluation of an injury is critical to diagnosis and management. A health care provider will do an initial assessment (evaluation) of the injury. In an assessment, the provider performs a physical examination; during this process, the provider asks questions regarding the date and mechanism of injury (MOI; how the injury occurred); location of pain; presence of swelling, redness, and bruising; ability to bear weight and pursue normal functions; and the effects on dance moves. Musculoskeletal and neurological assessments include objective measurements that will be used over time as a measure of progress and advancement in abilities. Strength, joint range of motion (flexibility), balance, agility, cardiorespiratory endurance, and trunk strength are some of the measures that may be assessed. For a dancer, one of the most important evaluations is assessing dance technique to determine which movements are contributing to the injury. Ongoing technique assessments throughout rehabilitation support clear communication about when and what to modify in class (Sabo, 2013). Initial goals are to decrease swelling, protect the injury, address pain, and design the plan of care. Long-term goals are to safely and gradually progress intensity of movement, restore function, and return the dancer to their physical and emotional preinjury state.

Conditioning

Cardiorespiratory conditioning and core stability need to be maintained while your injury continues to heal. Deconditioning (the loss of strength and aerobic capacity) can occur after an injury. Cardiorespiratory training can help reduce both physical and mental stress associated with injury. The heart, lungs, and blood vessels work together to deliver needed oxygen to all areas of your body. Conditioning the cardiorespiratory system will increase oxygenated blood flow to the injured area and promote healing. Improvement in mental health also is a well-known benefit of physical exercise. Your health care providers can design the appropriate program for you depending on the injury. Swimming is one of the best forms of nonweight-bearing exercise (figure 10.8*a*). You could do

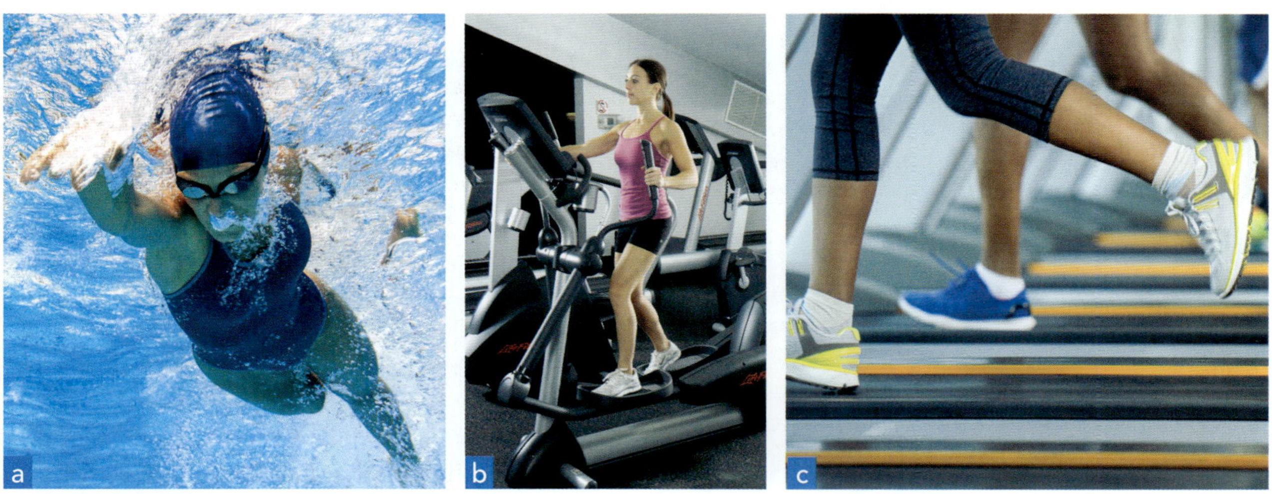

Figure 10.8 Maintenance of physical fitness, including aerobic capacity, is important whenever you are confronted with an injury. Doing so protects the injured body region from reinjury; at the same time, it keeps you trained and better prepared for resumption of full dance activity after healing.

A: microgen/Getty Images/iStockphoto; C: RuslanDashinsky/iStockphoto/Getty Images a barre series in a pool while you recover. Guided elliptical training can be effective (figure 10.8*b*) and intervals of different walking speeds on a treadmill also help maintain aerobic fitness (figure 10.8*c*). Exercise-induced fatigue is associated with injury, and maintaining optimal levels of aerobic fitness can reduce it. An in-depth discussion of physical conditioning appears in chapter 5.

Decreased core stability is a risk factor for injuries, particularly those in the lower extremities (Rickman, 2012). The deep and superficial muscles that make up the core are very important in their role of supporting the spine because the spine may become unstable due to the demands of dance participation. The core muscles also contract prior to lower-extremity movement. Therefore, maintaining strength, endurance, and activation timing of the deep and superficial muscles of the core must receive attention during injury recovery and beyond. Rehabilitation professionals should incorporate into a treatment program a healthy progression of exercises for the core.

Rehabilitation Progression

The progression of your rehabilitation program relates to the tissue healing process and how you respond to treatment. Your health care providers may include supplementary exercise programs that correlate with your injury-specific rehabilitation to improve balance, coordination, and neuromuscular control. Participating in a Pilates-based program can be a safe non-weight-bearing intervention to promote core strength and muscular balance (figure 10.9). Chapter 5 contains guidance about Pilates exercises.

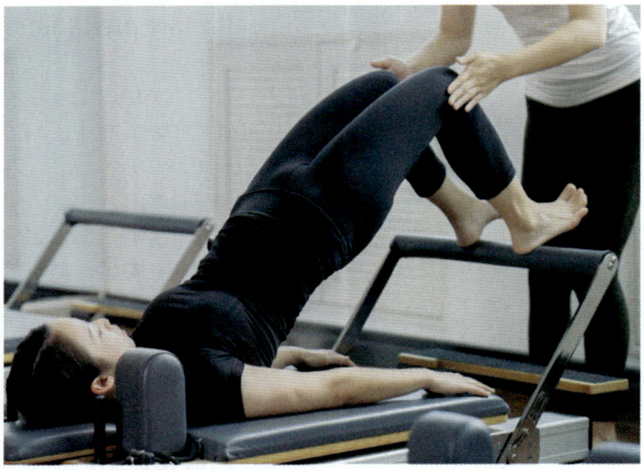

Figure 10.9 Pilates training is a helpful method of reconditioning following an injury.

Nicholas Fu on Pexels

Some clinicians use floor barre in addition to therapeutic exercise to perform non-weight-bearing exercises and to simulate dance movement patterns. Gyrotonics, yoga, and somatic exercise methods can be beneficial for injury recovery and overall conditioning. Somatic exercises use the mind–body connection to improve awareness of pain or muscle imbalance. Somatic practices include the Alexander Technique and the Feldenkrais Method, which promote mindful movement, alignment, and body awareness.

Rehabilitation phases consist of the protected phase, motion-controlled phase, and return to function phase (Potts, 2001). As shown in table 10.3, each of the phases coordinates with the healing process. It is tempting to rush through rehabilitation to get back to class and rehearsal; however, for optimal healing, the body must go through the inflammatory, repair, and remodeling stages described earlier. Not respecting the entire healing process risks inadequate recovery, possible reinjury, chronic inflammation, impaired function, and lingering pain.

Once your injury is healing and you can begin to progress to more challenging dance-related movement, it is important to have a detailed progression of exercises that uses pain as the guide for how much to try. Your health care team will direct you in moving from basic to more advanced combinations while assessing your technique. Dance exercises should progress from slow to quick and from two legs to one. Jumping exercises should start at the barre, then move to the center, and then progress from two legs to one. Health care providers can discuss the appropriate levels of activity and necessary modifications with your dance instructors when you return to class and rehearsal.

Healing Environment

Creating an optimal **healing environment** is crucial for injury recovery and successful return to dance. Healing is the process of becoming free from injury, restoring health and wellness, and reestablishing wholeness. An ideal healing environment addresses the six dimensions of wellness that were presented in chapter 1. An integrated approach is needed to heal, repair, and recover from injury. To facilitate healing, one must address four healing environments: internal, behavioral, external, and interpersonal (DuBose et al., 2018).

Table 10.3 **Phases of Rehabilitation for Facilitating Gradual Progress and Injury Reduction**

Phase	Objectives
Protected phase	Provide patient education. Control pain and swelling. Possibly immobilize injured region. Perform gentle passive movements. Preserve conditioning. Maintain function of uninvolved areas.
Motion-controlled phase	Continue patient education. Promote healing. Possibly use taping or functional bracing. Move from passive to active movements. Progress to strengthening exercises. Perform proprioceptive training upon weight bearing. Continue conditioning.
Return to function phase	Continue patient education. Increase soft tissue and joint mobility. Progress strengthening exercises. Develop muscle endurance. Accelerate functional training. Incorporate dance-specific activities.

Internal: Psychological Awareness

The internal environment includes psychological and self-efficacy awareness. Many dancers struggle with anxiety and depression, particularly during injuries. Unfortunately, the history of dance culture has promoted injury intolerance. Healing can benefit from reducing personal stress and anxiety as well as improving mood (Pollitt & Hutt, 2021). Learning to adapt to situations and changes related to injury also helps build a better healing environment. In addition, in search of wholeness, you will need to address the emotional responses that follow injuries. Chapter 8 is an exceptional resource on the mental health aspects related to dance.

Behavioral and External: Integrated Health Care

Focusing on quality **integrated health care** consists of collaboration between members of a trusted health care team who support the dancer's behavioral and external environments. This team can be composed of several specialists from different disciplines within the health care field. Every injury is unique; your team will create a plan of care that best suits your needs and promotes healing. Overall, your behavioral decisions can produce optimal or suboptimal healing depending on the choices made. Health care providers will guide and assist; ultimately, however, you have to make wise decisions to promote your recovery.

Integrated health care ideally includes a lead physician with dance-specific knowledge to best understand your needs and provide diagnostic tools and procedures. The team may also include physical therapists, occupational therapists, or athletic trainers who will focus on musculoskeletal injury assessment, management, recovery, and return to dance. Management strategies include taping, manual therapy, and various modalities to assist your body in healing damaged tissue. Chapter 15 explores the various types of health care professionals that dancers might consult.

Attaining an optimal healing environment might also include a food and nutrition expert, such as a registered dietitian experienced in working with dancers and athletes to address inadequate eating habits and dehydration that could delay tissue healing. Nutrition impacts recovery; therefore, a well-designed diet will support the healing process. Hydration is another factor that can impact recovery. Lack of adequate hydration is a common reason cell recovery is disrupted. See chapter 7 for a full discussion on nutrition for dancers.

Additional providers to support the integrated health care approach may include a massage therapist, chiropractor, or acupuncturist. In addition, injuries and injury rehabilitation are physically and mentally challenging. A sport psychiatrist, psychologist, or counselor also can be enlisted to promote healthy coping strategies, such as cognitive and motivational imagery. If they are familiar with dance and dancers, they can be even more helpful as you face the emotional stressors that could impair recovery and healing.

When the high demands of dance and university life are combined with an injury, it can lead to sleep disturbances, too. Lack of sleep can deplete your immune system and interrupt healing time. Growth hormones that enable proteins needed to repair damaged muscles, tendons, and ligaments are released when you are in a deep sleep. The more hours of quality sleep you receive, the greater the production of growth hormones to improve healing.

Some dancers use tobacco, alcohol, or caffeine to cope with their injury. These practices do not support an ideal healing environment for injury repair and recovery; in fact, they may impede healing. Ballet dancers have been known to smoke cigarettes in an attempt to suppress their appetite to reach a thin body aesthetic. Tobacco use is also associated with binge drinking (Stein et al., 2016), and it is known to disrupt tissue healing following surgery (Beahrs et al., 2019). Nicotine and caffeine are vasoconstrictors (they reduce blood flow in tissues); vasoconstriction undermines the healing process. Binge drinking can also decrease production of proteins needed for wound repair (Jung et al., 2011).

Interpersonal: Social Support

Addressing the interpersonal domain relates to social support. Encouragement from dance instructors, family, and peers is important in promoting healing. Feeling stress or pressure to return to the studio before you have fully recovered—whether you place that burden on yourself or others do—can put you at risk for reinjury. Some dancers have been known to hide their injury due to fear of losing their spot in an ensemble; they continue to dance through the pain despite the likelihood of increasing the injury's severity and delaying its recovery. Certainly, this practice is not encouraged.

Feelings associated with pain include fear, shame, and guilt. When these factors are combined with injuries, emotional stress—and its negative impact on your immune system—increases the risk for injury and illness. Moreover, cortisol is a hormone your body releases when you are under stress. Elevated levels of cortisol can interfere with the healing aspects of the inflammatory process, thus hindering progress. In addition, stress has been known to cause poor compliance with attending rehabilitation appointments.

In general, much of the negative consequences discussed in this section stem from the lack of adequate social support that results in increased stress. Moreover, negative judgment from family, peers, and teachers can impede healing and recovery. A supportive social environment will help buffer the impact stress has on your recovery. Creating a safe space for healing requires a balance of body, mind, and psychosocial cohesion to give you the best opportunity for restoration and return to dance.

Conclusions and Practical Relevance

Injuries are inherent to any physical endeavor. Learning basic injury concepts, including anatomy, types of injuries, mechanisms of injury, and injury management, can help you if you experience a dance injury. This information will better equip you not only to manage the injury immediately but also to play a key role in forming an alliance with your health care team; ultimately, it will lead to an optimal recovery and to the quickest possible route back to the studio.

Discussion Questions

1. A 19-year-old ballet dancer slips while performing a pirouette en pointe, resulting in rolling and twisting the right ankle and then falling to the floor. The dancer is unable to stand on the right foot, and swelling and bruising are evident on the outside (lateral) part of the ankle. Is this injury acute or chronic? What types of structures could be injured? Describe what types of injuries may have occurred. What would be the best course of action for immediate treatment?
2. Describe the attributes of each rehabilitation phase and how they coordinate with the physiological stages of healing.
3. Think about a time when you needed to visit a health care professional for a dance-related injury. Do you consider the care you received to have been delivered by an integrated health care team? Why or why not? What are the specific characteristics of the care you received that either were or were not helpful in moving you forward toward returning to dance?
4. Analyze the optimal healing environment by describing how both the internal and interpersonal domains relate to each other for a positive impact on injury recovery.

WWW Go to HK*Propel* to access supplemental information and activities connected to chapter content.

Part III

Common Dance Injuries

Dance Injuries in the Lower Extremity

Amanda Blackmon, PT, DPT, OCS, CMTPT
Nancy Kadel, MD
Meg Schneider, MS, ATC

11

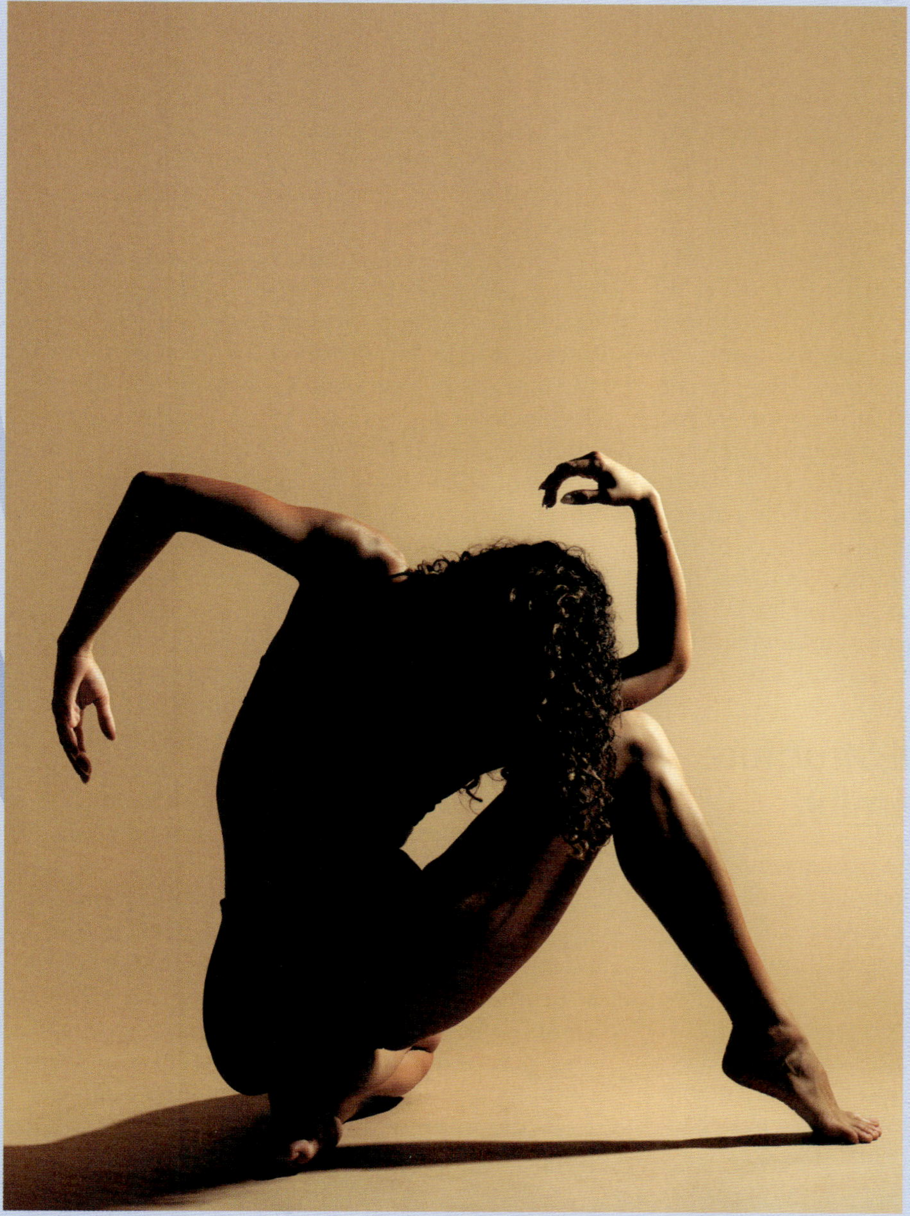

Photo: Claire Imler; Dancer: Makaila Teagle

Considering all dancers in all genres of dance, the lower extremity sustains more injuries than any other part of a dancer's body. Because your foot is both your physical and your artistic connection to the floor, you must pay close attention to this important region.

Key Terms

- Achilles tendon
- anterior cruciate ligament (ACL)
- anterior talofibular ligament (ATFL)
- anterior tibiofibular ligament
- athlete's foot
- bunion
- calcaneus
- calcaneofibular ligament (CFL)
- chondromalacia patella
- cuboid syndrome
- deltoid ligament
- dorsiflexion
- eversion
- fibularis longus and brevis
- hallux valgus
- iliotibial band (ITB)
- inversion
- medial collateral ligament (MCL)
- meniscus
- neuroma
- patella
- phalanges
- plantar fascia
- plantar flexion
- posterior talofibular ligament (PTFL)
- pronation
- Q angle
- sesamoids
- supination
- talus
- valgus
- varus

WWW *Additional key terms are boldface in the chapter and defined in the glossary. A full list of key terms is available in HK*Propel*.

LEARNING OBJECTIVES

After completing this chapter, you will be able to do the following:

- Identify anatomical structures of the thigh, knee, ankle, and foot.
- Describe common dance injuries to the lower extremity.
- Explain structural pathologies of the lower extremity.
- Implement measures to reduce the risk of lower-extremity injuries.
- Implement techniques for self-care of foot and toe issues related to dance shoes.

Injuries are common among dancers of all levels and styles. Annual incidence may range from 67 to 95 percent, depending on a variety of factors and surveillance techniques utilized. A study of preprofessional modern dancers reports that approximately 65 percent of injuries occur in the lower extremity (Bronner, 2021). While most dance injuries are from overuse, approximately 28 to 35 percent are traumatic in nature (Ekegren et al., 2014; Campbell et al., 2019). It is important for the university dancer to recognize potential injuries and be able to respond accordingly to an overuse versus a traumatic onset of pain and dysfunction.

This chapter introduces basic anatomy of the lower extremity, explains common injuries and musculoskeletal complaints, describes initial care for injury, and guides the dancer in understanding how and when to seek further medical care.

Basic Anatomical Structure of the Lower Extremity

The lower extremities have three primary functions: supporting the weight of the body, locomotion, and maintenance of balance (Dalley & Agur, 2023). They are often called the legs; however, anatomically, the leg is the region between the knee and the ankle. The lower extremity has six primary regions: the gluteal and hip region, the femoral (thigh) region, the knee, the leg (lower leg), the ankle, and the foot. The hip and its injuries are explored further in chapter 13; the other five regions are described next.

Thigh

The femur is the longest bone in the body, and it joins with the pelvis to make the hip joint. Many of the muscles that act on the hip are located in the thigh, and some also work across the knee joint. These muscles can be divided into five major groups: hip flexors, quadriceps femoris, abductors, adductors, and hamstrings (figure 11.1). The hip's external rotator muscles form a sixth group that is discussed in chapter 13.

The hip flexors comprise primarily the psoas major and the iliacus. Other weaker hip flexors include the sartorius, **tensor fasciae latae (TFL)**, and pectineus. The hip flexors bring the leg up toward the torso as in a forward kicking motion (flexion). Tightness in these muscles may restrict a dancer's ability to extend (opposite of flex) the hip, as in an arabesque. The quadriceps femoris group (quads) covers the anterior surface of the femur; it includes the rectus femoris (also a weak hip flexor), vastus intermedius, vastus lateralis, and vastus medialis. The quads act to extend the leg at the knee joint. They are very important for walking, running, jumping, and landing as the muscle group both generates and absorbs large amounts of forces. Its four parts join to insert onto the **patella** (kneecap) and then travel downward to an insertion point on the upper portion of the tibia (shin bone). You can feel the prominence of this insertion below the bottom of the patella.

The posterior thigh contains the hamstring group: biceps femoris, semitendinosus, and semimembranosus. Collectively, these muscles extend the hip and flex the knee. The hip abductors are composed of the gluteus maximus, gluteus medius, and gluteus minimus. Located on the outer portion of the pelvis, these muscles move the thigh away from the midline of the body (abduct). They are important for stability and control, especially when standing on one leg, walking, running, or jumping. The adductor group is made up of the adductor magnus, adductor longus, adductor brevis, and gracilis muscles, all of which are located along the inner thigh. They work opposite the abductor group as they pull the thigh toward the midline of the body (adduct). They also are important for stabilization and balance.

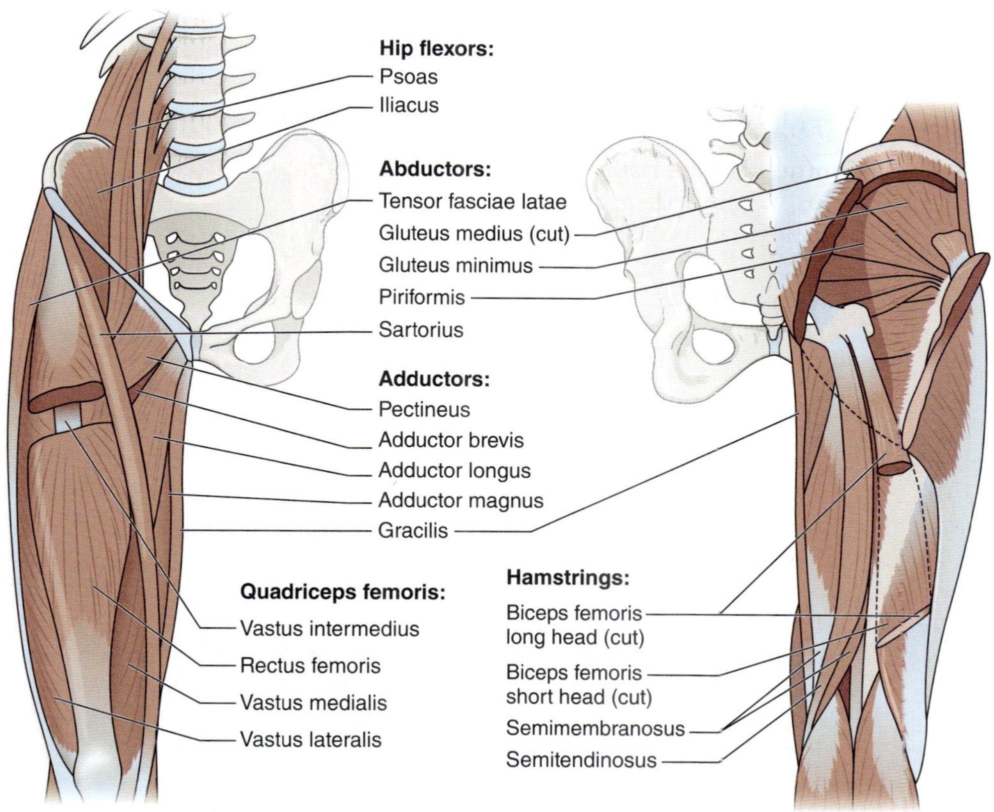

Figure 11.1 Five major muscle groups that act on the hip are the hip flexors, quadriceps femoris, hip abductors, hip adductors, and hamstrings.

Knee

The femur and tibia join together to form the knee joint, with the fibula situated laterally alongside the tibia. The patella on the front of the knee joint offers increased mechanical advantage and leverage for the quadriceps pulling across it. Inside and outside the knee, four main **ligaments** work together to stabilize the joint. These ligaments are the **anterior cruciate ligament (ACL)**, the posterior cruciate ligament (PCL), the lateral collateral ligament (LCL), and the **medial collateral ligament (MCL)**. The medial **meniscus** and lateral meniscus are horseshoe-shaped pads that act as cushions between the bones of the femur and the tibia. They also add stability to the joint by serving as saucer-like pads that hold the rounded portions of the femur, which rest on the flat top of the tibia.

Leg

The leg (commonly called the lower leg), contains the long tibia and fibula bones, which are connected by a strong, fibrous sheet termed the **interosseous membrane**. The muscles of this region are divided into four compartments and can be categorized by function. The calf includes the gastrocnemius and soleus muscles of the superficial posterior compartment. These muscles are considered the primary plantar flexors of the ankle that point the foot. They come together behind and above the ankle to form the **Achilles tendon**. Deep in the calf, there are three long muscles in the deep posterior compartment that act as weak plantar flexors, toe flexors, and inverters (turn the sole inward) of the foot; they are the tibialis posterior, the flexor digitorum longus (FDL), and the flexor hallucis longus (FHL). The anterior compartment encompasses three muscles that dorsiflex the ankle (pull the foot upward) and extend the toes: tibialis anterior, extensor digitorum longus (EDL), and extensor hallucis longus (EHL). The lateral compartment includes the fibularis longus, fibularis brevis, and (in some individuals) the fibularis tertius; these muscles act to evert the foot (turn the sole outward). The tendons of the brevis and longus pass behind the outside ankle bone (the lateral malleolus at the end of the fibula); they attach at the base of the fifth metatarsal and under the arch of the foot at the base of the first metatarsal, respectively.

Ankle

The ankle joint is where the distal ends of the tibia and fibula meet the **talus** bone. This joint has some innate bony stability but is significantly reinforced by a large number of ligaments and connective tissue. Most dance forms require large range of motion from this joint in multiple planes. The ankle joint and foot can move in four directions, as shown in figure 11.2; **dorsiflexion** (pulling the foot and toes upward), **plantar flexion** (pointing the foot downward), **inversion** (moving the sole of the foot inward toward the midline of the body), and **eversion** (moving the sole of the foot outward away from the midline of the body). Technically, inversion and eversion occur at the subtalar joint, a joint of the foot located below the ankle joint.

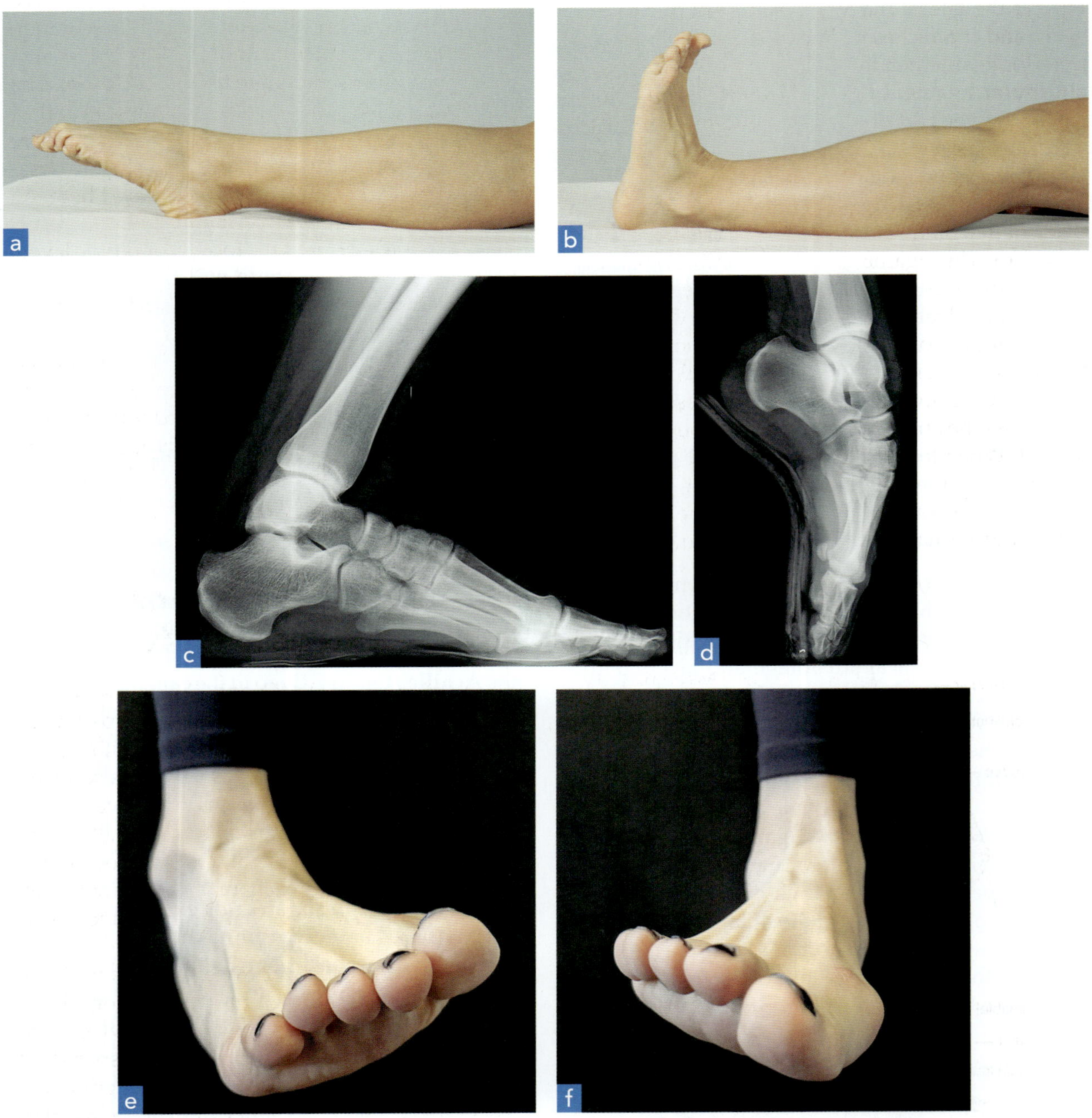

Figure 11.2 *(a)* Plantar flexion of the foot that occurs at the ankle. *(b)* Dorsiflexion of the foot that occurs at the ankle. *(c)* X-ray of a dancer in demi-plié (dorsiflexion). *(d)* X-ray of a dancer en pointe (plantar flexion). *(e)* Inversion of the foot that occurs at the subtalar joint. *(f)* Eversion of the foot that occurs at the subtalar joint.

C/D: Peter Lewton-Brain. E/F: Dr. Jeff Russell

Several ligaments hold the ankle joint's structures in place (figure 11.3). On the lateral (outside) area of the ankle, three main ligaments support the joint. The **anterior talofibular ligament (ATFL)** gets its name from its position at the ankle and its attachments. It is anterior to the lateral malleolus of the fibula (the bony protrusion on the outside portion of the ankle), and it runs between this structure and the talus. Moving posteriorly, the next ligament is the **calcaneofibular ligament (CFL)**. The CFL starts at the lateral malleolus just posterior to the ATFL, and it attaches on the **calcaneus**. The most posterior ligament in the ankle joint is the **posterior talofibular ligament (PTFL)**. The PTFL runs from the back lower part of the fibula into the back portion of the talus.

On the medial side of the ankle, the main ligament is the **deltoid ligament**, a strong, triangular ligament that binds the base of the tibia to the bones of the foot. This ligament lays in a fanlike position, and it comprises several deep and superficial ligaments; however, for the purposes of this book, consider it to be one structure in its relationships to the joint and injuries sustained in the ankle.

Most of the lower-leg muscles discussed previously cross the ankle in some manner and insert on the foot. When looking at muscular and structural injuries to the lower leg, ankle, and foot, the anatomy should always be viewed as a whole, rather than as individual joints or pieces. Often an injury to one of the leg, ankle, or foot structures can lead to secondary injury to other structures in the area.

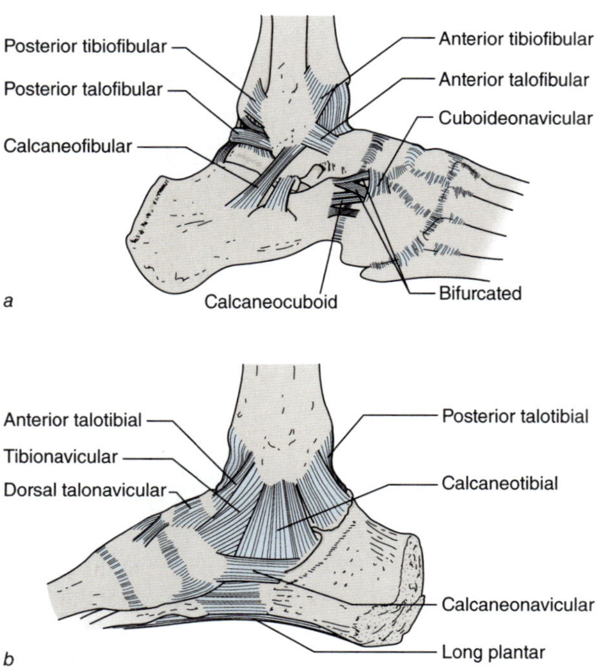

Figure 11.3 The lateral *(a)* and medial *(b)* ligaments of the ankle.

Foot

The foot is divided into three regions: the rearfoot (also called hindfoot), the midfoot, and the forefoot (figure 11.4). The rearfoot is made up of the talus and calcaneus bones. Its position and mobility are very important for proper walking, running, and jumping mechanics. The midfoot is made up of five bones: the navicular, the cuboid, and three cuneiform bones. The structure and mobility in this area can determine arch height in the dancer's foot. The forefoot contains 5 long bones (metatarsals) and 14 small bones that make up the toes; these bones are the **phalanges**. The two small, bean-shaped sesamoid bones (**sesamoids**) also are located here, on the undersurface of the first metatarsal.

The plantar surface of the foot has multiple layers of muscles. Together, these muscles support the arch of the foot; offer support and stability; move the toes; and contribute to walking, running, and jumping. The **plantar fascia** is a thick, fan-shaped band of fibrous connective tissue running along the bottom of the foot. It is intertwined with the foot muscles, and it has connective, supportive, and shock-absorbing functions. The plantar fascia is also important for helping to maintain the primary arch of the foot.

Anatomical Variations in the Lower Extremity

The quadriceps angle (**Q angle**) is a measure of the angle formed between the quadriceps muscle and the patella. The anterior superior iliac spine (ASIS) on the pelvis is used as a landmark for the measurement. Because females often have a wider pelvis than males, their Q angle is typically larger than that of males (figure 11.5). An increased Q angle may contribute to biomechanical alterations at the knee joint, which may result in injury (Daneshmandia et al., 2011).

In different people, the knee displays variation in angular alignment from a frontal view. These variations are termed genu **varus** (bowlegs) and genu **valgus** (knock-knees). Figure 11.6 depicts both variations with an example of typical alignment in the center. Extremes in either direction may place excessive forces across the tendons and ligaments around the knee, which may lead to injury.

Many dancers exhibit some degree of genu recur-

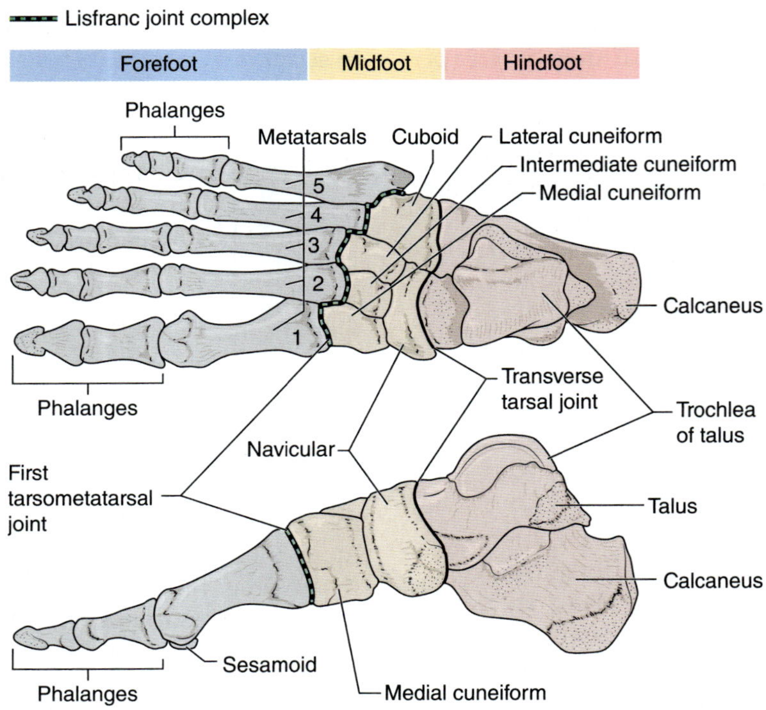

Figure 11.4 The regions and bones of the foot.

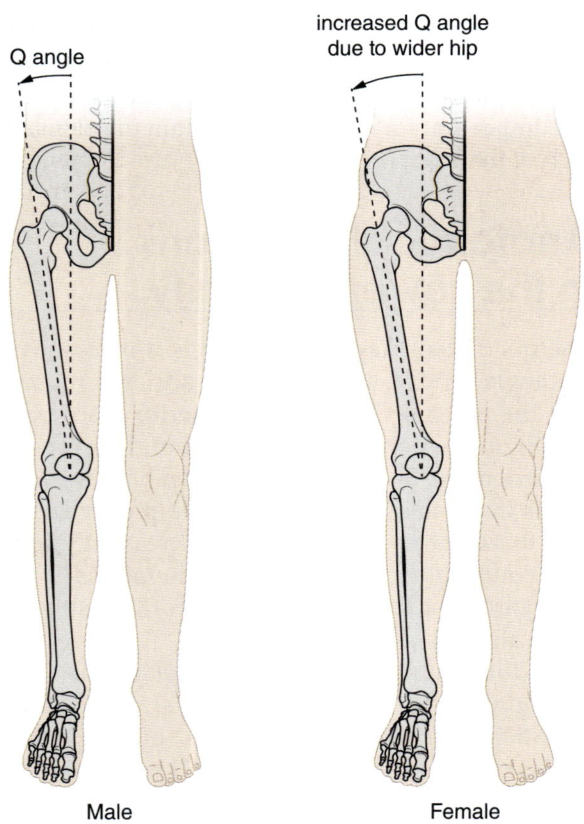

Figure 11.5 The Q angle is usually wider in females than in males because females typically have wider hips than males. Notice how the wider pelvis changes the position of the femur and thus the angle at which the femur approaches the knee.

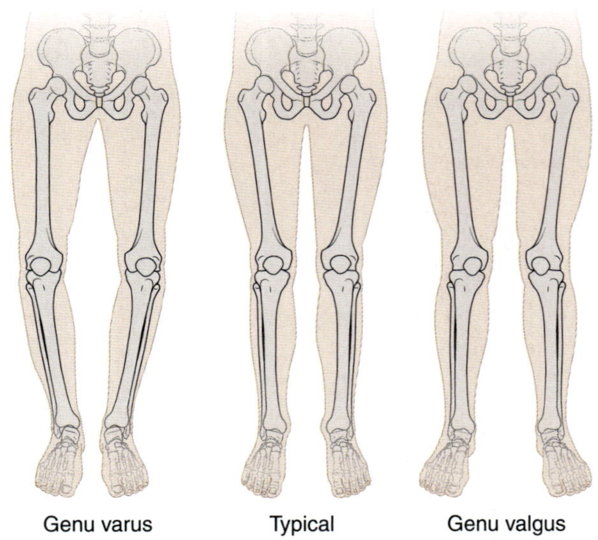

Figure 11.6 A comparison of genu varus (bowlegs), typical knee alignment, and genu valgus (knock-knees).

vatum (knee hyperextension); examples are shown in figure 11.7. This variation may be considered aesthetically pleasing in many dance styles. However, as with varus and valgus, without proper muscular control and stability, genu recurvatum may lead to increased forces across the back of the knee, which can cause injury (Campbell et al., 2019).

When describing the foot, it is helpful to use some common anatomical terms. Feet come in many shapes and sizes. As seen in figure 11.8, they vary from extremely high-arched (pes cavus) to very low-arched (pes planus). In addition to variations in the natural structure of the foot, a dancer may have altered alignment due to training, injury, or habits. A dancer's alignment of the foot and ankle when standing in a parallel position is important for assessing these deviations. High-arched feet may stand in **supination** (with the weight distributed to the outside border of the foot), whereas low-arched feet may stand with **pronation** (rolled in, with the weight along the inside border of the foot) (figure 11.9). Dancers who force their turnout may stand in pronation no matter what arch height or foot type they have; this habit creates undue stress along the medial arch.

Hallux valgus is an atypical deviation of the great toe away from the midline of the body (toward the smaller toes of the foot), which may result in a **bunion** and become painful (figure 11.10). A **bunionette** (also called a *tailor's bunion*) is a painful condition when the fifth (pinky) toe joint becomes enlarged and painful. This deformity originates from either an enlargement of the fifth metatarsal head or a change in the angle of the bones of the fifth toe.

Injuries to the Lower Extremity

The lower extremity is your connection to the floor, so its proper function is of utmost importance. When an injury occurs in the lower extremity, the dancer–floor interaction is disrupted; the likely result is compromised dancing. While many injuries can beset a dancer, some of the most common ones—injuries that should be part of your knowledge toolkit—are presented next.

Thigh and Knee Injuries

Among the most common injuries in the lower extremities are muscle strains in the quadriceps, hamstrings, and adductor muscle groups. Muscle **strains** are acute, painful injuries resulting from partial or full tearing of muscle fibers, often near the musculotendinous junction (where a muscle starts to become more tendinous in nature as it nears its insertion to a bone via a tendon) or in the mid-muscle belly (Sueki & Brechter, 2010). Muscle strains can happen with quick takeoff and lifting motions, or with stopping and lowering motions. Damage to the muscle fibers may result in swelling, warmth, redness, bruising, and pain. The pain is often worse

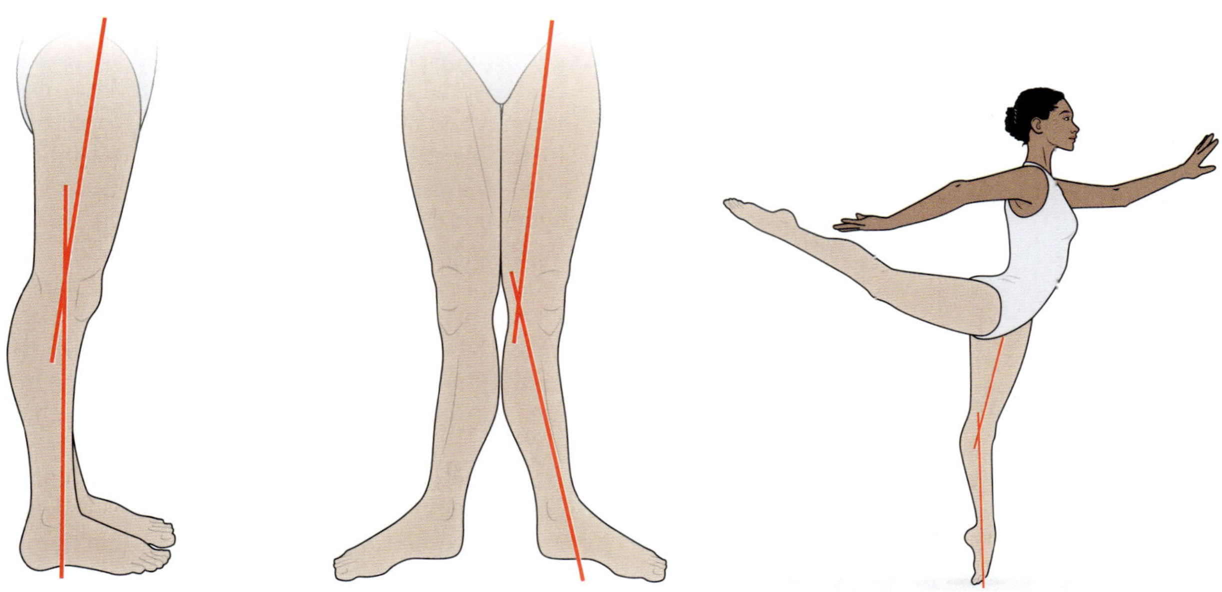

a b c

Figure 11.7 When the knees are locked to full extension in someone with genu recurvatum, the knees show hyperextension (back knees). *(a)* Side view; *(b)* dancer in first position; and *(c)* dancer in arabesque.

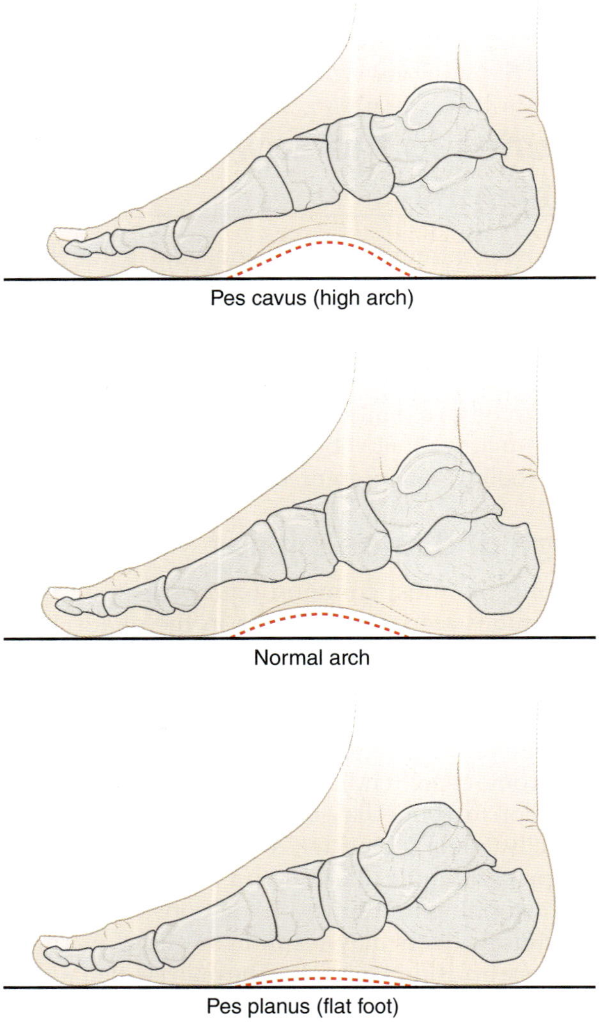

Figure 11.8 Configurations of the three types of arches: pes cavus, typical arch, and pes planus.

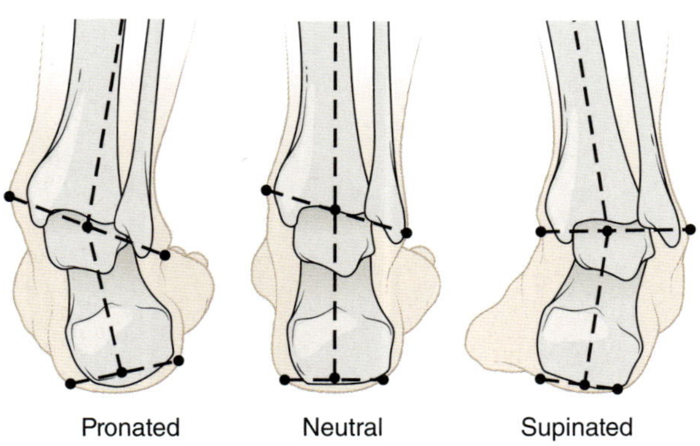

Figure 11.9 Looking from behind the leg, the heel and foot will exhibit one of these three arrangements. Pronated feet are usually associated with pes planus, while supinated feet typically occur with pes cavus.

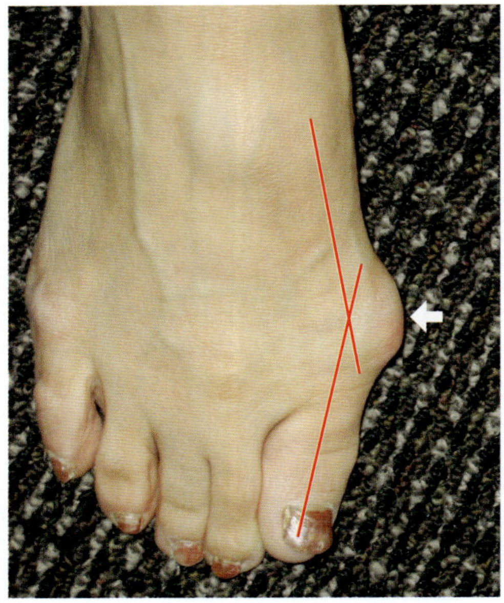

Figure 11.10 Extreme angulation between the first metatarsal in the foot and the great toe can create a bunion, as indicated by the white arrow.

Dr. Jeff Russell

with movements that cause the muscle to contract or stretch. For example, a strain to the quadriceps will be most painful with movements that involve active knee extension or passive knee flexion.

Muscle strains are graded I, II, or III depending on the severity of the injury and amount of damage to the muscle tissue. A grade I strain has stretched muscle fibers with tiny tears. A grade II strain exhibits tearing through some part of a muscle, and a grade III strain involves complete tearing of a muscle. Muscle strains, especially grades I and II, often can be treated conservatively with rest, ice or heat, gentle massage, and taping or compression garments. A dancer should consult with a healthcare professional for timing of these interventions and recommendations for over-the-counter medications, including aspirin, acetaminophen, and NSAIDs. Also, aggressive massage should not be used on an acute muscle strain because it may increase tissue damage and prolong healing time. Chapter 10 provides more specific insights into treating injuries.

Abnormal mechanics or muscle imbalances around the hip or knee may contribute to **iliotibial band (ITB)** syndrome. Pain from dysfunction in this area may occur at the lateral hip (covered in chapter 13) or at the lateral knee. The ITB is a thick band of fascia running down the outside of the thigh and connecting the gluteal muscles, the TFL, the quads, and the hamstrings to the knee. Dysfunction may result from variations in knee alignment, weakness in the gluteal muscles, overworking of the quadriceps, or tightness in the ITB (Sueki & Brechter, 2010). While foam rolling of the lateral thigh is often recommended for treatment of this condition, compression and trauma to the tissues may actually worsen the pain; it depends on the root cause of the pathology. A dancer suspecting ITB syndrome should seek proper examination, evaluation, and treatment from a qualified health care practitioner.

Although injuries to the patella may often be associated with sports, such as soccer or basketball, they are common in dance and other performing arts, too (Peng et al., 2015). Many of the movements associated with sports—such as jumping, landing, and deep knee bends (pliés)—are also common in most forms of dance. As addressed previously, the upper muscles of the thigh and the ITB have a significant impact on the patella and how it interacts with the groove of the femur in which it rests.

One of the most common injuries pertaining to the patella is caused by improper sliding in its groove. When it rides to one side (almost always laterally), a condition known as **chondromalacia patella** can develop. Chondromalacia is the roughening of the normally smooth cartilage behind the patella. Contributing causes of chondromalacia may include weakness in the medial quadriceps muscle, tightness in the quadriceps or ITB, and a large Q angle. All of these factors can lead to the patella being pulled laterally which, in turn, increases its pressure against its groove. Dancers tend to describe chondromalacia pain as a grinding sensation as the patella rides against the outer part of the patellar groove. One analogy for how chondromalacia feels is when a car is driving on a highway and it veers toward the side of the road, hitting the rumble strip (a series of rough grooves designed to alert drivers) (figure 11.11).

Initial treatment for chondromalacia is relative rest and ice. A patellar tendon strap or taping may

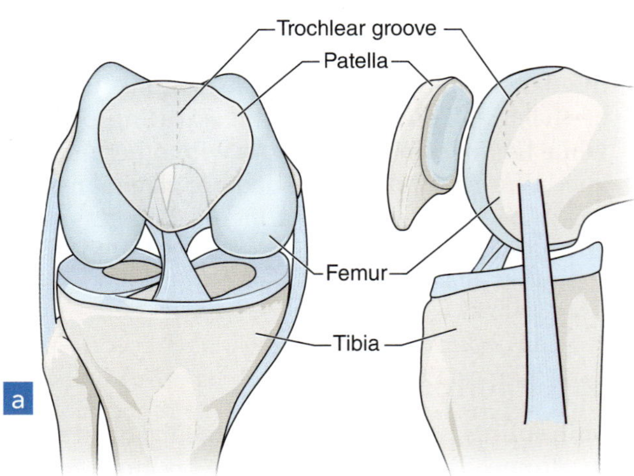

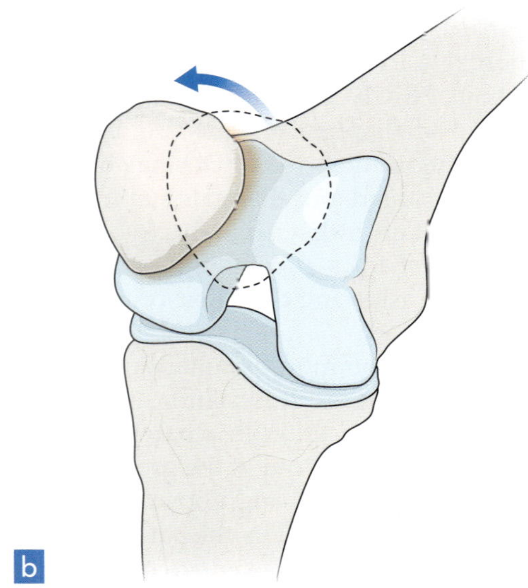

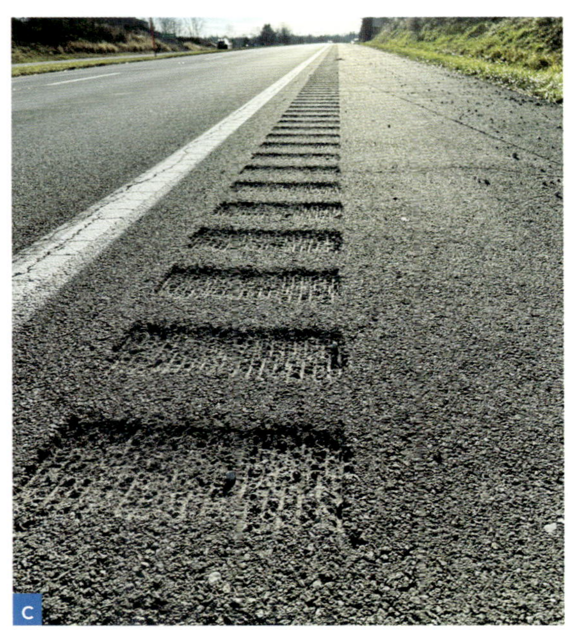

Figure 11.11 *(a)* The patella has a ridge on its posterior side from top to bottom. This ridge fits into a groove on the femur, which allows the patella to slide up and down. *(b)* Sometimes the patella sits too far to one side of its groove (almost always the lateral side), which can create pain. When it is not in its groove, the smooth back of the patella can become rough, or its groove can become rough, or both. *(c)* This positioning may create a grinding sensation that is similar to a rumble strip on a highway that alerts a driver that their vehicle is drifting off the side of the road.

C: Dr. Jeff Russell

be recommended for maintaining proper alignment of the patella, but it should be applied under the guidance of a trained health care professional. Long-term care of chondromalacia is usually managed by assessing the biomechanics of the knee and incorporating rehabilitative exercises for factors such as tight thigh muscles, muscle weaknesses, or imbalances between muscles. The goal for all of these treatments is to restore nonpainful tracking of the patella in its groove.

Other injuries associated with the patella include patellar tendinopathies, subluxations, and dislocations. Patellar **tendinopathy** can be acute or chronic in nature, and it may be associated with variations in alignment of the patella. *Tendinopathy* refers to a condition that creates pain in a tendon. Self-care for patellar tendinopathy is similar to that for other knee injuries; it should be treated with PRICE (protection, rest, ice, compression, elevation); more details about PRICE and other injury treatments are provided in chapter 10. Nonsteroidal anti-inflammatory medications (NSAIDs) may be helpful if they are warranted, but these are not innocuous drugs to be taken indiscrimately. Evaluating a dancer's biomechanics and thigh muscle flexibility may help in assessing the cause of the patellar tendinopathy.

Although less common, patellar subluxations and dislocations can result in significant pain and dysfunction for a dancer. With a **patellar subluxation**, the kneecap slides out of the groove (almost always to the lateral side) and pops right back in. With a full patellar dislocation, the patella typically slides all the way out of its groove and may not return to position without applying manual force. Both of these injuries should be assessed by a medical professional; they will require rehabilitation to return to dance. Often, chronic patellar subluxations can lead to patellar dislocations; once one dislocation happens, subsequent occurrences are more likely. As with all knee injuries, alignment, strength, and flexibility in the thigh should be addressed to reduce the risk of reoccurrence.

Injuries may also happen to the four main ligaments of the knee (ACL, PCL, MCL, and LCL). Liederbach and colleagues (2008) report that the two most commonly injured ligaments in dancers are the ACL and the MCL. Injury to the ACL in a dancer can occur similarly to an ACL injury in other athletes. However, ACL injuries are less common in dancers than they are in traditional sports (Liederbach et al., 2008). This lower rate is most likely attributed to the aesthetic nature of jump landings that dancers must execute compared to how jump landings are performed in sports such as basketball or volleyball. In dance these landings are typically choreographed and practiced repeatedly, whereas in jumping sports they often are instinctual and unplanned in response to the action of a game or match.

Often the mechanism of injury (MOI) is a planting and twisting motion in the knee joint or is related to poor landing mechanics. Many athletes state that they experience a popping sensation when this injury occurs, followed by pain and swelling in the knee joint. The knee may also hyperextend with walking, or it may feel unstable. A suspected injury to the ACL should immediately be assessed by a medical professional. Often, a severe injury to the ACL will result in surgery and/or an extended time for rehabilitating the knee and lower extremity.

The other commonly injured ligament in the medial portion of the knee is the MCL. Like the ACL, this ligament can be injured with a twisting motion or a force applied from the lateral side of the knee that forces the MCL to elongate or tear. Most injuries to the MCL do not require surgery, but rehabilitation is essential to reduce the risk of further damage to the MCL and other structures of the knee joint.

The medial and lateral menisci may also be injured. Although chronic deterioration of the meniscus may occur in older dancers, a more common injury in younger dancers is a meniscus tear. This injury can cause pain and discomfort for the dancer, and it frequently leads to complaints of clicking or locking sensations during pliés or while landing from a jump. As with other internal knee injuries, injury to the medial or lateral meniscus must be assessed by a medical professional. Treatment plans for the meniscus tend to focus on symptom relief. This injury may or may not require surgery.

Leg Injuries

Shin splints is a general term for medial tibial stress syndrome. Shin splints may have multiple causes: inflammation of the thin membrane covering the tibia; trigger points or overuse of the soleus, flexor digitorum longus (FDL), or posterior tibialis muscles; or fascial tightness in the calf. Dancers may experience generalized pain along the back, front, or inside of the lower leg along the tibia. Shin splint pain may be an early warning sign of faulty biomechanics that can lead to more serious injuries such as stress fractures and chronic exertional compartment syndrome (CECS).

A **stress fracture** is the term for microdamage to the bone. It is the result of repetitive stress forces, often accompanied by poor technique or biomechanics with running and jumping. Lack of rest is one factor that may lead to the injury. University dancers are more likely to experience a tibial stress fracture in the upper third of the bone (Sueki & Brechter, 2010). Pain usually occurs on the front of the bone in a very localized spot, and it gets worse with running and jumping. In addition, a dancer with a stress fracture may complain of throbbing pain at night and while resting. Female dancers, as well as those with disordered eating or nutritional deficiencies, are more likely to develop stress fractures of any type. Dancers with tibial stress fractures may be put on a non-weight-bearing status to allow the bone to rest and heal. Stress fractures can accompany relative energy deficiency in sport (REDs), a nutritional condition discussed in chapter 7.

Fibular stress fractures are similar to those in the tibia; however, the pain is on the outside of the leg and usually closer to the ankle. All suspected stress fractures should be evaluated by a health care provider. They may use a tuning fork, ultrasound, bone scan, X-ray, MRI, or CT scan to determine the presence of this injury. Dancers with achy bone pain should avoid medications until medical evaluation is completed because certain medications may delay bone healing.

Chronic exertional compartment syndrome (CECS) is a condition in which increased pressure within a confined space disrupts muscle, nerve, and/or circulatory function. CECS may be felt as shin or calf pain, and it occurs when the muscles swell inside the restricted space of their compartments. While compartment syndrome can be caused by direct trauma to the leg—which, if severe enough, can create a medical emergency—dancers are more likely to experience the chronic form. Symptoms tend to appear gradually at a predictable time during dance; they may include weakness, pain, numbness, tingling, tightness, and swelling. In CECS, symptoms resolve with stopping dance and elevating the leg, but they return when dance is resumed. Often CECS can be treated conservatively; it should be evaluated by a medical professional. Some patients require surgery to make a small cut in the fascia and relieve the pressure in the muscle compartment (Sueki & Brechter, 2010).

A strain to the calf muscles is similar to a strain in the thigh muscles (as previously addressed). Muscle strains in this area may happen with takeoff or landing movements because of the high muscle forces applied to accelerate or decelerate the body. Pain is worse with dance movements such as single-leg relevé, plié, or other movements requiring weight-bearing plantar flexion.

Ankle and Foot Injuries

One of the most common injuries to the lower extremity is a lateral ankle **sprain** (injury to a ligament); this trend is the same in dancers as it is with nondancers (Hamilton, 1982; Prakash, 2017; Ramkumar et al., 2016). A variety of factors could contribute to ankle and foot injuries in dance, including ankle instability, shoe design, choreographic requirements, or dance surfaces. Some of these factors, such as shoe type, may be outside the dancer's control. Strengthening the muscles around the ankle joint can reduce injury risk.

Lateral ankle sprains occur with a roll onto the outside of the foot (inversion injury)—often while en pointe or demi-pointe—or in a missed landing from a jump (Kadel, 2014). This movement can be relatively small for someone dancing barefoot or large in a dancer wearing a high-heeled character shoe or a pointe shoe. Ankle sprains can be acute or chronic in nature, and treatments vary based on type. For many performers, their first acute ankle sprain may be significant; it should be rehabilitated properly so that it does not become a long-term chronic or recurring injury (Russell, 2010).

An acute sprain on the lateral side of the ankle is the most common type and may be associated with one or more lateral ankle ligaments (ATFL, CFL, PTFL). The grade indicates the severity from a stretch (grade I) to a complete tear (grade III). Injury to the lateral ankle often results in pain, swelling, bruising, and limping. Other injuries may accompany sprains; therefore, ankle sprains should always be evaluated by a health care professional. Proper rehabilitation of the ankle is important for decreasing the risk of sustaining repetitive ankle sprains and chronic ankle instability. These conditions result from reinjury to the area, poor strength, poor proprioception, and naturally loose ligament tissue (Lin et al., 2011; O'Loughlin et al., 2008; Steib et al., 2013).

Although less common than lateral ankle sprains, medial ankle sprains do occur in performers (Waterman et al., 2011). Medial ankle sprains occur when the foot is rolled away from the midline of the body (everted) and the deltoid ligament is injured. The deltoid ligament—with its multiple layers—tends to provide more stability and is less likely to be injured than the lateral ligaments. Sprains to the medial side of the ankle often take longer to heal, and other injuries to the surrounding areas are common. With all injuries to the ankle, medical evaluation should be a top priority to ensure a speedy recovery.

A third type of ankle sprain is a **high ankle sprain**. This type of sprain causes damage to the ligaments that hold the tibia and fibula together. The **anterior tibiofibular ligament** runs between the front of the tibia (at the top of the ankle) and the fibula. An injury to this ligament and the interosseus membrane is often caused by a twisting force in the lower leg with the foot planted on the floor. High ankle sprains may be very painful. Insufficient rest and rehabilitation for this injury can result in chronic pain, instability, dysfunction of the muscle and tendon structures in the lower leg and foot, and an extended return to dancing.

The tendons of the lower leg, ankle, and foot of a dancer are susceptible to injury from overuse, poor mechanics, and other external factors. The **Achilles tendon** is the largest and strongest tendon in the body; it connects the calf muscles to the calcaneus. The Achilles tendon is subject to extremely high forces with jumping, running, and relevé. Lack of strength and endurance of the calf muscles may lead to Achilles tendon dysfunction (Mahieu et al., 2006). Dancers who force their turnout or don't put their heels down when landing jumps are also at risk for Achilles tendon injury.

A dancer with Achilles tendinopathy usually has pain, stiffness, swelling, and tenderness in the back of the heel or just behind the ankle joint. This pain is often worse at the beginning of activity, and it may improve as the dancer warms up. Relative rest, contrast baths, gentle stretching, and strengthening of the calf muscles can improve the symptoms. In ballet dancers, modifying the placement and tightness of pointe shoe ribbons may provide some relief. If pain persists, evaluation and treatment by a health care practitioner is needed. Rehabilitation with manual techniques, use of a night splint for sleeping, and calf strengthening exercises may help.

Flexor hallucis longus (FHL) tendinopathy is seen most frequently in the female ballet dancer; it is often described as *dancer's tendinopathy*. The repetitive motion at the foot and ankle when moving from plié to relevé (or to en pointe position) can lead to inflammation and swelling of the FHL tendon as it passes through a tunnel just under the medial ankle. When the tendon is swollen, dancers may feel pain and popping or catching behind or under the medial ankle bone, especially with takeoff from jumps, rising to the en pointe position, and even in grand plié. Since the FHL tendon attaches to the bone at the end of the great toe, the toe may lock because the tendon does not slide properly through its tunnel. Relative rest, reducing relevés, taking a break from pointe work, rehabilitation exercises, and taking anti-inflammatory medication (NSAIDs) usually resolve the problem. Inattention to this injury typically worsens the problem until the lubricating **synovial sheaths** in which the tendon travels become inflamed. This condition, called **tenosynovitis**, is much more difficult to treat. Since the FHL is such an important tendon for dancers, it is important to seek medical treatment, particularly in those dancers whose symptoms persist and those with restriction of movement in the great toe.

The **fibularis (or peroneus) longus and brevis** tendons can be injured acutely during an ankle sprain. Pain, swelling, or popping along the lateral ankle that is worsened with winging the foot may indicate irritation to these tendons. Sometimes after an ankle sprain, the tendons can sublux (slide or pop from their normal position behind the lateral ankle bone) with ankle movement. Avoidance of painful movements, using ice or contrast baths, taking NSAIDS, and participating in rehabilitation may help. A health care professional should be consulted if symptoms continue.

Anterior ankle impingement, felt as a pinching in the front of the ankle, may be the result of swollen soft tissues or small protrusions of bone in the front ankle joint. Symptoms include pain with landing jumps, along with restricted and painful plié and demi-plié. Swelling may or may not be visible. To reduce the symptoms, dancers can try avoiding jumps, avoiding forced pliés, and adding heel lifts to their shoes. A health care professional should be consulted if the symptoms persist. Brief use of a walking boot and a night splint may help alleviate pain and inflammation. Rehabilitation with a specialist will address technical errors and foot alignment issues. If pain persists, injections and surgical treatments may be helpful (O'Kane & Kadel, 2008).

Posterior ankle impingement is characterized by pain in the back of the ankle during plantar flexion (figure 11.12). This condition is found commonly in dancers; it occurs because of compression of bony or soft tissues in the back of the ankle between the end of the tibia and the calcaneus (Russell et al., 2010). Stiffness, limited mobility, and pain with relevé and pointe work are the typical symptoms. A dancer may find they cannot fully plantar flex,

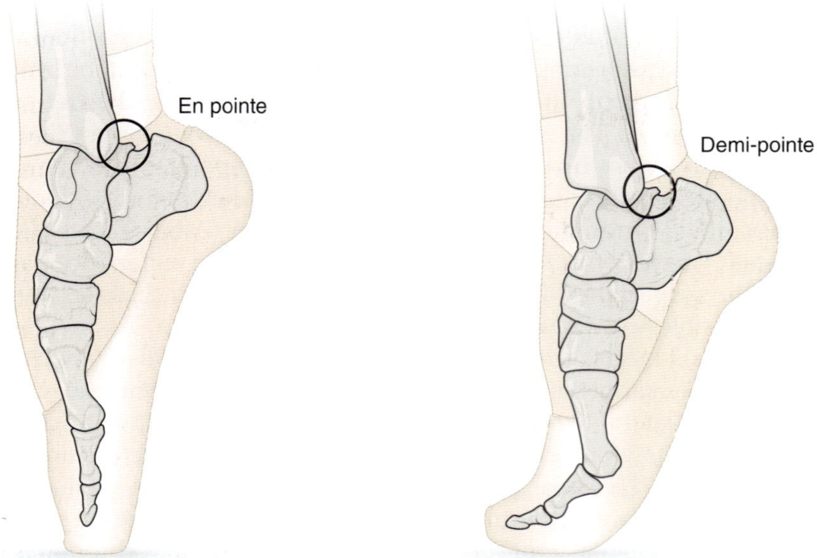

Figure 11.12 Diagram showing the areas where posterior ankle impingement occurs. Within the encircled areas, the bones of the ankle and foot come together, thus increasing the possibility of bone or soft tissue becoming entrapped there.

Adapted by permission from J.A. Russell, "Pathoanatomy of Posterior Ankle Impingement in Ballet Dancers." *Clinical Anatomy*, 23, no.6 (2010): 613-621. doi: 10.1002/ca.20991.

achieve three-quarter pointe, or get onto the box of their pointe shoe. Pain is usually felt in the posterior ankle, just in front of the Achilles tendon and slightly toward the outside. When the pain occurs toward the inside of the ankle, posterior impingement and FHL tendinopathy may be occurring together. The dancer should limit painful activities (including pointe work) and seek medical advice for strengthening and mobilizing the ankle joint. Use of a night splint may help to reduce stiffness and inflammation. In some cases, surgery may be necessary to remove the bone or soft tissue that is being compressed at the back of the ankle.

WWW Go to HK*Propel* to read the supplemental content "Inside Views of the Ankle and Foot en Pointe" and "Evaluating Readiness for Dancing en Pointe".

A **Lisfranc sprain** is an injury to the ligaments of the midfoot joints, which are called Lisfranc's joints. These ligaments support the arches of the foot. Injury to the Lisfranc joints may occur with a fall off the pointe position, a missed jump landing, a takeoff for a jump, or an over-arching of the foot. A severe Lisfranc injury causes significant swelling and bruising on the bottom of the foot. Most dancers cannot bear weight following a severe midfoot sprain. If the ligaments are fully torn, the foot becomes very unstable; severe Lisfranc injuries require surgery and recovery is usually prolonged. It begins with non-weight-bearing activities for 6 to 12 weeks to allow for healing; then, focused rehabilitation of the entire kinetic chain of the lower extremity is needed to return the dancer to full performance (Kadel & Donaldson-Fletcher, 2004).

An **accessory navicular** is an extra bone that forms a bump on the navicular bone. It is located at the top of the arch on the medial foot, where the posterior tibialis tendon attaches to the foot just below and forward of the ankle. It is considered a normal anatomical variation, and is present in 4 to 21 percent of the population (Kalbouneh et al., 2017; Kelikian & Sarrafian, 2011); it does not create problems in most people. Accessory navicular syndrome describes when this bump becomes painful. Often, pain occurs after twisting the foot, falling, or spraining the ankle. The area over the irritated accessory navicular may be tender, swollen, or red. Initial treatments for the pain can include a heel wedge in the shoes, taping, over-the-counter arch supports, NSAIDs, and rehabilitative exercises. If these measures do not resolve the pain, physician evaluation is needed because surgical treatments may be recommended (Nwawka et al., 2013).

The cause of **cuboid syndrome** (also called cuboid subluxation) is poorly defined. It is likely a joint dysfunction of the lateral midfoot, where the oblong cuboid bone can slide or rotate from its normal position. Symptoms of this condition include lateral foot pain with weight bearing and an inability to roll through the foot correctly to achieve demi-pointe or full pointe position. The pain can develop gradually (especially when repetitively doing relevés or hops en pointe) or after a traumatic event (e.g., ankle sprain). Cuboid syndrome may be difficult to identify clinically or even with X-rays or other imaging. Dancers who suspect they have this injury should whenever possible find a health care provider who is familiar with dancers. The condition responds well to manual treatments, taping, and padding. Tightness of the lateral leg muscles should be addressed, and pointe work or jumps may need to be limited (Durall, 2011; Kadel, 2014).

Metatarsal stress fractures in the foot are the most common stress fractures reported in dancers. They often occur at the base of the second metatarsal near the midfoot (Albisetti et al., 2010). Complaints include throbbing, dull, or toothache-like pain at the end of class or with specific activities (e.g., jumps). If untreated, pain and swelling may worsen and become more constant, presenting at rest or at night. When dancers develop midfoot pain, they should avoid anti-inflammatory medications until a diagnosis from a health care provider has been made, as these medications may inhibit bone healing. Medical imaging and other techniques may be needed to fully diagnose a stress fracture.

Casting or surgery is usually not necessary for foot stress fractures as long as the dancer can avoid painful activities. If walking in supportive sneakers is painful, the dancer should use crutches or a walking boot until the symptoms improve. Conditioning can be maintained with floor barre, Pilates, pool exercises, or non-weight-bearing cardio exercises if they cause no pain in the area of the stress fracture. Rehabilitation includes gradual return to class with avoidance of pointe work, jumps, turns, and demi-pointe until healing is complete and the foot is no longer tender (Albisetti et al., 2010).

Dancers often experience pain in the ball of the foot. Causes may include sesamoiditis, plantar plate injury, or neuroma. As mentioned earlier in the chapter, the sesamoids are two tiny bones under the head of the first metatarsal. Much like the patella in the knee, the sesamoids act to improve the function of the tendons across the great toe joint. They are very important in push-off with walking and jumping, as forces that are several times the dancer's body weight go through the joint with these activities. The sesamoids may become inflamed or fractured with overuse or trauma. Sesamoid injury may cause a dancer to experience pain with relevé. Relative rest, padding, taping, and modification of activity are important ways to manage this condition.

The **plantar plate** comprises the ligamentous structures supporting the joints that connect the toes to the foot. Dancers may sprain or tear these structures, especially under the second metatarsal. This injury may be traumatic in nature (e.g., from a hard landing from a jump), or it may be an overuse injury. Significant trauma to the plantar plate or to the other ligaments of the toes may also result in toe dislocation. Any injuries to this area should be assessed by a health care professional; they may be treated with or without surgery.

Dancer's Feet and Legs Self-Care Toolkit

The following collection of widely available products will help dancers keep their feet and legs in excellent condition.

- Pinky ball, lacrosse ball, or avocado ball (for rolling out trigger points in smaller areas)
- Foam roller (for rolling out trigger points in broader areas)
- Ice pack (refreezable)
- Stretching strap
- Exercise band
- Pumice stone or emery boards
- Pedi-shaver
- Moisturizer

A final cause of symptoms in the forefoot may be a **neuroma**, a benign mass, swelling, or thickening caused by irritation of one of the tiny nerves between the metatarsals that provide sensation of the toes. Pain is typically between the second and third toes, or the third and fourth toes; the syndrome is termed Morton's neuroma (Sueki & Brechter, 2010). Symptoms may include sharp or burning pain in addition to numbness and tingling. Tight-fitting shoes, trauma, overuse, or variations in alignment may contribute to a neuroma. This condition is often treated conservatively with taping, padding, or shoe adaptations.

Plantar fasciitis is inflammation of the plantar fascia. Clinical evidence shows that many patients have plantar fascia pain without inflammation. The injury is typically caused by overuse. It may be accompanied by microtears in the plantar fascia or bone spurs on the underside of the calcaneus. Pain may also occur because of **myofascial trigger point** referral from the gastrocnemius or soleus muscles (figure 11.13). Trigger points are localized, tender spots of hyperactive, hypersensitive muscle and fascia tissue.

Factors such as body weight, shoe wear, jumping, or limited ankle flexibility may all contribute to plantar fasciitis. Pain often increases with standing, walking, running, and any other activity requiring repetitive use of the foot. However, a telltale sign of true plantar fasciitis is heightened pain first thing in the morning or after a prolonged period of sitting. Dancers with suspected plantar fasciitis should seek an evaluation with a rehabilitation professional to thoroughly assess potential causes of their pain and to receive corrective treatments and exercises.

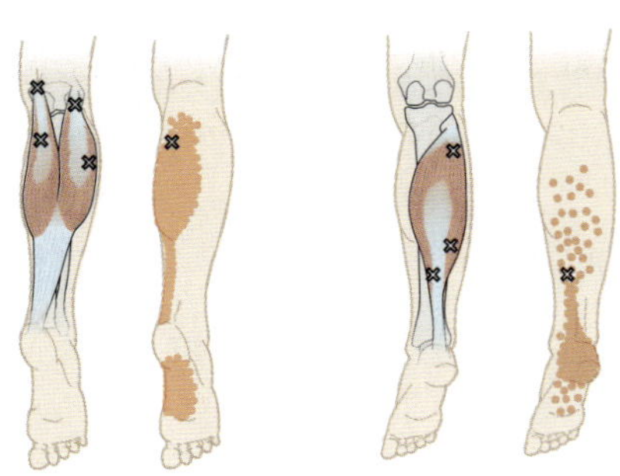

Figure 11.13 Myofascial trigger point (x) pain can be referred to the plantar fascia on the bottom of the foot by trigger points in both the *(a)* gastrocnemius and *(b)* soleus muscles.

Other Common Conditions of the Feet

As a dancer, your feet are not only your main mode of transportation but a critical part of your craft and art form. Therefore, caring for your feet must be a high priority. This care should include the skin in and around the feet, the nails, and the nail beds. This section covers conditions associated with these parts of the feet and provides prevention strategies to reduce their occurrence.

Fissures, cracks, and splits are terms used to describe openings in dancers' feet; they often occur under or between the toes, or under thick calluses. These openings can be difficult to heal; if not treated, they may bleed and become infected. Washing the feet daily with soap and water and drying them thoroughly between the toes may prevent splits. Keeping the feet dry is important because soft, moist skin tears easily.

Calluses are thickened areas of skin that develop in response to pressure (from dancing barefoot or from shoes). Some callus formation is protective; however, it is important to use an emery board, foot file, or pumice stone to reduce the callus layers if they become thick and dry. A build-up in these layers can lead to fissures. Keeping calluses moisturized may also be helpful. Occurrence of redness, swelling, increased pain, or drainage may indicate an infection for which the dancer should seek medical advice. See the sidebar titled Dancer's Feet and Legs Self-Care Toolkit on the previous page for a list of helpful preventive products for dancers.

Athlete's foot (medical name: tinea pedis) is an itchy, scaly foot rash caused by a fungus; the rash usually starts between the toes. It is common in people who have sweaty feet and wear tight-fitting shoes (a familiar scenario for many dancers). It is a contagious condition that can spread to your fellow dancers through contaminated towels, socks, shared shoes, and floors. Keeping the feet clean and dry, changing sweaty socks and shoes as soon as possible, and rotating your use of several pairs of shoes can help prevent the spread of infection. Use of an over-the-counter antifungal cream may clear up the symptoms. If not improved after these measures, a health care provider's advice is needed.

Blisters happen to almost everyone, and they are common in dancers. Contributing factors include new shoes, ill-fitting shoes, excessive sweating, and high friction points between the skin and shoe. A blister may start as a hot spot or an area of the skin that is red and irritated. It is important to notice these spots and try to cover them prior to the skin breaking. If left untreated, continued friction occurs and the skin may tear, leading to more pain, redness, and bleeding (figure 11.14). Once the skin is broken, the area must be properly cleaned and dressed to prevent infection.

Preventing blisters is always the best practice. Dancers who wear shoes should examine them prior to rehearsal, feeling for any areas on the shoe that are tight or that may cause pressure. New shoes may require stretching or break-in time, so dancers should allow for this time in their rehearsal and performance schedule. If a dancer tends to have sweaty feet, frequent changes of socks or stockings may help. For those who dance barefoot, proper preparation of areas in contact with the floor may prevent blisters. Multiple products are on the market (e.g., tapes, bandages, blister pads, donut pads, and gel spacers) that can be wrapped and applied to the foot and toes to prevent friction and blisters (see sidebar titled Blister Self-Care Toolkit). Similar to breaking in new shoes, the dancer should practice using these products prior to starting rehearsal.

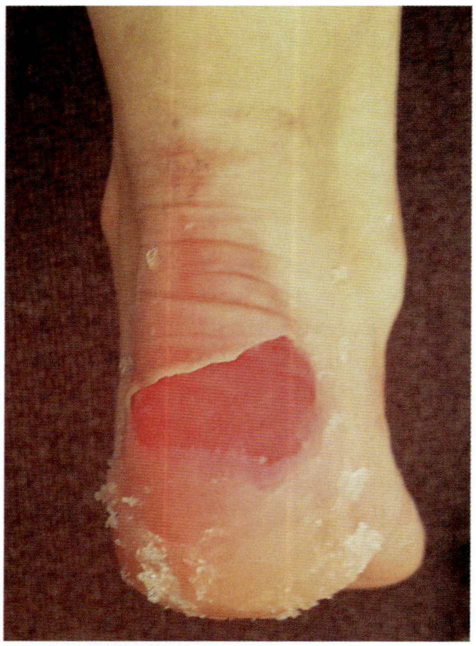

Figure 11.14 A blister can be surprisingly debilitating, especially if not treated properly.

Meg Schneider

Nail problems can affect dancers regardless of whether they perform in bare feet, pointe shoes, or heels. Ingrown toenails are a common problem. Stubbing the toe or having the toe stepped on may lead to an ingrown nail. However, the most common cause is trimming the nails too short. Nails should be trimmed straight across and square shaped. The corners should not be cut to follow the shape of the toe as the tapered edges may encourage the toenail to grow into the skin of the toe. Tight shoes and sweaty feet can contribute to the problem. Redness, pain, and swelling at the edge of the nail are the first signs of infection. Warm epsom salt soaks may help, but if symptoms worsen or persist, consult a podiatrist for treatment. Antibiotics may be prescribed.

A bruised toenail (subungual hematoma) is bruising and bleeding under the nail. Dropping a heavy object on the toes or being stepped on by someone can cause this condition; however, in dancers, a bruised toenail is usually the result of repeatedly jamming the toe into the toe box of a pointe shoe or another tight shoe. Throbbing pain of the toe is the first symptom, followed by discoloration under the

Blister Self-Care Toolkit

These items are a helpful collection of widely available products that will help dancers prevent and treat blisters (see corresponding numbers in figure 11.15).

1. Tape assortment, including adhesive and nonadhesive stretch tapes
2. Adhesive padding assortment in donut shapes
3. Water-based gelatinous friction pads
4. Silicone or gel toe spacers
5. Bandage assortment

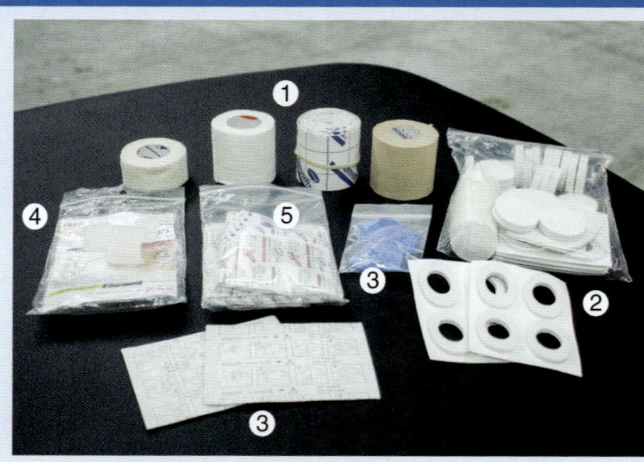

Figure 11.15 Blister kit.

Meg Schneider

nail. Icing the toe may be helpful for the pain, but treatment by a podiatrist is recommended to prevent worsening of the condition and loss of the nail.

Dance Shoes and the Feet

In the performing arts world, artistic directors and company managers often make determinations about footwear and costume choices. Not every dancer has the same size or shape foot, but performers are frequently required to wear uniform footwear to maintain the integrity of the costume appearance and the desired aesthetic. Attempting to force one's foot into a shoe that does not fit properly can result in many short-term issues mentioned previously, such as blisters and nail problems. Long-term use of ill-fitting footwear can also lead to chronic injuries such as plantar fasciitis or tendinopathy. Many options are available to the artistic team and the dancer to help alleviate some of these issues and to obtain a better fit for dancers. Consulting a health care professional accustomed to working with dance footwear may be helpful.

Many dance shoes lack proper arch support for maintaining stability during use. Using off-the-shelf arch supports is a great way to add additional support to a heeled or flat dance shoe. Another helpful product is a rubber or felt arch support that can be taped into the sole of the dance shoes. However, a medical professional should place them to ensure proper fit and support because often when external items, such as tape or arch supports, are added to a shoe, the shoe may feel too tight and create pressure points on the foot. Pressure points may also occur due to a dancer's natural anatomy, such as a bunion or a wide forefoot. In this instance, shoe alterations may be recommended by a health care provider.

Dancers should also be mindful of their footwear outside the studio or rehearsal space. Although flip-flops or sandals may feel great on the way to and from the studio to allow the feet to breathe, they provide virtually no support or protection. After a class, rehearsal, or performance, the legs and feet may be fatigued; in this instance, supportive shoes should be worn to protect the feet on the way to the next destination. Generally, athletic sneakers or similar shoes should be worn as much as possible outside of dancing to provide adequate support and rest for the feet.

Conclusions and Practical Relevance

Numerous lower-extremity injuries could occur in dancers of all dance genres. Therefore, knowing basic anatomy and giving attention to proper mechanics and preventive measures will prove extremely beneficial to anyone involved in dance. If a dancer sustains an injury, timely evaluation by a health care professional will speed recovery; moreover, it may keep an injury from becoming worse. Treating an injury early in its stages often results in less time off from dance and fewer compensations that could lead to further injury. Overall, there are many ways that you, the dancer, can take responsibility for keeping yourself performance-ready.

Discussion Questions

1. A director selects a new performance shoe, and several dancers start having lower shin pain and excessive blisters. What are some ideas for helping these performers?
2. You are a dancer. A new piece is set, and the decision is made to perform it in bare feet. What are some helpful strategies to help you protect your feet?
3. You are a dance teacher. A dancer comes to you complaining of medial knee pain along with lateral hip pain. Explain what anatomical structures should be addressed when dealing with this injury.
4. You are a choreographer. A female performer informs you that she has not had a menstrual cycle in over 2 years, and she is now having chronic foot and ankle pain. Discuss the steps and guidance you would give to this performer.
5. As a dancer, what are some of the initial treatments you can do on your own for tendon pain? What are those treatments for pain at the hip, at the knee, and at the ankle and foot?

WWW Go to HK*Propel* to access supplemental information and activities connected to chapter content.

Dance Injuries in the Upper Extremity

Steven J. Karageanes, DO, FAOASM
Amanda M. Donahue, MS, ATC
Lynnette Khoo-Summers, PT, DPT

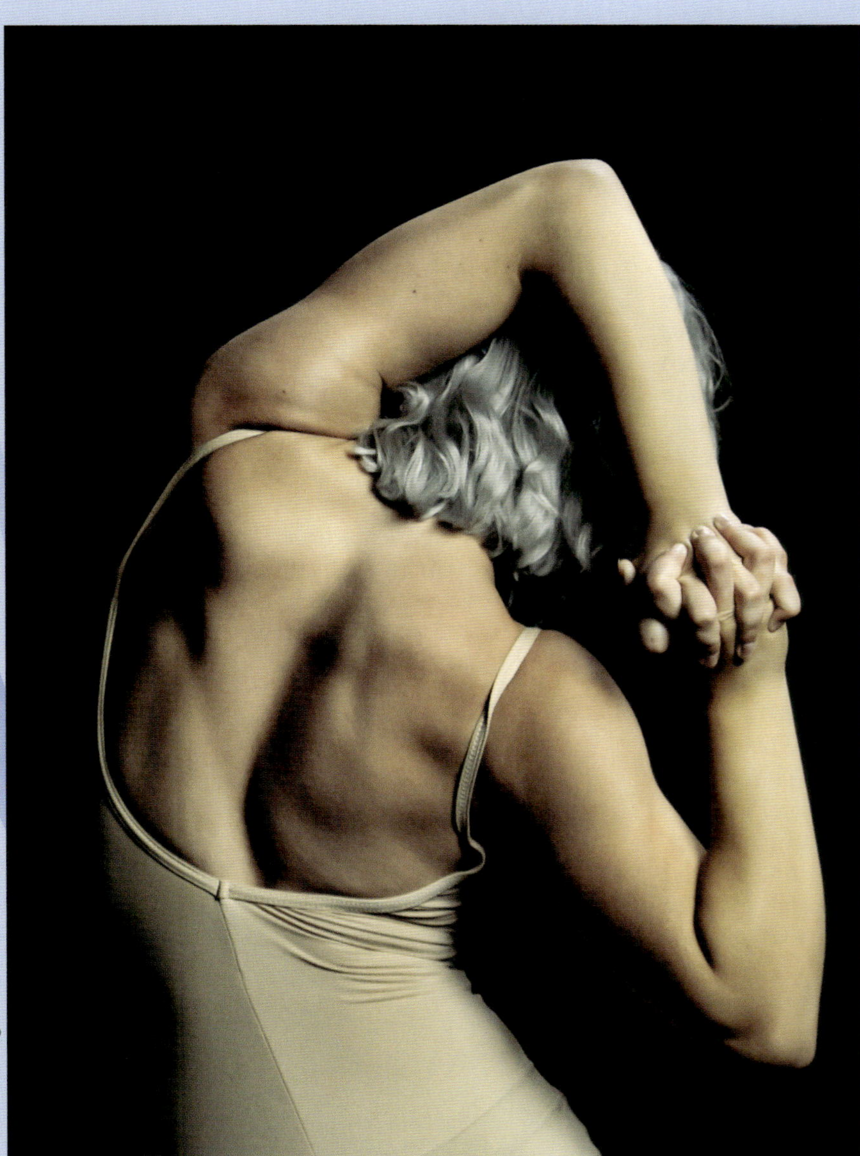

Dr. Steven Karageanes

Your upper extremities play both functional and aesthetic roles in dance. While they are not connected to the floor as much as your lower extremities, you often ask your upper extremities to bear weight, such as when you lift or hold something or someone, or when you use them to support your body on the floor. Therefore, they are prone to injury, and they need your close attention and care.

12

Key Terms

- anatomical snuffbox
- arthroscopic surgery
- bursa
- bursitis
- deep extensor compartment
- deep flexor compartment
- dislocation
- growth plate
- impingement
- joint capsule
- labrum
- repetitive overuse injury
- rotator cuff
- scapular dyskinesis
- shoulder instability
- stress fracture
- subluxation
- superficial extensor compartment
- superficial flexor compartment
- tendinitis
- traumatic injury
- triangular fibrocartilage complex (TFCC)

LEARNING OBJECTIVES

After completing this chapter, you will be able to do the following:

- Identify anatomical structures of the shoulder, elbow, wrist, and hand.
- Describe common dance injuries to the upper extremity.
- Explain structural pathologies of the shoulder, elbow, and wrist.
- Implement measures to reduce risk for shoulder and elbow injuries.
- Implement self-care strategies for issues related to the shoulder.

Dance is a unique activity in that the dancer often uses the entirety of their anatomy to perform, from the fingertips to the toes. Performing anything from floor work to acrobatic techniques, the upper extremity undergoes a large range of stress and repetitive use. Although upper-extremity dance injuries are less common than those to the lower extremity, the incidence is still significant. Research suggests that 63.3 percent of all injuries in collegiate dancers involve the lower extremity, while 17.7 percent occur in the upper extremity (Sides et al., 2009). Sides and colleagues (2009) also found that upper-extremity injuries required 16.5 percent of all health care visits. Since dancers sustain many upper-extremity injuries, understanding the anatomy and injury mechanisms of the upper extremity aids injury prevention and management. This chapter discusses these issues and describes specific injuries.

The two primary types of injuries are traumatic injuries and repetitive overuse injuries. **Traumatic injuries** (also called acute injuries; see chapter 10) are caused by a sudden external physical force to the body. This force can come from a blunt object, another person, a slip and fall, or an unexpected physical load. These acute injuries usually require immediate treatment. **Repetitive overuse injuries** (also called chronic injuries; see chapter 10) have a proposed mechanism where repeated movements and sustained postures of daily activities (e.g., self-care, household chores, and dance) lead to musculoskeletal pain and dysfunction. These faulty or impaired positions and movements lead to stress being placed on the dancer's body. When these movement impairments are not addressed with rest and proper recovery, they proliferate and become chronic injuries.

Basic Anatomical Structure of the Upper Extremity

Educating yourself about anatomy is crucial because anatomical knowledge can lead to comprehending what parts of the body are injured and why. In addition, learning the relationships between the various anatomical structures will increase your appreciation for the mechanics of the body. Beyond all these practical applications, the human body is fascinating in its design and function, all of which allows you to dance.

Shoulder Anatomy

The shoulder bones comprise the humerus, scapula (shoulder blade), and clavicle (collarbone), as seen in figure 12.1. The scapula is the foundation of the shoulder. This broad bone is held against the thorax (rib cage) by muscles, ligaments, and fascia. It glides in multiple directions through the scapulothoracic articulation where the scapula rests against the thorax.

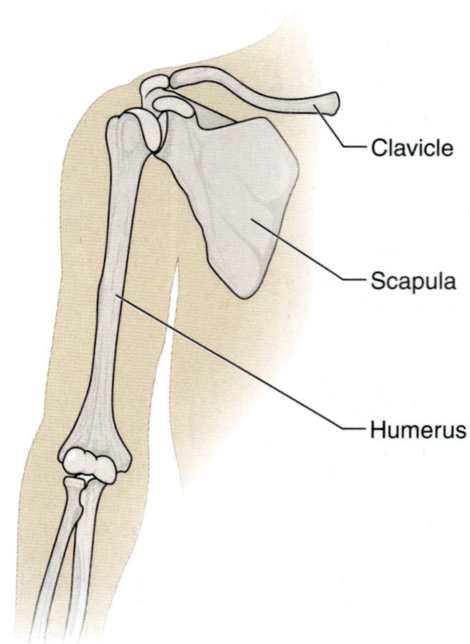

Figure 12.1 The humerus, scapula, and clavicle are the bones providing structure to the shoulder region. Note the irregular—but well-designed—shapes of the scapula and clavicle that, with the humerus, form the very mobile architecture required for upper-extremity movements.

Movements of the Scapulothoracic Articulation

The scapulothoracic articulation is a surprisingly complex region in the shoulder. Several motions occur along this flat, broad area where the scapula and thorax meet. They are listed and defined as follows:

- *Elevation*—Sliding upward.
- *Depression*—Sliding downward.
- *Abduction*—Moving away from the spinal column.
- *Adduction*—Moving toward the spinal column.
- *Upward rotation*—Bottom tip of the scapula rotates outward and upward.
- *Downward rotation*—Bottom tip of the scapula rotates inward and downward.
- *Internal rotation*—Edge near the spinal column moves away from the thorax.
- *External rotation*—Edge away from the spinal column moves away from the thorax.
- *Anterior tilt*—Bottom tip moves away from the thorax.
- *Posterior tilt*—Bottom tip moves toward the thorax.

The clavicle attaches to the top of the scapula to form the acromioclavicular (AC) joint. The ball of the humerus attaches to the scapula at the glenohumeral (GH) joint; the flattened socket located on the scapula is called the glenoid fossa. The GH joint is capable of flexion and extension (moving arms forward and back), abduction and adduction (lifting arms overhead to the side and back down), horizontal adduction and abduction (horizontal motion from behind the body toward the front and returning to the back), and internal and external rotation (inward or outward rotation of the humerus).

The **rotator cuff** is a group of four muscles (supraspinatus, infraspinatus, teres minor, and subscapularis that originates on the scapula and inserts around the rounded portion of the upper humerus (called the humeral head), resembling a shirt cuff (figure 12.2). They control the movement of the humeral head within the glenoid fossa. They have two main tasks: 1) create rotational movement, and 2) add stability to the joint by holding the humerus close to the glenoid fossa. The other muscles that affect movement at the shoulder joint and scapula are the pectoralis major and minor, deltoid, biceps brachii, latissimus dorsi, teres major, rhomboid major and minor, trapezius, levator scapulae, and serratus anterior.

The glenohumeral joint has ligaments that strengthen and stabilize the **joint capsule**, which is the ligamentous casing surrounding the joint.

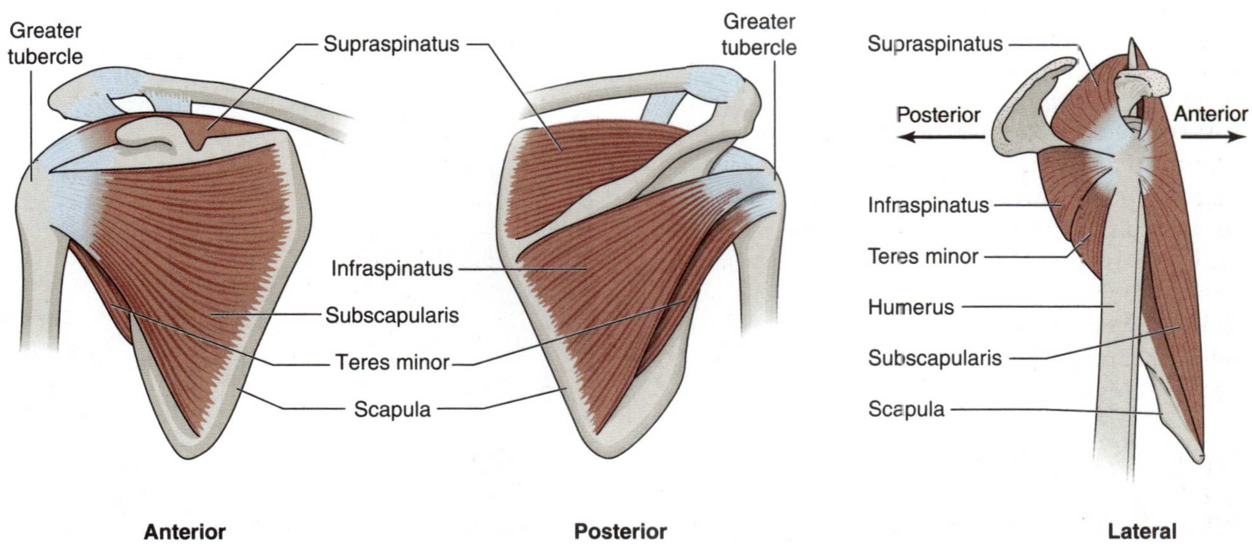

Figure 12.2 The insertions of the four rotator cuff muscles surround the humerus at the shoulder joint as the cuff of a shirt surrounds the lower forearm near the wrist.

Within the capsule is the glenoid **labrum**, a ring of elastic-like cartilage that runs around the perimeter of the glenoid fossa. It aids the rotator cuff in stabilizing the humerus as it moves. Another kind of cartilage, smooth articular cartilage, lines the bony surfaces of the GH and AC joints. Injury to or loss of this joint cartilage leads to degenerative osteoarthritis.

Elbow Anatomy

The elbow region contains a hinge joint (the elbow joint itself) and a pivot joint (the radioulnar joint) that link the upper arm and forearm (figure 12.3). It comprises three bones: the humerus (upper arm), the ulna (forearm), and the radius (forearm). The upper end of the ulna is called the olecranon, which is the point of the elbow. The bony prominence on the inner part of the elbow is called the medial epicondyle, while the outside prominence is the lateral epicondyle. Both are sites of common injuries.

Multiple muscles connect around the elbow to allow it to flex and extend like a hinge and to rotate. The biceps brachii, brachialis, brachioradialis, and extensor carpi radialis longus muscles flex the elbow, while the triceps brachii extends it. The pronator teres and quadratus turn the palm inward or downward (pronation), while the supinator and biceps brachii rotate the palm outward or upward (supination).

The elbow is held together on the sides by the collateral ligaments. The ulnar collateral ligament is on the inside of the elbow, and it absorbs significant stress in activities requiring overhead throwing. The radial collateral ligament stabilizes the part of the elbow toward the outside. The annular ligament wraps around the upper end of the radius and holds it against the ulna, allowing rotation as the radius turns inward and outward in pronation and supination.

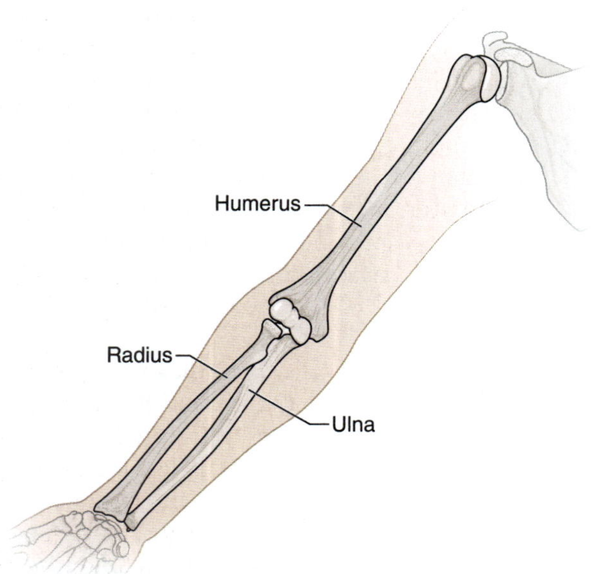

Figure 12.3 The bones of the arm and forearm, along with the elbow joint.

While several nerves pass through the elbow region, the ulnar nerve deserves special mention. You have likely heard of hitting your *funny bone.* It is not a bone, and it isn't funny when you accidentally hit it; rather, the odd pain you feel is an impact to the ulnar nerve, which passes through a bony groove behind the medial epicondyle of the elbow. You can easily find this location and press on the nerve, possibly getting it to send twinges toward your fingers. The nerve's lack of protection in its groove near the skin surface makes it vulnerable to trauma.

Elbow extension usually reaches 0 degrees; in other words, when the elbow is extended completely, the upper extremity is completely flat. However, some people have elbows that bend backward naturally, sometimes between 10 and 20 degrees beyond 0; this range of motion is called elbow hyperextension (figure 12.4). Measuring this hyperextension is part of an assessment for joint hypermobility known as the Beighton scale (Beighton et al., 1973). This is indeed seen in hypermobile dancers and is considered desirable in some cases. Although many do not have symptoms, some hyperextending elbows can be painful and should be evaluated.

Forearm Anatomy

The forearm consists of the radius (laterally, or thumb side of the forearm) and ulna (medially, or little finger side) running from their articulations at the elbow down to the wrist (figure 12.5). At the elbow, the ulnar end is large and gives the elbow its point (the olecranon), while the radius has a smaller head attached to the ulna by the semicircular

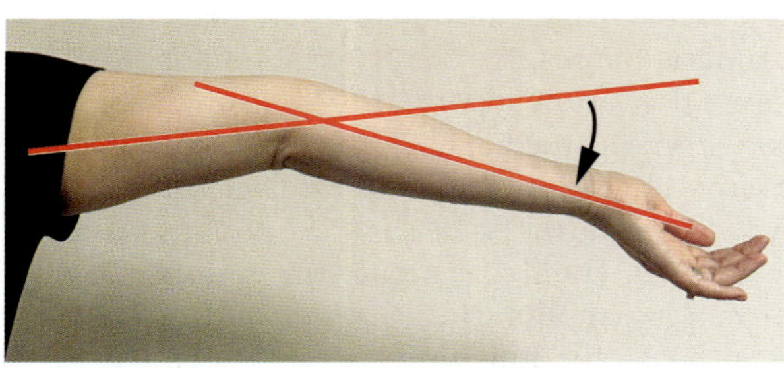

Figure 12.4 Elbow hyperextension occurs when an elbow is able to extend past the so-called straight (0°) position.
Amanda M. Donahue

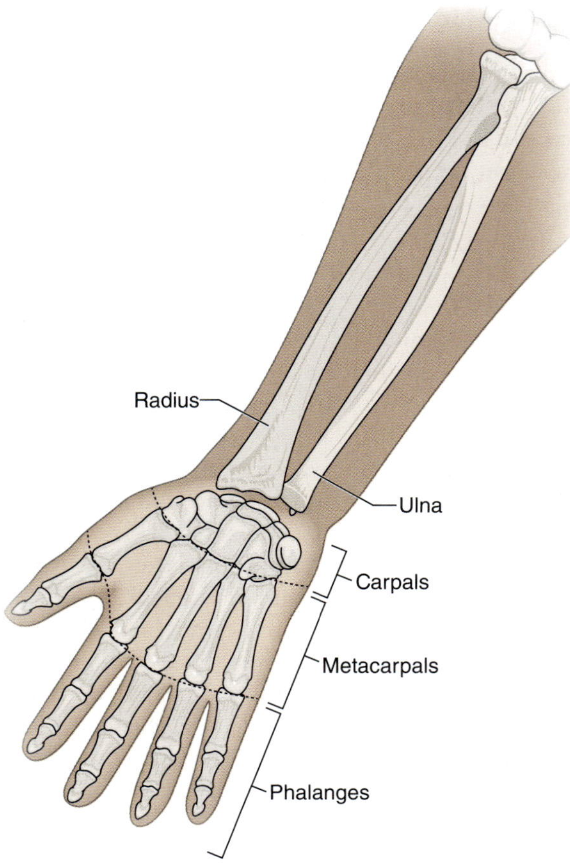

Figure 12.5 The main anatomical features of the forearm, wrist, and hand.

annular ligament. The radius also rests against the end of the humerus. Down at the wrist, the radius is much larger and connects to the wrist joint, while the ulna is much smaller and more slender; it does not touch the bones of the wrist.

The forearm has two main compartments: anterior (flexor) and posterior (extensor). Twenty different muscles reside in these compartments, which are divided into superficial and deep compartments. The **superficial flexor compartment** contains the pronator teres, the flexor carpi radialis longus, the palmaris longus, the flexor carpi ulnaris, and the flexor digitorum superficialis—all of which originate from the medial epicondyle. The **deep flexor compartment** consists of the flexor digitorum profundus, the flexor pollicis longus, and the pronator quadratus. The flexor digitorum superficialis and profundus run along together to digits two through five to flex the fingers. The **superficial extensor compartment** consists of the brachioradialis, the extensor carpi radialis brevis, the extensor carpi radialis longus, the extensor digitorum, the extensor digiti minimi, the extensor carpi ulnaris, and the anconeus. All but the brachioradialis originate from the lateral epicondyle. The **deep extensor compartment** contains the adductor pollicis longus, the extensor pollicis longus and brevis, the extensor indicis, and the supinator.

Hand and Wrist Anatomy

The anatomy of the hand and wrist is complex; it is designed to maximize the ability to grasp and manipulate objects. Twenty-nine bones create the numerous joints in the fingers and wrist. The most important structures for dancers to know are covered in this section.

Each of the fingers is made of three bones (the proximal, middle, and distal phalanges) while the thumb has only two (a proximal and distal phalanx). The palm has five metacarpal bones to which the fingers attach. The wrist contains eight carpal bones that fit together like a puzzle. The base of the hand joins the distal row of the trapezium, trapezoid, capitate, and hamate. The radius of the forearm and the distal radioulnar joint connect to the proximal row of the scaphoid, lunate, triquetrum, and pisiform (figure 12.6). These eight carpal bones are formed into a semicircular configuration known as the carpal tunnel. Four tendons from each of the flexor digitorum profundus and the flexor digitorum superficialis, the flexor pollicis longus tendon, and the median nerve all run through this area; the transverse carpal ligament covers them, thus creating the tunnel (figure 12.7).

The extensor tendons are divided between six compartments that run along the back of the hand and thumb. Each tendon is surrounded by a synovial sheath, which provides lubrication and reduces friction as the tendons slide back and forth during finger movements (figure 12.8). On the palmar side is one main compartment with a superficial and deep layer of flexor tendons. As noted previously, the tendons and their synovial sheaths run through the carpal tunnel to the fingers and attach to the distal phalanges. The tendons and sheaths are held against the fingers by bands of tissue that act as pulleys.

Two other areas of the wrist deserve special mention: the anatomical snuffbox and the triangular fibrocartilage complex (TFCC) (figure 12.9*a* and 12.9*b*). The **anatomical snuffbox** is located at the base of the thumb; it is created by the tendons of extensor pollicis longus on one side and the extensor pollicis brevis and abductor pollicis longus on the other. You can easily see the snuffbox and feel these tendons by holding one of your hands with

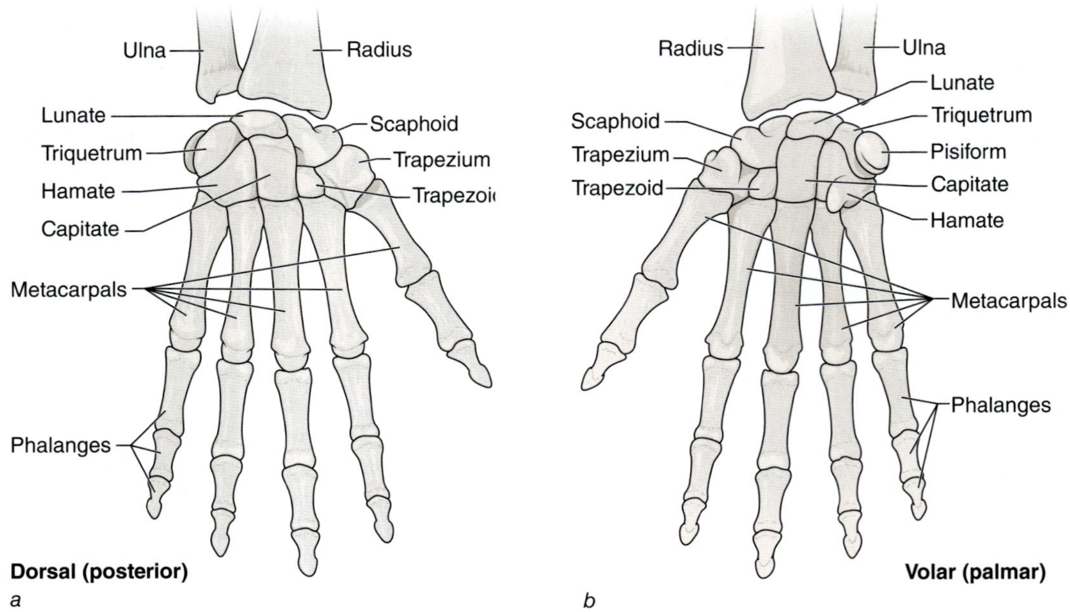

Figure 12.6 The array of bones forming the right wrist and hand. *(a)* Front view; *(b)* back view. Note that the distal radius—but not the ulna—articulates with the wrist bones.

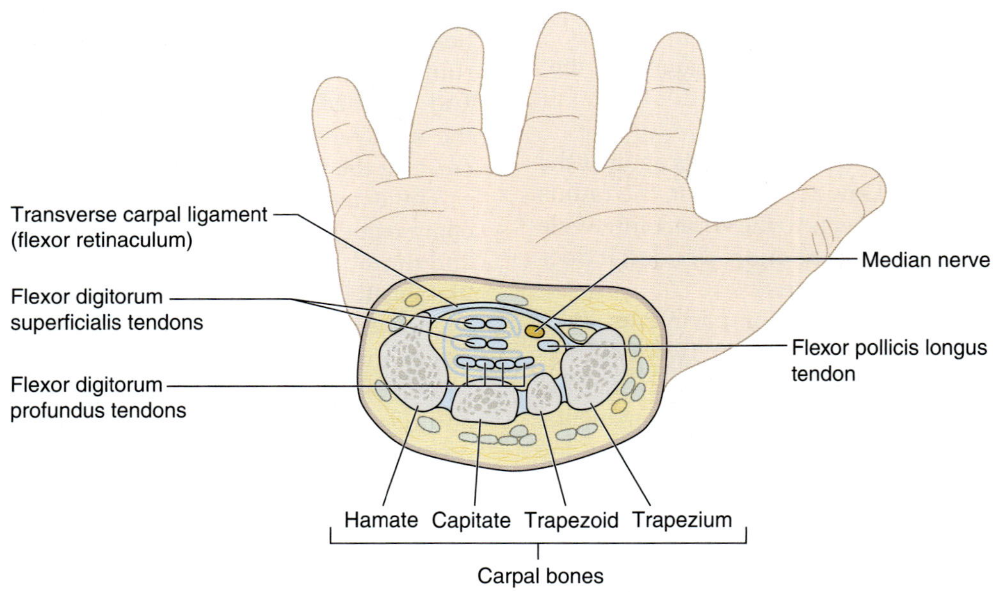

Figure 12.7 The carpal tunnel is created by the semicircular shape of the carpal bones and the transverse carpal ligament that contains the 10 structures that run through the tunnel.

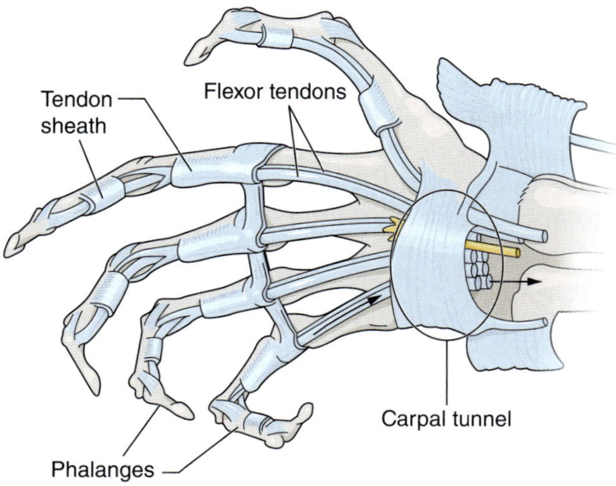

Figure 12.8 A typical finger flexor tendon complex contains two flexor tendons; these tendons are surrounded by a synovial sheath that is held in place by pulleys made of ligamentous bands. This is the palmar view.

the thumb upward while spreading your fingers. Inside the snuffbox lies the scaphoid bone. Pain with pushing on this area could be from a scaphoid fracture. (This injury is presented later.)

The **triangular fibrocartilage complex (TFCC)** is a load-bearing structure between the lunate, the triquetrum, and the ulna. There is a gap between the end of the ulna and the carpal bones of the wrist. The function of the TFCC is to act as a stabilizer for the ulnar aspect of the wrist. The TFCC is at risk for either acute or chronic degenerative injury.

Common Injuries in the Upper Extremity

Upper-extremity injuries (both traumatic and nontraumatic) typically occur less often in dance than do lower-extremity injuries. This difference makes sense because so much of dance requires movement across a floor. However, the incidence of dance injuries in the upper extremity varies by style of dance (Sides et al., 2009). A U.K. study of 320 hip-hop dancers found the prevalence of injuries to the arms and hands was 40.6 percent, while the prevalence of shoulder injuries was 35.9 percent, which was the highest of any single body site (Tsiouti & Wyon, 2021). Another study of 312 hip-hop dancers found that upper-extremity injuries in breakdancers accounted for 34 percent of all injuries. In poppers and lockers, they accounted for 25 percent and in new schoolers, 12 percent (Ojofeitimi et al., 2012). Meanwhile, a systematic review reported that 3.0 to 3.9 percent of all injuries in 1,365 amateur dancers occurred to the upper extremity, and 3.0 to 14.4 percent of all injuries involved the upper extremity in 900 professional ballet dancers (Smith

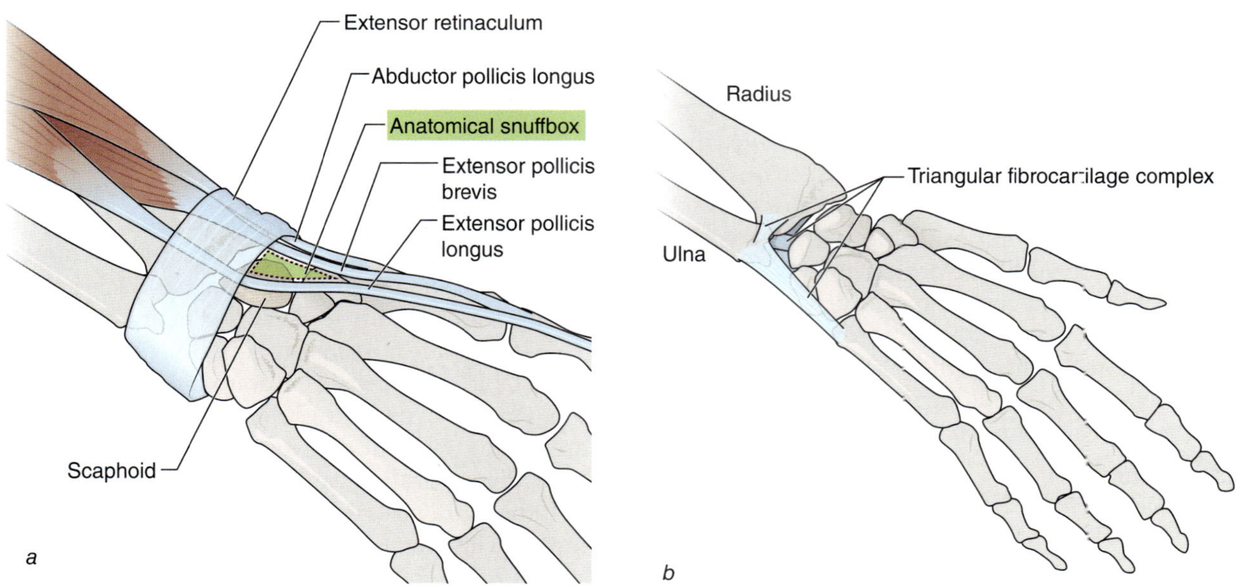

Figure 12.9 Two important areas of the wrist that are prone to injury from falls onto the outstretched hands: *(a)* The scaphoid bone inside the anatomical snuffbox, a common site of a fracture; and *(b)* the triangular fibrocartilage complex. Note the triangular piece of cartilage that can be torn.

et al., 2015). These figures highlight the importance of understanding specific styles of dance when evaluating injury risk and occurrence. Throughout the following sections, some basic treatment guidelines are offered for the musculoskeletal injuries that are described; however, additional management concepts for injuries are presented in chapter 10.

Traumatic Injuries to the Shoulder

Overall, upper-extremity traumatic injuries are relatively uncommon in dance. In a study of 210 dancers in Sweden, 101 of the 337 injuries dancers experienced were traumatic. However, only 12 involved the upper extremity, compared to 67 in the foot and lower leg (Leanderson et al., 2011). According to Wanke, Arendt, and colleagues (2014), the two most common factors leading to traumatic injuries are a dance partner and the dance floor. These injuries usually occur by falls or direct contact between dancers. Many other intrinsic and extrinsic factors affect the probability of traumatic dance injury incidence overall (Wanke, Mill, et al., 2014).

Fractures

Any trauma to the upper extremity that transmits sufficient force has the potential to fracture a bone. Adult bones fracture when a traumatic force causes a break through their walls. Young dancers (less than 16 years old) typically have skeletally immature bones with growth plates that are weak compared to the stronger ligaments, tendons, and muscles. **Growth plates** are areas where bone growth occurs as an individual matures. Trauma to a growth plate can cause a growth plate fracture without any apparent bony disruption on X-rays. However, more severe growth plate fractures can be seen on X-rays. Growth disturbance of a limb is one possible consequence of these injuries, so proper management by a qualified health care professional is essential.

One of the most common sites of fracture in the shoulder and upper arm region is the proximal humerus (toward the shoulder). Symptoms include a severely swollen shoulder, limited shoulder movement, and severe pain. The other common shoulder fracture occurs to the clavicle. This fracture can happen when a dancer falls on the side of their shoulder. These injuries occur most often in the middle portion (figure 12.10*a* and *b*). Fractures near either end of the clavicle are less frequent. Symptoms of a clavicle fracture may include sagging of the shoulder downward and forward; inability to lift the arm because of pain; a grinding sensation when raising the arm; deformity or a lump over the fracture site; and bruising, swelling, or tenderness over the clavicle. Most clavicle fractures can be treated without surgery using sling immobilization or a figure-8 sling (figure 12.10*c* and *d*). Surgery is necessary when a compound fracture has broken through the skin or the bone is severely out of place.

Scapular fractures are rare; they usually result from a direct blow to the scapula itself or a fall from a substantial distance. Symptoms include pain around the back of the shoulder, swelling, and severe bruising. Treatment usually involves immobilization with a sling or shoulder immobilizer, icing, and pain medications. See chapter 10 for specific guidance about appropriate treatment methods.

Sprains

Ligaments are connective tissue structures that connect bone to bone. A sprain is a disruption or tear of this tissue, usually due to trauma that stretches (grade I), partially tears (grade II), or fully tears (grade III) a ligament. Grade III tears of a ligament—such as an anterior cruciate ligament (ACL) tear in the knee—are unlikely in the shoulder except at the acromioclavicular (AC) joint. Most sprains are grade I, which rarely (if ever) require surgical intervention.

The most common sprain in the shoulder region occurs to the AC ligament at the AC joint. This injury is caused by a traumatic force against the joint, such as falling on the top or side of the shoulder or being struck directly on the AC joint. The injury is commonly called a shoulder separation. If the force is strong enough, one also can disrupt the ligaments underneath the clavicle, causing it to separate from the scapula. A small bump on the shoulder is commonly seen in mild cases, while a larger bump, called a step-off deformity, can be seen with more severe separations (figure 12.11). Symptoms include pain at the AC joint, pain with lifting the arm overhead, and swelling. Treatment is usually a sling, pain medication, and icing while resting the extremity to allow the ligaments to heal. This injury rarely needs surgery unless the clavicle is unstable and it causes chronic pain with everyday movement. Even though the joint and ligaments are small, the pain and disability associated with shoulder separation can be significant.

Other sprains of the shoulder involve the glenohumeral ligaments. These ligaments are the support structures at the front of the shoulder joint; along with the rotator cuff muscles, they restrain the humerus from shifting out of joint. They are usually sprained during shoulder dislocations or when the arm is suddenly thrust backward. Complete tears of these ligaments or resulting shoulder instability

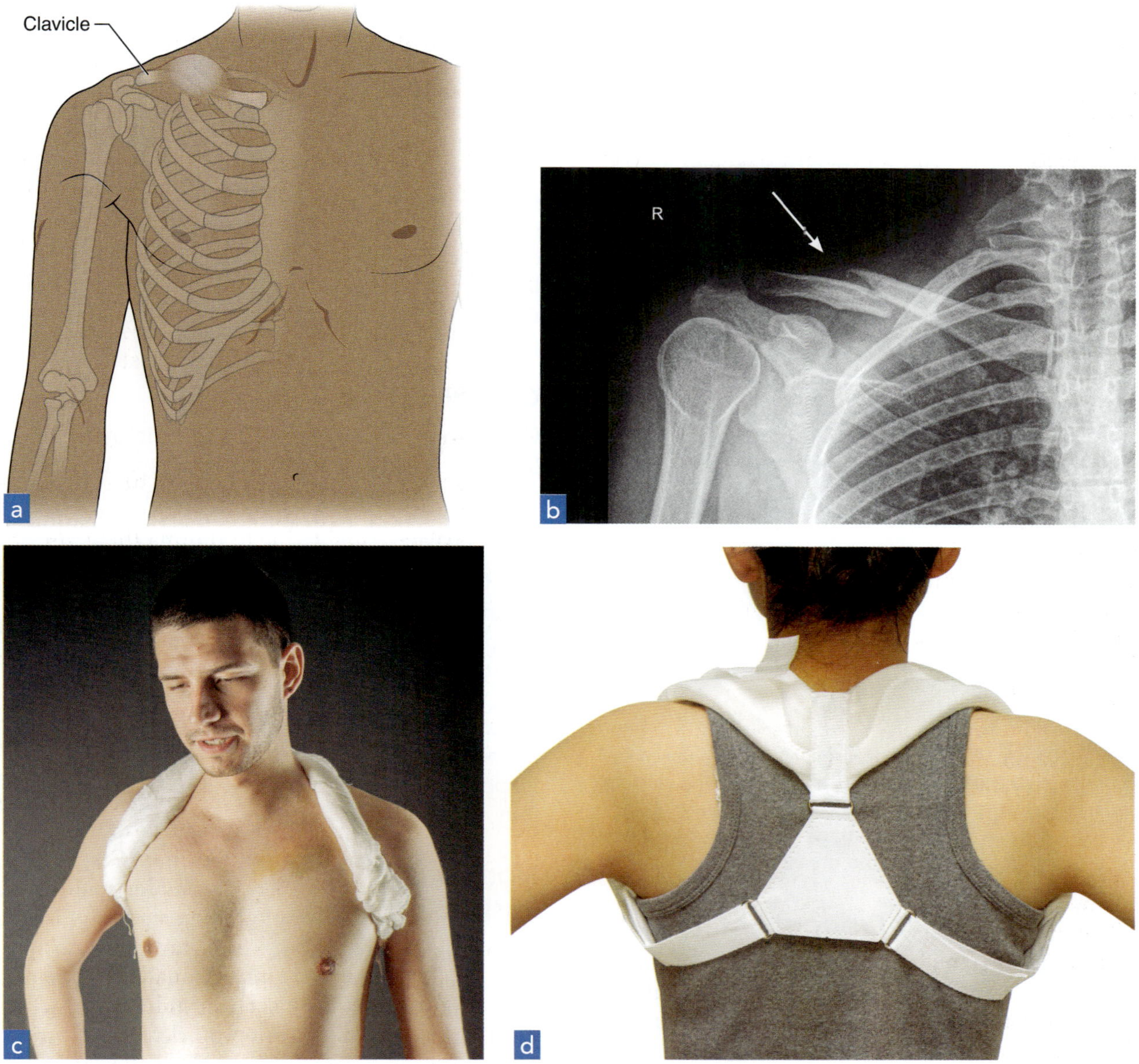

Figure 12.10 Clavicle fracture. *(a)* Appearance of the skin over the fracture site. *(b)* X-ray showing the fracture. *(c)* Anterior and *(d)* posterior views of a figure-8 splint to stabilize the fracture ends and allow healing.

B: MedPhotoStudio/stock.adobe.com; C: kroko21/stock.adobe.com; D: praisaeng/stock.adobe.com

could require surgery, while all others typically heal with rest and short-term shoulder immobilization.

Strains

Strains are injuries to muscles or tendons. Tendons are built similarly to ligaments, but they connect muscle to bone, thus bringing about joint movement. Similar to sprains, muscle and tendon strains are graded as mild (grade I), moderate (grade II), or severe (grade III). Grade III strains are complete tears, such as an Achilles tendon rupture or a complete hamstring tear.

In the upper extremity, strains usually result when too much force is applied to muscles or tendons during movement, or when they are suddenly overstretched. The recommended treatment for a strain is the same as for a sprain; again, chapter 10 provides specific advice. Treatment should be followed by formal rehabilitation to relieve pain and restore mobility, strength, and flexibility, as well as to guide your successful return back to dance without movement impairments. Surgery is not common for strains, except in cases of severe tears of muscles or tendons.

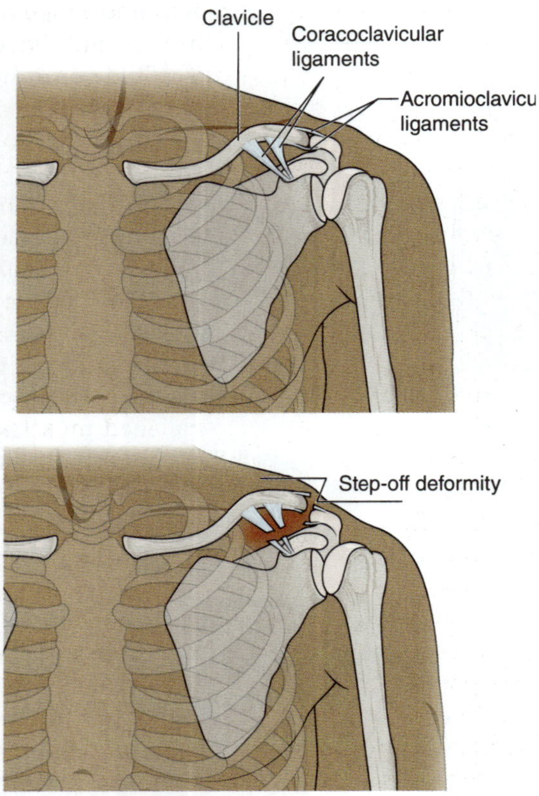

Figure 12.11 A step-off deformity (a larger than typical bump, or step, seen at the AC joint end of the clavicle) is one indicator of a significant AC joint injury. Usually, the greater the ligament damage around the joint and at the end of the clavicle, the greater the step.

Subluxations and Dislocations

The shoulder is the most mobile joint in the body. However, the more mobile a joint is, the less stability it enjoys; therefore, the shoulder is prone to subluxations and dislocations. A **subluxation** occurs when the humeral head shifts or slides partway out of joint but pops right back in. A **dislocation** occurs when the humeral head slides all the way out and stays out. Either one can be painful when it first occurs. Traumatic incidents such as these often lead to recurring episodes because the soft tissues responsible for stabilizing the shoulder become stretched.

Dislocations most often occur with trauma when the arm is in the throwing position (the glenohumeral joint is abducted and externally rotated). The joint can dislocate forward, downward, or backward; forward dislocation is most common. Although the joint can relocate spontaneously—especially with repetitive episodes because the stabilizing tissues become stretched—many dislocations require assistance in getting the humeral head back to its normal position in the joint. Considering the likelihood of significant injuries to structures around the shoulder joint, repositioning a dislocated shoulder should be performed only by a qualified health care provider.

Following initial treatment to reset the humeral head in its socket—which may require an emergency room visit and possibly some form of anesthesia—rest and immobilization are prescribed. The dancer should begin doing rehabilitative exercises once the pain subsides. Recurrent dislocations may benefit from a brace. If conservative measures do not improve the instability, the shoulder may need surgery.

Overall Safety

Given that many upper-extremity injuries occur because of falls, attention to safety is an important risk reduction measure. The use of mats and other equipment may help reduce the risk of injuries during some types of dance training. Dancers who are new to movements such as inversions, handstands, stunts, and aerial work should be taught the proper way to perform these movements, and spotting by their instructors is necessary. When using equipment such as poles or silks for aerial work, safety checks should be implemented prior to each use. In addition, floor surfaces should be inspected for any foreign objects or wet spots that may cause falls.

Nontraumatic Injuries to the Shoulder

Most nontraumatic dance injuries are repetitive overuse injuries. These injuries occur gradually; they may first be perceived as only an annoyance, then become more painful and disabling with repeated activity. When an activity is repeated without allowing enough time for recovery or for correcting an improper or impaired movement, tissue damage occurs and further compensation patterns develop that alter normal dance biomechanics. These adaptations make it possible for dancers to perform through pain and disability, but recovery is complicated.

Overuse injuries affect all types of tissue, including bones (and growth plates in young dancers), muscles, ligaments, and tendons. Symptoms of overuse injuries include pain, swelling, changes in form or technique, and decreased interest in practicing. Pain often increases with activity and decreases with rest. Poor movement mechanics and muscular imbalances that occur during daily functional tasks and dance can increase the chances of developing injuries. Different dance styles put different loads and stresses on the upper extremity, so understanding the volume and variety of dance training is necessary to optimally treat any injury.

The occurrence of repetitive overuse injuries in children has significantly increased in recent years. This phenomenon is well documented in the sports world as workloads and specialization in sports have increased over the years. The American Academy of Orthopaedic Surgeons recommends against children playing one sport year-round (Popkin et al., 2019). In fact, athletes who specialize in one sport too soon are at risk of physical, emotional, and social problems (Brenner, 2016). Although similar research is limited in the dance world, the norm has long been that dancers specialize in dance at very early ages and log many hours in the studio to the exclusion of other activities. Some researchers and dance medicine physicians have openly endorsed limiting hours of dance training and integrating other activities such as volleyball, tennis, or swimming in order to limit overuse injuries (Henderson, 2021).

Recall that the rotator cuff tendons originate from the scapula and attach to the humeral head to stabilize it in the socket. **Bursas** are lubricating pads that protect the tendons from rubbing against bones when the arm is moved. Ordinarily, the shoulder structures all function smoothly together for strength, stability, and mobility. When a dancer uses the arm repetitively at or above shoulder level, more pressure and stress are placed on the tendons and bursas, which can cause microtears and irritation. If these changes are not allowed to heal, the damage lingers and increases, leading to more pain, rotator cuff muscle weakening, and changes in shoulder mechanics.

The rotator cuff can cause pain due to the following conditions:

› ***Tendinopathy***—Irritation of the rotator cuff tendons.
› ***Bursitis***—Inflammation and swelling of a bursa that hurts when compressed or pinched by movement.
› ***Impingement***—Compression of the tendon and bursa between the humerus and the underside of the acromion when raising the arm above shoulder height.
› ***Strain***—Damage to the tendon fibers, which rarely occurs in young dancers.

Early-stage symptoms include minor pain with activity and rest, pain radiating to the front and side of the arm, and sharp pain with lifting and reaching. As a condition progresses, pain occurs more often at night, the shoulder loses strength and range of motion, and movements behind the back and above the head become increasingly difficult to perform.

Treatment usually requires multiple approaches. Anti-inflammatory drugs such as ibuprofen or naproxen reduce pain and swelling, and they can be used effectively and safely for a short duration. The offending activity needs be modified to avoid further irritation; seeing a rehabilitation specialist can help. Rehabilitation is key to returning to dance by correcting the movement impairments that stress the soft tissues. Also essential are patient education about faulty movement patterns and how to correct them; exercises to strengthen weakened muscles; and stretches to improve mobility throughout the shoulder joint, scapula, thorax, and neck. Therapeutic modalities and taping are other ways to decrease inflammation and pain. If a condition does not improve, anti-inflammatory steroid injections may be effective, particularly into a bursa. If all conservative treatment fails, **arthroscopic surgery** (surgery using a slender telescopic instrument) can be performed to create more space for the rotator cuff. If the tendon is torn (rare in young dancers), the surgeon can repair the tendon at the same time.

Biceps tendinitis is inflammation of the slender tendon of the long head of the biceps brachii located directly in front of the shoulder. (There also is a short head of the biceps muscle.) The tendon acts as a stabilizer of the humeral head. A sheath surrounds the tendon, which helps protect the tendon from abrasive damage as it moves and glides along the humerus inside a tunnel formed by a ligament (figure 12.12). Both the tendon and its sheath can be irritated from repetitive shoulder forward flexion and overhead lifting. Over long-term use, degeneration can cause the tendon to thicken and increase the chance of further inflammation.

Symptoms of biceps tendinitis are pain in the front of the shoulder that increases with overhead lifting or reaching behind the back, pain or ache that radiates down the arm, and a snapping or catching sensation in the shoulder. Treatment is similar to rotator cuff impingement; it includes rest from the offending activity, icing, anti-inflammatories, and rehabilitation. Exercises guided by a rehabilitation professional will modify how you move your shoulder and scapula and decrease the stress placed on the tendon. If the biceps tendon breaks down and ruptures, surgery is rarely done to fix it as long as the second (short) head of the muscle is intact.

Scapular dyskinesis is a condition in which the scapula's position is altered at rest or in movement;

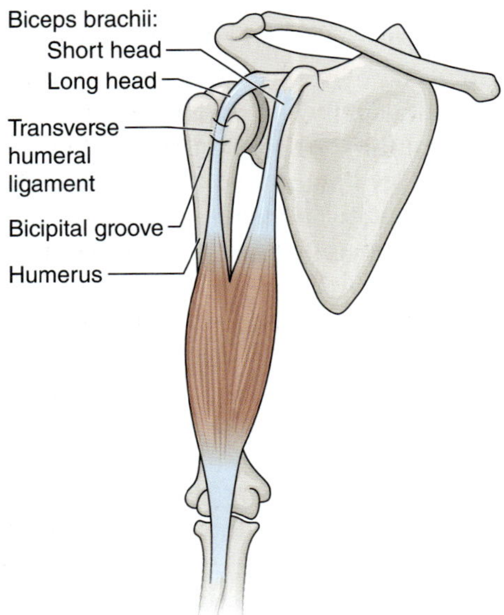

Figure 12.12 The long head (tendon) of the biceps brachii muscle travels through a synovial sheath inside a groove on the anterior humerus that is covered by the transverse humeral ligament. The tendon plays a major role in stabilizing the humeral head and keeping it against the glenoid fossa.

symptoms are created by faulty range of motion. Because the scapula has numerous muscle attachments and performs many complex movements, abnormal motion can cause pain in the back, neck, or shoulder. A normal scapula moves in harmony with the glenohumeral joint. This rhythm can be disturbed by inappropriate muscle activation (too fast or too slow) or inappropriate force of muscle contraction (too strong or weak) (Burn et al., 2016).

One of the signs of dyskinesis is the medial border (toward the spine) of the affected scapula being more prominent than the lateral side (figure 12.13). This position may cause an audible crunching (called snapping scapula). Once the impaired motion of the scapula is corrected, the snapping should resolve (Panagiotopoulos & Crowther, 2019). Dancers are prone to developing this type of condition if they are hypermobile and their movements do not allow the muscles in the shoulder and scapular region to work in an ideal manner. Scapular winging—where the medial edge of one or both scapulae protrudes significantly away from the thorax—may be more prominent when moving or holding the arms at chest level or above. Since dance requires smooth and graceful movements as well as transitions from one position to the next, scapular dyskinesis can negatively affect performance.

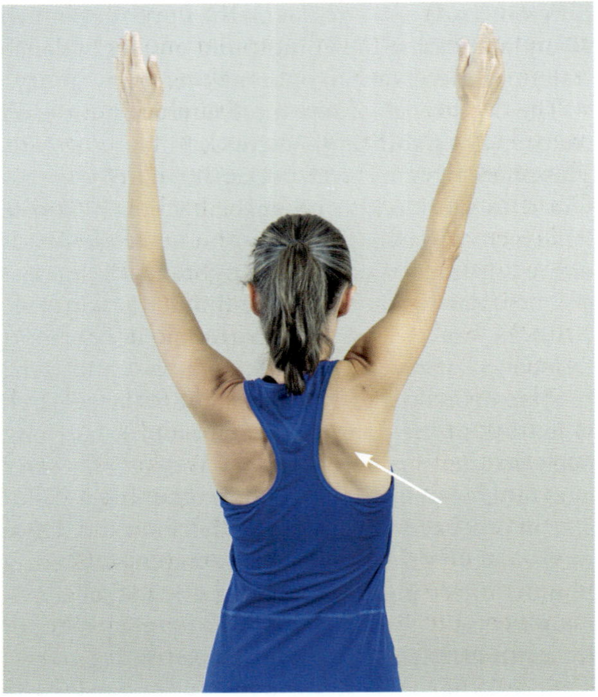

Figure 12.13 Scapular dyskinesis of the right scapula. The scapula is not sitting against the thorax as it should; this alteration in position is caused by neurological inhibition, or by muscular weaknesses or imbalances. Movement of this right shoulder would demonstrate further abnormalities of the scapula's position as it tries to glide smoothly along the thorax.

Most Common Signs and Symptoms of Scapular Dyskinesis

Scapular dyskinesis does not allow the shoulder complex to operate with its usual smooth gliding mechanism. When this condition occurs, several common signs and symptoms may be noted (Kibler & Sciascia, 2017):

1. Pain or tenderness around the scapula
2. Weakness or fatigue in the affected arm with repetitive activities, especially overhead movements
3. Difficulty moving the arm overhead
4. Crunching or snapping sensation with movement
5. Protrusion of the scapula
6. Drooped or forward-tilted upper-back and shoulder posture on the affected side

Customary dancer cues also may play a role in developing atypical scapular movement. For example, one common cue is *Bring your shoulders away from your ears* to create a desirable long, downward-sloping line from the neck to the fingertips. This maneuver requires use of the rhomboids and latissimus dorsi muscles of the back. However, if a dancer holds this position for an extended time, these muscles stay active and tighten. This tightening restricts upward movement of the scapula and reduces its ability to move harmoniously with the humerus (Schaeffer, 2022).

The muscles most responsible for dyskinesis are the upper and lower trapezius and the serratus anterior (Paine & Voight, 2013). Weakness of these and other scapular stabilizers can occur from muscle or nerve injury. The nerves in the shoulder region can be injured from stretching or compression, or the nerve roots connected to the spinal cord can be pinched in the neck. Pain or injury in the AC or glenohumeral joint also can cause dyskinesis (Burkhart et al., 2003).

Chronic scapular instability may stretch and distort the fascia that surrounds and supports the scapula, thus making recovery more challenging. Perhaps the most correctable cause of scapular dyskinesis is a slouched posture that leads to core muscle imbalances. These imbalances, in turn, alter normal spinal curvatures and soft tissue tensions (Crosbie et al., 2008). In general, attention to scapular dyskinesis in dancers is important for aesthetic reasons, particularly when dance performance wardrobing reveals the contours of a dancer's upper back.

Due to the complexity of scapular dyskinesis, treatment should begin with proper evaluation by a qualified health care professional (e.g., physician, physical therapist, athletic trainer) to identify specific contributors to the condition. Rehabilitation is usually necessary to treat scapular dyskinesis and its associated factors. Most cases do not cause significant problems in the neck, shoulder joint, or nerves, but scapular dyskinesis is more difficult to treat if any conditions in surrounding tissues go unidentified and untreated. A period of relative rest may be needed if pain and inflammation impede movement. Anti-inflammatory medication can help with pain and inflammation. Surgery is rare; it is reserved for when a specific condition, such as a labral tear in the shoulder joint, is present.

Additionally, dancers must be instructed about how to properly move the scapula and shoulder by using various verbal and manual cues. These exercises are then performed throughout the day, from reaching overhead into a cabinet to doing port de bras in dance class. Posture corrections are necessary for any painful positions, including sleeping. Exercises also are provided to improve muscle action, strengthen weak and overstretched muscles, stretch muscles that are shortened and stiff, accentuate breathing mechanics, and stabilize the trunk.

Shoulder instability refers to problems with the ball-and-socket mechanics of the shoulder. As mentioned earlier, the shoulder is the most mobile joint in the human body, which also makes it the least stable. Traumatic injuries to the shoulder can cause the humeral head to slide out of joint. However, the shoulder can become unstable without trauma. In dancers who have naturally loose ligaments and, therefore, excess joint mobility (often called being *double-jointed* despite the individual having only one joint the same as everyone else), instability in more than one direction may occur. (Saccomanno et al., 2013).

Dancers with hypermobile joints are more prone to chronic shoulder instability. Since the socket of the shoulder joint is more like a shallow saucer than a socket, the ligaments, capsule, cartilage, and muscles must act as stabilizers. Dancers who do excessive overhead motions or stretch their shoulders too far and too often to increase range of motion may experience more instability and some limitations in their dancing. Moreover, if the scapular and rotator cuff muscles are weak, episodes of instability become more frequent, especially with pushing off (as in getting up from the floor) or pushing or lifting overhead.

Symptoms of shoulder instability include pain deep in the shoulder joint, repeated sensation of giving way or dislocation episodes, and a persistent sense of the joint feeling loose or slipping out of place. This loose sensation can be worse when the arm is at or above shoulder height. Imaging studies (e.g., X-rays, ultrasound, and MRI) may be ordered to look for damage to the bones, shoulder capsule, ligaments, cartilage, and rotator cuff tendons.

Treatment for shoulder instability focuses on stabilizing the shoulder region through rehabilitative exercises that are very similar to scapular dyskinesis rehabilitation. The typical way the humerus subluxes (partially dislocates) or dislocates from the glenoid fossa is when the dancer pulls the scapula downward excessively for aesthetic purposes. This downward motion blocks the preferred movement of the humeral head and forces the shoulder to pop out when the dancer moves their arm upward. Minimizing scapular depression during all arm motions will decrease the incidence of subluxation occurring. Anti-inflammatories can be used to control symptoms; however, rehabilitation to improve the shoulder's stability is crucial. If imaging shows damage to the ligaments or capsule, surgery can repair them (Fares et al., 2023). However, dancers who are generally hypermobile, but especially in the shoulder joint, do not respond well to surgery in the long run.

Traumatic Injuries to the Elbow

The majority of traumatic elbow injuries are from blunt forces such as falls or hitting the arm against a hard object. The elbow joint can be dislocated by a blow to the back of the completely extended elbow, or by falling with the hand planted on the ground, thus driving the forearm and elbow backward (e.g., certain hip-hop maneuvers, figure 12.14). Complex dislocations may also include bone and ligament injuries (Englert et al., 2013). The elbow's bony architecture is very stable, so a dislocation is a significant injury that requires splinting and emergency attention.

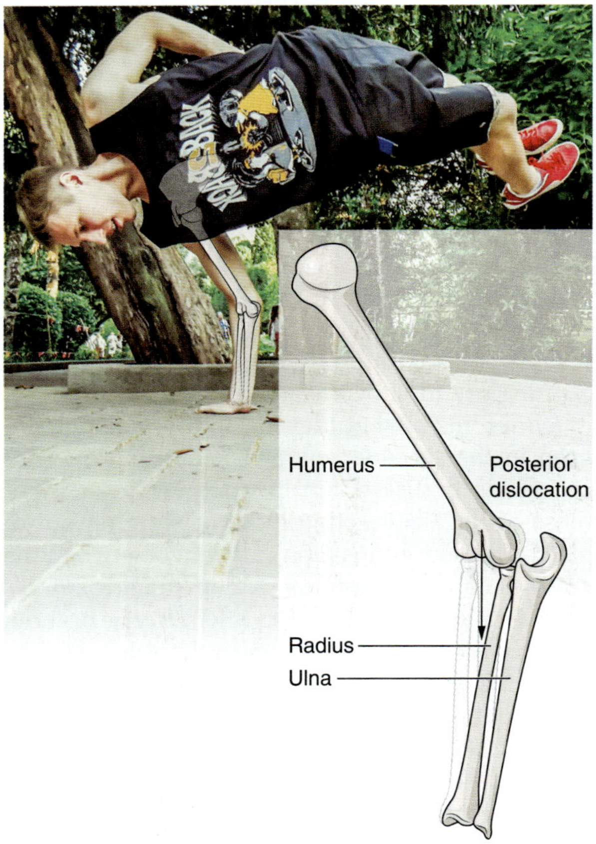

Figure 12.14 One mechanism of an elbow dislocation. The forearm and hand are stabilized by the ground—either purposely (in the case of a dance move on the floor) or during an accidental fall—while the weight of the body moves downward in the direction of gravity (black arrow), thus creating a posterior dislocation (inset).

Photo: Mike Shots on Pexels

Elbow sprains can result from falling on an outstretched arm. The ligaments that stabilize the sides of the elbow—particularly in activities such as acrobatic dance moves that load the arm—can be sprained. When loading the arm with the hand on the ground, any abnormal stress toward one side or the other can cause the elbow to buckle. This buckling is especially common on the inner portion of the elbow. Rest, ice, and compression are the important first steps in treatment. If the main stabilizing ligament tears completely, reconstructive surgery to restabilize the elbow may be recommended.

If an elbow hyperextends (straightens beyond its normal straight position), the capsule around the elbow can be sprained, and the tendons can be strained. This injury can occur during acrobatic dance moves in modern, hip-hop, and breaking styles, such as back walkovers, cartwheels, and various power moves. Dancers with elbows that hyperextend naturally are at higher risk. Symptoms include pain, swelling, stiffness, elbow deformity, weakness, and discoloration. Treatment includes rest and brief immobilization, icing and compression with a wrap, and pain medication. If any of the connective tissue tears fully, surgery may be needed to repair it.

A hard blow to the elbow can cause swelling of the olecranon bursa, a lubricating sac covering the olecranon (point of the elbow). The bursa can produce excess fluid when it is struck. Called olecranon bursitis, it is recognized by a prominent, relatively soft deformity; redness and warmth may develop. Infection can sometimes occur with this bursitis; however, if it is not infected, a dancer can treat a mild case by wearing elbow pads, avoiding repeated contact to the injury, and using a pain reliever. If the fluid does not subside in a few days, a health care consultation is needed.

A distal biceps or triceps strain can occur from a forceful load onto either muscle. It can occur in dancer fitness training, such as weight training or Pilates, or during more acrobatic moves with the hand loaded on the floor, such as back walkovers, cartwheels, and handstands. A strain can occur to the tendon itself or at the junction where the muscle and tendon come together. Initial treatment is protecting the area, rest, icing, a compression sleeve or wrap, and elevation (PRICE method, as described in chapter 10). Rehabilitation may be needed to build back strength and restore movement and function.

Other acute strains can occur at the medial and lateral epicondyles, especially in younger dancers with immature skeletal development. All of the wrist and finger extensor muscles begin with a tendinous attachment at the lateral epicondyle, while the flexor muscles have a similar origin at the medial epicondyle. Sudden wrist movements against resistance can strain these connective tissues or the muscles' fibers, usually causing pain with gripping or moving the wrist. Acute treatment is the same as for other muscle strains mentioned previously.

Nontraumatic Injuries to the Elbow

The majority of nontraumatic injuries to the elbow are caused by repetitive stress to the tendinous attachments of the muscles at the medial and lateral epicondyles. In adolescent dancers, these epicondyles have growth plates known as apophyses. Inflammation of these apophyses (called apophysitis) results from excessive pulling forces by the forearm muscles that put traction on them. In skeletally mature dancers, pain is caused by excessive tension on the tendons that attach to the epicondyles; this injury is called medial or lateral epicondylitis because the area around the epicondyle is inflamed. In dance, this injury can occur from repetitive acrobatic maneuvers in which the arm is loaded by body weight, such as back walkovers, cartwheels, and handstands. Excessive fitness training in both young and mature dancers can also play a role in this injury.

Treatment for these chronic injuries is first to reduce the problem forces by resting the elbow. A rehabilitation professional can help you correct your upper-extremity mechanics, modify workloads, and create a plan to return successfully to full dance activities. Pain medications and ice will help with pain and swelling. A brace or elastic sleeve will also control swelling and may help decrease tension on the elbow's musculotendinous tissues. A lateral or medial compression strap can be applied just below the elbow on the painful side (figure 12.15). This compression reduces the tension on the origin of the muscle group. Continued symptoms should be evaluated by a physician, and X-rays, musculoskeletal ultrasound, or MRI may be performed to rule out subtle conditions of the bone and soft tissue.

Cubital (meaning "elbow") tunnel syndrome occurs when the funny bone nerve (the ulnar nerve described earlier) that runs along the inside portion of the elbow becomes irritated or compressed in the tunnel that keeps the nerve in place. The classic signs that you are experiencing this condition are pain, numbness, and tingling down to the ring and little finger as well as weakness in those fingers. Anything that puts pressure on the ulnar nerve can cause the syndrome, such as leaning on the elbow for long periods or trauma that creates fluid buildup. In addition, repetitive and excessive bending can create inflammation that leads to swelling. In rare cases, the nerve repeatedly slips out of and back into the groove in which it sits; this movement can also inflame the nerve. Treatment includes modifying activity, splinting the arm at night to avoid excessive elbow bending while sleeping, anti-inflammatory medication, and nerve gliding exercises that rehabilitation personnel can perform. If the nerve is too compressed and symptoms worsen over time, surgery may be necessary.

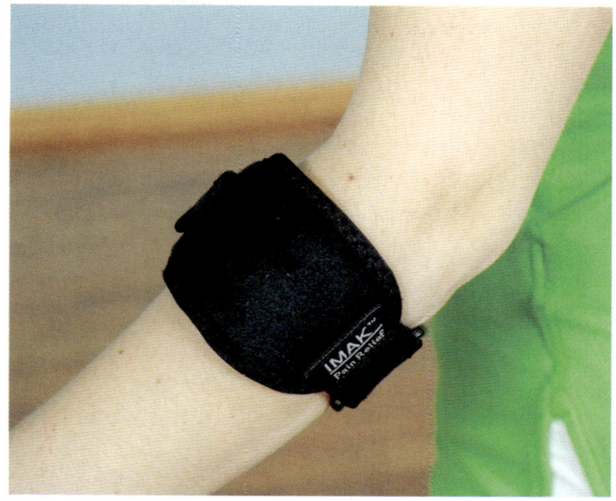

Figure 12.15 A compression strap placed on the lateral elbow (for lateral epicondylitis) or the medial elbow (for medial epicondylitis) may reduce tension of the muscles on the epicondyle. Note the placement of the pad portion of the strap; lateral compression is shown here.

Traumatic Injuries to the Hand and Wrist

Hand and wrist trauma most often occurs from falls on an outstretched hand and direct blows. These traumatic forces can cause fractures of several bones in this area. (General information about fractures appears in chapter 10.) Some of the more common ones and their signs are as follows:

- *Scaphoid fracture*—in the scaphoid bone at the base of the thumb. This fracture causes pain in the anatomical snuffbox (presented earlier). Delayed treatment can cause poor healing of the bone; such an occurrence may necessitate extended healing time and surgery.

- *Distal radius fracture*—in the wrist region at the end of the bone on the thumb side of the forearm. In young dancers, the bone can have a torus fracture, or buckle fracture, in which the bone bends but does not break all the way through.
- *Metacarpal fracture*—in one of the five long, slender bones in the palm of the hand. A common metacarpal fracture is called a boxer's fracture. This fracture occurs near the end of the fifth metacarpal toward the pinky finger, usually caused by hitting something hard with a fist.

Treatment for any fracture involves immobilization in a cast or splint for 3 to 6 weeks; longer casting may be required for scaphoid fractures because they take longer to heal than most other fractures. Wrist fractures usually need casting or substantial splinting, while fingers may require removable splints or buddy taping to the next finger; it depends on the amount of fracturing present. Hand and wrist stretching and other exercises can begin after removal of the cast or splints. A rehabilitation professional such as an athletic trainer or physical therapist can guide you to recovery.

A sudden force that pulls the thumb backward or away from the hand can overload its ulnar collateral ligament, spraining its fibers; a grade III sprain can destabilize the thumb. This injury is called gamekeeper's thumb or skier's thumb (DeFroda, 2018). Symptoms include pain, swelling around the thumb base, discoloration, and difficulty grasping objects between the thumb and fingers. X-rays are needed to rule out a fracture. Treatment for mild sprains includes protection, rest, ice, compression, and elevation (PRICE). Splints can be used to support healing and allow better function of the thumb in daily activities. Complete tears may require a cast for at least 6 weeks; they may even require surgery to restabilize the joint (Schroeder & Goldfarb, 2015).

Fingers can sustain a similar overload as what has been described for the thumb, resulting in a sprain of its collateral, or side, ligaments, particularly when a dancer jams a pointed finger while moving to the floor, slips when doing maneuvers such as back walkovers or cartwheels, or has a finger twisted by a partner grabbing it. In addition, the ligaments that support the finger joints on their palmar surfaces (called volar plates) can be torn, especially if a finger is hyperextended (figure 12.16*a* and 12.16*b*). Unlike gamekeeper's thumb, traumatic finger sprains that do not show significant deformity can be managed with finger splints and buddy taping to the adjacent uninjured finger for 3 to 4 weeks. Gradual return of motion using finger exercises is allowed as long as the finger is protected.

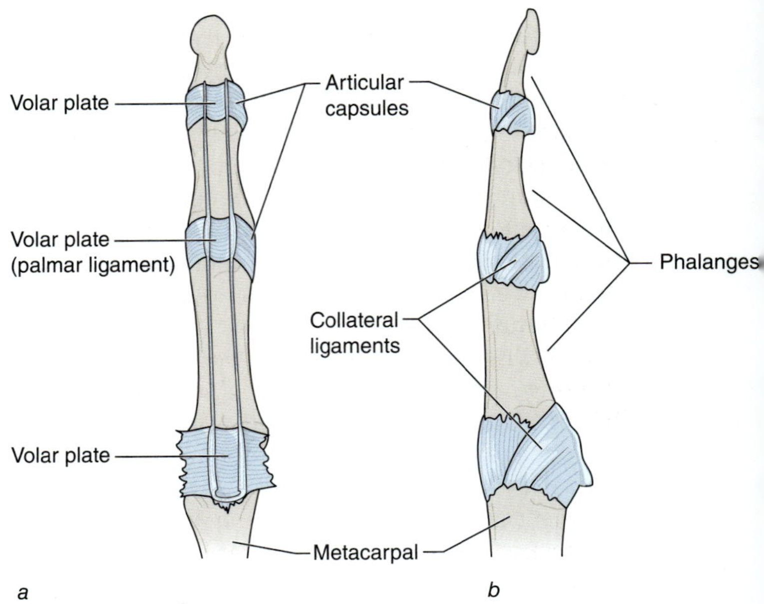

Figure 12.16 Main supporting ligaments of the fingers. *(a)* The volar plates that support the palmar part of each joint and prevent hyperextension *(b)* The collateral ligaments that support the sides of each joint.

Sometimes, the same forces that can fracture a finger or sprain its ligaments may cause a dislocated finger or thumb. This injury is unmistakable because of the pain, joint deformity, and swelling surrounding it. It may be tempting to just pull on the finger to realign the bones; however, doing so may cause more damage and prolong recovery. The appropriate treatment plan is to have a physician evaluate the finger and set it back in place. A dancer with this injury should immobilize the finger and seek care from their physician or an urgent care center. X-rays are usually performed to rule out a fracture. Treatment typically involves first splinting or buddy taping, then beginning therapeutic exercises when the pain and swelling subside. When a dislocated joint is unstable, surgery may be necessary.

As presented earlier, the ulnar side of the wrist is supported by the triangular fibrocartilage complex (TFCC). Falling on an outstretched hand or twisting the wrist while loaded with body weight (such as in modern or hip-hop floor moves) can tear the TFCC structures. Symptoms include pain with movement, clicking, and swelling in the pinky finger side of the wrist. Treatment includes rest and splinting. This injury is known to be difficult to manage. If the TFCC shows significant disruption of its ligaments or tearing of its cartilage, surgery may be needed to repair the damage (Casadei & Kiel, 2021).

Strains can occur in any of the many flexor or extensor tendons of the hand. A sudden pulling force on flexed fingers (e.g., when holding the hand of a dance partner) can excessively load a contracting muscle-tendon unit and damage the tissue by overly stretching it. As mentioned before, these injuries are categorized as grade I (stretched), grade II (partially torn), or grade III (completely torn). Initial treatment is protection, rest, ice, and compression, for 48 hours, then therapeutic exercises when pain and swelling are improved. Wrapping, taping, or splinting may be needed in grade II injuries. Grade III tears of the flexor or extensor tendons of the hand or wrist may require surgery. Both grade II and grade III strains should be evaluated by a physician.

Other traumatic tendon injuries of the hand have characteristic appearances; examples are shown in figure 12.17. Any of these injuries requires a physician to administer proper treatment to avoid permanent deformity. Mallet finger (figure 12.17*a*) is an injury to the extensor tendon attached to the end joint of the finger or thumb that causes the fingertip to droop. This can occur when a dancer hits a fingertip against an unyielding object, thus forcing the fingertip into flexion. This action disrupts the tendon attachment to the bone, resulting in loss of fingertip extension. Splinting the finger in a straight position is appropriate until a physician can be consulted.

A boutonnière deformity (figure 12.17*b*) is a rupture of part of a finger's extensor tendon and the slipping sideways of two other parts of the tendon. A force directed at a fingertip is the usual culprit. The word *boutonnière* is French for "buttonhole," as in a boutonnière flower often worn in the buttonhole of one's coat at a formal event. The damage to the extensor tendon complex creates a slot that the first knuckle of the finger slides through as a button slides through a buttonhole. As with the mallet finger, splinting the finger in a straight position and a physician visit are necessary responses to this injury.

Another traumatic finger injury is known as jersey finger. This name comes from the typical mechanism of a football player grabbing another player's jersey during a tackle and having the jersey then pulled forcibly from their hand. Generally, the injury occurs to a flexor tendon attached to the end joint of the finger or thumb when the digit is forced into extension from a flexed position, as when grasping something. This can happen when a dancer gets a finger caught in another dancer's costume or when grabbing any sort of implement, wardrobe piece, or equipment and then having that item forcefully removed from the clenched hand. The sudden pulling force disrupts the tendon attachment to the bone, making the fingertip unable to flex (de Villeneuve Bargemon et al., 2021). As with mallet finger and boutonnière deformity, this injury should be reported to a physician.

Nontraumatic Injuries to the Hand and Wrist

A ganglion cyst is a mass or lump that forms around a joint. This type of mass can be found throughout the body, but it is most common at the back of the wrist (figure 12.18). A wrist ganglion

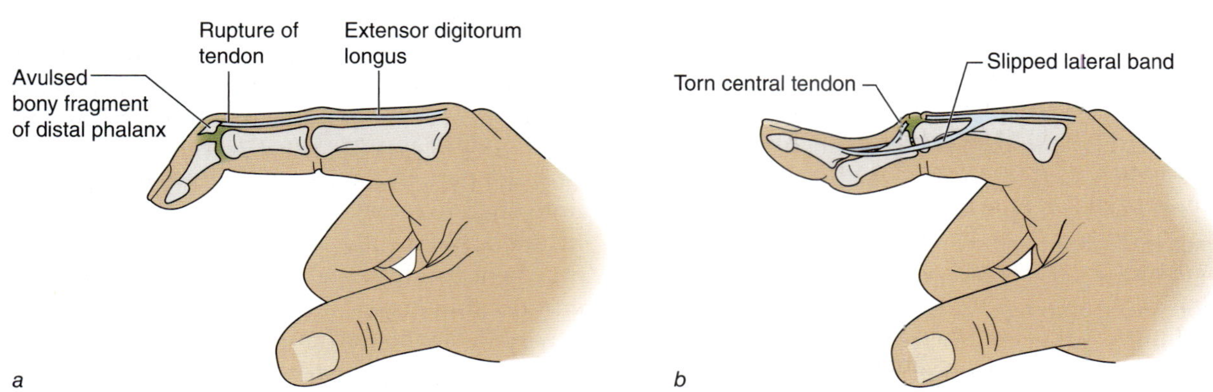

Figure 12.17 *(a)* A mallet finger caused by a tear of the finger extensor or the tendon pulling a piece from the bone in the fingertip. In either case, the muscle-tendon unit is not able to extend the fingertip, resulting in the mallet-like appearance. *(b)* A boutonnière deformity occurs when one part of an extensor tendon tears and two other parts of it split, thus allowing the middle knuckle of the finger to pop through the tendons. This causes flexion of the first knuckle of the finger and hyperextension of the second knuckle.

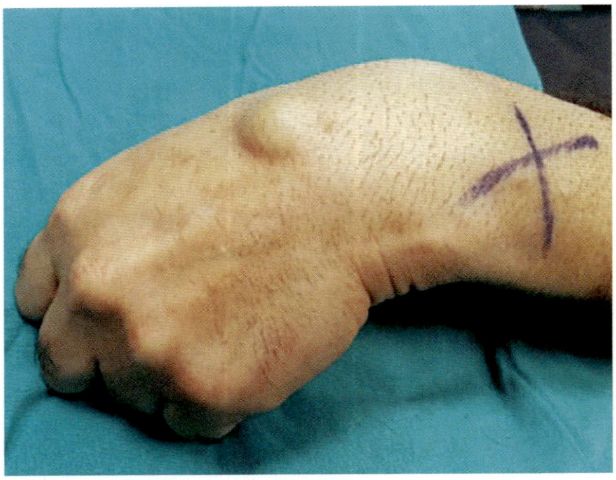

Figure 12.18 A ganglion cyst is a fluid-filled lump that appears most commonly on the back of the wrist.

cyst appears as a compressible lump that usually becomes more evident as the wrist is flexed in the palmar direction (i.e., wrist flexion). This condition is harmless, but it can cause significant pain when extending or loading the wrist. Ganglion cysts are most common in people between the ages of 15 and 40 years, and women are more likely to be affected than men. Ganglion cysts are common in gymnasts as well as in dancers who perform similar types of gymnastic or acrobatic maneuvers. Yoga, Pilates, and weight training can irritate a ganglion cyst and cause it to swell. Treatment is relative rest to allow the cyst's symptoms to calm down, immobilization with a splint for comfort, and having a physician drain the cyst (Head et al., 2015).

Dance choreography should be reviewed when a dancer suffers a ganglion cyst. In choreography for which a dancer must push off the floor repeatedly with the hands, the repetitive load can forcefully pinch the wrist's joint capsule and the cyst; this causes inflammation and swelling, thus enlarging the cyst. As the cyst takes up more space in the wrist region, more pain results. Exercises that strengthen the scapular stabilizers, deltoids, pectoral muscles, latissimus dorsi, and rotator cuff help decrease the load shift to the wrist, thus reducing the risk of worsening the condition and having it reoccur once it is treated.

Prevention of ganglion cysts starts with stability and strengthening of the shoulder girdle muscles. Dancers who are weak in these muscles tend to load the wrist with more force when doing exercises such as push-ups, downward-facing dog pose, and chest presses.

Carpal tunnel syndrome (CTS) causes numbness, tingling, and weakness in the hand. The carpal tunnel is a crowded space (see figure 12.7). CTS symptoms are caused by compression of the median nerve as it travels in the tunnel under the transverse carpal ligament in the palmar portion of the wrist. Most cases get progressively worse over time, so early treatment is important. Prolonged compression of the nerve can cause irreversible nerve damage (Wipperman & Goerl, 2016).

Causes of CTS include repetitive hand use (particularly with activities involving extreme extension or flexion for prolonged periods), resting the wrist on a hard surface for extended durations (such as when using a computer keyboard or mouse), pregnancy, inherited traits (e.g., a small carpal tunnel), and health conditions (e.g., diabetes, rheumatoid arthritis, and thyroid imbalances). Treatment includes bracing or splinting, exercises to stretch the transverse carpal ligament, anti-inflammatories, and activity modification. Steroid injections may be used to treat the inflamed nerve. Another procedure used to treat CTS is a technique called perineural hydrodissection (using fluid to expand tissue around a nerve). In this procedure, a solution of dextrose and water or saline is injected to make space for the nerve (Wu et al., 2019). If symptoms are severe enough despite conservative treatment, surgery is recommended to release tension from the transverse carpal ligament (Aroori & Spence, 2008).

Inflammation of the flexor digitorum tendon sheaths can create stiffness and catching when the fingers flex, causing a so-called trigger finger. A trigger occurs when the swollen portion of a tendon slips through a restricted area of the tendon's sheath, causing a popping sensation. This condition occurs more often in females than males, and causes can include activities that require repetitive gripping. Treatment includes nighttime splinting, stretches, anti-inflammatories, and rest from the irritating activity. Rehabilitation and corticosteroid injections may be prescribed for advanced cases (Armstrong & Hubbard, 2018). Severe cases that do not respond to conservative therapy may need surgery to release the tissue that restricts the tendon (Sarwark, 2010).

EXERCISES TO REDUCE THE RISK OF UPPER-EXTREMITY INJURIES

With the continued evolution of dance and choreography, numerous styles of dance (e.g., modern, jazz, and breaking) include increasing levels of partner work, floor work (including falls and handstands), and aerial work. In addition to these higher levels of upper-extremity activities, all forms of dance require some element of power, momentum, and aesthetic appearance through use of the arms. Thus, a full-body approach that includes upper-extremity cross-training should be considered for reducing the risk of injury and enhancing physical performance.

Assessing the upper-extremity strength of a dancer may help prevent many shoulder, elbow, and wrist injuries. Researchers have established normative baseline data for upper-extremity strength in collegiate dancers; they utilized the push-up to measure upper-body strength and endurance and the seated medicine ball throw to measure upper-body power (Coogan et al., 2021). These tests can easily be incorporated into dancer wellness screenings, preparticipation physical examinations, or personal assessments that provide data with which to create conditioning programs as described in chapter 5.

Specificity in exercise selection based on movement goals and demands is an essential consideration. In most dancers, the serratus anterior and the middle and lower trapezius are relatively weak muscles. Therefore, these muscles are addressed in the recommended exercises that follow. The following exercises are geared toward strengthening the upper extremity for dance technique and may help in reduction of injury; they focus on common errors and how to address them. Remember to breathe in and out while exercising to prevent passing out (known as vasovagal syncope) (Raut & Maheshwari, 2014).

EXERCISE 1: PLANK PLUS

Muscles involved: serratus anterior, rhomboids, middle and lower trapezius

The plank is a common upper-extremity exercise utilized in jazz and modern technique warm-up classes. It is an opportunity to practice proper alignment in the spine, scapulothoracic junction, and elbow joint. During this exercise, you will explore movement of the scapulae while training both the serratus anterior (movement of the scapulae away from each other) and rhomboids and middle trapezius (movement of the scapulae toward each other).

Exercise Instructions:

1. Start in a prone (facedown) position, then place your hands and knees with your hands on the floor under your shoulders and knees under your hips.
2. Straighten your knees so they are off the ground and you are supported by your hands and toes (figure 12.19*a*). Your body should form a straight line from head to toe (plank position).
3. Be sure to keep your elbows unlocked, but straight.
4. To create the *plank plus*, imagine pushing the floor away from you as your scapulas move apart from each other and your upper back lifts an inch or so upward toward the ceiling (arrow in figure 12.19*a*).
5. Maintain this position for 5 seconds, then slowly lower your upper back to the starting position. Repeat for 8 to 10 reps.

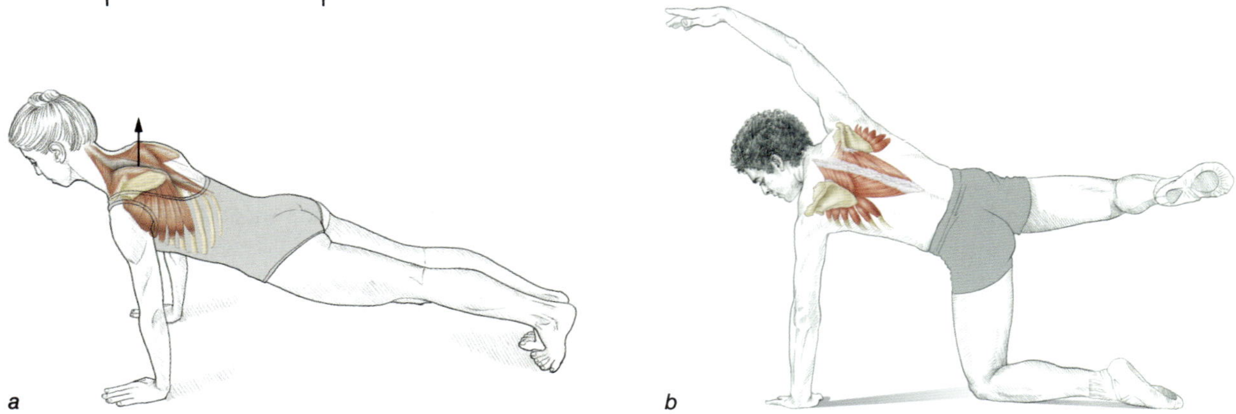

Figure 12.19 Plank plus exercise: *(a)* Proper starting positioning. *(b)* An example of how the muscles trained with this exercise are used in dance.

EXERCISE 2A: PRONE SHOULDER EXTERNAL AND INTERNAL ROTATION

Muscles involved: infraspinatus, teres minor, subscapularis, and trapezius

This exercise isolates your rotator cuff muscles for external rotation (infraspinatus and teres minor) and internal rotation (subscapularis) while engaging the trapezius to stabilize your scapulae. As you complete this exercise, try not to depress or elevate your scapulae.

Exercise Instructions:

1. Position yourself prone (face down) on an elevated surface such as a table or bed with the forearm of the upper extremity you will exercise over the edge. Prop yourself with pillows and towels as shown in figure 12.20 and be sure your shoulder girdle alignment is in its most ideal position.
2. Use external rotation in the shoulder joint to rotate the hand and forearm toward a position where the forearm is parallel to the floor (figure 12.20*a*). Then reverse to shoulder internal rotation and move your hand and forearm in the other direction (figure 12.20*b*) until the forearm is parallel to the floor. Perform 8 to 10 reps.
3. As you rotate your arm either externally or internally, do not lift your humerus off the supporting towel roll; doing so will cause you to substitute with your posterior deltoid muscle and will also change the position of your scapula.
4. To increase the exercise's difficulty and increase your strength, use handheld or wrist weights.

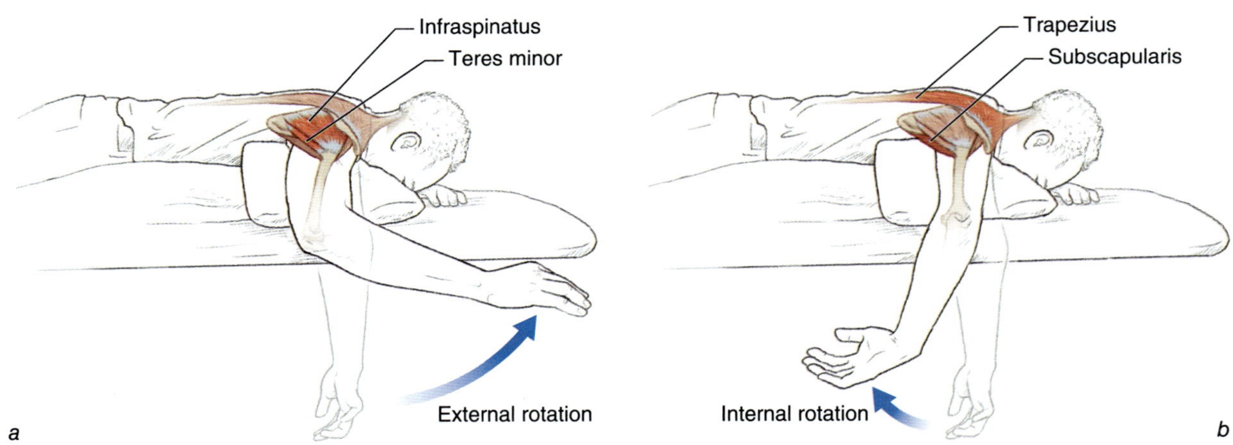

Figure 12.20 Proper positioning and movements for prone shoulder external and internal rotation exercise. *(a)* Movement of external rotation. *(b)* Movement of internal rotation.

EXERCISE 2B: SHOULDER EXTERNAL ROTATION AT 90/90

Muscles involved: deltoid, supraspinatus, biceps brachii, upper and middle trapezius, serratus anterior, and triceps brachii

If you struggle with the correction of keeping your shoulder blades down and back, or if you are training for partnering work, this exercise will help (especially when paired with exercise 2A). This movement will strengthen your rotator cuff and help keep the humeral head in its socket.

Exercise Instructions:

1. Start by standing feet shoulder width apart and lift your arms into a 90/90 position with your shoulders abducted and elbows flexed to 90 degrees. Both your upper arms and forearms should be parallel to the floor. Be sure to allow your scapulae to upwardly rotate (but not elevate; do not shrug your shoulders) as you lift to the 90/90 position.
2. Externally rotate from your shoulder joints by lifting your forearms (figure 12.21*a*). As you pull your forearms backward, exhale to engage your abdominals, being careful to not let your lower ribs flare. Drawing your navel slightly inward toward your spine will help. Perform 8 to 10 reps.
3. Once you are able to perform the exercise correctly with good shoulder and upper-extremity control, add a long elastic resistance band. Hold one end in each hand and stand on the middle of the band. The resistance will make the exercise more challenging and will help you develop more strength.

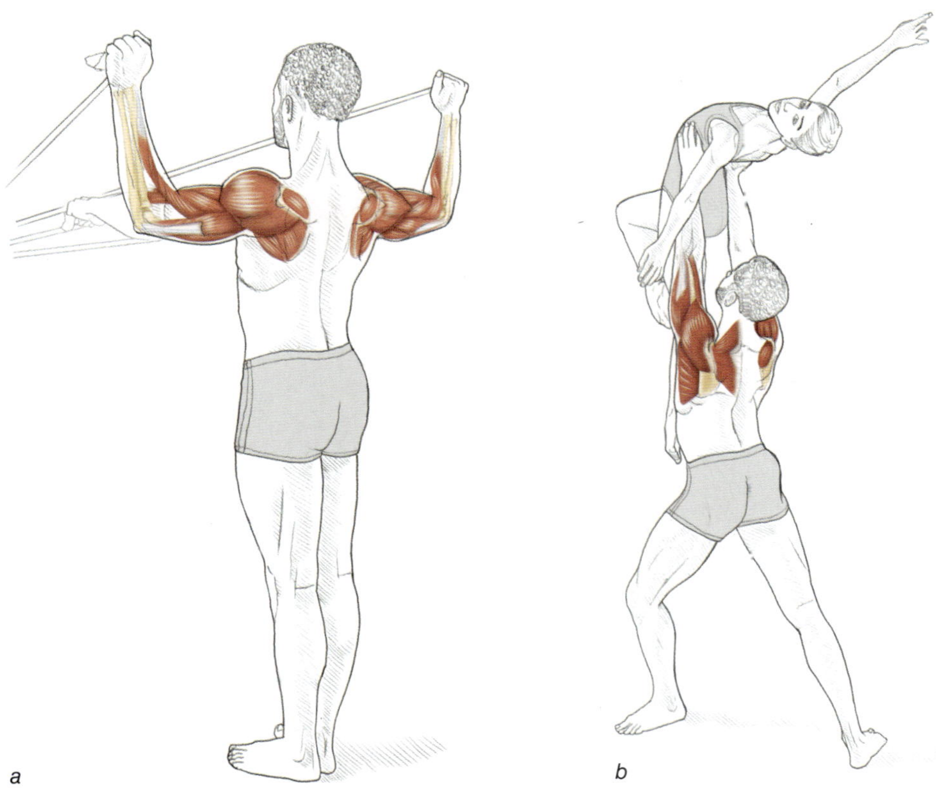

Figure 12.21 External rotation at 90/90 exercise: *(a)* Proper positioning. *(b)* An example of how the muscles trained with this exercise are used in dance.

EXERCISE 3A: PRONE V

Muscles involved: trapezius, and possibly internal and external rotators

Try this exercise as a way to isolate your trapezius as well as your shoulder external rotator muscles.

Exercise Instructions:

1. First, make sure you are propped with pillows and towels such that your shoulder girdle alignment is in its most ideal position while lying prone (face down) on an elevated surface such as a table or bed.
2. Extend your arms to the sides so your shoulders are slightly below 90 degrees of abduction, your elbows are flexed slightly more than 90 degrees, and your thumbs are pointing upward toward the ceiling (figure 12.22*a*).
3. Engage your trapezius muscle (upper back) first, but do not depress or elevate your scapulae.
4. Next, slide your hands forward past the top of your head (figure 12.22*b*) so your shoulders are in a V-shaped position (figure 12.22*c*). Then bring them back to the starting position while continuing to stabilize with your upper back muscles; in other words, do not let your arms drop. Perform 8 to 10 reps.
5. To make the exercise slightly more difficult, lift your hands first and then lift your elbows off the supporting surface prior to moving your arms forward into the V position. Adding weights will make this exercise even more challenging.

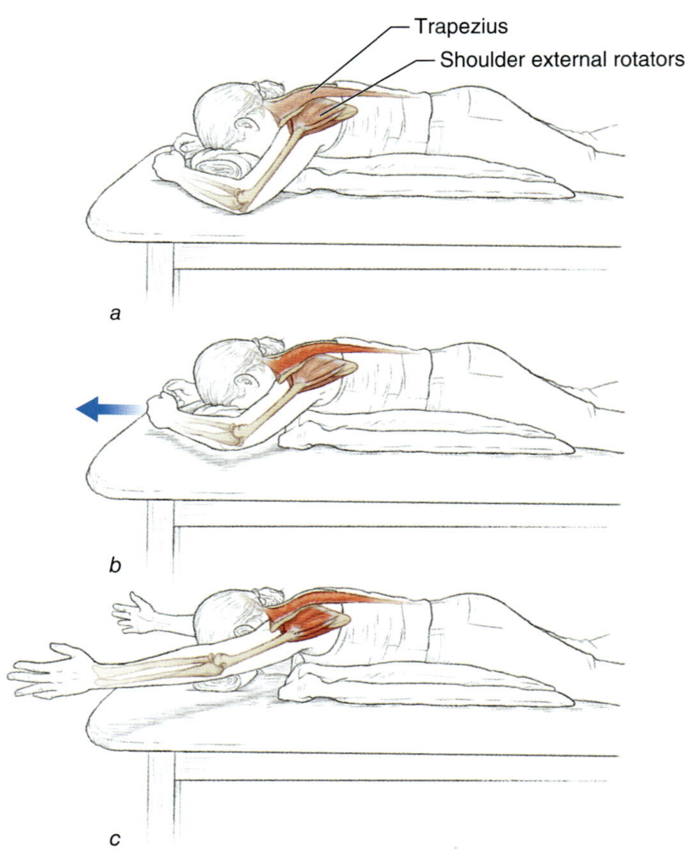

Figure 12.22 Prone V exercise: *(a)* Starting position. *(b)* Initiation of forward movement. *(c)* Ending position.

EXERCISE 3B: V

Muscles involved: middle deltoid, supraspinatus, serratus anterior, trapezius, pectoralis major, rhomboids, and levator scapulae

Dancers lift their arms overhead in many styles of dance; positions include high parallel, fifth position, or high V. When in these positions, some dancers may elevate the scapulae and overuse the upper trapezius muscle. This scenario may also occur in dancers with scapular dyskinesis who are unable to coordinate upward rotation of the scapulae without winging or elevating excessively. This exercise provides practice in maintaining control of your scapulae and trapezius.

Exercise Instructions

1. Start by sitting or by standing feet shoulder width apart with your arms by your sides with your thumbs pointing outward.
2. Draw your navel to your spine to stabilize your core, then exhale as you lift your arms to a V position while picturing your shoulder blades upwardly rotating along your rib cage (figure 12.23a). Imagine sending energy along the undersurface of your arms and through your pinky fingers to help create a beautiful arc of movement while keeping your upper trapezius calm. Concentrate on not shrugging your shoulders as you move your arms.
3. Inhale as you return to the starting position and repeat for 8 to 10 reps.

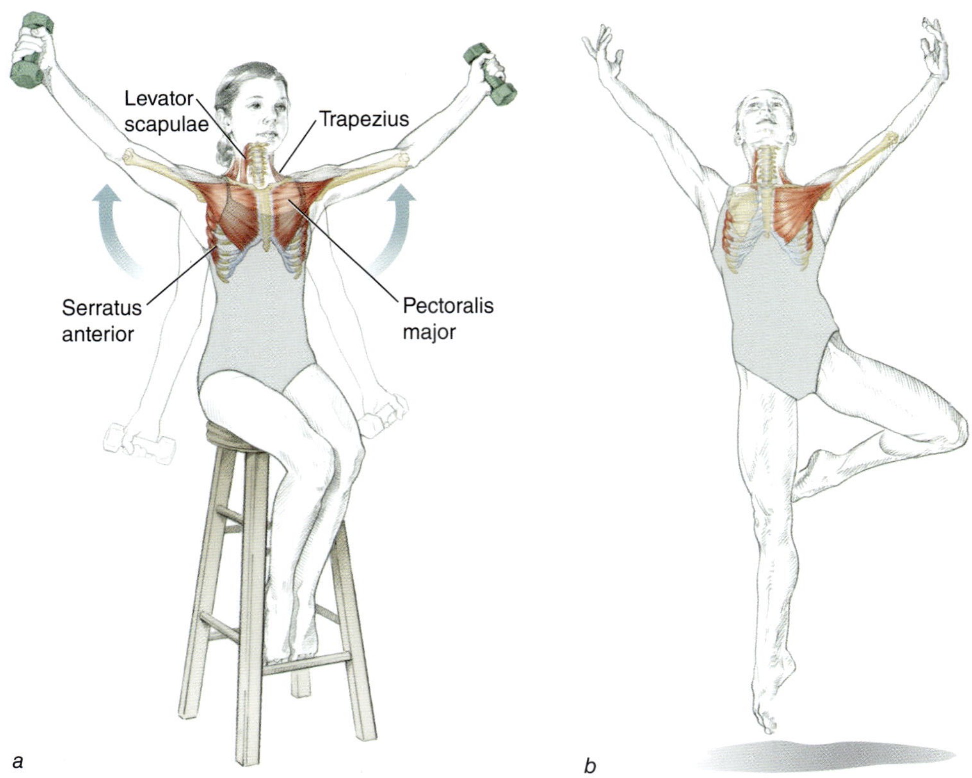

Figure 12.23 V exercise: *(a)* Proper positioning. *(b)* An example of how the muscles trained with this exercise are used in dance.

EXERCISE 4: NARROW ROWING

Muscles involved: lower and middle trapezius, rhomboids

Dance requires movements of the arms not only in front of the body but also back behind the body while opening the chest. Use an elastic exercise band to provide resistance; it must have enough resistance to make the exercise challenging. The narrow positioning of the arms means this exercise focuses on the scapular stabilizers, which are commonly weak in dancers.

Exercise Instructions:

1. Sit on a table or the floor. Grasp one end of an elastic resistance band with each hand and then anchor the band around your feet with your legs placed straight in front of you.
2. Sitting up tall with your shoulders back, draw your navel toward your spine to stabilize your core. Then exhale while you pull your elbows back along either side of your rib cage (figure 12.24*a*) using the muscles in your upper back. Be sure to keep your chest open and your core engaged during this movement.
3. Slowly return to the starting position while inhaling. Do not compensate by rounding your shoulders forward.
4. Perform 10 to 12 reps. This exercise can be made more difficult by using a thicker band to create more resistance.

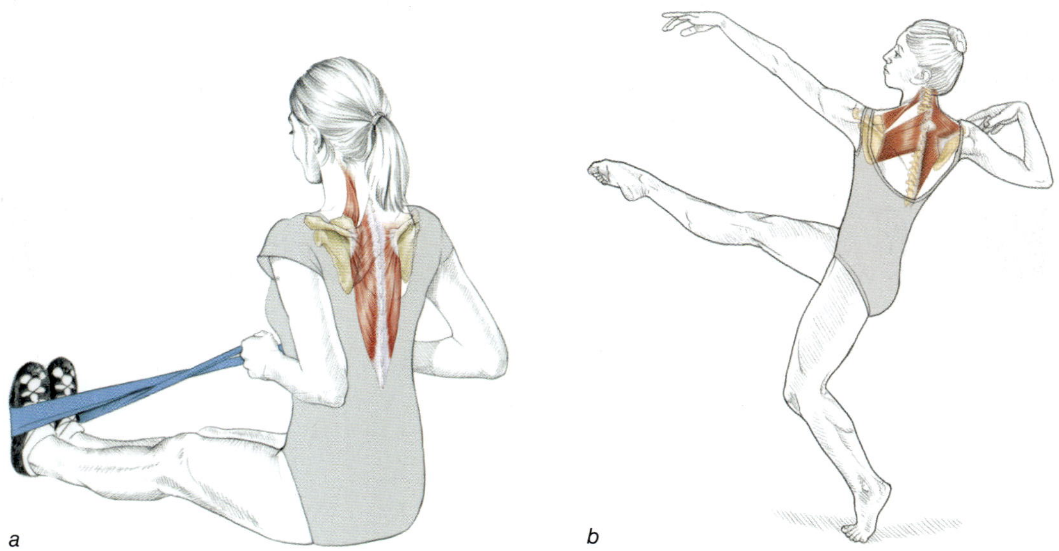

Figure 12.24 Narrow rowing exercise: *(a)* Proper positioning. *(b)* An example of how the muscles trained with this exercise are used in dance.

Conclusions and Practical Relevance

In dance, upper-extremity injuries are typically less common than injuries in the lower extremity; however, many of these injuries can occur in dancers, particularly those who dance in genres emphasizing weight bearing on the hands or supporting loads with the upper extremities. Learning the anatomy of the upper extremity and the exercises that improve muscle strength and endurance in the shoulders and arms can help you optimize scapular biomechanics, improve aesthetic performance, and reduce the risk of injury. Taking a whole-body approach to training is important for any dancer's overall health and performance. Seeking medical evaluation early for signs of pain or dysfunction—especially to further understand your scapular mechanics and posture—may help sustain your dance career.

Discussion Questions

1. You are regularly getting corrections in ballet class to lower your shoulders when holding your arms in fifth position and you frequently experience neck tightness. What may account for your symptoms, and what are some exercises you would consider to address the issue?
2. You have been given the opportunity to teach a contemporary dance class, and your choreography includes many repetitive overhead movements. Your most flexible dancer complains of daily shoulder soreness after your class. The contours of the dancer's shoulder blades look uneven from behind. What could explain this unevenness? What exercises would be beneficial for this dancer?
3. One of your dance classmates complains of pain and numbness in the hand—especially on the palm of the thumb and first two fingers—when holding a plank position on the floor or using a computer for a while. What might account for these symptoms? What advice can you offer?

WWW Go to HK*Propel* to access supplemental information and activities connected to chapter content.

13

Dance Injuries in the Lumbar Spine, Pelvic Floor, and Hips

Lauren Elson, MD
Brooke Winder, DPT
Susan Mayes, PhD, AM

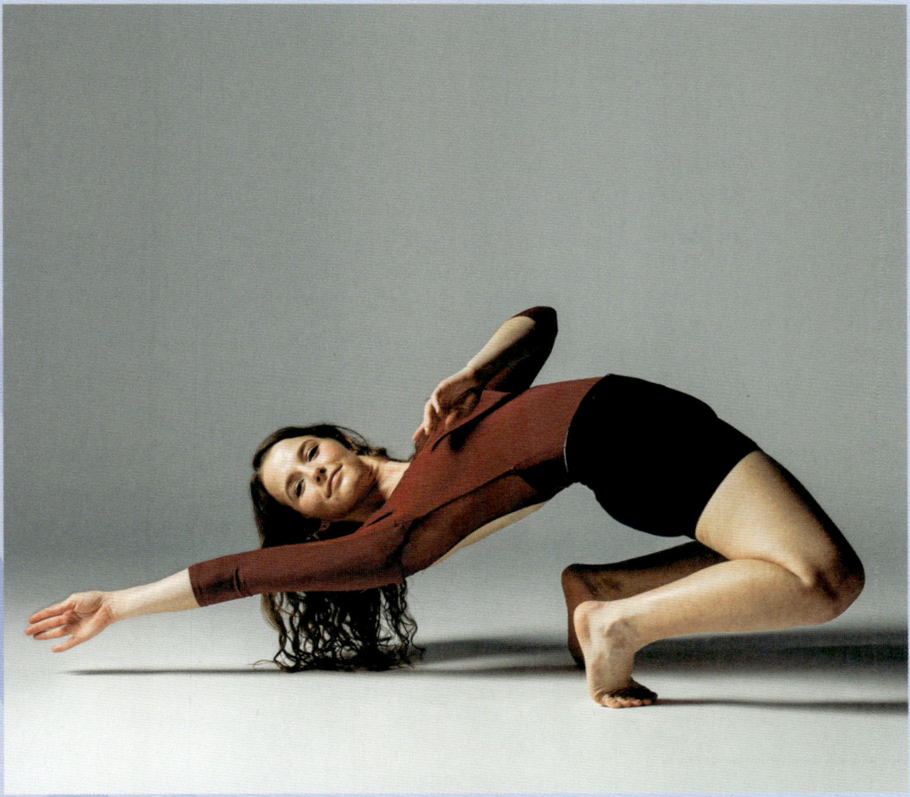

Belhaven University Dance Department, Jackson, Mississippi. Photo: Fluid Frames Dance Photography; Dancer: Olivia Holland

The lumbar spine, pelvic floor, and hips are areas that do not receive enough attention; nevertheless, if they are not working well, they can negatively affect virtually everything a dancer does. These areas are absolutely crucial to success in dance because they provide a solid base (or, if not cared for properly, a wobbly one) for movement and stability of the entire body. Just as a strong foundation in a building provides the support it needs to avoid toppling over, these areas provide the support your body needs to dance.

Key Terms

apophysitis
avulsion
cancellous bone
coccydynia
continence
core stability
form closure
incontinence
intra-abdominal pressure (IAP)
pelvic floor muscles
pelvic ring
pubic symphysis dysfunction
sacroiliac
sphincter
spondylolisthesis
spondylolysis
synovium
vertebra

LEARNING OBJECTIVES

After completing this chapter, you will be able to do the following:

- Describe the anatomy and mechanics of the lumbar spine in relation to common injuries in this region.
- Describe the anatomy and function of the pelvic floor in relation to common injuries in this region.
- Explain and apply basic interactions in breathing, pressure-management, and core control to develop optimal core stabilization.
- Describe the anatomy and mechanics of the hip in relation to common injuries in this region.

The lumbar spine, pelvis, and hip regions interact closely to form a stable, powerful base for the production of movement in dance. Most dance forms place a large range of motion demand on the lumbar spine, pelvis, and hips while requiring coordinated strength, endurance, and control of these regions. Developing a thorough understanding of how to efficiently stabilize and optimally move the spine, pelvis, and hips—while integrating optimal breathing and management of pressure—can help dancers set a good foundation for progressing their technique and artistry. Dancers also benefit from understanding common injuries in each of these areas and how these injuries are typically managed.

Bones and Joints of the Lumbar Spine

As shown in figure 13.1, the spine has 32 vertebrae (the singular is **vertebra**), and they are divided into five regions: cervical (neck), thoracic (midback, attached to the ribs), lumbar (lower back), sacral (lower back, attached to the pelvis), and the coccygeal (tailbone). Each region is composed of vertebrae with a unique shape that allows for the specific motions of that region. The lumbar, sacral, and coccygeal regions are the areas of focus in this chapter.

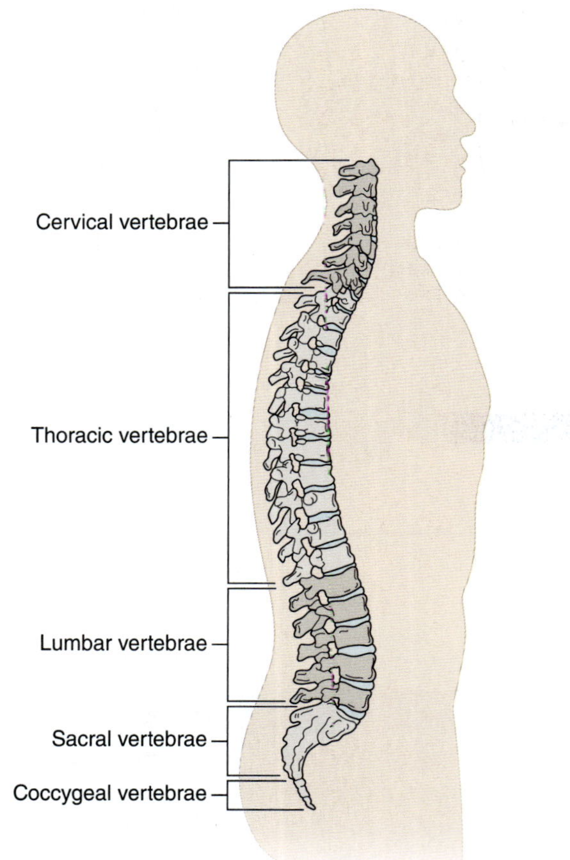

Figure 13.1 The five regions of the human spinal column.

Most people have five lumbar vertebrae; however, it is not unusual to have six. These vertebrae have no ribs attached to them (as in the thoracic spine); therefore, the lumbar region is very flexible, allowing for movement in several planes, including flexion (forward bending), extension (backward bending), and lateral flexion (side bending). The vertebral body (figure 13.2) is the major weight-bearing surface of the bone. Both the spinous processes and the transverse processes have ridges for the attachment of ligaments and muscles, facilitating movement and control of the spine. The superior (upper) and inferior (lower) articular processes form the joints between two adjacent vertebrae. In the lumbar spine, relative to the other regions, the articular processes have a vertical orientation that prevents rotation (Waxenbaum et al., 2022).

The inferior articular process of the lowest lumbar vertebra (usually L5) articulates with the sacrum, the wedge-shaped bone that connects the two sides of the pelvis posteriorly and serves as the back of the pelvic ring. Intervertebral discs are the shock-absorbing cushions between each pair of vertebral bodies. Completing the bony ring of the vertebrae are the pedicles; they connect the posterior structures (attachment sites for the muscles) with the vertebral body. This ring of each vertebra protects the spinal cord. Nerves that branch from the spinal cord exit the vertebral column to transmit signals to and from the pelvis and lower extremities, thus allowing for movement of your legs, sensation of your lower body, proprioception in the lower body, and control of the pelvic floor muscles and **sphincters** (figure 13.3).

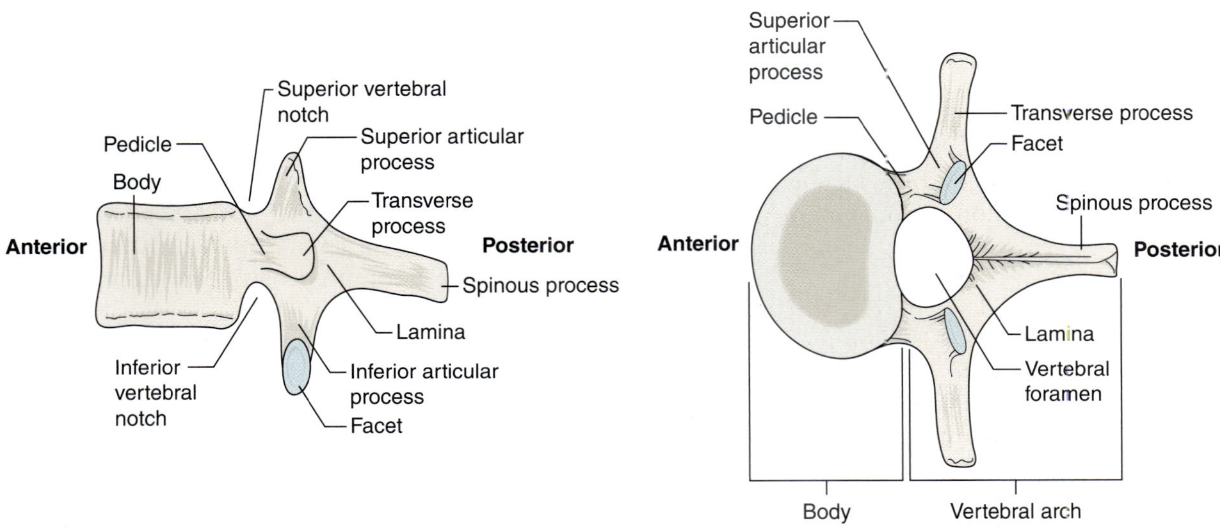

Figure 13.2 The anatomy of a typical vertebra.

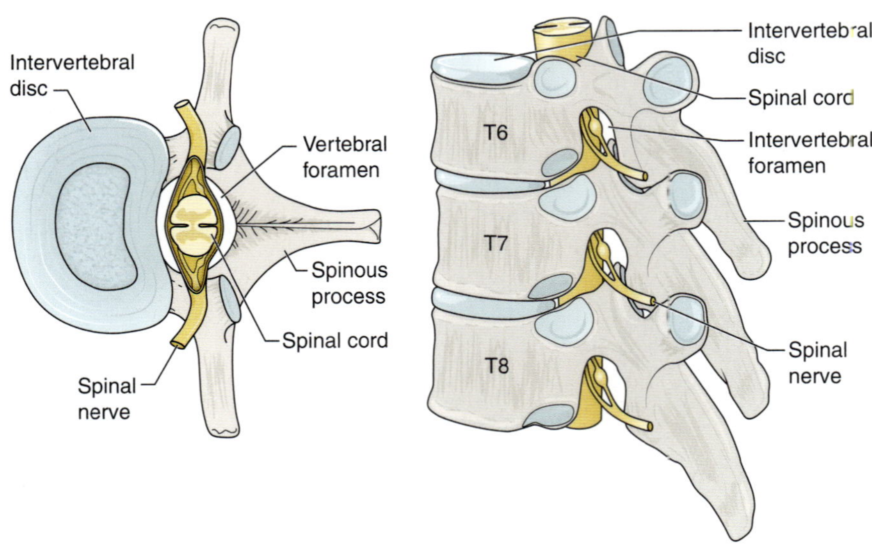

Figure 13.3 Each vertebra is designed to fit together with the one above and the one below. The column of assembled vertebrae forms a tunnel that protects the spinal cord. Each pair of spinal nerves exits between two adjacent vertebrae to provide sensory and movement capability for the body.

Lumbar Ligaments and Muscles

Many strong ligaments attach to and surround the spine, and they have several functions (figure 13.4). They help maintain alignment, prevent excessive motion, and protect the discs. They are uniquely designed to allow necessary mobility of the individual pieces of the spine without jeopardizing the discs and the spinal cord.

Several layers of muscles control the movement of the lumbar spine. Perhaps the most important is the transversus abdominis. Like a corset, it surrounds the entire abdomen; it attaches superiorly to the ribs, inferiorly to the pelvis, and posteriorly to the lumbar spine at the back. When engaged, it primarily functions to stabilize the lumbar spine, providing a solid base of support and control. For dancers, this support is particularly important because it allows for a solid central anchor around which the limbs move more freely (figure 13.5).

The internal oblique, external oblique, and rectus abdominis are three more broad, flat muscles of the trunk (figure 13.6). The muscular layer that directly overlays the transversus abdominis is the internal oblique, named because of its oblique (diagonal) fibers. Over the internal oblique is the external oblique, with its fibers oriented in the opposite diagonal direction. Both of these muscles contribute to increasing intra-abdominal pressure, such as with the Valsalva maneuver (bearing down, e.g., as during a bowel movement) as well as during breathing. However, their main function is spinal rotation (twisting of the trunk). The internal oblique creates trunk rotation to the same side, and the external oblique rotates the trunk to the opposite side. For example, rotating right would primarily involve the right internal oblique and the left external oblique.

The rectus abdominis—the so-called six-pack muscle—is the most superficial, anterior (outermost) layer of the abdominal muscles. It is actually more of a 10-pack. This appearance comes from the fascia bands that cross it to create its characteristic bulges; six of these bulges are the easiest to see. This muscle runs from the pelvis to the bottom of the sternum and cartilage of the lower ribs. Its main role is to flex the trunk. Although it is a strong, powerful muscle, it is not the most important for maintaining stability. Therefore, the sit-up (which targets this muscle) is not a comprehensive core-strengthening exercise.

Although primarily a hip flexor (discussed in detail next), the psoas major muscle (figure 13.7) also affects the movements of the lumbar spine. It

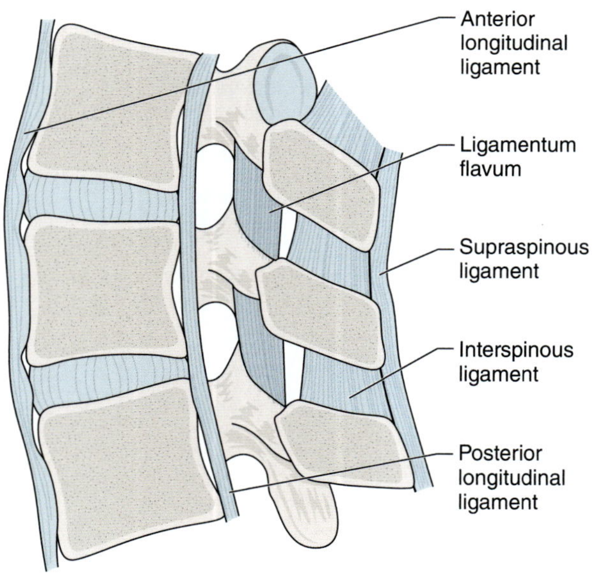

Figure 13.4 Several ligaments run the length of the spine to stabilize the vertebral column, thus reducing the chance of injury to the intervertebral discs.

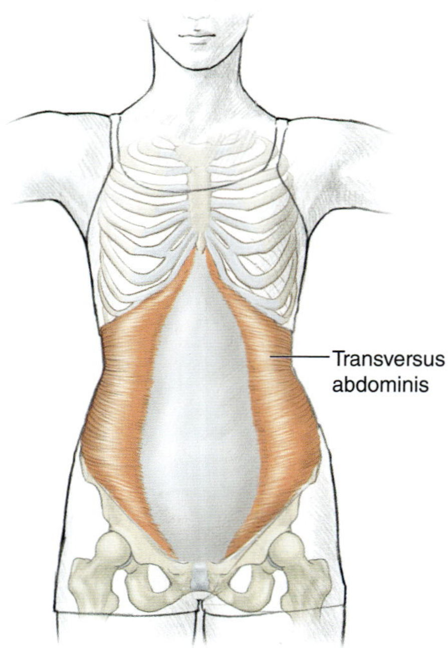

Figure 13.5 The transversus abdominis muscle is a key to providing the anchoring support needed for a dancer to successfully use the upper and lower extremities during dance.

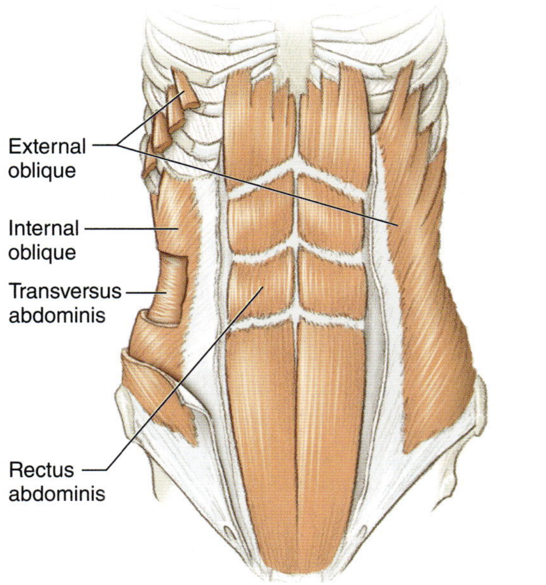

Figure 13.6 The layers and fiber directions of the muscles that surround the lower portion of the trunk. (Fascia is shown in the light color.)

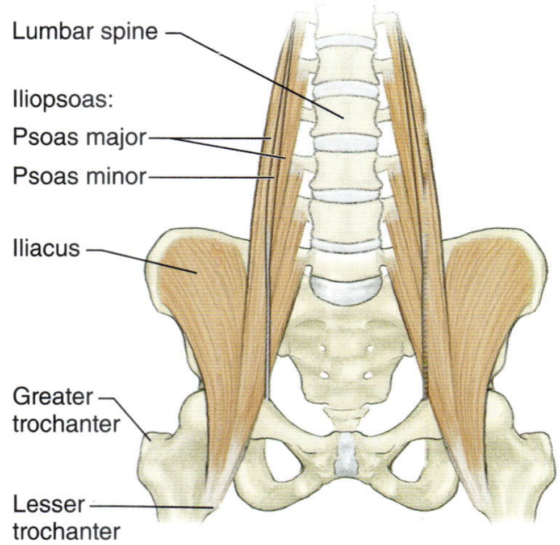

Figure 13.7 The course of the psoas major muscle positions it for hip flexion, but it can also pull the lumbar spine forward because of its attachments there. At its distal end, it joins the iliacus muscle. The pair together are called the iliopsoas muscle.

attaches to the sides and front surface of thoracic vertebra 12 and the lumbar vertebra and joins with the iliacus muscle in the pelvis to attach to the femur.

Several layers of muscles on the back of the vertebrae produce trunk (spine) extension and help keep you upright. Each muscle has a slightly different function, but they work together to stabilize the spine and facilitate movement while protecting the nerves. The deepest layer of muscles that help with spine extension includes the multifidus (figure 13.8*a*). The quadratus lumborum, another muscle in the deep layer, laterally flexes the trunk and assists with trunk flexion; because it attaches to the 12th rib, it also aids respiration (figure 13.8*a*). On top of that layer are the iliocostalis and the longissimus (figure 13.8*b*).

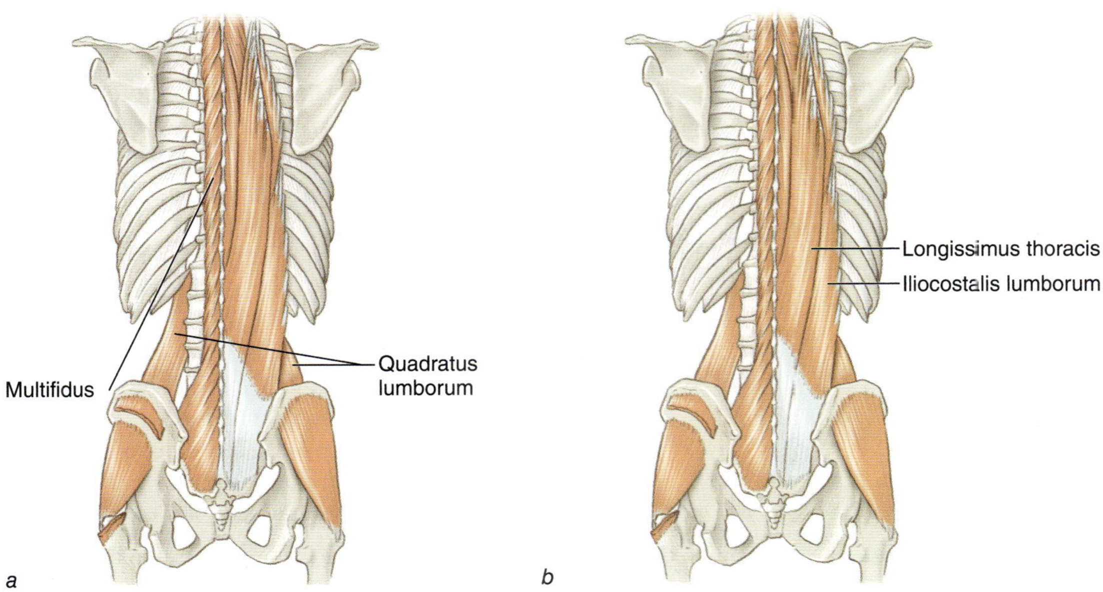

Figure 13.8 Muscles of the posterior trunk can make multiple contributions to movement. *(a)* The multifidus and the quadratus lumborum. *(b)* The longissimus and iliocostalis muscles, both of which have portions named for their vertebral attachments (e.g., longissimus thoracis, iliocostalis lumborum).

The thoracolumbar fascia (figure 13.9) is a thick sheet of connective tissue that covers the posterior muscles of the lower thoracic and lumbar spine. It is the attachment site for several large muscles, including the gluteus maximus and the latissimus dorsi. The latissimus dorsi is a powerful muscle affecting multiple body regions through its connections from the pelvis and spine (through the thoracolumbar fascia) to its attachment site on the humerus.

Mechanics and Function of the Lumbar Spine

The spine is designed to move through each vertebral level. If some levels are less mobile than others, the body may compensate by moving excessively at other levels. Restrictions may occur because of bony anatomy, improper alignment of the bones, and muscle imbalances.

Tight muscles in body regions surrounding the lumbar spine can cause abnormal forces through the lumbar spine, leading to dysfunction and pain. For example, a weak or tight psoas muscle can impair spinal movement, particularly limiting spinal extension at its levels of attachment. Low-back pain also can be caused by strength imbalances, tightness, or muscle pain referred from the gluteal muscles or the latissimus dorsi, since these muscles all attach to the spine via the thoracolumbar fascia.

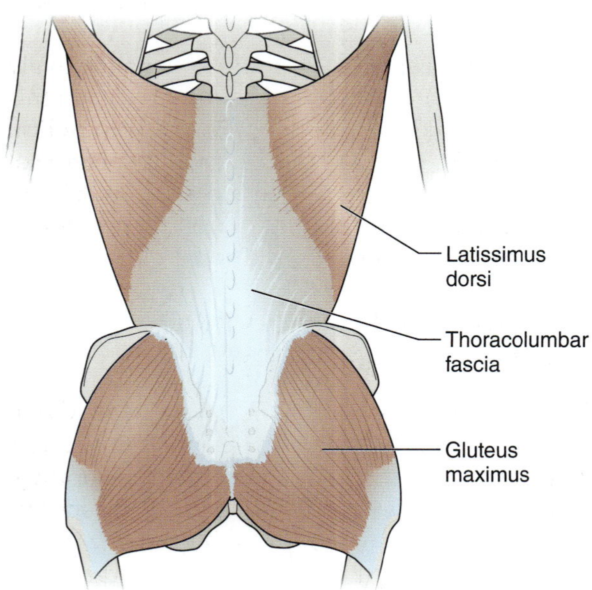

Figure 13.9 The thoracolumbar fascia encloses a large portion of the lower back, including the important latissimus dorsi muscle. The latissimus dorsi originates at the pelvis, thoracolumbar fascia, lower ribs, and thoracic vertebrae; travels upward to form the posterior wall of the armpit; and inserts to the humerus of the upper arm.

Lumbar lordosis is the natural curve of the lumbar spine. In the ideal posture (figure 13.10*a*), the muscles around the spine are balanced; they both support the spinal structures during extreme range of motion and provide a firm base of support around which the limbs can freely move. Too much (hyperlordosis; figure 13.10*b*) or too little (hypolordosis; figure 13.10*c*) curvature loads the structures of the spine less efficiently and makes the spine and core less stable. As a result, balancing and turns are more difficult to accomplish, potentially leading to injury. Risk factors for hyperlordosis include tight hip flexors, weak or impaired use of the lower abdominal muscles (especially the transversus abdominis), and forcing turnout. Gripping through the gluteal muscles and hip flexors can lead to hypolordosis.

Lumbar Dysfunction and Injury

Lumbar injury occurs when the lumbar spine is subjected to abnormal forces, which are often caused by muscle imbalances. The prevalence of back pain is high in dancers; it is the second most prevalent region for dance injuries (Bowling, 1989; Swain et al., 2019).

Spondylolysis

Spondylolysis is a stress fracture of the pars interarticularis, a portion of the ring of a vertebra that encircles the spinal cord as well as forms part of the arch through which the spinal roots leave the spinal cord (figure 13.11). Many factors may lead to this injury in dancers. If repetitive lumbar flexion and extension are performed without adequate core stabilization by the surrounding muscles, this part of the bone is subjected to excess stress. Ideally, when extending the spine (for example, in a cambré derrière [leaning backward]), a dancer should move through the entire posterior chain.

Tight hip flexors and forced turnout (discussed later in this chapter) also cause excessive lumbar lordosis, in turn causing abnormal loads on the posterior portion of the spine that may cause pain and potentially lead to spondylolysis. With excessive lumbar lordosis, increased extension exists through one level as opposed to being evenly distributed among multiple levels. It also is evident when a dancer is in arabesque but does not lengthen the

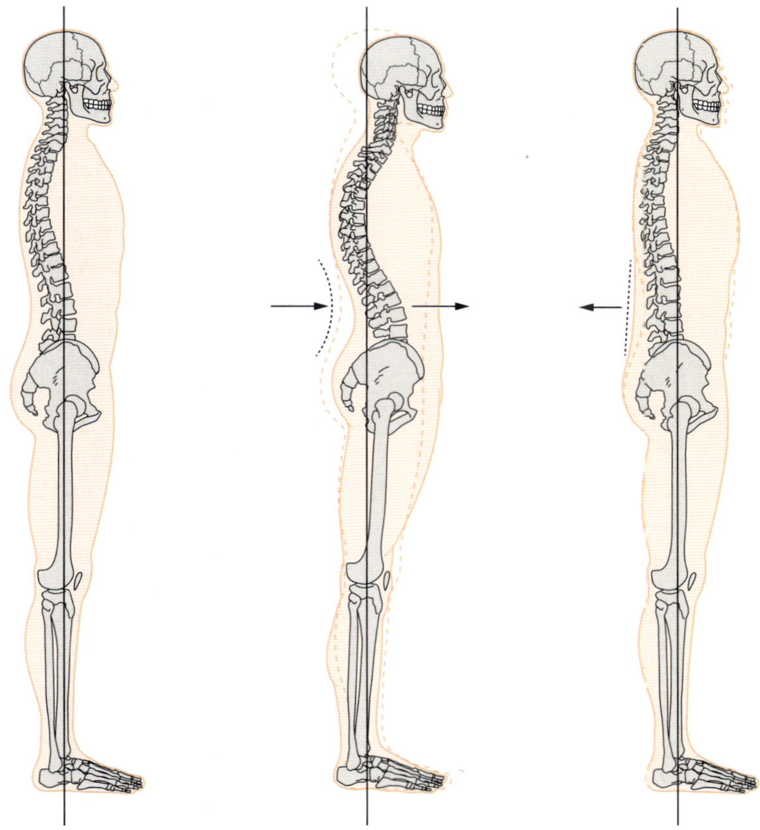

Figure 13.10 *(a)* The typical amount of lordosis seen in the lumbar spine. *(b)* Example of a spine with too much lordosis present. *(c)* Example of a spine with not enough lordosis, which can also create pain and decreased mobility.

torso. In such a situation (figure 13.12*a*), the dancer creates a right angle between the spine and the leg. Forced hyperextension during lifts can lead to similar stress patterns (figure 13.12*b*) (Gelabert, 1986).

Over time, the excessive forces on the bone cause breakdown of bone cells to occur faster than they can be rebuilt. This situation initially causes swelling and weakening of the bone, a pattern that eventually leads to spondylolysis, as mentioned previously, a stress fracture at the pars interarticularis. It can be seen on X-rays in what is known as the Scottie dog sign (figure 13.13*a*). In spondylolysis, the X-ray shows the Scottie dog with a collar (figure 13.13*b*).

Spondylolisthesis

Spondylolisthesis occurs when there is a spondylolysis of both pars interarticularis segments on one vertebra and they fracture through. This situation allows the vertebral body to slide forward and backward because it is no longer connected to the posterior portion of the vertebrae (Keim & Kirkaldy-Willis, 1980). On an X-ray, the vertebral bodies do not line up (see figure 13.13*c*). Although many soft tissues still can hold the bone relatively in place, abnormal movement of the bones in this region can affect the nerves, and it requires medical attention. The treatment depends on the degree of instability. At some point, treating both spondylolysis and spondylolisthesis requires optimization of the mechanics throughout the body.

Treatment of Spondylolysis and Spondylolisthesis

The most important factor in treating spondylolysis and spondylolisthesis is resolving the biomechanical imbalances that led to the development of the fracture. Relative rest (avoiding the specific movements that cause pain) is important. If pain occurs with activities of daily living, a brace can be prescribed for temporary use until the pain improves. Anti-inflammatory medications are typically avoided with this injury because they can mask the pain (thus preventing the dancer from knowing when to avoid particular movements). Moreover, regular use of these medications can prevent bone healing.

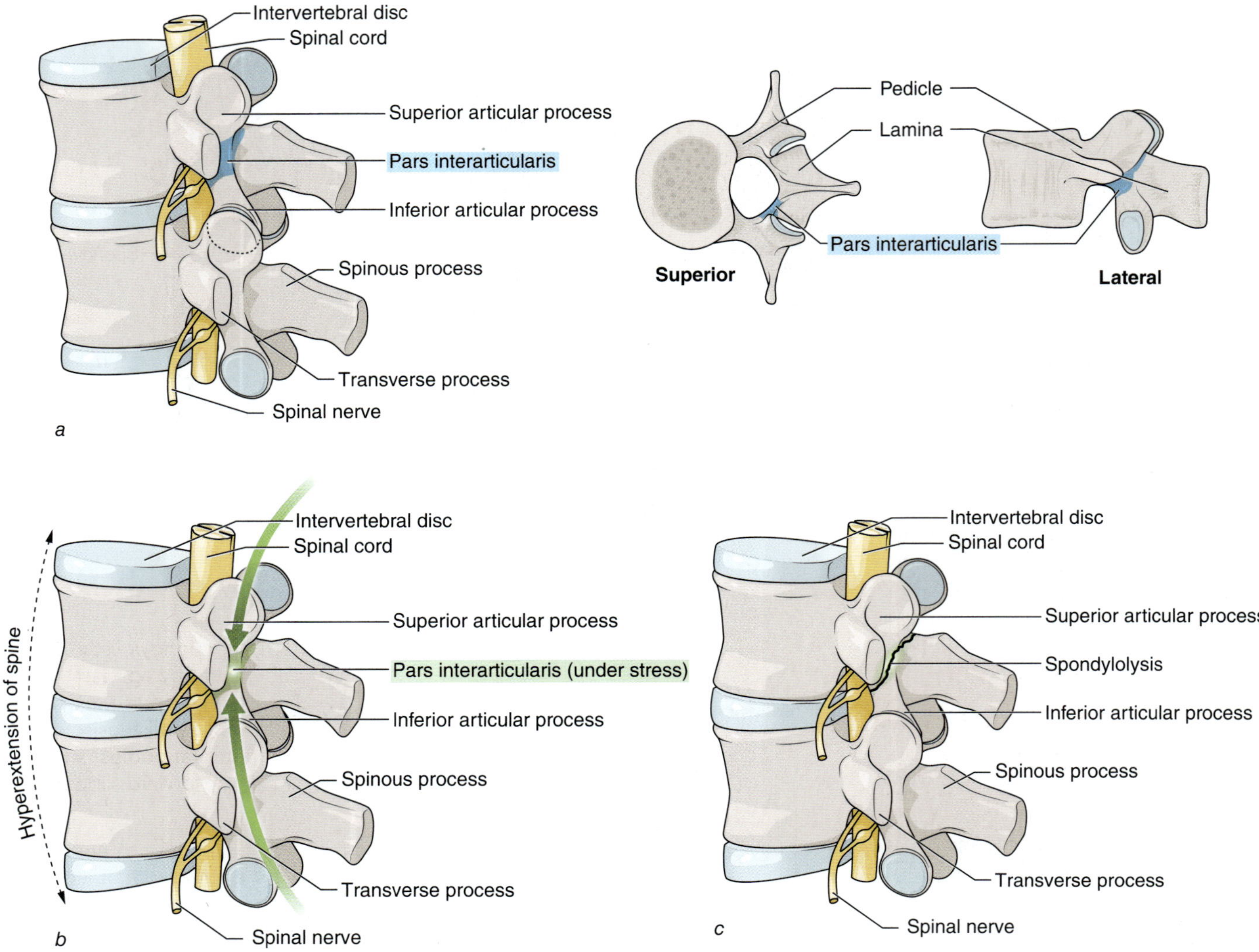

Figure 13.11 *(a)* The pars interarticularis is a small, but important, part of a lumbar vertebra. *(b)* When hyperextension of the lumbar spine creates hyperlordosis (dashed black arrow), excessive stress can be exerted at the pars interarticularis (green arrows). *(c)* These mechanical forces can create the stress fracture known as spondylolysis.

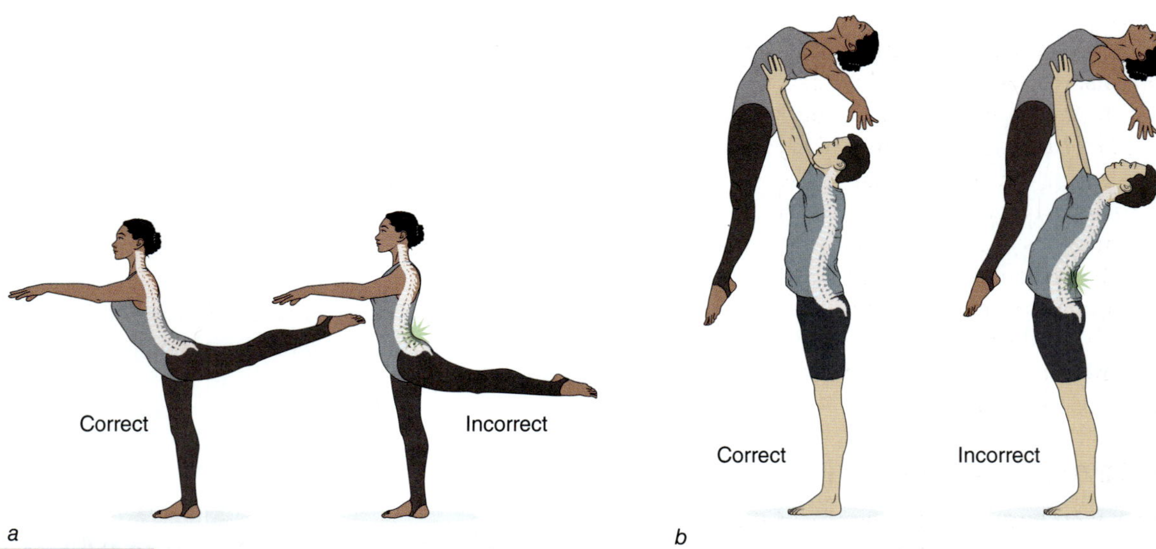

Figure 13.12 *(a)* An improper arabesque technique can create undue hyperextension stress in the lumbar spine. *(b)* Incorrect form in lifting a partner can exert similar hyperextension forces on the lumbar spine.

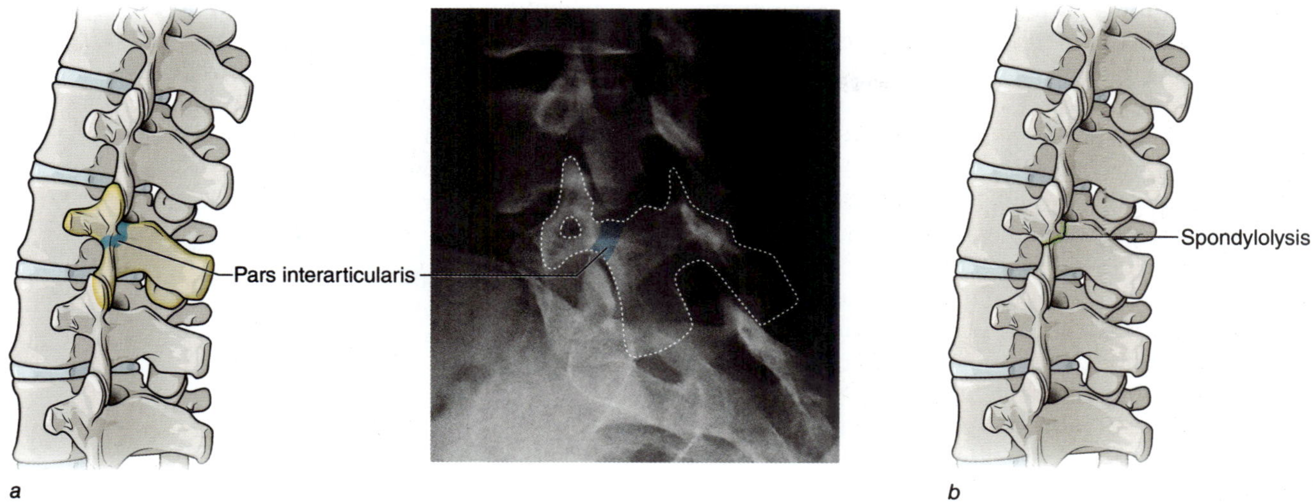

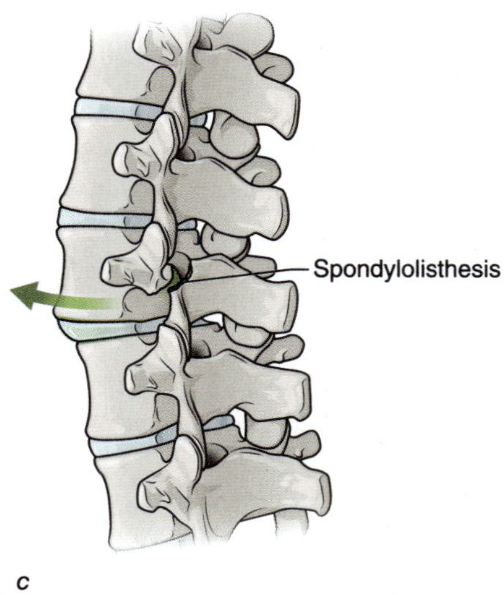

Figure 13.13 Comparison of spondylolysis and spondylolisthesis. *(a)* Lumbar spine X-ray showing how the bone anatomy appears like a Scottie dog. *(b)* Spondylolysis in the lumbar spine seen as the Scottie dog with a collar. *(c)* The Scottie dog sign in spondylolisthesis, where the dog's head appears detached and the vertebral bodies' anterior edges do not line up. This condition is caused by forward slippage of the vertebra with the fracture.

A: X-ray courtesy Steven J. Karageanes

Facet Inflammation

Facet inflammation (figure 13.14) is caused by the same risk factors and movements that contribute to spondylolysis. It also generates low-back pain that can spread to the gluteal region. Usually, the pain is worsened by lumbar extension. This injury is less common in young dancers; it is usually experienced by aging dancers (Grierson, 2019). As in the previously mentioned syndromes, facet inflammation resolves with correction of the movement patterns. A physician may recommend anti-inflammatories for a short duration or another intervention that breaks the inflammatory cycle once a stress reaction of the bone has been ruled out.

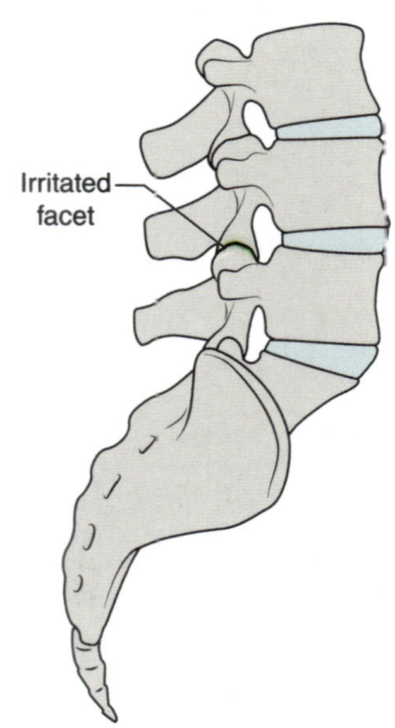

Figure 13.14 Too much repetitive loading at the facet joint where an upper and lower vertebral pair meet creates inflammation that manifests in low-back pain.

Sacral Stress Fracture

The sacrum is integral to the anatomy of the lower abdomen, trunk, back, and hips; thus, sacral stress fractures can cause low-back pain, gluteal pain, or both in the dancer. The pain also can radiate to the groin and into the thighs. Stress fractures in any region of the body occur either because of suboptimal loading through normal bone or normal loading through weakened bone (Longhino et al., 2011).

Bone is constantly remodeling—breaking down and rebuilding. Load-bearing activities are good for bone because they stimulate the remodeling process. However, if excessive stress is put on the bone, the bone breaks down faster than it can remodel. Complicating this situation, if a dancer has low energy availability (either because of suboptimal nutrition or an endocrine disorder), bone cannot repair itself quickly enough for the demands of dancing. In one study of stress injuries in ballet dancers (Kadel et al., 1992), the dancers with stress fractures were more likely to have been dancing longer than 5 hours per day (high load) or to have prolonged absence of their period (typically resulting from suboptimal hormone function and energy balance). The bone in the sacrum is particularly vulnerable to such stressors because it is made up of **cancellous bone** (spongy bone), which turns over more quickly in its breakdown and build-up cycle (figure 13.15).

If a dancer has low energy availability from suboptimal nutrition, the bone becomes less resilient (low energy availability's negative effects on the body are discussed in detail in chapter 7). Slight functional imbalances that might not impact most dancers can cause stress reactions and fractures in dancers whose nutrition is impaired. Treatment for sacral stress fracture involves optimizing the load through the region in addition to ensuring adequate nutrition. Relative rest is important to allow bone healing. The dancer's care team can develop individualized rehabilitation protocols to prevent deconditioning while at the same time preventing overstress of that region.

Sacroiliac Joint Dysfunction

Sacroiliac joint dysfunction can cause low-back pain in dancers that radiates to the gluteal region and sometimes down the leg. The two sacroiliac joints are located on the right and left sides where the sacrum and the ilium of each pelvic half meet (figure 13.16). Pain in the sacroiliac joint is thought to arise from asymmetric forces across the lumbar spine and pelvis that cause strain in the region where the sacrum and ilium meet (d'Hemecourt & Luke, 2012). Potential pain generators include the joint itself and the vast network of ligaments that stabilize the joint. The sacroiliac joint is unlike a shoulder or knee joint in that it is not designed for significant motion. Treatment involves working with a health care professional who is skilled in sacroiliac care to identify the imbalances contributing to the suboptimal forces and to provide rehabilitation to improve biomechanics.

Pelvic Floor Anatomy

The pelvic floor refers to the region of muscles, ligaments, and other tissues spanning within the base of the pelvic bones and supporting the pelvic

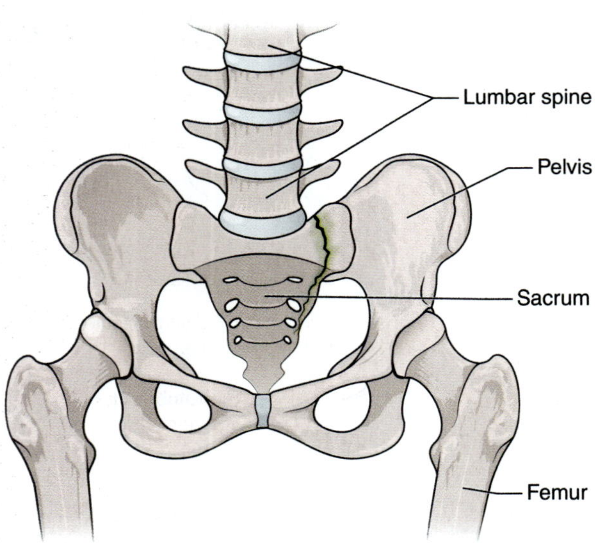

Figure 13.15 The areas of the sacrum where a stress fracture usually occurs. Notice the tight relationship of the sacrum to the pelvis and where the sacrum is positioned compared to the lumbar spine, hips, and lower abdomen.

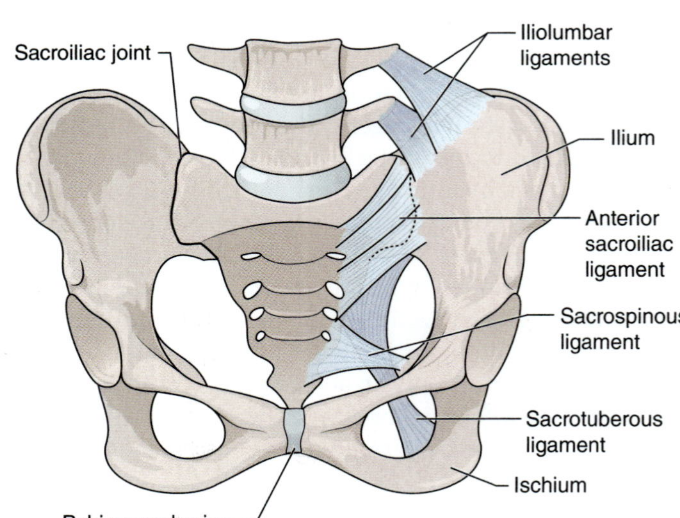

Figure 13.16 The sacroiliac joint is a relatively immovable joint because of its bony anatomy and the array of ligaments that bind the bones together.

organs. Understanding the anatomy in this body region can significantly help dancers in training, performance, and daily life.

Bones and Joints of the Pelvis

The pelvic bones are known as the ossa coxae. Each pelvic bone (os coxae) consists of three fused portions: ilium, ischium, and pubis. The right and left pelvic bones join anteriorly via the pubic symphysis joint. At the pubic symphysis, a fibrocartilage pad is located between the pubic bones to hold them together, and it absorbs forces at the front of the **pelvic ring**. The ischium's two large, downward protruding portions bear much of a person's sitting weight. For this reason, they are also known as the sitting bones, sit bones, or sitz bones. Figure 13.17*a* shows the parts of the pelvic anatomy.

As mentioned previously, at the back of the pelvis, the right and left ossa coxae join the triangular-shaped sacrum via two sacroiliac joints. Several strong ligaments bind the sacrum to the pelvis at the sacroiliac joint, including the sacrotuberous ligaments, sacrospinous ligaments, iliolumbar ligaments, and posterior and anterior sacroiliac ligaments (figure 13.17*b*). The shape of the wedgelike sacrum fitting against the two sides of the pelvis at the sacroiliac joint, along with the support created by the ligaments, helps to create stability through **form closure**. Distally, the tailbone connects to the sacrum at a joint known as the sacrococcygeal joint. The tailbone is known as the coccyx; it consists of three to five fused segments (Lewis et al., 2017).

The pelvis forms a bowl-like shape that is generally wider at the top than its narrower base. Genetic variation exists between pelvises such that some dancers have broader pelvic structures, while others have narrower or taller pelvic structures. The unique anatomical shape of your pelvis can contribute to variations in hip structure that are discussed later in this chapter. The pelvic bones also contain the socket for the hip joint known as the acetabulum; this will be discussed later.

Pelvic Floor Muscles

The muscular support located at the base of the so-called pelvic bowl is known as the pelvic floor. Three layers of **pelvic floor muscles** span from the pubic bone anteriorly to the coccyx posteriorly, as well as side-to-side from sitting bone to sitting bone. The pelvic floor acts as a hammock across this region, serving as the true dynamic floor of a dancer's core.

The most superficial layer and the middle layer of the pelvic floor consist of muscles that serve mainly as sphincters, including the external urethral sphincter and external anal sphincter (figure 13.18). These muscles help close the openings of the body (the urethra and rectum) to control the flow of urine and feces. The sphincters relax to allow comfortable urination and bowel movements (Eickmeyer, 2017).

The deepest (closest to the abdominopelvic cavity) pelvic floor layer consists of the muscles known as the pelvic diaphragm; they include the levator ani (pubococcygeus, puborectalis, and iliococcygeus) and the coccygeus. These muscles serve as the deep support for the organs of the pelvis, much like a hammock or basket. The portions of

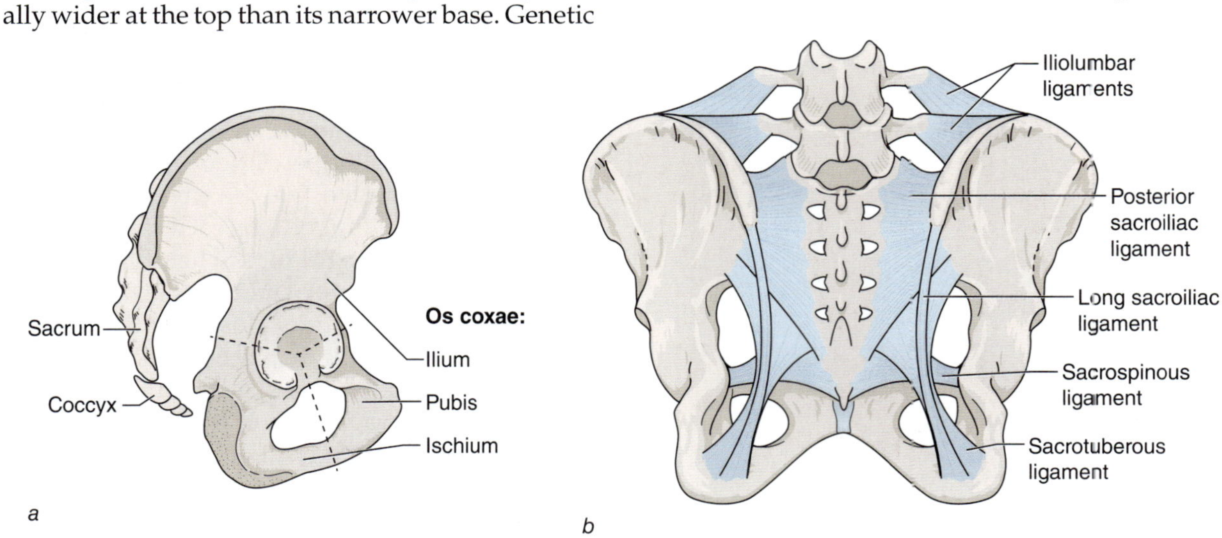

Figure 13.17 *(a)* The pelvic ring consists of the two pelvic halves (ossa coxae) and the sacrum. The ossa coxae are each formed by three portions. The anterior portion (pubis) of each os coxae meets the other at a joint known as the pubic symphysis. The coccyx extends from the bottom of the sacrum. *(b)* The ligaments of the pelvis and sacrum are strong, and they provide excellent stability.

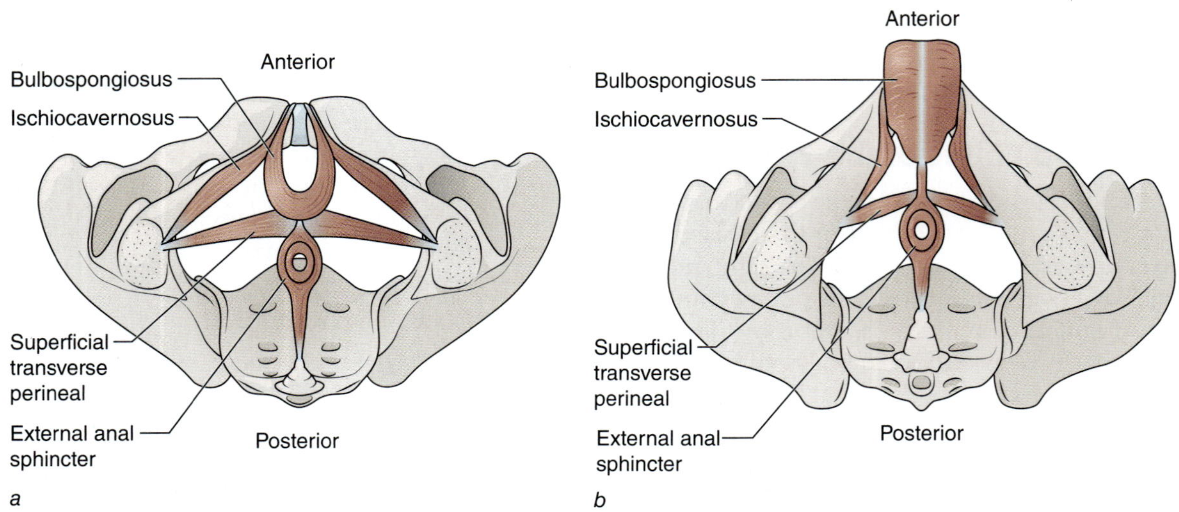

Figure 13.18 Superficial (outer) view, from below, of the pelvic floor muscles of a *(a)* female and *(b)* male.

muscle that attach to the coccyx help *tuck the tail* (flex the coccyx slightly forward) and allow the tailbone to gently tilt backward when relaxing during bowel movements (figure 13.19).

Organs within the pelvis (bladder, rectum, uterus, prostate) are suspended and held in place by the pelvic floor muscles as well as by a vast network of ligaments and fascia. The organs and muscles of the pelvic floor are fed by a complex supply of blood vessels and nerves. Of interest to dancers' pelvic well-being is the connection between the nerves of the pelvic floor and the autonomic nervous system, which is one of the parts of the nervous system that controls homeostasis, a physiologically balanced state. In order to optimize pelvic floor wellness, dancers must manage the balance between their stress response system (called fight, flight, or freeze) and their relaxation system (called rest and digest) (Prather et al., 2009; Quaghebeur et al., 2021). When

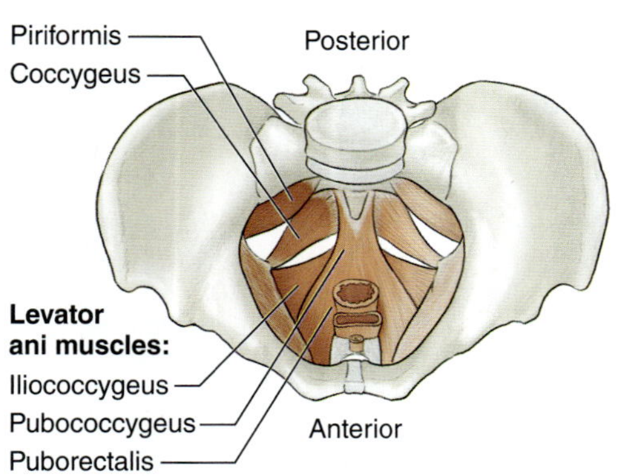

Figure 13.19 The deep layer of the pelvic floor muscles, viewed from above (from inside the abdominal cavity).

the stress response system overpowers other systems that regulate the body, dancers can experience excessive tension—or even pain—in the pelvic floor muscles.

Another significant point about the pelvic floor muscles that dancers should know is the anatomical connection between the muscles of the pelvic floor and a very important hip muscle: the obturator internus (figure 13.20). The obturator internus begins at the inner obturator foramen of the pelvic bone—the large hole in each os coxae—and wraps behind the hip to attach to the greater trochanter of the femur. It serves as one of the six deep outward rotators of the hip that are used consistently to produce turnout. The inner part of the obturator internus muscle attaches directly to the levator ani muscles of the pelvic floor via a ligamentous structure known as the arcus tendineus levator ani (ATLA). Therefore, when you contract your turnout muscles, you also produce force along the pelvic floor. Armed with this anatomical information, you can envision the pelvic floor muscles as a sling between each hip joint, spanning directly between the hips to help absorb forces from the large hip range of motion that dancers use.

The pelvic floor works closely with the main muscle of breathing, the diaphragm. The diaphragm is a dome-shaped sheet of skeletal muscle that sits in the lower thoracic region of the body, above the abdominal contents (figure 13.21). It attaches to the lower six rib cartilage sections and the first three lumbar vertebrae; it has attachments to many organs as well as the iliopsoas and quadratus lumborum muscles. During an inhalation, the diaphragm contracts and moves downward to allow air into the lungs, while the pelvic floor muscles lengthen

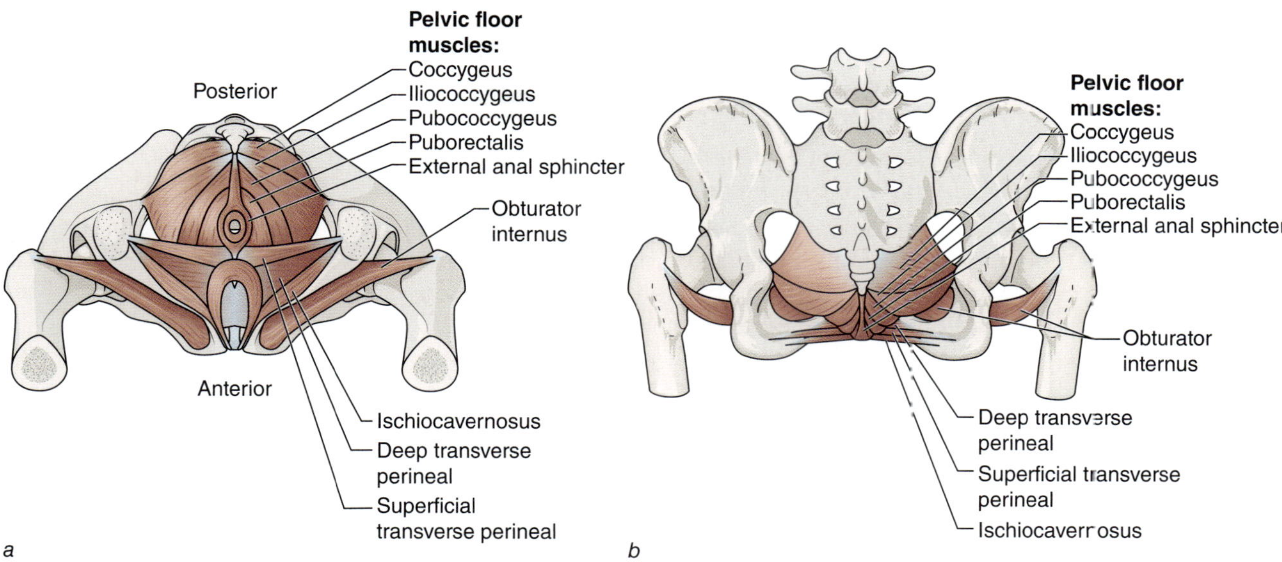

Figure 13.20 Views of the pelvic region showing the obturator internus muscle's relationship to the pelvic floor from *(a)* an inferior view and *(b)* a posterior view. Note that the ATLA (not shown) connects the obturator internus muscle to the pelvic floor muscles.

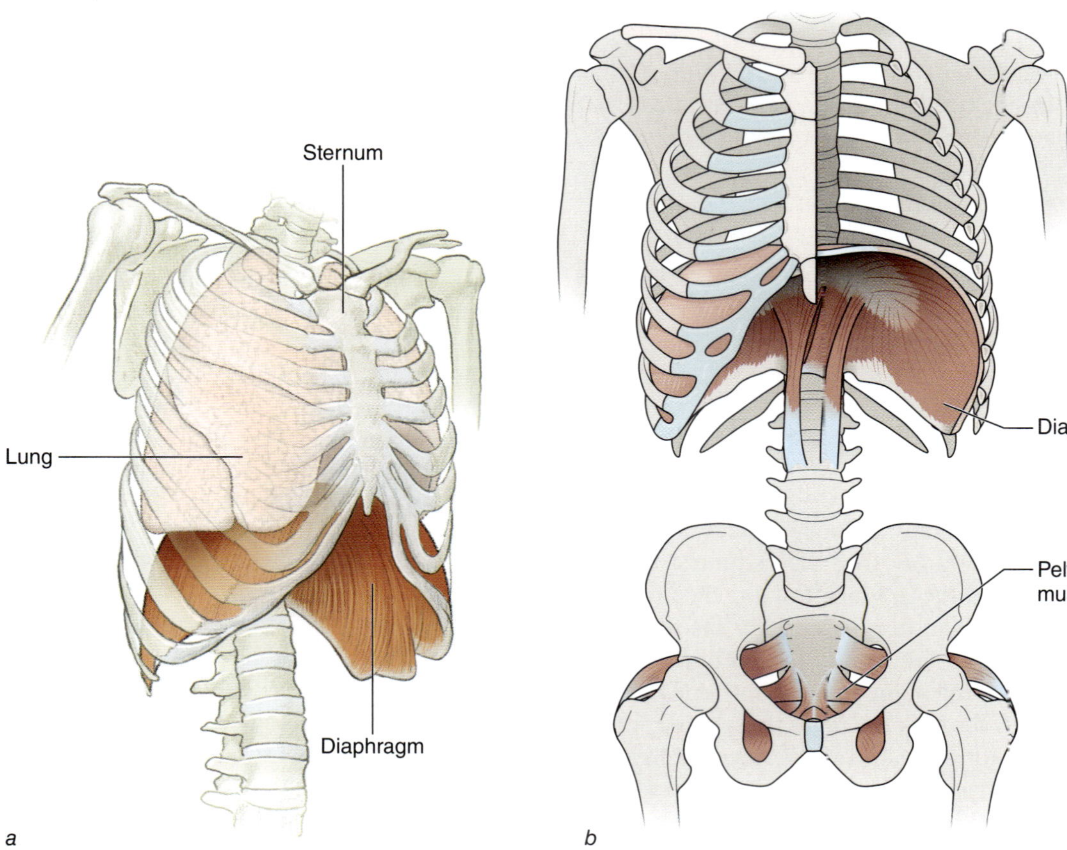

Figure 13.21 The anatomy of the diaphragm showing *(a)* its position and attachments and *(b)* its relationship to the pelvic floor muscles. The diaphragm can be considered the roof of the abdomen, while the pelvic floor muscles can be considered the foundation.

Mechanics and Function of the Pelvic Floor

The Five S Functions of the Pelvic Floor

The pelvic floor muscles are important for several reasons, and they are crucial to the successful functioning of a dancer's body. The pelvic floor has five major roles, each beginning with S:

- *Sphincteric*: The pelvic floor muscles help close the urethra and rectum to preserve **continence** (retaining urine and feces during most of the day or night). The pelvic floor muscles maintain some resting tone and contract with coughing or sneezing to manage pressure and prevent leakage. These sphincters relax to allow for urination and bowel movements.
- *Sexual*: The pelvic floor muscles are important for genital and sexual function.
- *Support*: The pelvic floor muscles serve as a hammock of support, along with ligaments and fascia, for the organs and the pressures from above.
- *Stability*: The pelvic floor muscles help provide stability across the bones of the pelvis.
- *Sump pump*: The pelvic floor acts as a muscular pump, assisting blood and lymph movement from the lower body up toward the heart.

Two More Important Functions Not Starting With S

You have clearly seen the importance of the pelvic floor musculature to many significant mechanisms of the body. Beyond the five S functions, it also serves these two important roles:

- *Breathing*: As mentioned earlier, the pelvic floor muscles move in sync with the diaphragm to control breathing. They expand and lower with inhalation, and they lift slightly with exhalation.
- *Intra-abdominal pressure management*: The muscles sit at the base of the trunk canister; thus, they receive increases and decreases in pressure from above. They automatically respond to and manage pressure throughout the trunk to optimize several functions, including coughing, sneezing, jumping, laughing, and lifting.

downward at the same time. During an exhalation, the diaphragm relaxes and moves upward to expel air from the lungs, while the pelvic floor lifts (Kocjan et al., 2017; Talasz et al., 2011).

Experience Pelvic Floor Muscle Contraction in a Lift

In order to feel the pelvic floor muscles contract, it can be helpful to know that they squeeze to close the openings and lift upward toward the crown of the head. The sensation is essentially the feeling as if you tried to stop the urine flow while urinating. (Note that stopping your urine flow repeatedly is not advised.) Exercises to create these contractions when not urinating are known as Kegel exercises.

An easy way to feel these muscles contract is to first sit comfortably on the floor or on a chair. Take note of the borders of your pelvis where the pelvic floor muscles connect; remember that the muscles span front to back from pubic bone to tailbone, and side-to-side between your sitting bones. If you like, you can place a small folded towel under your pelvic floor muscles to help provide more feedback.

To feel the contraction of these muscles, begin by inhaling while allowing the pelvic floor muscles to soften and relax into the floor (or chair, or towel) beneath you. Then, as you gently exhale—with lightly pursed lips, as if blowing out a candle or through a straw—feel the muscles pull together toward the center (as they close the openings). Then, lift them up toward your ribcage, as if sliding the pelvic floor muscles up the center pole of a circus tent.

Here are some other helpful images to help you complete a Kegel exercise:

- Imagine the muscles closing around a straw and sucking up a thick milkshake.
- Imagine picking up a tiny blueberry with these muscles and lifting it upward, inside the body, toward the crown of your head.
- Imagine closing a zipper from your back passage (anus) to your front passage (genitals). The space you are zipping up between these two areas is known as the perineum.
- Lift your muscles as if to prepare for a cough or sneeze.

› Pull the muscles upward, away from your sitting surface.

You should practice feeling this lift without moving the bones of the pelvis (i.e., do not let your pelvis tilt forward or rock back into a tucked position), without clenching your buttocks, and without holding your breath. You may feel some gentle abdominal contraction; that contraction is fine as long as you are not sucking in so much that you restrict your breathing.

After the contraction, focus on letting these muscles fully relax or on gently dropping them toward the floor. Remember that the relaxation is just as important as the contraction. Many dancers have difficulty feeling the length and relaxation of the pelvic floor, especially if they have a habit of lifting up and in or working in turnout for most of their dance practice. If dancers learn how to only pull the pelvic floor muscles up without learning how to also lengthen and relax them, it can contribute to tension and pain in the pelvis and hip.

Experience Pelvic Floor Relaxation and Lengthening

To practice a full relaxation and lengthening of the pelvic floor muscles, yoga postures (e.g., child's pose, happy baby pose, supported deep squat) can be helpful. Common images to encourage pelvic floor muscle relaxation include the following:

› Soften the muscles of the pelvic floor like a flower gently blooming and opening its petals.
› Imagine your sitting bones gently spreading apart.
› As you inhale, allow the pelvic floor muscles to expand outward like a balloon filling up.
› Send your inhalation all the way to your tailbone.

Pelvic Floor Dysfunction and Injury

If pelvic floor dysfunction arises, dancers might experience one or more of the issues detailed below. All of these are manageable, however. Consult a health care provider skilled in treating pelvic floor conditions for assistance.

Incontinence

Incontinence is the involuntary loss of urine or feces. Leaking urine while dancing or during daily activities is not as uncommon as you might think. In fact, roughly 30 percent of female athletes and about 14 percent of male athletes in impact sports (sports involving jumping or landing forces) experience urine leakage—even at relatively young ages such as late adolescence (de Mattos Lourenco et al., 2018; Pires et al., 2020; Teixeira et al., 2018). These rates are similar in professional dancers (Winder et al., 2023).

There are different types of urine leakage, or urinary incontinence (UI). Stress UI occurs when urine leaks during coughing, sneezing, laughing, or exercise; it is the most common issue experienced by athletes and dancers. Stress UI usually occurs due to an imbalance between the pressure from above and the resistance provided by the pelvic floor; this imbalance could be due to a combination of factors, including too much squeeze pressure from the trunk canister above (sucking in the abs too much, too much breath holding, or poor general trunk strength and stability), poor coordination and strength of the pelvic floor muscles, or a combination of the two. Urge UI, on the other hand, occurs when one experiences a strong urge to urinate, and urine leaks before they can make it to the toilet. Some athletes experience mixed UI, a combination of stress UI and urge UI (Haylen et al., 2010).

Pelvic floor rehabilitation is considered the first line of treatment for urinary incontinence (Dumoulin et al., 2018; Sorrigueta-Hernández et al., 2020). Common pelvic floor interventions for incontinence may include pelvic floor muscle relaxation, coordination, strengthening, and endurance training; core training; and hip strengthening. Helping dancers learn to distribute load optimally and efficiently throughout the feet, legs, hips, pelvis, and trunk while using appropriate breathing, pressure-management, and strength activities also is paramount.

Overactive Bladder

Increased urinary frequency—called overactive bladder—typically manifests as having to urinate more often than every 2 to 4 hours during the day and more than once per night. Symptoms may include feeling as though you have not completely emptied your bladder or you need to urinate again within a few minutes of voiding. Some people may feel as if they have a urinary tract infection in the absence of a true infection.

All of these symptoms can be related to overactive pelvic floor muscles, the bladder muscle (called the detrusor) contracting at inconvenient times, chronic stress responses, or improper bladder habits. Good bladder habits for decreasing the likelihood of urinary frequency or bladder irritation including getting adequate hydration by drinking plenty of water (a hydrated bladder is a happy bladder), managing stress, practicing slow and relaxed breathing, training yourself to listen to the true call of your bladder (instead of going to the bathroom just in case you might need to go), and practicing pelvic floor relaxation and lengthening. If you are preparing for an upcoming performance, and know you need to hydrate more in anticipation of increased fluid loss from sweating, it can help to focus on increasing fluid intake bit by bit earlier in the day instead of all at once. Before performances, you may also want to decrease the intake of liquids or foods that can increase bladder irritation (bladder irritants are highly individual, but some common examples are coffee, carbonated beverages, teas, or acidic or spicy foods).

Constipation

Many factors can cause constipation, but the pelvic floor can play a role, particularly when pelvic floor muscles have difficulty lengthening or relaxing. Chronic constipation (typically meaning fewer than three bowel movements per week), frequent straining, and hard and lumpy stools also can cause abdominal, pelvic, or low-back pain. Constipation may make urinary leakage or urinary frequency feel worse, often because a full rectum places pressure on the nearby bladder.

Constipation is not unusual in athletes or dancers. There are many ways to improve constipation, including adequate hydration, pelvic floor lengthening and relaxation training, abdominal massage, and stress management. Consulting a registered dietitian is an important way to ensure you consume adequate levels of food (including optimal fiber) while managing existing food sensitivities or allergies.

Pelvic Floor Myofascial Pain

Pelvic floor myofascial pain is typically related to overworked, overly tensioned, or chronically irritated pelvic floor muscles or nerves. Symptoms can include pain in the genitals, perineum (the fleshy area you sit on between the sitz bones), pubic bone, rectum, or tailbone. Pain from the pelvic floor muscles can also be felt in the muscles of the lower abdomen, low back, groin, buttocks, or posterior thigh (Meister et al., 2019; Prather et al., 2009).

Pelvic floor myofascial pain can occur in dancers for many reasons. It can be a compensation or guarding response to an injury in a nearby area (e.g., the hips or low back), a stability compensation for hypermobile hips, or a response to trauma to the pelvis (e.g., a fall). Excessive tension and pain in the pelvic floor is not uncommon in dancers who tend to experience intense overtraining stress combined with habits such as constantly gripping the muscles of the pelvic floor, abdomen, or hip. Management of pelvic floor myofascial pain can include pelvic floor relaxation exercises and myofascial release, meditation or mindfulness activities, abdominal relaxation exercises, stress management techniques, exercises to improve hip mobility or hip strength, and pelvic floor rehabilitation.

Coccydynia

Coccydynia refers to pain at or around the coccyx (tailbone). The most common cause for it in dancers is a fall onto the tailbone or posterior pelvis. Resulting pain after the trauma can make sitting very painful—especially sitting and leaning back, which increases pressure on the coccyx (Lirette et al., 2014). The muscles attached to the coccyx are often overactive; therefore, pelvic floor rehabilitation focused on relaxation and myofascial release to the surrounding muscles and the sacrococcygeal joint can be helpful.

Pubic Symphysis Dysfunction and Osteitis Pubis

Pubic symphysis dysfunction—often resulting from excessive stress or movement at the pubic symphysis joint—can include burning, shooting, grinding, or stabbing pain at or near the pubic symphysis with walking, stair use, standing or weight bearing on one leg, or transitional movements such as rolling over in bed. *Osteitis pubis* is the medical term for inflammation that occurs at the pubic symphysis.

This issue is a common occurrence during pregnancy, but nonpregnant dancers, too, can be susceptible. The large range of motion demanded at the hips and pelvic joints as well as the high rate of hypermobility in dancers can increase the risk of pubic symphysis dysfunction. In addition, excessive stresses transferred across the pelvis may irritate the adductor or gracilis muscles at their pubic attachment points (Elattar et al., 2016).

Tips for Pelvic Floor Health in Dancers

- Hydrate! Drink enough water to match your activity level.
- Manage stress levels to make sure you keep your nervous system in balance. Meditation, mindfulness, and slow breathing techniques (e.g., box breathing) can calm the nervous system to help decrease bladder irritation, pelvic floor muscle tension, and constipation. See *Mental Health Tools and Self-Care Measures* in chapter 8 for more suggestions for dealing with stress.
- Work on pelvic floor and core strength and stability as well as pelvic floor muscle lengthening and relaxation.
- If you dance in forms involving repetitive turnout, also work on strength and mobility in the opposite range of motion (hip internal rotation).

Treatment for osteitis pubis may include temporary use of pelvic stability belts, supportive taping, core and hip muscle strengthening, pelvic floor muscle strengthening, and pelvic floor myofascial release. Stress fractures can occur at the pubic area of the pelvis; therefore, they should be considered during assessment by a health care professional. This injury must be confirmed with an X-ray, MRI, or bone scan. In the case of a stress fracture, management will include rest to allow healing, then a progressive return to dance.

The Core and Pressure-Management System

Now that you have a basic understanding of the anatomy of the spine and trunk, pelvis and pelvic floor, and diaphragm, you can begin to visualize how this anatomy functions to control your core. To better understand core function, this section first addresses the concept of **intra-abdominal pressure (IAP)**. IAP is the pressure within the abdominopelvic cavity (Milanesi & Caregnato, 2016). The abdominopelvic cavity can be visualized as a can of soda pop; the can's top represents the diaphragm, the can's bottom is the pelvic floor, the front wall of the can is the abdominal wall and musculature, and the can's back wall is the spine and spinal extensor muscles (figure 13.22). Of course, the muscles of the core also wrap around the sides of the trunk, just as a can has enveloping sides. In reality, remember that the inside of your can is not empty, nor does it contain bubbly liquid; it is filled with organs, blood vessels, fascia, and fluid. Moreover, the pressure inside this canister is not static; in other words, it changes in response to movement, breathing, impact, load, coughing, sneezing, and vocalization (using your voice).

An easy way to understand this concept of IAP is to experience changes in pressure produced by the muscles that surround the canister. For example, feel the extent to which your abdominal or pelvic floor muscles need to work when you are lying on your back or sitting and relaxing. During these activities, the pressure inside the canister is relatively low and the surrounding muscles do not contract much. Tiny changes in pressure naturally occur with each of your inhalations and exhalations.

Now, try any of the following:

- Sing or yell loudly.
- Practice blowing up a balloon or pretend you are blowing out a big candle.

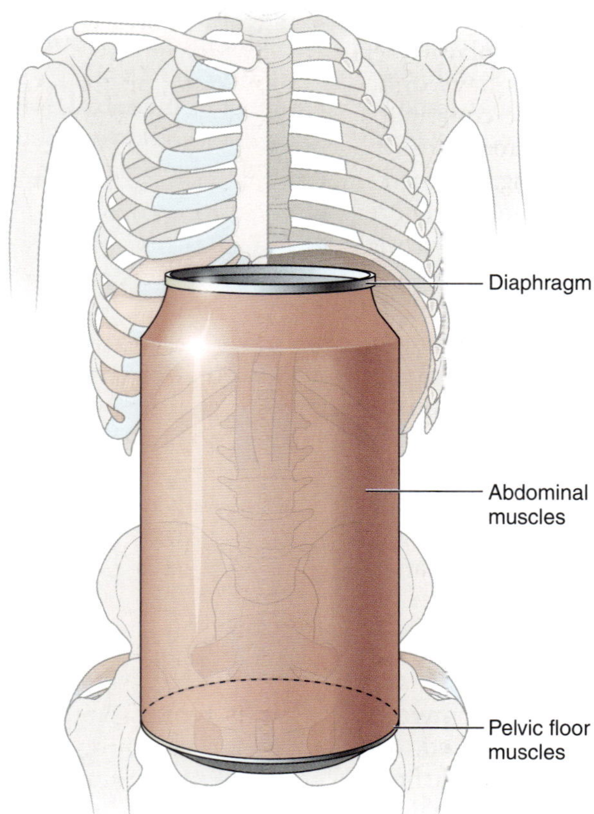

Figure 13.22 Think of the core of the body as a soda pop can, with a top, bottom, front, back, and sides.

› Lift something relatively heavy off the floor.
› Push a heavy door closed.
› Cough.

Do you notice that when you do each of these activities, you feel a natural increase in the muscle tension of your trunk muscles, particularly across your abdominals and pelvic floor? Those muscles increase the pressure inside the canister to push air upward for a yell or a cough, or to increase spinal stiffness in order to create a stable base for lifting, pushing, pulling, or other body movements (Hodges et al., 2005; Stokes et al., 2010). IAP created by balanced contractions of the diaphragm, pelvic floor, abdominals, and back extensors helps increase stiffness and stability that unloads pressure on the spine.

Dancers must learn how to control this pressure system efficiently to create a powerful and stable base for movement of the limbs (Frank et al., 2013). This skill is often called **core stability** or spinal stability. Developing good core stability is akin to building a strong foundation before adding the rest of the structures to build a house. Without a strong and stable foundation, the entire house is more susceptible to the stresses of the surrounding environment. Think about how powerful your dancing could be if you were adept at keeping your spine and pelvis strong and stable while moving your arms and legs. If you had a cannon and wanted to shoot a cannonball from it as far and powerfully as possible, would you shoot it from a rocking boat on unpredictable ocean waters or from stable, dry land? That dry land and the strong foundation of the house both represent the core stability that is your key to producing efficient movement when you dance.

To learn how to efficiently produce core stability, dancers should work on exercises that train this skill. In simplest terms, core stability exercises involve keeping the spine neutral and very still while moving the limbs or while pushing, pulling, or lifting weight. Core stabilization exercises can be performed in many positions (e.g., supine, prone, quadruped, side-lying, side-propped, plank positions, half or full kneeling, during squats or deadlifts, and while balancing on one leg). Many Pilates-based exercises focus on core stabilization as well as strengthening of the abdominals, back extensors, diaphragm, and pelvic floor. Examples of core stabilization exercises—including Pilates—can be found in chapter 5.

No matter the position or task involved in core stabilization training, you should keep these principles in mind to enhance performance:

› Keep your head, neck, rib cage, and pelvis aligned (figure 13.23) in neutral as you perform movements of the arms or legs, you hinge the hips, or you push or pull a weight. As you maintain this alignment, you should feel your cylinder-like trunk canister tension evenly. Maintaining this even tension means you shouldn't be pushing your abdominal

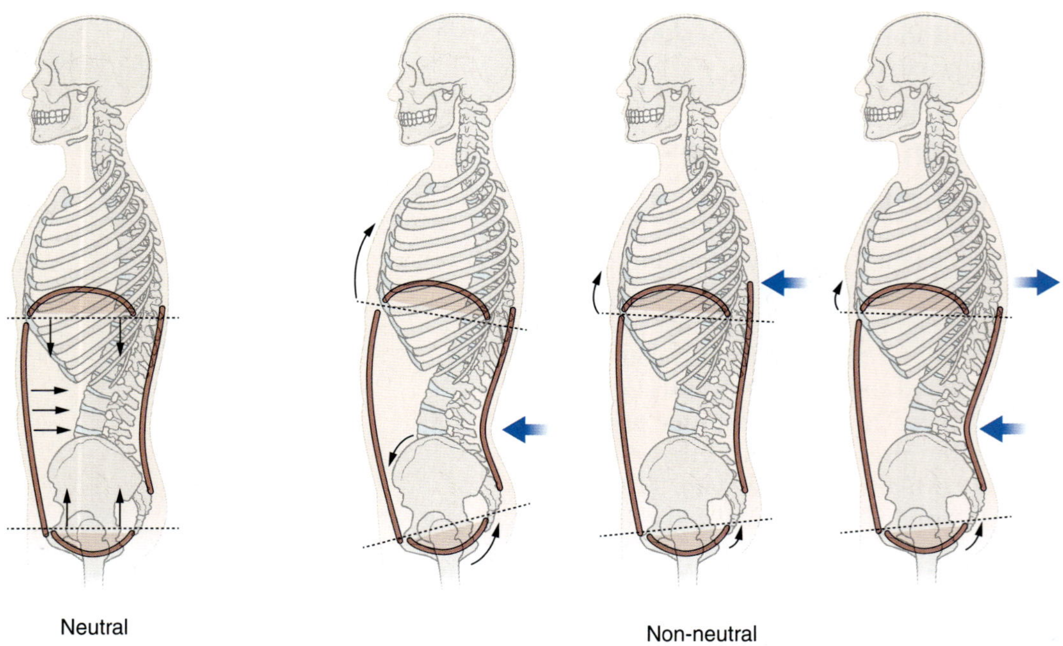

Figure 13.23 During any core stabilization activity or exercise, a neutral spine must be maintained to maximize the benefit.

muscles outward or sucking them way inward; instead, just feel a stiffening of the trunk muscles (along with a lengthened spine) naturally occur in response to the task.

- Be sure to breathe. Holding your breath should only occur if you are doing a maximal lift of heavy weight as a means to stabilize your core and spine. Otherwise, inhaling and exhaling should be maintained throughout the movement.
- Your neck and shoulder muscles should be fairly relaxed.
- The amount of tension and pressure produced in your trunk should match the difficulty of the task. For example, if you are lying on your back doing simple marching of the legs, you might not be working too intensely in the trunk; therefore, you may not need to minimize spinal movement. However, if you are performing single-leg extensions while in a plank, you will feel your trunk muscles naturally contract more intensely to keep your spine and pelvis stable. Part of your job in any core stabilization activity or exercise is to teach your trunk muscles and pressure-management system to automatically control different intensities of movement.

Understanding how to keep your spine stable during multiple types of challenges can help you develop strength, endurance, and stability as well as provide protection to your spine for lifting and supporting other dancers during partner work. Core stability can help prevent technique issues that may result from moving, twisting, or arching your low back too much or too soon with leg movement. It also helps prevent too much compression on the joints of your lower back. Optimal core stabilization can help you balance and find your center more easily, unload an overly tense or irritated neck, and create a stable launching base for increasing the height of your leg extensions. When you are considering cross-training and conditioning programs, do not skip the core stabilization practice; it is your home base for efficient and powerful dancing.

Hip Anatomy

The anatomy of the hip joint is designed to absorb and transmit load between the trunk and pelvis complex and the ground during weightbearing. The hips also can move into extreme ranges of motion during dance as they control a supporting leg or a gesture leg.

Joint Structure

The hip is a ball-and-socket joint (figure 13.24) formed by the cup-shaped acetabulum of the pelvis and the spherical femoral head of the femur. Both the acetabulum and femoral head are lined with hyaline articular (joint) cartilage that is nourished

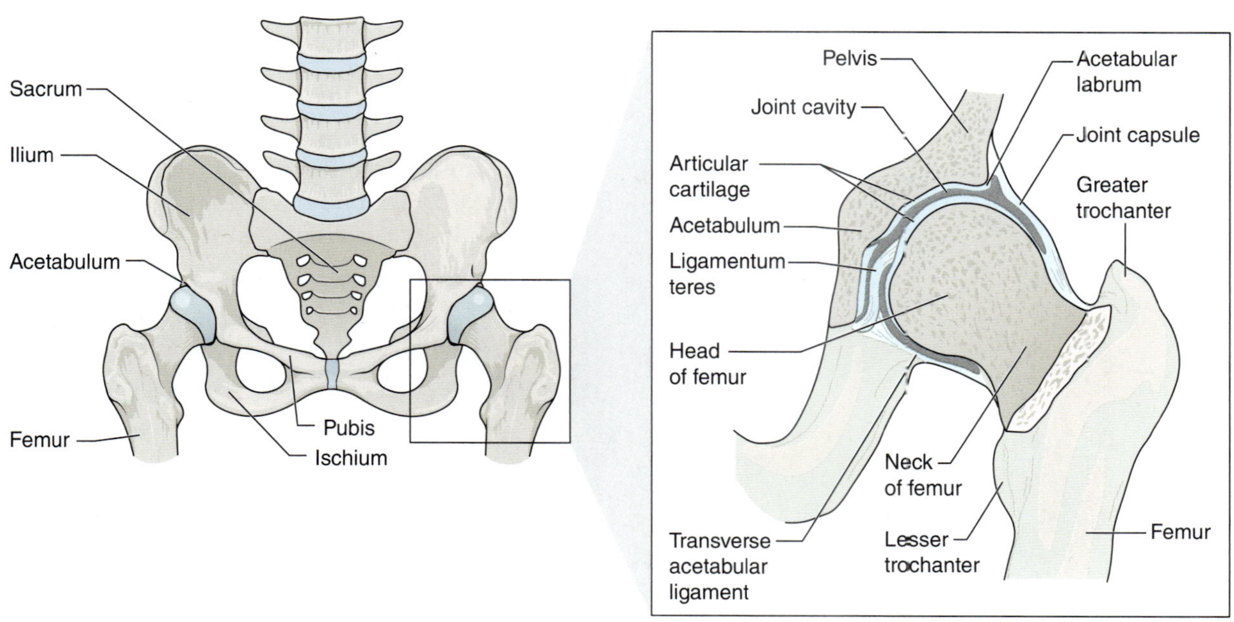

Figure 13.24 Significant anatomical structures of the hip. Note that the acetabulum usually faces slightly forward. All the anatomical features of the hip, as in the rest of the body, vary from individual to individual.

with a very slippery liquid called synovial fluid. The acetabulum, a relatively deep socket, usually faces slightly forward, a position called anteversion; it covers the femoral head to form a very stable joint.

Everyone has their own unique hip bony anatomy. Elite ballet dancers tend to have bony anatomy that allows them to move their hips through extreme ranges of movement (Mayes et al., 2017). They have spherical femoral heads with narrow femoral necks, the angle between their femoral necks and the femoral shaft is large, their acetabulum faces more sideways than forward, and some may have a shallow acetabulum (acetabular dysplasia) (Harris et al., 2016; Mayes et al., 2017). This unique bony anatomy may explain why dancers tend to have greater passive hip external rotation, abduction, flexion, and extension range of motion compared to nondancers (Mayes et al., 2017).

The acetabulum is deepened by the acetabular labrum, a fibrocartilage lip that attaches to the edge of the acetabulum; it is triangular in cross-section and made of fibrous cartilage (figure 13.25). The labrum also enhances joint stability. It protects the smooth (hyaline) cartilage of the hip joint by maintaining a synovial fluid seal around the joint that suctions the femoral head into the acetabulum. If the femoral head is distracted (pulled away from the socket), a pop may be felt as the negative intra-articular pressure that suctions against the femoral head is released. Although the hip may feel freer than usual for a short time, maintaining the negative intra-articular pressure is important for joint stability.

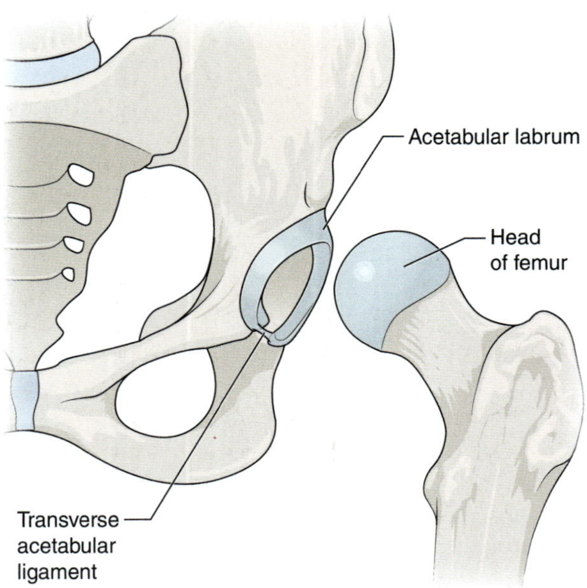

Figure 13.25 The labrum of the acetabulum forms a lip around the edge of the acetabulum's socket.

The capsule and ligaments surrounding the hip joint provide stability in all directions of movement. The joint capsule is reinforced by four ligaments: the iliofemoral, pubofemoral, and ischiofemoral ligaments and the zona orbicularis (annular ligament). Some components of these ligaments are taut in all ranges of movement (van Arkel et al., 2015), thus adding to the hip's stability. The ligamentum teres is a pyramid-shaped ligament within the joint that originates from the acetabulum and inserts into the femoral head. The ligamentum teres supports the role of the capsular ligaments, and it limits rotation in hip flexion and abduction. The ligament is tensioned if the hip is subluxated or dislocated; it likely limits the extreme ranges of movement used in dance (Mayes et al., 2016a).

Often dancers have a condition that affects their joint movements; it is known as generalized joint hypermobility (GJH). GJH is an inherited trait that could be considered an asset because it allows extreme joint range of movement due to laxity of the soft tissues such as the capsule and ligaments. GJH has been associated with injuries in dance; however, in a study of professional ballet dancers, Mayes, Smith, Stuart, and Cook (2021) found that dancers with GJH showed that they were less likely to have hip joint injury and were not at risk of developing hip pain over 5 years. These dancers engaged in hip-strengthening exercises upon employment that may have protected their lax hips from injury. Therefore, it is important that any dancer who exhibits this type of joint flexibility engage in an appropriate strengthening program so that the more-flexible-than-typical joints have strong musculature to support them. Chapter 6 introduces GJH (see the section *Hypermobility*) in the context of flexibility, while chapter 5 explains the principles of conditioning.

WWW Go to HK*Propel* for supplemental content on hypermobility that discusses this condition in more detail.

Muscles

The passive stabilizers of the hip joint (e.g., acetabulum, labrum, and ligaments) are dynamically supported by musculotendinous structures surrounding the hip joint. They are presented in the following section, where they are grouped according to function.

Hip Flexors

The iliopsoas is the main hip flexor. It provides support to the front of the hip joint (figure 13.26). It is a key muscle for dancers; a strong iliopsoas allows high and powerful elevations of the gesture leg to the front and to the side, and it decelerates the leg in extension movements such as a grande battement derrière (moving the leg backward). The iliopsoas is larger in elite ballet dancers compared to other athletes, and it is larger in ballet dancers who have been training professionally for more years than those with less experience (Emery et al., 2019; Gildea et al., 2013). The iliopsoas originates from the bodies of the last thoracic and lumbar vertebrae and inserts into the lesser trochanter of the femur; therefore, it also provides trunk stability. The rectus femoris, pectineus, tensor fasciae latae, and sartorius also flex the hip. The rectus femoris and sartorius cross both the hip and the knee, and they are less effective hip flexors when the hip joint is in high elevations. The sartorius holds the leg in an attitude devant (leg in front of you with the hip externally rotated and the knee bent) position.

Hip Abductors

The gluteus minimus, gluteus medius, gluteus maximus, and tensor fasciae latae all abduct the hip (move the leg away from the midline of the body); they have been found to be larger in elite ballet dancers compared to other athletes (Emery et al., 2021; McMillan, 2023). Dancers use these muscles to lift the gesture leg, and they are also important stabilizing muscles for the hip of the supporting leg. On the supporting leg, they tilt the pelvis to allow increased height of the gesture leg and to limit excessive hip adduction (movement toward the midline of the body) when landing from jumps. The hip abduction musculature is shown in figure 13.27.

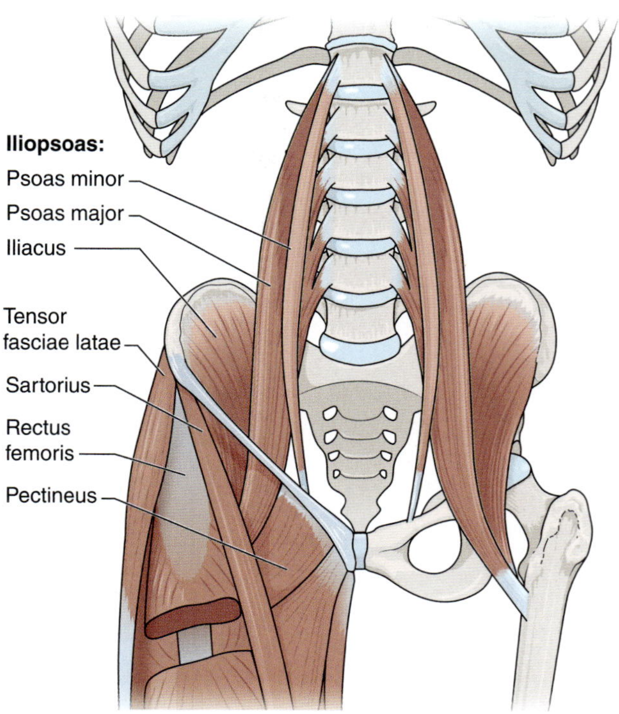

Figure 13.26 The primary muscles of hip flexion.

Hip Adductors

Adductor longus, adductor brevis, adductor magnus, gracilis, and pectineus adduct the hip. Normally the hip abductors (ABD) and adductors (ADD) are of approximately equal strength (ABD:ADD strength ratio = 1), but Hamilton and colleagues (1992) reported that ballet dancers tend to have stronger abductors than adductors (ABD:ADD ratio > 1). The adductors have an important role in decelerating hip abduction, such as when performing a deep squat, split jump, or penché.

Hip Extensors

The gluteus maximus is the largest and strongest hip muscle, and it is the main hip extensor (moves the leg backward). The gluteus maximus provides power and height to explosive jumps, and it works eccentrically (contracting while lengthening) to control landings. The gluteal muscles work with the hamstrings to decelerate the gesture leg when it moves into flexion (e.g., in a grand battement devant or a split jeté), and they eccentrically control hip flexion (e.g., lowering the body over the supporting leg in a penché). The adductor magnus also acts as a hip extensor, and it works with the gluteus maximus to support partnering of another dancer. Figure 13.28 shows the hip extensor muscles.

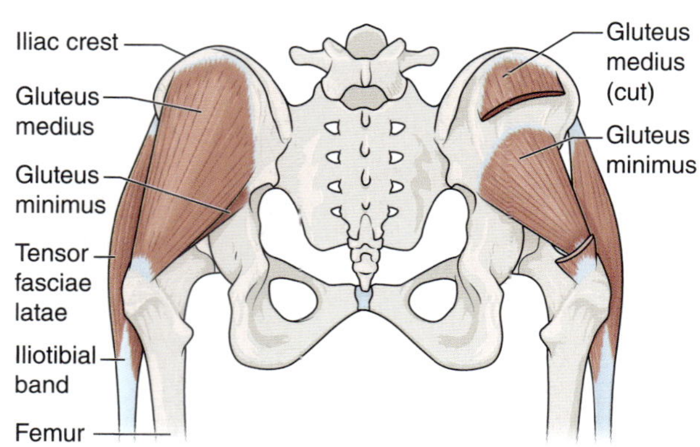

Figure 13.27 The posterior view of the primary muscles of hip abduction.

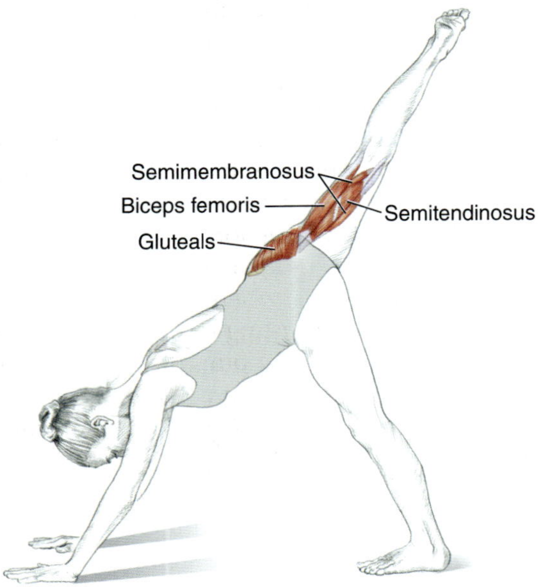

Figure 13.28 The primary muscles of hip extension.

Hip Rotators

Most of the hip muscles have a secondary rotation action; generally, the anterior muscles internally rotate the hip, while the posterior muscles externally rotate the hip. When the hip moves into flexion, some posterior muscles, such as the gluteus medius and the underlying piriformis, change their action from external to internal hip rotation. The deep hip external rotator muscles include the obturator internus, obturator externus, gemellus inferior, gemellus superior, and quadratus femoris (figure 13.29). You might assume that ballet dancers have more-developed hip external rotator muscles due to working in turnout; however, when compared to other athletes in research studies, only the obturator externus was larger in dancers versus athletes (Emery et al., 2021; Mayes et al., 2018). The obturators are the largest of the deep external rotators; obturator externus can externally rotate the hip in high ranges of hip flexion (Mayes et al., 2018). Because these muscles are close to the center of rotation of the hip joint, they may play an important role in hip joint stability.

Hip Mechanics

The range of motion (ROM) of the hip joint is determined by the bony anatomy as well as the flexibility of the capsule, ligament, tendon, and muscle combined with the strength and control of the surrounding muscles. The extreme ROMs required in many forms of dance may be safely achieved with the combination of optimally shaped bones, flexible soft tissues, strong muscles, skilled proprioception, and neuromuscular control. Dance movements that involve extreme hip ROM (e.g., développé or splits) can result in impingement between the femoral head and neck junction and the rim of the acetabulum (figure 13.30) with subluxation (partial dislocation) of the femoral head from the acetabulum (Charbonnier et al., 2011; Mitchell et al., 2016). As the hip moves into extension and external rotation during an arabesque, the femoral head moves forward in the acetabulum, and it may compress the labrum and cartilage at the front of the joint. *Impingement* is the term for these structures contacting one another this way. Muscle strength is required to control and decelerate these movements at their end range to minimize the impact on the cartilage, labrum, and bone.

Overall, your posture and the position of your pelvis impact hip mechanics. Excessive anterior pelvic tilt and lumbar lordosis may result from forcing hip external rotation or turnout. In such an instance, the acetabulum rotates closer to the

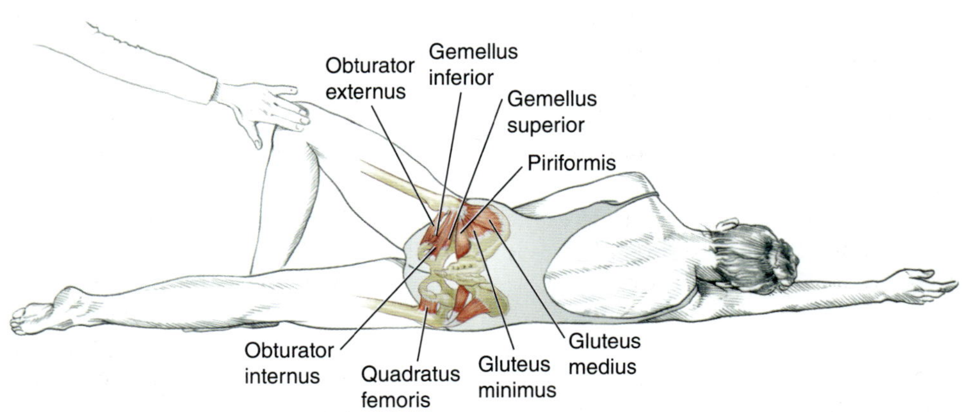

Figure 13.29 Primary muscles of hip rotation.

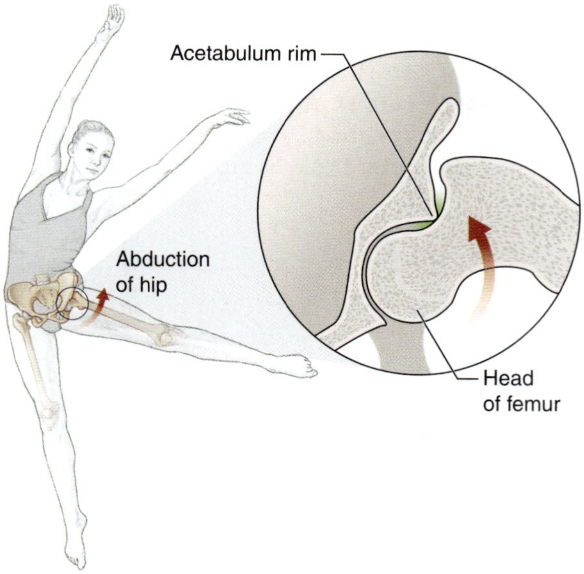

Figure 13.30 When a dancer moves into the extremes of hip flexion, extension, or abduction, the portion of the femur where its head and neck meet can collide with the acetabulum's rim and the portion of the labrum located there.

femur than usual, thus causing impingement to occur earlier in the ROM during flexion movements. Standing or dancing with excessive posterior pelvic tilt is another common fault. Posterior rotation of the acetabulum diminishes the coverage of the femoral head, which in turn increases the hip joint's compressive forces and stretches the passive and dynamic stabilizers at the front of the hip. This compensation may lead to the femoral head sliding anteriorly, potentially resulting in instability.

If a dancer has a weak iliopsoas muscle and attempts to lift the leg into retiré (lift leg with a bent knee), they may excessively or prematurely tilt the pelvis upward with the gesture leg to allow other, less efficient hip flexors to compensate. As a dancer extends the leg into a développé, the pelvis needs to gradually tilt upward to prevent impingement. Attempting to keep the pelvis *square* (a teaching cue to level the two sides) may prevent full elevation and lead to impingement injury.

During ballet movements that require extreme hip ROM, skilled dancers combine hip and pelvic motion, a strategy that allows greater overall ROM while reducing the need for extreme hip joint movement (Krasnow et al., 2011). During an arabesque, expert dancers extend the trunk and hip of the gesture leg with a smooth motion. In contrast, novice dancers focus predominantly on moving the hip with less trunk motion or smooth action (Krasnow et al., 2011), potentially increasing the forces on the hip joint. It is biomechanically impossible to keep the pelvis square in arabesque; to prevent excessive hip joint impingement and instability, the pelvis must tilt anteriorly and rotate as the hip extends in a smooth, coordinated action.

Excessive hip adduction and internal rotation of the supporting leg when performing a fondu (bending on the supporting leg) or landing from a jump also could lead to impingement and excessive loading of the acetabulum. Strong hip abductors and external rotators—with adequate hip joint balance and proprioception—are required to control this motion.

Turnout

Turnout involves external rotation of the lower limbs, and it is the foundation of all ballet movements. Turnout has an aesthetic and mechanical role. Hip external rotation allows extreme abduction ROM by rotating the greater trochanter of the femur posteriorly to avoid impingement with the acetabular rim (figure 13.31). Strong hip external rotators are required to minimize impingement in these positions.

Dancers have greater passive ROM and greater strength in hip external rotation than nondancers; however, if a dancer has insufficient hip external rotation, they may compensate by rotating their knees, ankles, and feet outward (Khan et al., 1997). Several methods are available to measure turnout (table 13.1; figures 13.32 to 13.34). Standing functional turnout (table 13.1, figure 13.33) ROM ranges from 129 to 134 degrees (Quanbeck et al., 2017; Washington et al., 2016). A study on professional ballet dancers found that the hip joint contributed 76 percent to the total turnout ROM, with only 24 percent coming from rotation at the knee and ankle or foot (Washington et al., 2016). In contrast, a study on a younger cohort performing active standing turnout on low-friction discs found a fairly equal contribution to total ROM between the hip (36%), knee (32%), and ankle or foot (32%) (Quanbeck et al., 2017). Dancers vary in how they achieve turnout; however, with training, they can increase their functional turnout by increasing hip external rotation strength, thus reducing the need for external rotation of the joints below the hip (Khan et al., 1995; Khan et al., 1997).

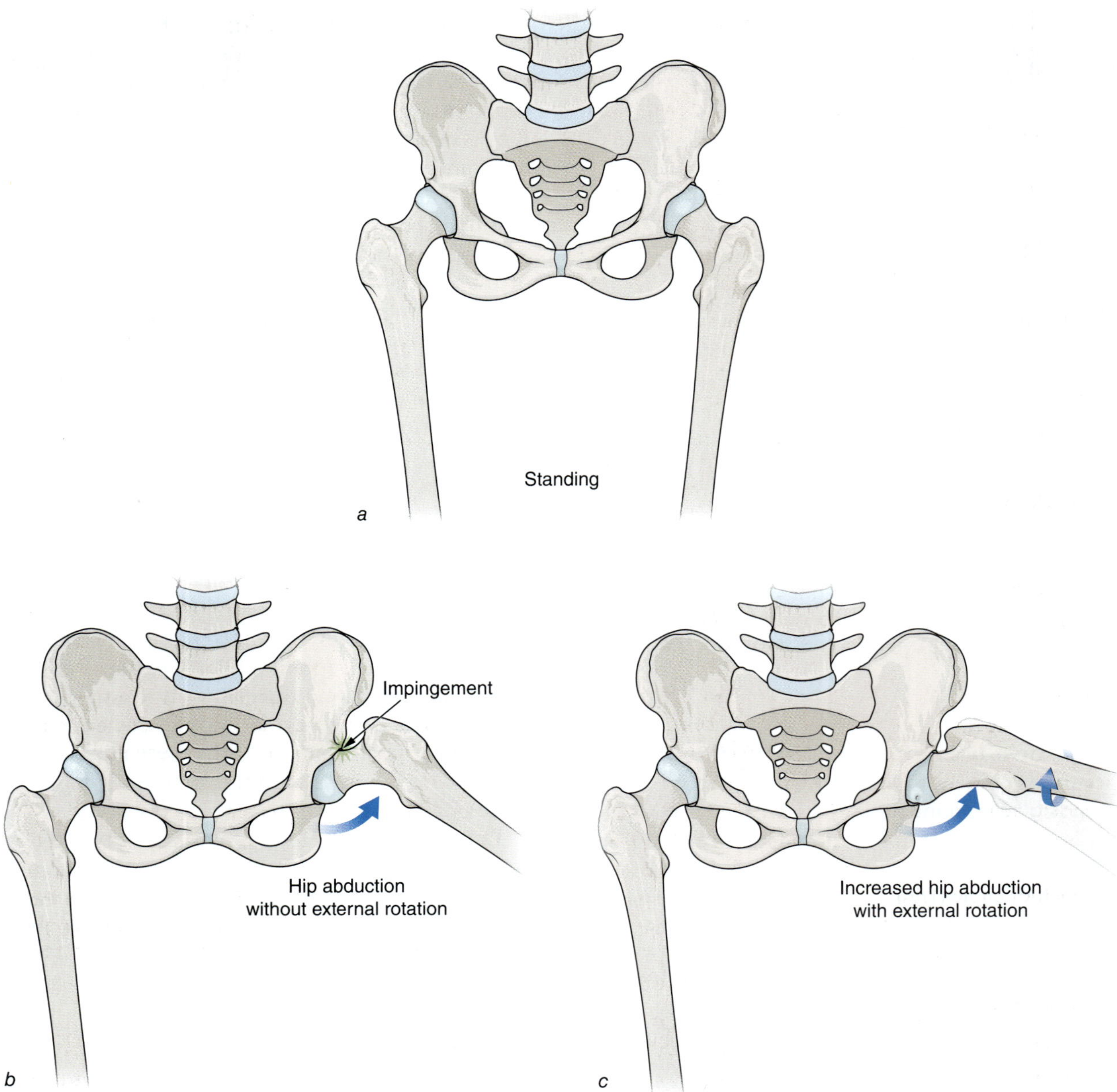

Figure 13.31 Anterior and lateral view of the hip. *(a)* Standing. *(b)* Hip abduction without external rotation of the femur. *(c)* Hip abduction with external rotation of the femur to increase abduction ROM and prevent impingement.

Hip Injuries in Dance

Thirteen percent of all injuries in professional dance occur in the hip region; up to 60 percent of dancers report hip pain, and 10 percent report chronic hip pain (Duthon et al., 2013; Vassallo, 2017). According to Smith and colleagues (2017), 10 percent of dancers felt that a hip injury was the worst injury they had experienced. Although the hip joint is not the most prevalent site of injury in dance, an injury in this area can interfere with a dancer's career; in some cases, it can lead to early retirement or long-term symptoms (Smith et al., 2017). Dancers are at no greater risk of hip injury and pain compared to other athletes (Mayes et al., 2016b; 2016c), especially if they commit to keeping their muscles strong to cope with the demands of dance. Reducing your risk for hip injuries should be a primary goal for you as you study this book and throughout your dance career.

Hip injuries may develop gradually due to an accumulation of high levels of hip joint loading or suddenly with an acute impingement or joint sprain. Any structures around the hip can be

Table 13.1 **Summary of Terms and Positions Used in Assessing Turnout**

Turnout measure	Definition
Passive external rotation (ER) range of motion (ROM)	Passive* ER ROM tested in supine (back-lying) or prone (front-lying) position with hips in neutral or at 90° and the knees at 90° (figure 13.32).
Active ER ROM	Active** ER ROM tested in positions as above.
Active ER lag	Active ER lag = passive ER ROM − active ER ROM
Functional turnout (FTO)	Total static turnout of both lower limbs (usually tested in standing first position, but other positions of the feet have been tested). Dancer stands heel-to-heel, externally rotates feet maximally, and the angle between the long axis of both feet (heel midpoint to second metatarsal shaft) represents FTO (figure 13.33).
Dynamic turnout	FTO measured after landing from a jump.
Static–dynamic discrepancy	Static–dynamic discrepancy = FTO − dynamic turnout
Compensated turnout (CTO)	CTO measures the nonhip component of turnout. CTO = Functional turnout − active or passive ER ROM Also known as below-hip ER or nonhip ER.
Total turnout (TTO)	TTO measures passive or active ER of all joints of the lower limb (hip, knee, foot and ankle complex). In supine, with hip and knee in neutral, the entire lower limb externally rotates. The angle between the long axes of the feet represents TTO (figure 13.34).
Standing active turnout	Active TTO is measured on reduced-friction discs to eliminate assistance from friction between the foot and floor.
Thigh–foot angle (TFA)	Angular difference between the long axis of the thigh and foot, measured with the dancer kneeling on a table with the hip neutral and knees flexed 90°. A joint angle measurement device (goniometer) is placed along the second metatarsal, and the other arm is aligned with the thigh (figure 13.35).

*Passive ROM is measured when a clinician moves the dancer's limb into the desired position.

**Active ROM is measured when a dancer moves their limb into the desired position without assistance.

Adapted from L.M. Champion and S.J. Chatfield, "Measurement of Turnout in Dance Research: A Critical Review," Journal of Dance Medicine & Science 12, no. 4 (2008), 121-135.; J.A. Coplan, "Ballet Dancer's Turnout and its Relationship to Self-Reported Injury," Journal of Orthopaedic and Sports Physical Therapy 32, no. 11 (2002), 579-584. Doi:10.2519/jospt.2002.32.11.579; W.G. Hamilton, L.H. Hamilton, P. Marshall, and M. Molnar, "A Profile of the Musculoskeletal Characteristics of Elite Professional Ballet Dancers," American Journal of Sports Medicine 20, no.3 (1992), 267-273.; J.B. Jenkins, M. Wyon, and A. Nevill, "Can Turnout Measurements Be Used to Predict Physiotherapist-Reported Injury Rates in Dancers?" Medical Problems of Performing Artists 28, no. 4 (2013), 230-235.; V. Negus, D. Hopper, and N.K. Briffa, "Associations Between Turnout and Lower Extremity Injuries in Classical Ballet Dancers," Journal of Orthopaedic and Sports Physical Therapy 35, no. 5 (2005), 307-318. doi:10.2519/jospt.2005.35.5.307; D.C. Reid, R.S. Burnham, L.A. Saboe, and S.F. Kushner, "Lower Extremity Flexibility Patterns in Classical Ballet Dancers and Their Correlation to Lateral Hip and Knee Injuries," American Journal of Sports Medicine 15, no.4 (1987), 347-352.; K. Sutton-Traina, J.A. Smith, D.N. Jarvis, S.P. Lee, and K. Kulig, "Exploring Active and Passive Contributors to Turnout in Dancers and Non-Dancers," Medical Problems of Performing Artists 30, no. 2 (2015), 78-83. doi: 10.21091/mppa.2015.2013.

injured, including the labrum, cartilage, ligaments, muscles, **synovium**, bones, and nerves.

Hip Joint Injury

Hip joint injury causes pain in the front, the side, and sometimes the back of the hip. Although injury to any of the hip joint structures can lead to pain, it is often difficult to diagnose exactly which structure is causing symptoms. Hip joint pain can be dull or sharp; it can spread into the thigh, and it can even spread down to the knee. Clicking, catching, locking, giving way, and stiffness are other symptoms commonly experienced with hip joint injury.

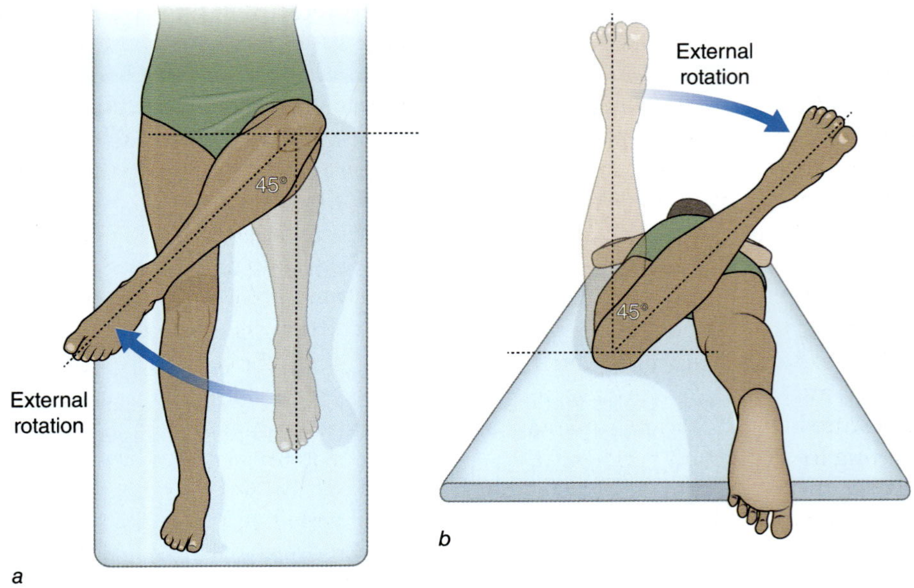

Figure 13.32 Measurement of passive hip external rotation with the dancer lying on a table. *(a)* Hips at 90 degrees. *(b)* Prone, with hips in neutral position.

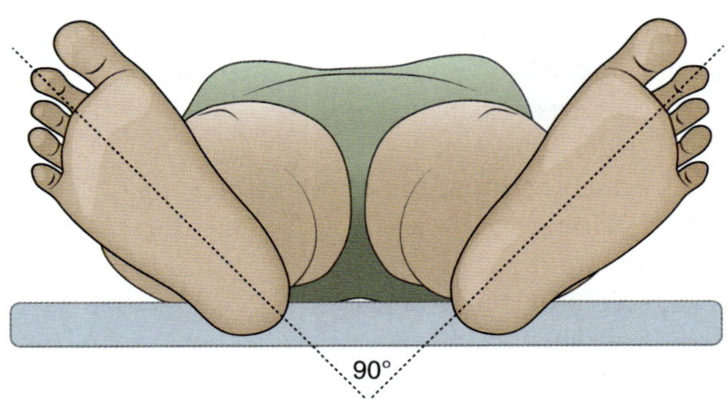

Figure 13.34 Measurement of total turnout (TTO).

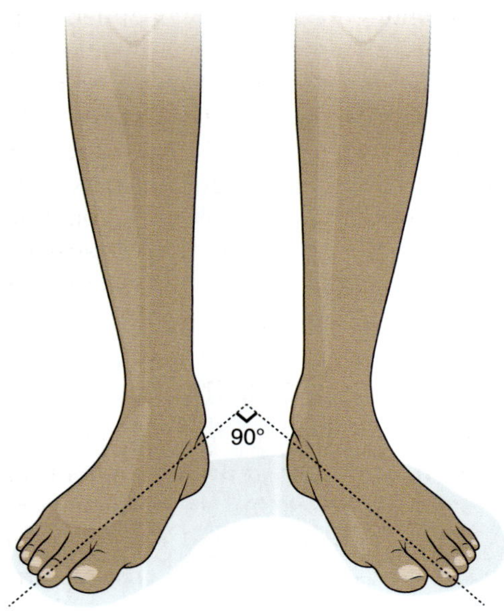

Figure 13.33 Measurement of functional turnout (FTO).

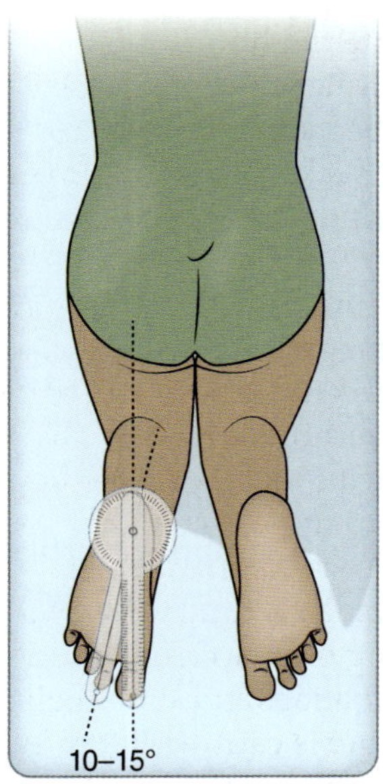

Figure 13.35 Measurement of thigh–foot angle (TFA).

Most hip joint injuries can heal completely, especially if you report the most minor symptoms to your health care provider as early as possible and start rehabilitation according to their guidance. Complete rest usually is not beneficial; if all movements in dance are painful, immediately starting an exercise program prescribed by your practitioner is recommended. Strengthening all the hip, trunk, and pelvic muscles is key to recovery, and it can prevent reinjury of your hip. The muscles must be strong enough to decelerate your femur in extreme ROMs to limit joint impingement. To speed up recovery, avoid painful activities such as holding your gesture leg in elevation, forcing your turnout, and sitting for prolonged periods. As your hip muscles strengthen, you will be able to hold your leg in high elevations without experiencing pain; the key is to gradually increase the height and duration of the sustained holds. Take care with activities such as fast walking and swimming until your hip flexors are strong enough, as these activities are considered high load. You may be able to continue activities such as vertical jumping if they are pain free, as the hip flexors do not work as hard in vertical movements.

Stretching the front of the hip can feel good, but avoid doing so; it may lengthen the important hip joint stabilizers, including the iliopsoas and joint capsule, and lead to labrum and bone impingement. Not all sensations of tightness are due to short muscles. A muscle that feels tight or is not lengthening may be a sign of weakness and fatigue, and strengthening is often the best method to manage tight muscles. Sitting in splits or the frog position, especially for long periods, can impinge and partially dislocate the hip, potentially leading to hip joint injury (Mitchell et al., 2016). Popping the hip should also be avoided; it disrupts the stabilizing vacuum that sucks the femur into the acetabulum, and it can irritate the tendons around the hip and pelvis.

Hip joint imaging, such as X-rays or magnetic resonance imaging (MRI), may be necessary to detect serious conditions that need special management. These techniques, especially MRI, are excellent for showing detailed anatomy. Interestingly, atypical anatomy is commonly found in people who have never experienced hip symptoms, and therefore, these structural variants may never be an issue. Imaging of dancers with hip pain can show numerous variations and abnormalities, but finding which structure is causing the pain is not possible with imaging alone. Such tests should never be interpreted without special tests, such as hip ROM and strength assessment, as well as a thorough discussion between the health care practitioner and the dancer about the dancer's pain.

It can take as long as 6 weeks to start to feel improvements in hip pain during rehabilitation, and full recovery can take up to 12 months. Rehabilitation and massage can help restore movement in stiff joints and release tension in muscles to facilitate the strengthening process. Surgery to repair injured joint structures may be required occasionally. Surgery should be considered only if a dancer has failed to improve following at least 3 months of rehabilitation (Kemp et al., 2020), unless there is a serious condition that requires immediate intervention. Hip surgery followed by thorough rehabilitation can be effective, but not all dancers recover fully after surgery; moreover, some potential complications of surgery can be career threatening.

Acetabular Labral Tear

The labrum can be injured if it is impinged by the femur in extreme ROMs. This can occur in all directions of movement. Damage to the labrum usually occurs gradually with repeated impingement, but can occur suddenly if the force applied to the hip joint is high enough. Labral tears are common in dancers and other athletes, but not all labral tears cause symptoms. In fact, many dancers with a torn labrum shown on MRI don't experience hip pain (Mayes et al., 2016c). A torn labrum can lose its stabilizing and protective role, potentially leading to cartilage damage. Improving the strength and function of the surrounding muscles can compensate for a torn labrum.

Articular Cartilage Injury

Like labral tears, damage to hip joint cartilage is common in dancers' and athletes' hips (Mayes et al., 2016b). Elite ballet dancers do not appear to be at risk of cartilage injury that deteriorates over time, especially if they engage in a regular hip-strengthening program (Mayes, Smith, Stuart, Semciw, & Cook, 2021). The articular cartilage does not have a nerve supply; therefore, cartilage damage is often not painful. Injury to cartilage starts to become painful when the underlying bone swells. Cartilage damage causes swelling or synovitis (inflammation of the membranes that produce joint lubricating fluid) in the joint, and the swollen joint can then become painful. Cartilage injury can eventually lead to osteoarthritis in some individuals, but it is still unclear why only a small percentage of people with cartilage injury eventually develop osteoarthritis.

Ligamentum Teres Tear

A tear of the ligamentum teres is much more common in dancers than other athletes. According to Mayes and colleagues (2016a), it is likely that the extreme ROMs used in dance can lead to injury of this ligament, either by overstretching it or impinging it in the joint. In addition, risk of developing a ligamentum teres tear is higher as dancers age. Although common, most dancers with a ligamentum teres tear do not experience pain or loss of hip rotation ROM (Mayes et al., 2016a). Other stabilizing components, such as the capsule, strong hip muscles, and the joint suction force, can compensate for a ligamentum teres tear. The ligamentum teres is surrounded by synovium that can become inflamed and painful. Your doctor may prescribe medication to reduce the inflammation, and you should avoid painful positions that impinge the ligament so that the inflammation has a chance to subside.

Synovitis

Synovitis (inflammation of the synovial lining or membrane) in the hip joint is painful, and it appears to be the most common cause of hip joint pain in dancers (Mayes et al., 2020). Excessive movement of the joint or impingement of the synovium that lines the inside of the capsule surrounding a joint can cause synovitis. Prescribed medication and decreased activity to reduce the joint swelling may be required initially. Strong muscles with good balance and proprioception are necessary for prevention and management of synovitis because they control excessive movement or instability of the hip joint. Exercises should start slowly through small ROM and then gradually increase in ROM and speed. You should avoid extreme ROMs (positions of impingement) initially, then gradually increase your ROM once your muscles are strong enough to control the positions.

Osteoarthritis

Osteoarthritis is a disease of an entire joint; it affects all the joint structures, including the cartilage, bone, synovium, and labrum. Osteoarthritis can affect any joint in the body, but hip and knee osteoarthritis are the most common. It can result in severe pain, disability, and eventual joint replacement. Despite the extreme hip joint loading in ballet, hip osteoarthritis is no more common in dancers than nondancers (Teitz & Kilcoyne, 1998; van Dijk et al., 1995). Prevention of pain and disability can be achieved with exercises that promote good joint health. Dance can be an ideal form of exercise for hip joint health if supported with education, active full ROM, muscle strengthening, and balance exercises.

Femoroacetabular Impingement (FAI) Syndrome

Femoroacetabular impingement (FAI) syndrome is a common cause of hip pain in young and middle-aged adults. FAI syndrome is diagnosed in someone with all of the following: hip pain, symptoms that are reproduced with clinical tests (e.g., hip ROM tests), and specific findings on imaging. For example, a cam morphology (figure 13.36) is a bony bump at the head–neck junction of the femur (Griffin et al., 2016). Cam morphology can cause impingement of the neck of the femur with the acetabulum, thus limiting hip ROM, and can cause injury to the labrum, cartilage, and synovium. Cam morphology is less common in elite dancers compared to other athletes (Mayes et al., 2017). Dancers with FAI syndrome should expect that certain ROMs may be limited; these positions should not be forced, and the dancer should strengthen their muscles to prevent excessive impingement.

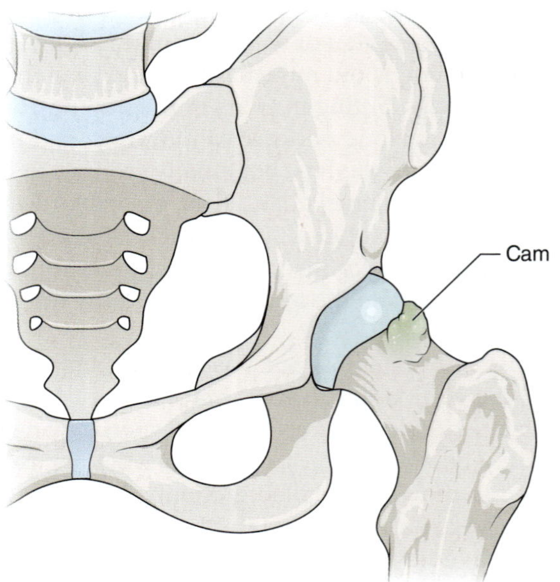

Figure 13.36 A cam morphology is a bump that forms where the head of the femur joins the femoral neck. This bump can impinge against the acetabulum during hip movement.

Acetabular Dysplasia

Acetabular dysplasia is common in elite ballet dancers and may allow excessive hip ROM (Harris et al., 2016). In a hip with acetabular dysplasia, the acetabulum is shallow with less coverage of the head of the femur, resulting in instability, greater ROM, and sometimes pain and clicking or a feeling of the hip giving way. Acetabular dysplasia is usually detected in babies when they are born using special hip ROM tests, but the condition can be missed. Acetabular dysplasia in adults is diagnosed with X-rays. This condition can lead to osteoarthritis if it is severe; in that case, surgery may be required to prevent osteoarthritis. In less-severe cases, strengthening the stabilizing muscles of the hip, avoiding stretching or popping the hip, and balance exercises can help stabilize the hip.

Snapping Hip Syndrome

Painful snapping hip is common in dance, especially during adolescence, when a dancer is still developing muscle strength around the hip and pelvis. Snapping is categorized as either external or internal. The external cause is usually the iliotibial band sliding across the prominence of the femur's greater trochanter. It may also occur posteriorly when a hamstring tendon flicks across the ischial tuberosity where the hamstrings originate.

Internal causes of snapping hip are typically much more bothersome for dancers. A torn labrum—where the torn portion is caught in the joint and then snaps back into its original position—is a less common but particularly noteworthy cause. It must receive attention from a health care professional to avoid increasingly serious damage to the hip joint.

The most common cause of snapping results from the iliopsoas tendon snapping off the iliacus muscle onto the pelvis (Deslandes et al., 2008). As the leg is moved into a retiré position, the iliopsoas muscle rotates, and the iliacus muscle rolls under the psoas major tendon. When the leg is returned to neutral, the tendon can snap off the iliacus muscle onto the pubic bone. A snapping hip is often painless, but the tendon can become irritated and cause pain.

Another common reason for a dancer's internal snapping hip is the iliopsoas tendon snapping over the anterior ridge of the head of the femur or along the front of the pubic portion of the pelvis as the hip is moved through the ROM required in dance. In addition, the iliopsoas tendon's movement is lubricated by a bursa (fluid-filled sac) that sits between the front of the hip joint and the iliopsoas tendon. The bursa protects the tendon from compression and friction during hip movements. It can become inflamed from the snapping, excessive compression, or friction of the iliopsoas tendon as the tendon moves across the front of the hip. It may cause pain and limit hip movement. Figure 13.37 shows a variety of the sources of hip snapping.

A snapping hip originating from the iliopsoas or bursitis is best managed with strengthening of the hip and pelvic muscles. The iliopsoas should be strengthened rather than stretched because the compression of the tendon across the front of the hip with a stretch can irritate both the iliopsoas tendon and the bursa. The iliopsoas may become tight if it is weak, so strengthening can improve the control of the muscle-tendon unit, thus reducing the tight feeling and improving the snapping sensation.

Dancers with a snapping hip or bursitis often have poor pelvic control and a weak core; resulting excessive movement of the pelvis could lead to tension and snapping of tendons around the pelvis. A posterior pelvic tilt can cause tension in the iliopsoas and compression of the tendon against the bursa and the head of the femur. Excessive anterior pelvic tilt may impinge the iliopsoas tendon or bursa and compress the hamstring tendon against the ischial tuberosity (figure 13.38), thus allowing the pelvis to drop. Adducting the hip of the supporting leg can create tension of the iliotibial band against the greater trochanter and lead to lateral hip snapping.

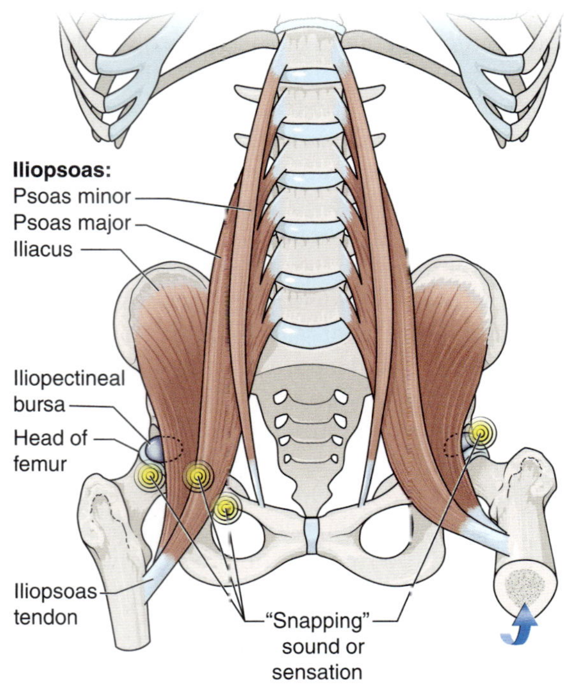

Figure 13.37 Internal snapping hip is common to dancers, and it has a variety of sources.

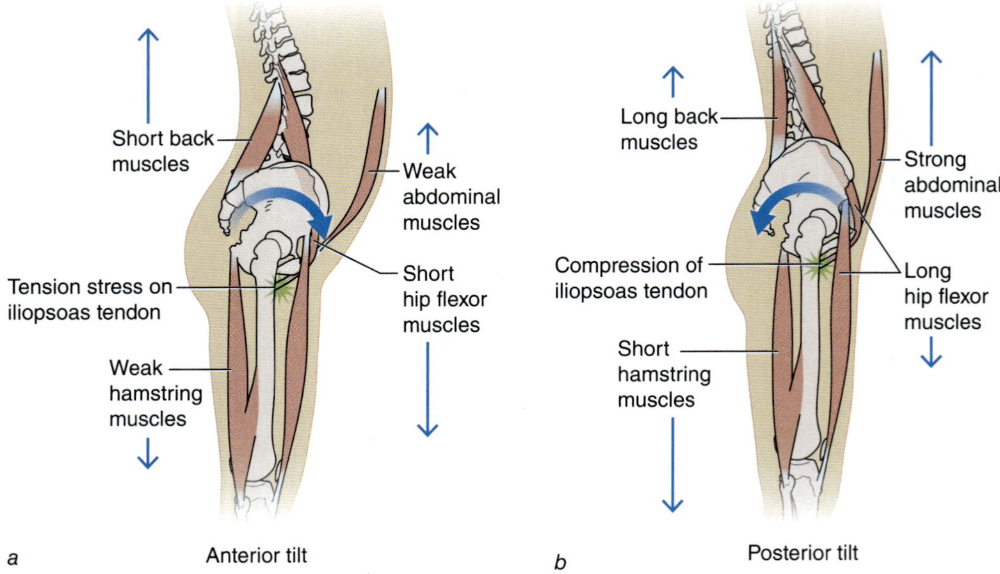

Figure 13.38 The biomechanics of the pelvis are important to the overall health of the iliopsoas tendon and its bursa. Note how the relative lengths and strength or weakness of the hamstrings, gluteus maximus, and rectus abdominis affect the *(a)* anterior tilt *(b)* and posterior tilt of the pelvis. When the pelvis tilts too far anteriorly, the iliopsoas tendon can be impinged. In neutral position and posterior tilt, the tendon can be compressed against the anterior pelvis and femoral head. Any compression of the iliopsoas tendon also results in compression of the underlying bursa.

Improving pelvic stability, including strengthening the abdominal and hamstring muscles, can reduce compression of the tendons around the pelvis and prevent snapping.

Capsular Ligament Sprain

The iliofemoral ligament is one of the capsular ligaments of the hip (figure 13.39). It is very strong, but it can become stretched and weakened with excessive stretching, excessive posterior pelvic tilt, or dynamic dance actions involving hip extension and external rotation (e.g., grand jeté). If a dancer is not warm enough or prepared for a grand jeté or grand battement derrière, these actions could tear the iliofemoral ligament, thus causing a sudden, sharp pain at the front of the hip. When the iliofemoral ligament is sprained, a dancer experiences pain with hip extension. They should keep the injured gesture leg low in arabesque and avoid grand jetés until the ligament heals. Strengthening the muscles that support the iliofemoral ligament and capsule (e.g., the iliopsoas) and avoiding prolonged, passive stretching of the front of the hip may help reduce the likelihood of iliofemoral sprain.

Muscle and Tendon Injury

Any of the hip muscles and their tendons can be injured in dance, especially as a dancer's muscles work eccentrically to decelerate the femur in extreme ranges of motion. If a dancer is not accustomed to the demands placed on their muscles or the muscles are not strong enough for those demands, the risk of muscle or tendon injury can range from delayed-onset muscle soreness (DOMS) to tendinopathy to tearing and rupture.

The most common muscle or tendon injuries around the hip in dance include the iliopsoas, hamstrings, and adductors. Allowing time for a muscle or tendon to recover is essential, but complete rest will only weaken the structure further. Gentle contraction with a light load, such as slowly performing an isometric contraction (a contraction against an immovable object so there is no movement), could be a starting point. The next step is to gradually build the load with a resistance band or light weights while slowly increasing the ROM, then progress to building the speed of the movement. The final step is to make the movement more complex and functional to meet the demands of dance.

A young dancer may be at greater risk of injuring a bone's growth plate where a tendon inserts into the bone than sustaining a muscle tear. **Apophysitis** is inflammation of a growth plate of this type (called an apophysis); this area typically is weaker than muscle and tendon. Apophysitis may occur in many places around the pelvis and hip during adolescence (figure 13.40). Excessive stretching or

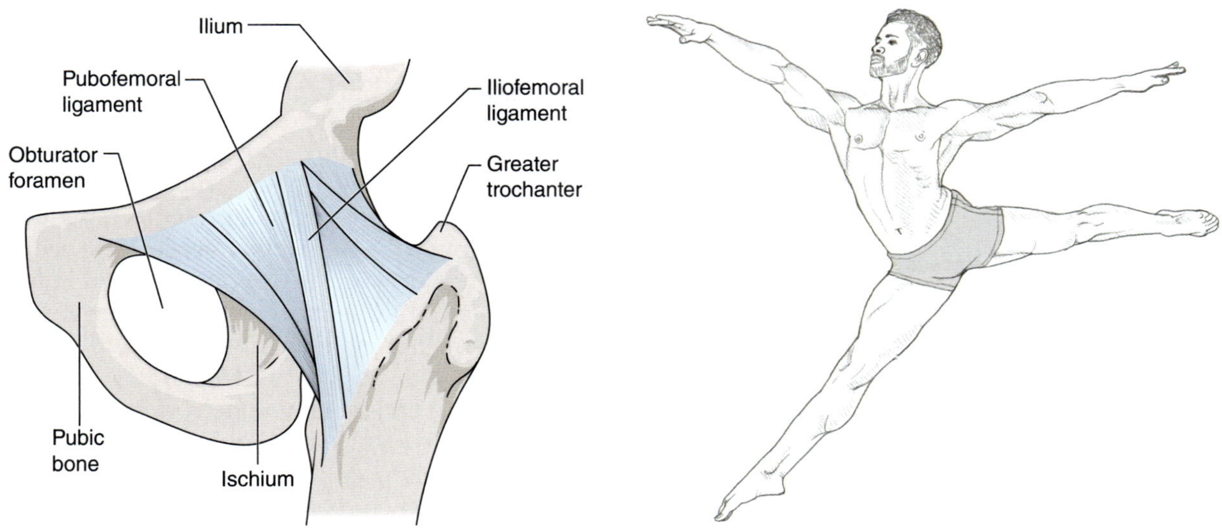

Figure 13.39 The strong iliofemoral ligament secures the hip joint with twisting fibers around the acetabulum, femoral head, and femoral neck. This ligament can be injured in the hip of the rearward extended leg during a grand jeté, among other dance movements.

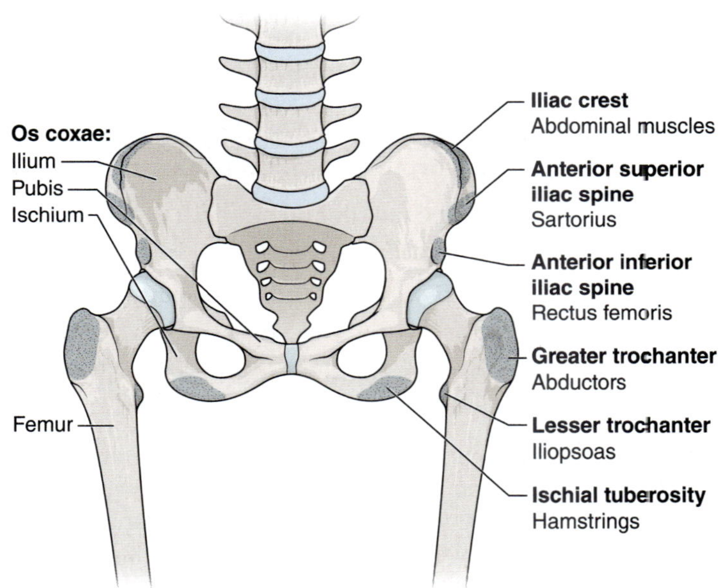

Figure 13.40 Locations of the apophyses (plural of apophysis) in the pelvis and hip, including the tendons of the muscles that attach at each one.

muscle contractions irritate the growth plate by placing traction on it.

An effective warm-up that activates the muscles prior to dance training can help prevent apophysitis. Participation in dance and sports activities should be modified to allow reduction of the apophysitis and its pain. Growth plates throughout the body fuse at different ages of skeletal maturity, and these ages can vary significantly between individuals. Some growth plates in the pelvis do not fuse until individuals are in their twenties.

Fractures and Stress Fractures

The most common stress fracture around the hip occurs at the neck of the femur, but this injury is uncommon in dance. More frequent in dancers is an **avulsion** fracture that occurs at the ischial tuberosity where the hamstrings attach to the pelvis. An avulsion fracture may follow a strong contraction of the hamstrings, resulting in the tendinous attachment of the muscle pulling a piece of the bone away from the pelvis where the tendon attaches. A fast and powerful front kick or slipping into the splits are examples of mechanisms that can cause this injury.

An avulsion fracture can occur at other sites, too, such as the tendon attachments of the rectus femoris, sartorius, iliopsoas, and abdominal muscles. Avulsion injuries may also occur in young dancers at any of the apophyses described earlier, again because an apophysis is a relatively weak link in the muscle-tendon-bone chain. All of these injuries require relative rest and a progressive return to activity under the guidance of a medical professional.

Conclusions and Practical Relevance

You have now gained important knowledge regarding how the lumbar spine, pelvis, and hips interact with dance movement, stability, and control. These extremely important regions undergo repetitive stresses through the demands of dance. Knowledge of common injuries, related symptoms, and injury management in these areas will empower you to reduce the risk of injuries. It will also help you to sense when your body is not responding the way you want it to and when you need to seek professional care. This knowledge should inspire you to be diligent in working on proper strength, mechanics, and stability to help your lower back, pelvis, and hips work well together for your success as a dancer.

Discussion Questions

1. Move your body in a way that accentuates motions in the lumbar spine. As you do, recognize the number of muscles required for successful trunk movement. How is the lumbar region of your spine designed to help you move this way? What would be the result if you had only one tall lumbar vertebra instead of a set of five? What if you did not have intervertebral discs between each pair of vertebrae—how would that affect lumbar spine and trunk movement?
2. Explain the anatomical reason why the length and strength of the iliopsoas muscle affects the position—and therefore the health—of the lumbar spine and pelvis.
3. How would you explain the pelvic floor muscles and their function to a dancer who has never heard of this region before?
4. Describe four major concepts to keep in mind when performing core stabilization exercises that create and support efficient technique.
5. Reflect on the importance of the hips to your dancing (not only in ballet). Discuss any modifications to your dance practice you feel would be helpful to ensure that your hips stay as healthy as possible in order to serve you well. If you are in a situation where your hips are not healthy and are affecting your overall wellness, what steps will you take to change this pattern?

WWW Go to HK*Propel* to access supplemental information and activities connected to chapter content.

14

Head Impacts, Whiplash Injuries, and Concussions in Dance

Lauren McIntyre, ATC
Kathleen L. Davenport, MD

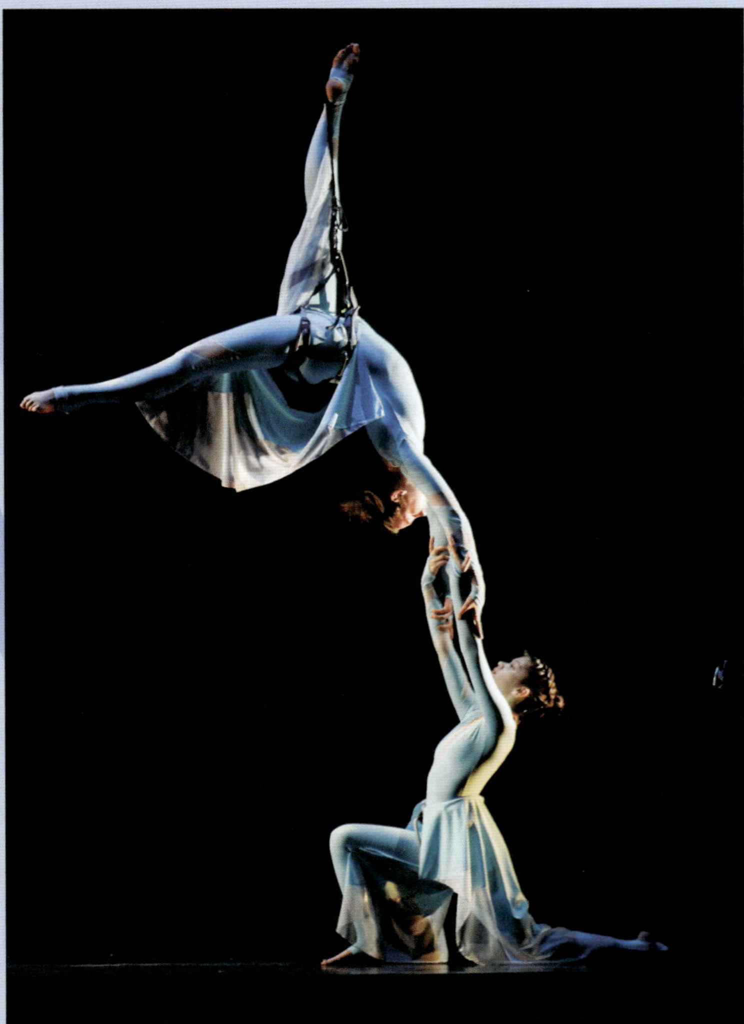

University of Wyoming, Department of Theatre and Dance, Laramie, Wyoming. *Sastrugi*, choreographed by Margaret Wilson, University of Wyoming. Photo: David Andrews Photography; Dancers: Brittany Schoer and Brittany Ching.

Key Terms

baseline testing
central nervous system (CNS)
cerebrospinal fluid
concussion
contrecoup injury
coup injury
cranium
hematoma or hemorrhage
meninges
postconcussive syndrome or persistent postconcussion symptoms
skull fracture
subconcussive impacts
subsymptom threshold aerobic exercise training
traumatic brain injury (TBI)
vestibular and ocular rehabilitation
whiplash

You only get one brain, so you must take as good care of it as possible. Head injuries get a lot of attention in sports; unfortunately, they don't get that same level of attention in performing arts. It is crucial that dancers possess up-to-date knowledge about head impacts, whiplash injuries, and concussions and take responsibility for their brain health.

LEARNING OBJECTIVES

After completing this chapter, you will be able to do the following:

- Outline the basic anatomy and function of the skull, brain, and supporting structures of the central nervous system.
- Improve concussion reporting by combining knowledge of potential head injury mechanisms and concussion symptoms with an understanding of the necessary initial steps to manage a concussion.
- Minimize the risk of prolonged concussion recovery by utilizing appropriate rest and gradual return to activity under the guidance of a health care professional.
- Compare the characteristics of concussion to those of other head and brain injuries.

The brain is your body's central nerve bank. It initiates and processes all the important signals for the entire body to function, which means that an injury to the brain can affect any and all functions of the body. It can cause pain, headaches, vision changes, and sensitivity to sound or other stimuli. It can also affect the body's physical functions, such as strength, coordination, balance, and sensation. An injury to the brain may alter emotions, sleep patterns, and memory. These alterations can have detrimental effects on dance because dancers require all aspects of the brain—from conveying emotions to coordinating the physicality of movement—to excel at their art form. This chapter describes the anatomy of the brain, explores injury to the brain, promotes the importance of early diagnosis and treatment in the event of brain injury, and discusses other injuries to the cranial region.

Basic Anatomy and Function of the Head and Brain

The brain and spinal cord make up your **central nervous system (CNS)**. The role of the CNS is to manage body movement and coordination, learning, and behavior. The adult human brain weighs just over 3 pounds (1.5 kg), and it is the most complex organ in the human body (Van de Graaff et al., 2013). In order to understand injuries to this intricate system, it is important to have basic knowledge of its anatomy.

The Skull

The bony skull is composed of 22 bones. Fourteen bones form the face, and eight comprise the **cranium**. Figure 14.1 illustrates the eight cranial bones. The cranial bones are separate at birth; they fuse together in childhood, forming immovable joints called sutures. The skull protects the brain, but its rigid structure can create problems in the event of swelling or blood in the cranium because little room exists for anything other than the brain and its supporting structures. For example, if swelling or blood pools around the brain from an injury, the brain has nowhere to go against the hard skull bones; therefore, it may be compressed and damaged.

The Brain

The main areas of the brain include the cerebrum, cerebellum, and brain stem. Each region executes specific functions.

The Cerebrum

The cerebrum handles many of the body's higher functions, such as memory and reasoning, and it makes up 80 percent of the brain's mass (Van de Graaff et al., 2013). The cerebrum is divided into a right hemisphere and a left hemisphere. The right

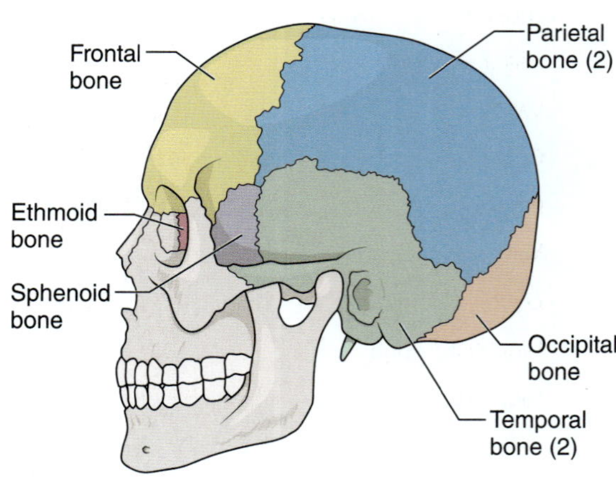

Figure 14.1 The cranial bones.

cerebrum controls the left side of the body and tasks related to spatial awareness, creativity, face recognition, and perception; the left cerebrum controls the right side of the body and tasks related to language, analysis, calculation, and sequencing (figure 14.2). The cerebrum is further divided into five lobes, each with a specific function (figure 14.3).

The Cerebellum

The cerebellum is located at the back of the brain, and it is the primary center for balance and coordination. It operates on a subconscious level, constantly communicating with the rest of our body to maintain balance (Van de Graaff et al., 2013). This area of the brain is crucial for dance because it allows dancers to excel in balancing, coordinated movement patterns, and controlling their movements. Injury to the cerebellum can cause uncoordinated movements, tremors, and impaired precision when directing the limbs in space. When damage occurs to the cerebellum, even walking and standing without falling can become major challenges, let alone advanced dance choreography.

The Brain Stem

The brain stem is divided into three regions: the midbrain, pons, and medulla oblongata. Like the cerebellum, the brain stem also operates on a subconscious level. Its role is to regulate basic life-sustaining functions, such as breathing, heart rate, and blood pressure—functions that are critical in physical activity such as dance (Van de Graaff et al., 2013). The midbrain is a major connection center between areas of the brain, and it helps control vision, hearing, memory, and movement. A severe injury to this area of the body can create permanent visual impairment, paralysis of nerve and muscle function, and memory difficulties.

The pons is also a connection center between areas of the brain, and it contains many important cranial nerves. It helps relay signals controlling sleep, vision, hearing, facial expressions, and other functions. Severe damage to the pons can result in a rare and devastating condition called locked-in syndrome; a person with this condition can perceive the outside world but has minimal or no ability to communicate or move. The medulla oblongata regulates essential functions for survival, such as heart rate, breathing, swallowing, and blood flow. Severe damage to this area of the brain is incompatible with life.

Supporting Structures

Cerebrospinal fluid is a clear fluid that surrounds the brain and spinal cord, allowing the brain to float within the bony skull. Although cerebrospinal fluid provides a protective cushion for the brain, it also permits the brain to move within the skull, which can result in injuries that are discussed later in this chapter.

The **meninges** are thin, connective tissue coverings over the brain and the skull that provide another layer of protection. The layers of meninges in the brain include the dura mater, arachnoid, and pia mater (Haines, 2015). Figure 14.4 illustrates the location of the three membranes in the skull. The dura mater is the outer (*durable*) portion. The arachnoid, named because of its spider-web-like

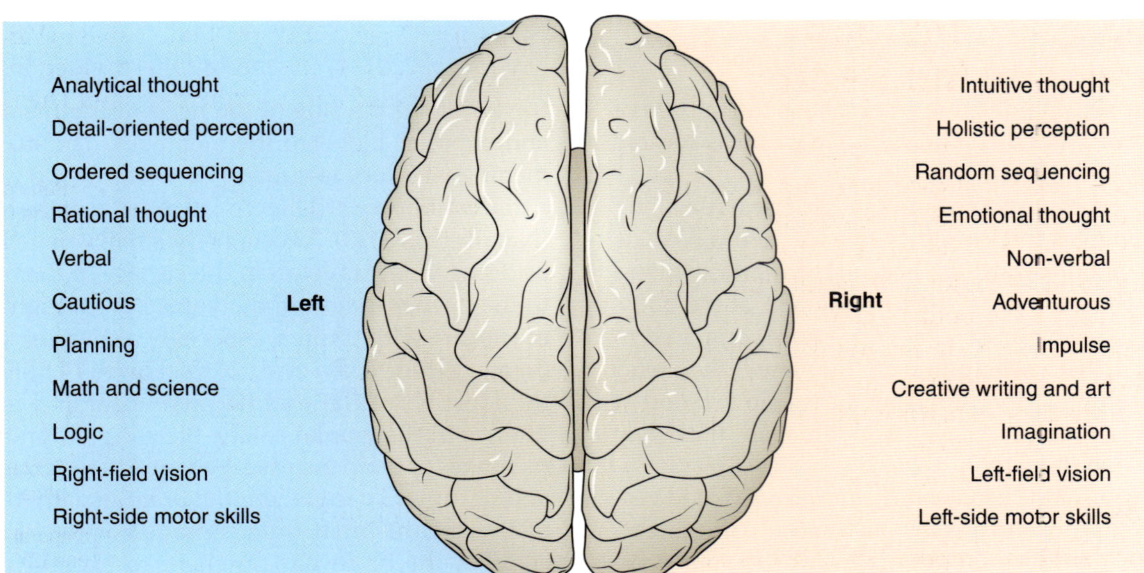

Figure 14.2 The cerebral hemispheres and their primary functions.

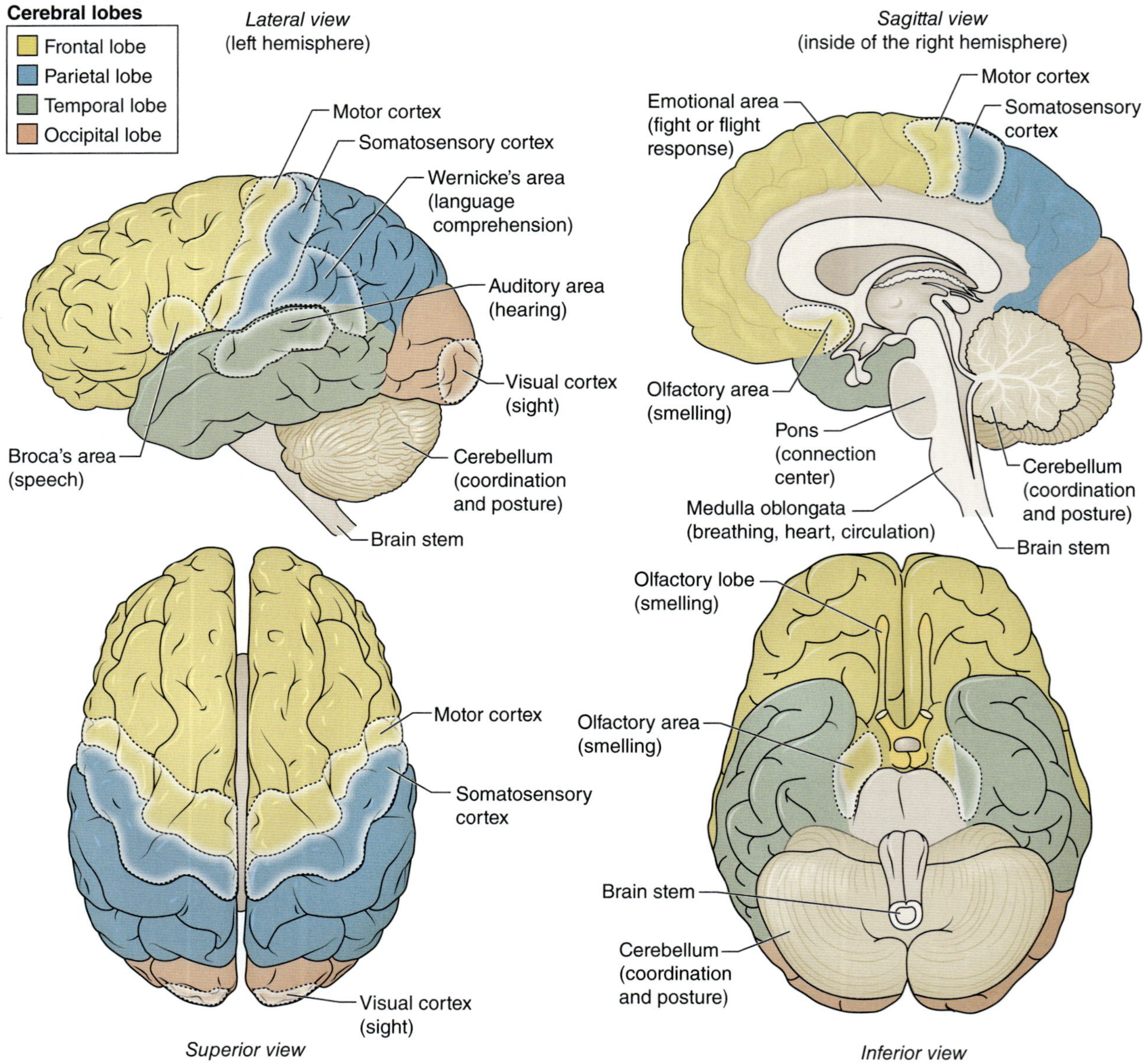

Figure 14.3 The five cerebral lobes and their corresponding functions.

appearance (spiders are *arachnids*) is the middle of the three layers. The delicate pia mater is located closest to the brain.

Blood vessels (both veins and arteries) run along the meninges and into other areas of the brain. Veins bring blood toward the heart; arteries carry blood away from the heart, toward the rest of the body. Veins move blood at a lower pressure compared to arteries; therefore, if they are damaged, they tend to ooze blood more slowly. Arteries move blood at a higher pressure; if they are damaged, they may lose blood quickly.

Trauma to the head or brain may cause blood vessels to rupture and bleed, which can be a life-threatening situation in severe cases. For example, an important artery called the middle meningeal artery travels along the side of the head inside the skull and supplies blood to the meninges. The middle meningeal artery is vulnerable to rupturing when a traumatic force is delivered to the side of the head (Natali et al., 2020). Additionally, small veins called bridging veins travel from the surface of the brain to the deeper tissues; these veins have a high risk of rupture with trauma, especially a shearing type of injury (Mortazavi et al., 2013). Figure 14.5 shows the location of the middle meningeal and other arteries in the cranial cavity. Bleeding around the meninges or brain increases pressure in the cranium and occupies space where the brain usually floats in its cerebrospinal fluid. Because of the skull's rigidity, the brain has nowhere to expand with the addition of more blood. Therefore, parts of the

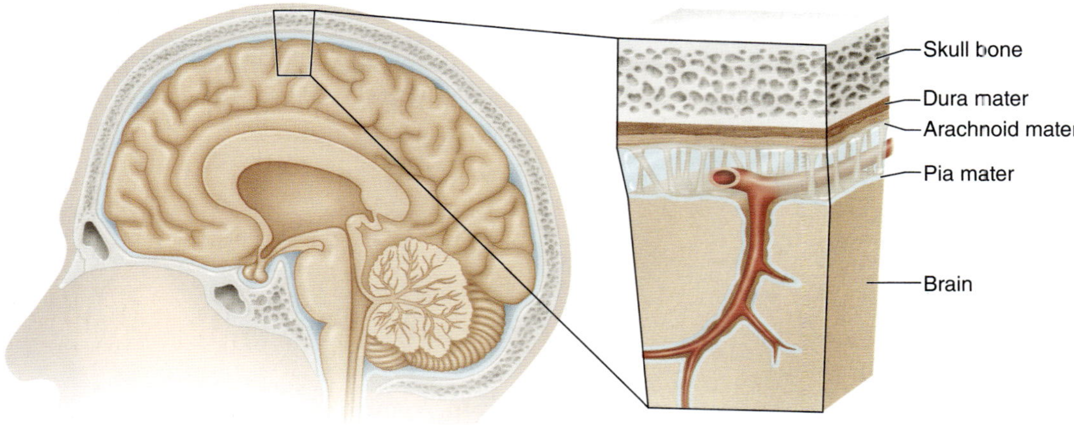

Figure 14.4 Meninges surrounding the brain.

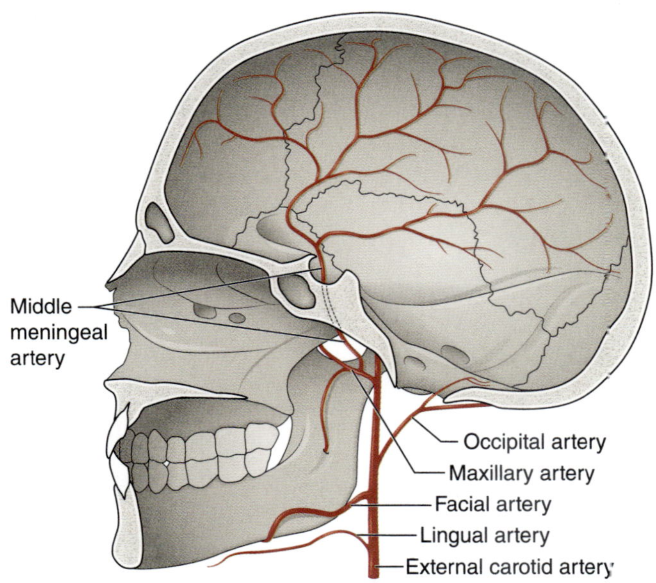

Figure 14.5 View of the inside of the skull with arteries (including the medial meningeal artery).

brain are compressed by the expanding collection of blood, resulting in possible damage to the brain and even in death.

Concussions

Concussions are mild traumatic brain injuries (mTBIs) caused by forces from an impact directly to the head or an impact elsewhere on the body that transmits a force to the head and brain (such as whiplash). These forces impair normal neurological function, causing the concussed individual to experience certain signs and symptoms (Patricios, Schneider et al., 2023). Table 14.1 lists some of the most common signs and symptoms that may be experienced with a concussion. Note that loss of consciousness is not a required symptom for a concussion diagnosis, but it does sometimes happen. In fact, the majority of concussions occur without any loss of consciousness. Concussion symptoms may be experienced immediately, or within minutes, or they may not appear for hours after a head injury occurs (Patricios, Schneider et al., 2023).

Not every impact to the head causes a concussion; however, because signs and symptoms can take time to evolve, it is important to report all

Table 14.1 **Common Signs and Symptoms of Concussion**

Observable signs	Symptoms felt by the individual
Balance difficulties	Headache or pressure in the head
Irritability	Drowsiness or fatigue
Confusion	Nausea
Increased emotionality	Blurred vision
Low energy	Light or noise sensitivity
Difficulty remembering and concentrating	Dizziness
Sadness	Neck pain

head impacts and to rest from dance until you have received clearance from a health care professional that it is safe to return (Patricios, Schneider et al., 2023; Stemper et al., 2019). Symptoms such as prolonged loss of consciousness, seizures, and tingling in the arms or legs could be signs of a more severe injury to the head or spine; these conditions require emergency transportation to a medical center. (Some of these more severe head injuries are discussed later in this chapter.) It is important to remember that concussions are a medical diagnosis; therefore, the assessment, management, and clearance to return to dance should be done by a health care professional with experience in treating concussions (Harmon et al., 2019).

Concussion Mechanisms in Dance

A dancer might sustain a concussion in two main ways: direct head or body impacts, or nonimpact forces such as during a sudden acceleration or deceleration of the head and neck (Hynes & Dickey, 2006). Dance-related movements with these types of forces include stunting, diving, flipping, accidental drops, slips and falls, direct blows to the head, collisions, and whipping the head and neck repeatedly (Russell et al., 2021). In addition, a concussion can occur from repetitive, symptomless head impacts and forces delivered over time. These **subconcussive impacts** may lead to gradual changes in the brain or cause a concussion to happen from a lower-than-expected force (Stemper et al., 2019). This chapter discusses both impact and nonimpact forces in more detail.

Head Impacts

As previously mentioned, the brain is floating in the skull, surrounded by a cushion of cerebrospinal fluid. When the skull is impacted two types of brain injuries can occur due to the floating nature of the brain. A **coup injury** is an injury to the brain next to the area of the skull that is hit. A **contrecoup injury** occurs to side of the brain opposite where the skull is impacted (Drew & Drew, 2004). For example, if a dancer is quickly bending forward and their head collides with another dancer's body, the site where their head hit the other dancer is where a coup injury would occur. Although the skull suddenly stops, the brain and cerebrospinal fluid continue to move, thus rebounding against the skull opposite from the impact. In this instance, the side receiving the rebounding blow is the site of the contrecoup injury (figure 14.6).

Nonimpact Forces

Sudden forces that occur during rapid head and neck accelerations or decelerations also can cause a concussion (Hynes & Dickey, 2006). These forces are similar to those that occur during whiplash. **Whiplash** is an injury that results from the neck being forcibly bent backward, sideways, or forward (Albano et al., 2014). Whiplash is common in contact sports, such as American football, rugby, and

Be Aware of Your Head

In an article by Kish and Koutures (2016), a dancer describes their concussion, which resulted from a class where they were doing a fast combination involving repetitive forward rolls. This dancer could not recall a moment when they hit their head, but they still developed symptoms after class. This situation demonstrates how important it is for dancers to be aware of both where their head is in their movement space and any unusual sensations that might indicate the brain has been affected. Every concussion is different because every dancer is different. In short, the opportunities for a concussion to occur in dance are plentiful and sometimes unexpected.

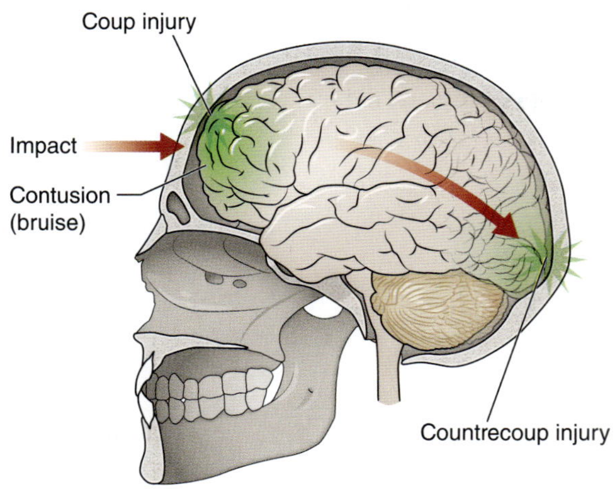

Figure 14.6 The difference between a coup and contrecoup injury.

Whiplash Injury

Hynes and Dickey (2006) followed 20 hockey teams to study the relationship between whiplash and concussion. They found that all injured athletes showed symptoms of both whiplash and concussion, regardless of whether they had a direct impact to the head or whiplash-like mechanism. None of the athletes showed isolated symptoms of one injury or the other, which means that it can be difficult to distinguish which injury has occurred without a thorough examination. In light of this information, dancers must recognize that any type of a whiplash movement may induce concussion symptoms and thus result in injury to the brain. When concussion symptoms appear, it is best to err on the side of caution and see a health care provider.

hockey, but dancers are at risk for whiplash injuries from movement that involves quick head and neck motions. For example, pirouettes require rapid turning of the head while spotting, and breaking power moves such as a flare require forceful spinning of the entire body (Prisk & Hamilton, 2008; Cho et al., 2009). Purposeful whipping of the head—such as is done to create dramatic effects with performers' long hair flying through the air—can also create a whiplash injury.

Whiplash often is associated with concussion, and both injuries have many similarities in their signs and symptoms, such as headache, neck pain, dizziness, fatigue, and cognitive impairments (Hynes & Dickey, 2006; Rebbeck et al., 2019). Because whiplash and concussion are difficult to distinguish, it is important to have both assessed in the event of a head impact or neck injury (Hynes & Dickey, 2006).

Incidence of Concussion in Dance

Since 2009, researchers have been studying the risk of concussion in dance. Table 14.2 includes a comprehensive list of studies and their results. These studies indicate that concussions can occur in classes, rehearsals, and performances. Researchers have not determined whether one type of activity or specific choreography puts you at higher risk for concussion.

Overall, initial data suggest that dancers are at relatively low risk for concussion; but this injury certainly does occur in dance, and it is neither uncommon nor insignificant. More studies are needed to establish injury rates across all genres of dance. Additionally, the rate of concussions in dance may be higher than reported in these studies because dancers are often hesitant to report injuries (Russell et al., 2021). Keep in mind that you can experience a concussion outside of the dance environment, and it will still affect your dance participation. Generally, it is important to seek professional health care advice from a provider who is well acquainted with treating concussions and to follow that provider's instructions. Once you are cleared to resume activities, you should slowly progress your dance activity regardless of how and where you were concussed. The next section provides more specific details about managing concussions in dance.

Management of Concussion in Dance

The best way to ensure that a concussion is appropriately managed is to have a plan in place prior to the injury. Similar to the emergency action plans (EAPs) mentioned in chapter 9, concussion management plans set a standard of care for the assessment and treatment of a dancer after a concussion. Specific components of a concussion management plan should include yearly concussion education, immediate removal from activity when a concussion is suspected, criteria for who can diagnose a concussed dancer and clear them for return to learning

Table 14.2 **Prevalence of Concussion in Dance**

Authors	Genre of dance	Participants	Concussions
Tsiouti & Wyon, 2021	Breakdancing	320 students, professionals, and recreational dancers	2.8% of dancers self-reported experiencing a concussion in the past 12 months.
Lee et al., 2020	Pole dancing	158 beginner through competition-level pole dancers	3 dancers self-reported a history of pole dance-related concussion.
Domene et al., 2018	Salsa	450 nonprofessional salsa dancers	2 dancers self-reported concussions over a year.
McIntyre & Campo, 2017	Ballet and modern dance	238 collegiate and professional dancers	5.5% of dancers self-reported a history of concussion.
Yau et al., 2017	Ballet and contemporary dance	480 high school and collegiate dancers	3% of dancers self-reported a history of concussion.
McIntyre & Liederbach, 2016	Ballet and modern dance	153 dancers aged 18-71 years	23.5% of dancers experienced a dance-related concussion at some point in their life.
Stein et al., 2014	Various styles, including ballet, modern dance, hip-hop, and acrobatic dance	3,011 concussion patients at a large teaching hospital	11 dance-related concussions occurred in a 5.5-year period.
Kauther et al., 2009	Breaking	40 professionals and 104 amateurs	6 dancers self-reported concussions.

and dance, and site-specific risk reduction (Buckley et al., 2017).

Baseline Testing

Although not required to appropriately manage a concussion, **baseline testing** is often a component of an organization's concussion management plan. Baseline testing can be used to help the health care team know if concussion signs and symptoms were present prior to the injury (Harmon, 2019). For example, balance difficulties are a sign of a concussion, but some dancers may have subtle impairments in their balance in the absence of a brain injury. Baseline testing can help identify these characteristics. It may be especially useful for dancers with a history of headaches, migraines, and psychiatric disorders such as depression because these conditions may affect the scores of a concussion exam, particularly the self-reported symptom section (Russell et al., 2021).

The symptoms of concussion are non-specific, thus making the diagnosis challenging (Patricios, Schneider et al., 2023). Illness, stress, certain medications, and even personality can influence the symptoms you experience on a day-to-day basis (Custer et al., 2016). For dancers, it may be especially important to evaluate concussion symptoms before an injury occurs. In a study of university and professional dancers, McIntyre and Campo (2017) found that although baseline cognitive, balance, and rapid number naming scores were similar to those in other athletes, the dancers' baseline symptom scores were elevated. Only 4.2 percent of the 238 participants in the study had zero concussion symptoms at their baseline evaluation.

What factors would elevate a dancer's baseline symptom score? The nature of dance training itself may be one reason. Student dancers must balance academic course loads on top of exhaustive training. This load leaves little time for adequate recovery; consequently, dancers can experience burnout or overtraining, particularly during exams and/or performance periods (Grove, 2013). Symptoms of fatigue, sleep disturbances, irritability, and difficulty concentrating are present in both burnout and concussion, creating the possibility for elevated scores in the absence of brain injury in this population (Grove, 2013).

Recognizing and Reporting Head Impacts and Concussion Symptoms

One of the cornerstones of concussion management is promptly recognizing the injury and notifying a health care professional. Prompt reporting to a health care provider any potential concussion mechanism or signs and symptoms of a concussion is essential. Research in other athletes shows this prompt attention is associated with lower risk of further catastrophic injury and a quicker recovery time (Kroshus et al., 2020). Because many dance environments do not have an on-site medical provider, concussion identification is the responsibility of the dancers themselves as well as parents, teachers, and choreographers (Russell et al., 2021). Resources such as the Concussion Recognition Tool 6 (Echemendia, Ahmed et al., 2023) are useful to help nonmedical persons recognize potential concussions, and they provide initial guidance on how to refer to a medical provider.

Unfortunately, delayed reporting is prevalent in athletes (Kroshus et al., 2020), and research suggests that it may be the same for dancers. As mentioned previously, dancers are hesitant to report injuries in general for a variety of reasons. In the case of a suspected concussion, a study found that the most common reason a sample of dancers did not report their concussion was underestimating the seriousness of the injury. This response is similar to concussion-reporting studies done in other athletes (McIntyre & Liederbach, 2016). How do people change the culture of reporting concussions in the dance environment? It may seem that educating dancers on concussion signs and symptoms—as well as the risks of continuing to dance with a concussion—would change behaviors, but research has shown that knowledge does not necessarily translate into action (Warmath & Winterstein, 2019). A study on the concussion knowledge and behaviors of dancers found that although 97 percent of participants had heard of concussions and they scored an average of 70 percent correct on a concussion quiz, 19 percent of them still had knowingly danced while concussed (McIntyre & Liederbach, 2016).

The answer may lie in a multifaceted approach. Empowering dancers to advocate for their needs, practicing the steps for reporting before injuries happen, and ultimately creating a culture of safety in the dance environment are all beneficial. Research shows that combining knowledge of concussion signs and symptoms with an understanding and rehearsal of each step in the reporting process increases the likelihood that people will tell someone about their concussion (Warmath & Winterstein, 2019). Additionally, if an injured dancer feels that their dance program prioritizes safety—and that their teachers, choreographers, and peers want them to speak up about a potential concussion—they are more likely to report it (Kroshus & Chrisman, 2019).

> **Safety Huddle**
>
> One way to consistently renew everyone's commitment to safety is to have a safety huddle prior to rehearsals, performances, and—at a minimum—the start of every university term. Dancers, choreographers, and staff can gather together briefly to reaffirm their commitment to each other's safety by promising to report injuries (including concussions), to identify unsafe conditions, and to generally support each other. The safety huddle also provides a great opportunity to review the emergency action plan (EAP) and steps for reporting injuries at that class, rehearsal, or performance location (Kroshus & Chrisman, 2019).

Concussion Evaluation

If a dancer is suspected of having a concussion, they must be examined by a medical professional to confirm the diagnosis, devise a recovery plan, and ultimately get clearance to safely return to dance. The two main types of evaluation are on-site and in-office. They are described next.

On-Site Evaluation

If a dancer has access to a medical provider at the time of injury, an immediate concussion evaluation can take place. In traditional sports, such as soccer, it is called a sideline evaluation; for the artistic athlete, it can be called an on-site or backstage evaluation. This evaluation is performed if a dancer is suspected of having a concussion or a more serious brain injury, and it helps the medical provider determine whether the dancer should be referred immediately to an emergency room, monitored with a follow-up at an in-office evaluation, or allowed to return to dance because a concussion has not occurred. If there is any doubt about the diagnosis, you must always assume that a concussion has occurred. Recall that signs and symptoms can be delayed, so the general rule is to never recommend a return to dance or other physical activity the same day that a suspected concussion occurs (Scorza & Cole, 2019).

Immediate on-site evaluations should be performed only by licensed medical professionals who are trained in the evaluation and management of concussion (Harmon et al., 2019). The first step in an on-site evaluation is to rule out life-threatening injuries. If the dancer is unconscious, or if a severe head, neck, or spinal injury is suspected, the health care provider will assess breathing, circulation, presence of a neck injury, and neurological health. Then, the dancer will likely be transferred to an emergency room or hospital. If this initial examination indicates that a concussion is suspected and a more serious injury has not occurred, then a concussion-specific evaluation is the next step.

Concussion is considered one of the most complex injuries to assess and manage. To make matters more difficult, there is no single best tool for diagnosing a concussion. For this reason, many providers use a combination of tests in both on-site and in-office evaluations. Most on-site evaluations include an assessment of the dancer's symptoms, cognition, and neurological function. One of the most commonly used on-site assessment tools is called the Sport Concussion Assessment Tool, 6th Edition (SCAT6). This validated exam takes about 20 minutes. It includes a symptom checklist, cognitive assessment, balance test, and rapid neurological screening (Echemendia, Brett et al., 2023).

In-Office Evaluation

An in-office evaluation often occurs a few days after a concussion, usually at the office of a physician who is trained in the evaluation and treatment of concussions. If you are unsure who to see for a concussion, a physician who has completed fellowship training in sports medicine is usually a good starting point. Often, a combination of examinations is used to monitor a dancer's progress and determine when they are able to return to dance activities. The SCAT6 may be used again to compare to the on-site SCAT6 evaluation (if it was done), and the doctor may add neurological tests, vision testing, neuropsychological testing, and stability and balance tests. The doctor may use the Sports Concussion Office Assessment Tool, 6th Edition (SCOAT6) (Patricios, Davis et al., 2023). As mentioned earlier, baseline tests (such as a beginning-of-the-academic-term SCAT6 evaluation) may also be used (if available) to compare the in-office results to the dancer's pre-injury state (Harmon et al., 2019). Medical imaging (e.g., X-rays, MRI, or CT scans) of the head or brain is not routinely necessary, but a physician may order it if recovery is prolonged (discussed later in this chapter) or if additional injury is suspected (Scorza & Cole, 2019).

Concussion Recovery

In most adult cases, concussion symptoms resolve within 10 to 14 days, and the vast majority experience recovery in 1 month (Patricios, Schneider et al., 2023; Iverson et al., 2017). Each concussion is unique; moreover, many factors influence an individual's recovery time, such as the severity of symptoms, prior mental health concerns, and a history of concussion (Iverson et al., 2017). Therefore, it is important to follow guidance from your medical provider about when it is safe to begin a gradual progression back to school, work, and dance activities.

Stage 1: Relative Rest

The first step in concussion recovery is a brief period of relative cognitive and physical rest and symptom-limited activities; it usually lasts for 24 to 48 hours. Relative rest can help alleviate initial symptoms and reduce the demand on the injured brain (Silverberg et al., 2020). This stage includes visual rest from screens, such as reducing phone and computer use (Leddy et al., 2023). Complete rest—including fully isolating a head-injured person or keeping them in a quiet, dark space—is generally not recommended. During this period, dancers may do activities of daily living and even some gentle stretching that does not exacerbate their symptoms (Leddy et al., 2023).

Stages 2 to 6: Return to School, Work, and Dance

As the concussion symptoms improve, your health care provider will begin to increase both your cognitive and physical activities. The progression will be individualized and gradual, ensuring that symptoms do not worsen as you move to the next stage. In general, it is advised to wait at least 24 hours before moving to the next stage (McCrory et al., 2017), but any advancement of activity should be systematic and monitored by a qualified health care professional (Patricios, Schneider et al., 2023). Key to success is establishing a partnership with a health care provider who is experienced in concussion management; they will be able to adjust your activities according to your clinical status, only clearing you for full return to dance when it is safe to do so. Remember, it is crucial that you care really well for your brain; it's the only one you've got, and it has to last for your lifetime.

Stage 2 Under the guidance of your health care provider, you may start some light aerobic exercise at an intensity that does not increase symptoms. This type of exercise is called **subsymptom threshold aerobic exercise training**. Research has shown that this type of training can safely speed the recovery process (Leddy et al., 2019). During this stage, you will also prepare to return to school and work (if applicable) by doing short bouts (5-15 min at a time) of cognitive activities such as reading, homework, or screen time (DeMatteo et al., 2019; Purcell et al., 2019).

Stage 3 During the next stage, you will return to school and work with accommodations depending on your symptoms. Commonly used accommodations to help concussed individuals tolerate a return to cognitive activities include the following (Purcell et al., 2019):

- Partial days and frequent breaks
- Modified assignments or workload
- Extended time for tests and assignments
- Environmental changes to improve focus and reduce distractions or stimulation

If it does not exacerbate symptoms, you may choose to watch dance classes with accommodations. You may only be comfortable watching for a short time, wearing earplugs if you experience noise sensitivity, or wearing sunglasses for light sensitivity. For physical activity, you may also begin some dance-specific training such as balance and stability work, gentle warm-ups, and even ballet barre (Russell et al., 2021).

Stage 4 During this stage, you will return to school and work full-time, gradually decreasing your accommodations. Dance activity will increase to noncontact choreography, including floor work, jumps, and (eventually) turns (DeMatteo et al., 2019; Russell et al., 2021). It is important to work with your health care team through this progression to address any deconditioning that may have occurred during your recovery. Additionally, the risk of musculoskeletal injury increases after a concussion; this increase is likely due to subtle, unresolved impairments in neural control. These impairments can affect postural stability, reaction time, and joint awareness, increasing your risk for injuries such as ankle sprains (McPherson et al., 2019).

Stage 5 At this point, your health care provider will clear you to dance with full effort in classes and rehearsals. Dancer-to-dancer contact also is introduced at this stage; in other words, you can return to partnering, contact improvisation, acrobatics, tumbling, and more intense floor work (Stein et al., 2014).

Pitfalls in Returning to Dance

Dance-specific pitfalls can occur when returning to full dance following a concussion, and certain potentially aggravating activities may be best saved until near the end of a recovery plan. These activities include repetitive turns (e.g., fouettés), stage lighting, loud music or percussion, movements requiring body inversion (e.g., shoulder stands), dancing on unstable surfaces (e.g., unique set pieces), or wearing cumbersome headgear in specific costuming. Extra caution and additional graduated return to these activities are essential.

Stage 6 The final stage of recovery is the return to full performance. Your medical provider should give clearance to dance without restrictions after you have successfully progressed satisfactorily through each prior stage. Complying with your medical provider's recommendations ensures that you do not return prematurely (while your brain is still recovering).

Prolonged Recovery

As mentioned, every concussion is unique and will recover in its own time frame. Research suggests that the average length of time for full return to activity is 19.8 days when a concussion is cared for properly (Patricios, Schneider, et al., 2023). However, a small percentage of cases require prolonged recovery. When concussion symptoms linger beyond 4 weeks, it is often termed **postconcussive syndrome** or **persistent postconcussion symptoms** (Leddy et al., 2017; Harmon et al., 2019). Some predictors of a prolonged recovery include a greater number and severity of reported symptoms, a history of prior concussion, and a history of mental health diagnosis (Iverson et al., 2017). Persistent symptoms do not necessarily mean continued injury to the brain. It is important to work with your health care provider to investigate reasons for continued symptoms and devise a treatment plan to address them (Harmon et al., 2019). Management of postconcussion syndrome or persistent postconcussive symptoms requires a multidisciplinary team and a variety of treatments and targeted therapies, such as the following (Ellis et al., 2016; Patricios et al., 2023):

- Subsymptom threshold aerobic exercise training
- **Vestibular and ocular rehabilitation**
- Physical therapy for the cervical spine
- Medications to manage headaches and migraines
- Psychological care

Minimizing Risk of Concussion in Dance

There is no single proven intervention to consistently eliminate the risk of concussion, nor has there been extensive research in this area on dancers (Waltzman & Sarmiento, 2019). Naturally, the best way to prevent a concussion is to avoid an impact to the brain. This approach includes proper technique during any movements with the potential for whiplash as well as awareness of your fellow dancers to avoid collisions, falls, and partnering errors. Maintaining a safe environment by monitoring the conditions of the floor (e.g., ensuring it is not slippery) and providing enough space for the number of people in the room are additional measures to prevent impacts to the head (Stein et al., 2014). Use of headgear (e.g., a helmet) has been extensively studied in high-risk sports. Although it is excellent at preventing skull fractures and brain bleeding, it does not significantly reduce concussion incidence (Harmon et al., 2019). Given that dancers rarely wear headgear, and certainly not routinely for class or rehearsal, it is not a recommended intervention.

Unfortunately, the greatest risk factor for a concussion is a history of previous concussion. Subsequent concussions carry additional risks such as a slower recovery time and concerns of cognitive decline, mood disorders, and degenerative disease in the brain (McAllister & McCrea, 2017). Future research is needed to establish the consequences of multiple concussions; nevertheless, is it critical to minimize additional concussion risk if you have a history of concussion (Abrahams et al., 2014). Following correct return to dance guidelines may decrease the risk for subsequent concussions (Harmon et al., 2019).

Common Head Injuries Other Than Concussions

Traumatic brain injury (TBI) is defined as a disturbance of brain function due to an external force. TBI can be caused by a wide variety of mechanisms within the brain itself (Khellaf et al., 2019). A wide range of mechanisms can disrupt normal brain function, including microscopic cellular damage and large collections of blood around the brain. A complete review of TBI is beyond the scope of this chapter; however, if a dancer experiences a head injury, it is important to recognize that more severe levels of brain injury exist beyond concussion.

Concussions are a type of mild TBI. However, concussions themselves are no longer categorized as mild, moderate, or severe because all concussions must be taken seriously and require appropriate medical attention. Brain injuries as a whole are diagnosed as mild, moderate, and severe, based on the following criteria (Lin & Wroten, 2022):

- Amount of time the person is unresponsive or has altered responsiveness
- Presence of bleeding within the cranium
- Presence of **skull fracture**
- Duration of hospital stay
- Glasgow Coma Scale score (figure 14.7)
- Ranchos Los Amigos Scale score (figure 14.8)

For example, a dancer with a mild brain injury, such as a concussion, may experience no or little time unconscious, no bleeding around the brain or fractures of the skull bones, no extended hospitalization, a Glasgow Coma Scale score of 12 to 15 (figure 14.7), and no need to be evaluated by the Ranchos Los Amigos Scale. Alternatively, a dancer with a

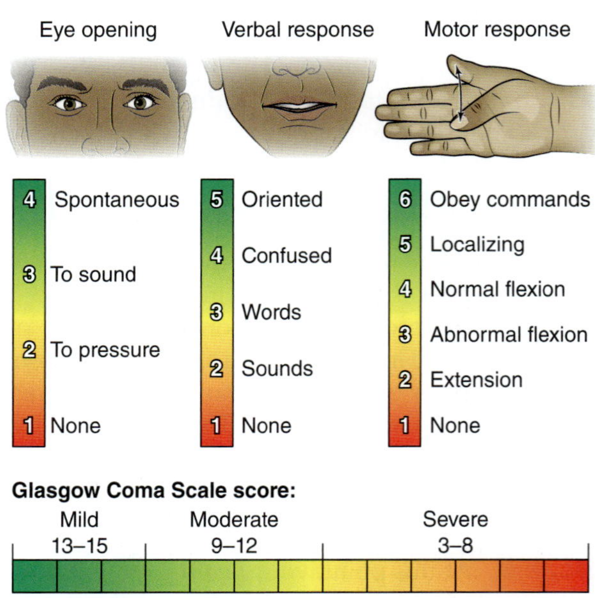

Figure 14.7 Glasgow Coma Scale, one of the tools used to diagnose the severity of a brain injury.

Level I
No Response:
Total Assistance

- No response to external stimuli

Level II
Generalized Response:
Total Assistance

- Responds inconsistently and non-purposefully to external stimuli
- Responses are often the same regardless of the stimulus

Level III
Localized Response:
Total Assistance

- Responds inconsistently and specifically to external stimuli
- Responses are directly related to the stimulus, for example, patient withdraws or vocalizes to painful stimuli
- Responds more to familiar people (friends and family) versus strangers

Level IV
Confused/Agitated:
Maximal Assistance

- The individual is in a hyperactive state with bizarre and non-purposeful behavior
- Demonstrates agitated behavior that originates more from internal confusion than the external environment
- Absent short-term memory

Level V
Confused, Inappropriate Non-Agitated:
Maximal Assistance

- Shows increase in consistency with following and responding to simple commands
- Responses are non-purposeful and random to more complex commands
- Behavior and verbalization is often inappropriate, and individual appears confused and often confabulates
- If action or task is demonstrated and individual can perform but does not initiate tasks on own
- Memory is severely impaired and learning new information is difficult
- Different from level IV in that individual does not demonstrate agitation to internal stimuli. However, they can show agitation to unpleasant external stimuli.

Level VI
Confused, Appropriate:
Moderate Assistance

- Able to follow simple commands consistently
- Able to retain learning for familiar tasks they performed pre-injury (brushing teeth, washing face) but unable to retain learning for new tasks
- Demonstrates increased awareness of self, situation, and environment but unaware of specific impairments and safety concerns
- Responses may be incorrect secondary to memory impairments but appropriate to the situation

Level VII
Automatic, Appropriate:
Minimal Assistance for Daily Living Skills

- Oriented in familiar settings
- Able to perform daily routine automatically with minimal to absent confusion
- Demonstrates carry over for new tasks and learning in addition to familiar tasks
- Superficially aware of their diagnosis but unaware of specific impairments
- Continues to demonstrate lack of insight and decreased judgment and safety awareness
- Beginning to show interest in social and recreational activities in structured settings
- Requires at least minimal supervision for learning and safety purposes

Level VIII
Purposeful, Appropriate:
Standby Assistance

- Consistently oriented to person, place and time
- Independently carries out familiar tasks in a non-distracting environment
- Beginning to show awareness of specific impairments and how they interfere with tasks, however, requires standby assistance to compensate
- Able to use assistive memory devices to recall daily schedule
- Acknowledges others' emotional states and requires only minimal assistance to respond appropriately
- Demonstrates improvement of memory and ability to consolidate the past and future events
- Often depressed, irritable, and with low frustration threshold

Level IX
Purposeful, Appropriate:
Standby Assistance on Request

- Able to shift between different tasks and complete them independently
- Aware of and acknowledges impairments when they interfere with tasks and able to use compensatory strategies to cope
- Unable to independently anticipate obstacles that may arise secondary to impairment
- With assistance, able to think about consequences of actions and decisions
- Acknowledges the emotional needs of others with standby assistance.
- Continues to demonstrate depression and low frustration threshold

Level X
Purposeful, Appropriate:
Modified Independent

- Able to multitask in many different environments with extra time or devices to assist
- Able to create own methods and tools for memory retention
- Independently anticipates obstacles that may occur as a result of impairments and take corrective actions
- Able to independently make decisions and act appropriately but may require more time or compensatory strategies
- Demonstrates intermittent periods of depression and low frustration threshold when under stress
- Able to appropriately interact with others in social situations

Figure 14.8 Ranchos Los Amigos Scale, which is used for patients with moderate to severe brain injury.

Adapted from Lin and Wroten (2022).

severe traumatic brain injury may be unresponsive for a long time and require emergency transportation to a nearby medical center; imaging may show fractures, bleeding, or both around the brain. This situation may require the dancer to undergo surgery or have a long stay in a hospital. They would have a Glasgow Coma Scale score of 3 to 8 and a Rancho Los Amigos Scale score of 1 to 5 at the time of injury, but they would hopefully move to a higher score as their condition improved.

Brain injuries have a wide spectrum of severity, and they can be unpredictable when first diagnosed. Although moderate and severe brain injuries are rare in dancers and traditional sports athletes, they are important to recognize quickly because they require different treatment than a concussion; moreover, they are considered medical emergencies. If a dancer is unconscious or unresponsive, has had a significant head injury, or is not responding with usual alertness, emergency medical services should be called immediately. Always keep in mind that any dancer suspected of having a major injury to their brain should also be suspected of having a serious injury to their cervical spine; therefore, anyone in their vicinity should use extreme caution in moving the injured dancer.

Skull Fracture

A skull fracture occurs when the force of the impact to the cranium is severe enough to cause a break in one or more bones surrounding the head. It may occur in any area of the skull, and it can result in additional injuries to structures nearby. For example, a traumatic force around the eye may cause a fracture to the eye socket, which could then result in altered function of the eye itself. This injury is called an orbital blowout fracture, and it requires immediate evaluation to ensure correct management that protects eye function (Boyette et al., 2015).

Hematoma or Hemorrhage

A skull fracture or traumatic brain injury can also result in bleeding in or around the brain, called **hematoma** or **hemorrhage**. Figure 14.9 shows hematomas in the brain. Because the bony cranium around the brain cannot expand, the blood causes pressure on the brain, which in turn may result in permanent damage to brain function and even in death. A subdural hematoma is caused by damage to the bridging veins, which can bleed slower than an artery. An epidural hematoma is caused by damage to the middle meningeal artery, which tends to bleed more quickly compared to a vein. Both of these conditions must be evaluated and treated urgently. As a general principle, if a dancer has a severe impact to their head and is unconscious or has altered responsiveness, emergency services should be immediately activated and the dancer should be transported to a hospital. These types of injuries require urgent diagnosis with imaging, and they may need surgery to relieve pressure on the brain before permanent damage or death occurs (Aromatario et al., 2021).

If a dancer drops to the floor and is unresponsive, it does not mean they have had a brain injury. Sudden collapse or altered consciousness can occur for many reasons, such as seizures, syncope (fainting), electrolyte and water imbalances, and conditions of the heart or blood vessels (Asplund et al., 2011; Maron et al., 2014). Any dancer who collapses and is not responding should be evaluated immediately by emergency medical services.

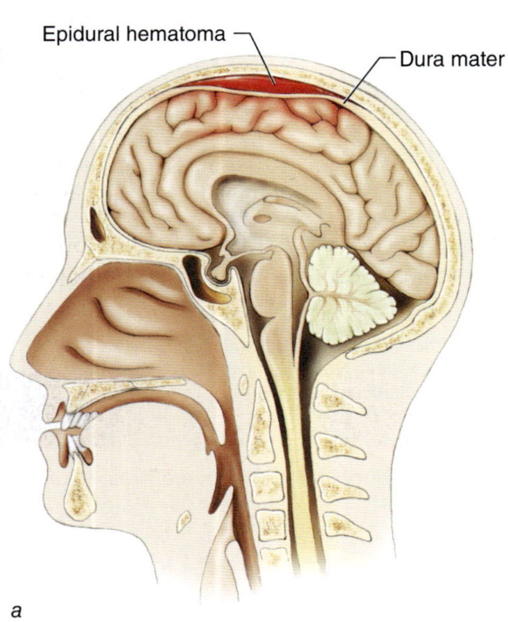

Figure 14.9 A hematoma is a collection of blood around the brain that can push inward against the brain because of the unyielding skull. *(a)* An epidural hematoma occurs outside the dura mater, between it and the skull. *(b)* A subdural hematoma occurs under the dura mater.

Conclusions and Practical Relevance

The brain is a complex organ with many supporting structures, and any injury to the head or brain can cause multiple challenges throughout the body. A concussion is a mild traumatic injury to the brain, and an impact to the head is not necessary for a dancer to have a concussion. It is important to not miss a concussion or a more serious brain injury; therefore, any possible concussion or brain injury should be taken seriously. If you suspect a concussion in yourself or another dancer, you should report the injury to someone in charge or to a qualified health care professional who can help you take appropriate steps toward diagnosis and correct treatment.

To minimize the risk of a prolonged recovery, a dancer must seek immediate evaluation and avoid returning to dance until cleared to do so by a licensed health care professional with training in managing concussions. Concussions should not be confused with other brain injuries, many of which can be very serious; thus, proper diagnosis and close monitoring are key. Any dancer suspected of having a more serious injury—or who is unresponsive—should be evaluated immediately at an emergency department or hospital. With correct diagnosis and treatment, dancers should expect to recover from a concussion and return fully to their activity.

Discussion Questions

1. What is the culture of concussion reporting in your dance environment? Can it be improved? What are ways that you, your institution, or your organization can encourage concussion safety and minimize risk?
2. What was your previous understanding of concussion symptoms before reading this chapter? Were you surprised that certain symptoms (e.g., loss of consciousness) do not necessarily occur with a concussion? What other points of interest did you find in this chapter? Do you think you could recognize the symptoms of a concussion in yourself or in a fellow dancer?
3. Discuss the relationship of a multisystem concussion assessment and the anatomy of the brain. What part of the brain anatomy and function did you find the most interesting? Why is it necessary to look at many different functions to determine the presence of a brain injury?
4. Have you ever experienced a dance-related concussion? Does the low rate reported in the scientific literature surprise you, or did you expect it? What would likely happen to that rate if dancers were in an environment where safety and reporting of concussions were prioritized and encouraged?
5. What styles of dance or movements do you think are most likely to cause a concussion? What ways can you identify to help prevent concussions in these movements or dance styles?
6. Do you know anyone who has experienced a serious brain injury? What should you look for to indicate that a dancer's injury may be severe? What should you do if you think someone has experienced a severe brain injury?

WWW Go to HK*Propel* to access supplemental information and activities connected to chapter content.

Part IV

Coordinated Safety and Wellness

15

Working Effectively With Health Care Professionals

Tina J. Wang, MD
Carina Nasrallah, MS, ATC, LAT, CISSN, PAM-C
Gayanne Grossman, PT, EdM, BFA, FIADMS
Jeffrey A. Russell, PhD, ATC

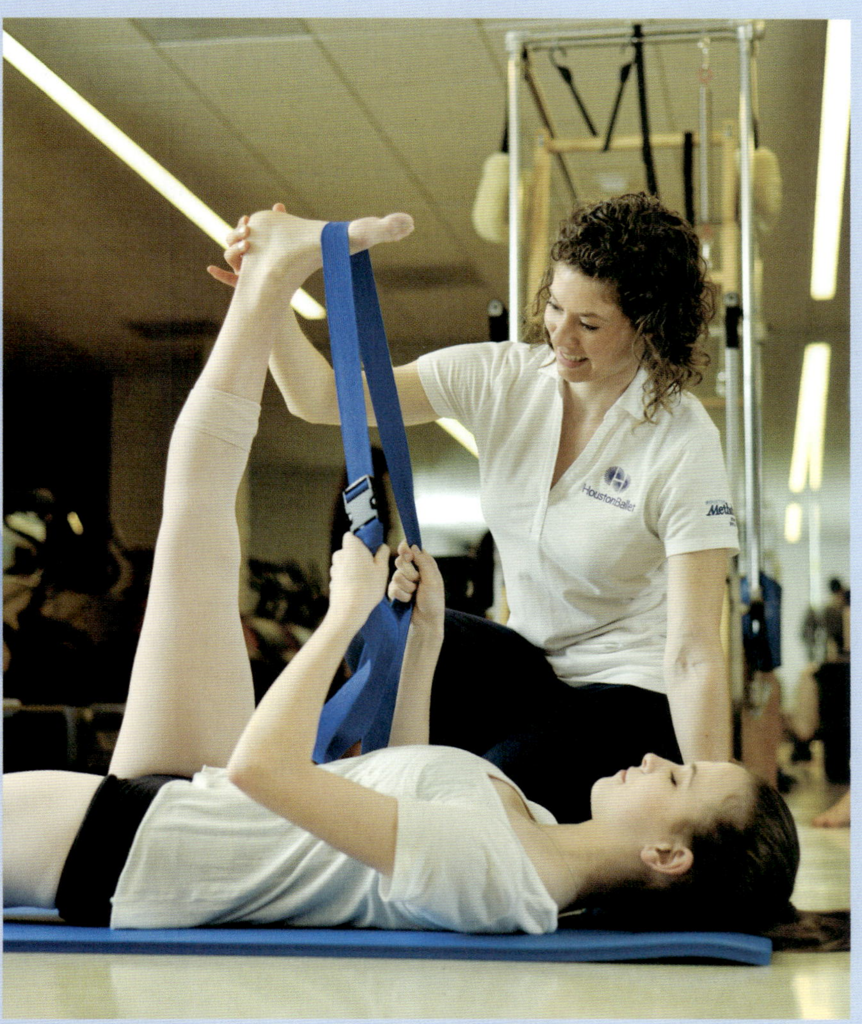

Houston Ballet, Houston, Texas. Athletic Trainer Carina Nasrallah working with dancer Claire Coffman. Photo: Carina Nasrallah.

Key Terms

- allied health professional
- emergency department
- clinical symptoms
- hospital-affiliated outpatient center
- performing arts medicine clinic
- private practices
- red flags
- student health center
- subclinical symptoms
- urgent care center
- walk-in clinic

One of the main reasons dancers don't like to report injuries is that they have a history of poor relationships with health care professionals. However, that situation does not have to continue. Many talented, compassionate health care professionals are willing to help dancers. In this chapter, you will learn how to better navigate the complex, often mysterious world of health care.

LEARNING OBJECTIVES

After completing this chapter, you will be able to do the following:

- Classify various health care practitioners and their areas of expertise.
- Describe different types of health care clinics and which is most appropriate for a given situation.
- Differentiate between subclinical and clinical symptoms.
- Appraise whether a cluster of signs and symptoms should be evaluated by a health care professional.

Dancers experience a high rate of injury (Rinonapoli et al., 2020; Russell, 2013); this high rate includes university dancers (Air et al., 2014; Wang & Russell, 2018; Weigert, 2005). Certainly, it is the goal of dancers and all who work with them to reduce the risk of sustaining injuries. However, when injuries do occur, determining when it is necessary to access health care is pivotal to ideal outcomes, and understanding how to communicate with health care providers reaps benefits for dancers who invariably want to return to dancing from an injury as quickly as possible.

A major barrier to adequate health intervention is prior negative experiences with the health care profession (Air et al., 2014; Thomas & Tarr, 2009; Wang & Russell, 2018). Nonetheless, dancers still need to access health care when they have injuries (figure 15.1). Being able to navigate the health care landscape—knowing when, where, and from whom to seek care—can help smooth out the experience and optimize care.

Types of Health Care Providers

As discussed throughout this book, dancers and dance teachers experience various types of injuries from minor to major. Some injuries can have serious consequences when they are not treated properly or in a timely manner; other injuries heal on their own. Dancers and teachers often wonder what type of health care provider to see for a correct diagnosis and treatment. How to take this first step is frequently complicated by what services are (or are not) available on campus, and by what you can (or cannot) access in the broader communities where you live, where your parents or caregivers live, or where you attend university. Some university dancers may choose to return to a trusted health care provider at home; others may not have that luxury. A basic understanding of how to navigate the health care system can save you time and money because obtaining a correct diagnosis allows treatment to begin sooner, thus aiding rehabilitation.

Several types of health care providers work with dancers, and they can provide needed services. Identifying every possible practitioner type and credential is not possible in this book; however, table 15.1 lists some of the ones most commonly encountered. Keep in mind that one can gain some very impressive-sounding credentials through relatively short, nonrigorous online or in-person courses. These types of courses are not necessarily bad or of low quality; however, the variability in educational pathways highlights the importance of researching the academic and clinical background of practitioners you consult. In the United States and most other countries, health care providers must have a license or registration in addition to academic degrees and qualifications.

Many variables and characteristics determine a professional's expertise and suitability for working with dancers, and they can be objective or subjective. Primary factors include university education, professional education, continuing education, background in the arts, length of experience caring for artists, and attitude and demeanor (i.e., bedside manner). Many health care providers fall short in the way they present themselves to patients who are dancers. Research by Wang and Russell (2018) reported that 55 percent of university dancers identified negative experiences with their providers. Of those dancers, 70 percent felt that their providers did not understand them, and 43 percent indicated that they received unhelpful advice. While this finding is somewhat discouraging, it supports the need for you to carefully select those professionals who care for you. Avoiding the opportunity to seek care for recurring pain or an injury should not be an option.

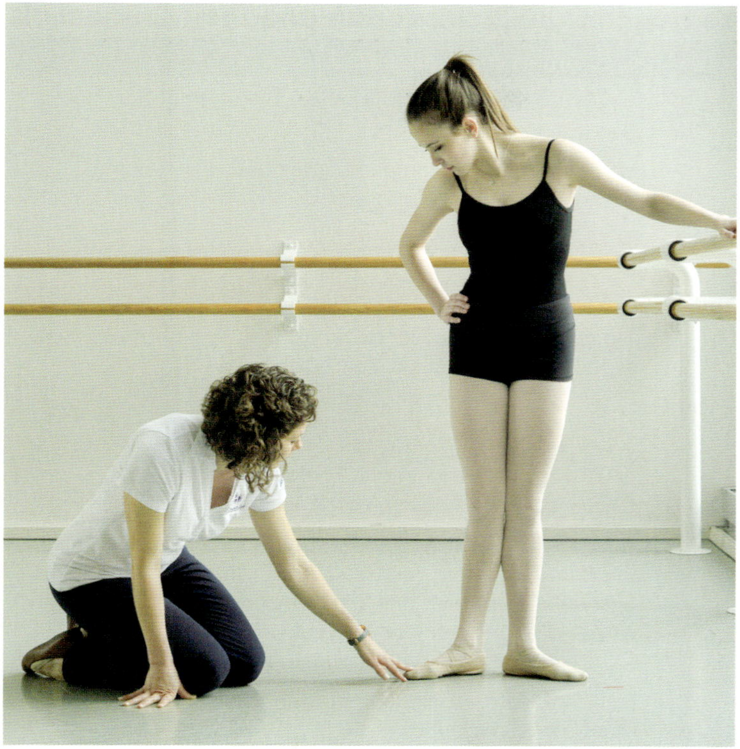

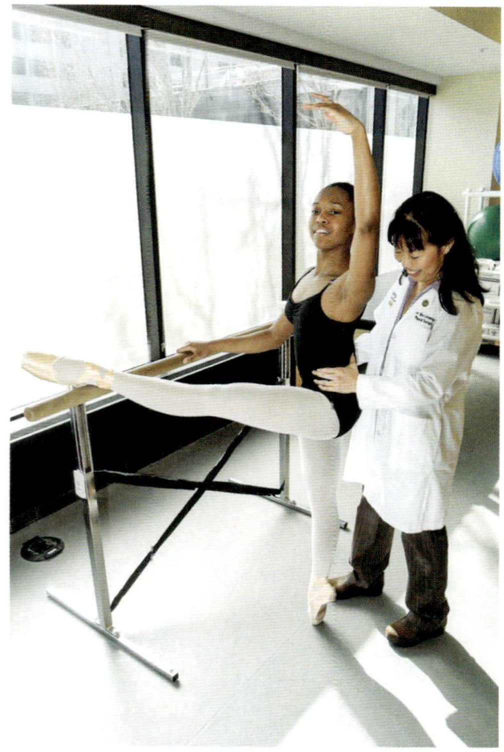

Figure 15.1 Finding a licensed health care professional who specializes in dance medicine or performing arts medicine can greatly improve a dancer's ability to receive the care necessary to return to dance.

(*a*) Dancer Claire Coffman with athletic trainer Carina Nasrallah. Photo: Carina Nasrallah. (*b*) Dancer Sylicia Gregory with physical therapist Lynnette Khoo-Summers. Photo: Washington University School of Medicine

Different health care professionals have different types of training, and each provider's scope of practice (the kinds of procedures they are licensed to perform) varies depending on that training. It is important that you be generally familiar with these different types of training. Thus, you can determine if a practitioner is qualified to perform the care you are seeking and whether it is within the guidelines, regulations, and laws of their professional associations and licensing bodies. They may have many impressive certificates hanging on the walls of their office, but it is you—the patient—who must verify that the practitioner is able and willing to communicate with you and provide the care you need. If not, seek someone who *is* able and willing.

MD and DO Physicians and Surgeons

Although many dancers seek advice from their teachers first (Air et al., 2014; Russell & Wang, 2018), dance teachers are not licensed to practice health care. Thus, your first step should always be a correct diagnosis from a qualified health care provider. Physicians and surgeons have the highest level of training and licensing. Often they are called doctors; however, be aware that many individuals may rightly be addressed as "Dr." (e.g., individuals with a doctor of philosophy, doctor of education, doctor of physical therapy, doctor of athletic training, or other doctoral degrees) without being physicians or surgeons. Note, too, that all surgeons may be called physicians, but not all physicians are surgeons. Surgeons have very specialized additional training to utilize invasive operative techniques as they care for patients. In some medical schools and countries, both labels may be employed, each for a specific type of doctor. Moreover, members and fellows of the Royal College of Surgeons are addressed as "Mr.," "Mrs.," "Miss," or "Ms." rather than as "Dr." To add to the confusion, outside the United States, a physician or surgeon who is a full professor at a university is properly addressed as "Professor" and not "Dr."

In the United States, physicians can be a Doctor of Medicine (MD) or a Doctor of Osteopathic Medicine (DO). These two degrees provide the same rights and privileges to practice medicine. DOs in the United States can also practice osteopathic manipulation. The practices of DOs in other countries are

Table 15.1 **Common Types of Dance Health Care Professionals and Their Credentials**

Type of professional	Credentials commonly used
Physicians and surgeons	
• Doctor of medicine	MD MBBS, MBChB (in some countries belonging to the Commonwealth of Nations)
• Doctor of osteopathic medicine (same rights, privileges, and responsibilities as MD in the U.S.)	DO
• Doctor of podiatric medicine (podiatrist)	DPM (Chiropodist is an older name for this type of professional, especially in Australia, Canada, and the UK)
Allied health professionals and nonphysician medical professionals	
• Athletic therapist (Canada and Ireland)	CAT(C) = Certified Athletic Therapist (Canada) CAT = Certified Athletic Therapist (Ireland)
• Athletic trainer (U.S. and select other countries, including Japan, Korea, and Taiwan)	ATC, AT, LAT, ATL, ATR (note that all except ATC usually refer to a U.S. state license or registration; ATC identifies one who has passed a U.S. national certification exam) DAT = doctor of athletic training
• Dietitian	RD = registered dietitian RDN = registered dietitian nutritionist LD = licensed dietitian
• Graduate registered sport rehabilitator (UK)	BASRaT-reg
• Massage therapist	LMT
• Nurse practitioner	NP-C, FNP-C, ANP-C, PNP-C (and several others, depending on their training) DNP = doctor of nursing practice
• Occupational therapist	OT; OTR OTD = doctor of occupational therapy
• Occupational therapy assistant	COTA
• Physical therapist (U.S.) • Physiotherapist/physio (outside U.S.)	PT, LPT, RPT DPT = doctor of physical therapy MCSP (UK)
• Physical therapy assistant	PTA
• Physician assistant • Physician associate	PA-C
Mental health professionals	
• Psychiatrist (physician)	MD, DO (U.S.), MBBS, MBChB
• Psychologist • Clinical psychologist • Sport psychologist	LP (Some do not use LP, but all licensed psychologists must hold a doctoral degree, such as a PhD or PsyD.)
• Professional counselor	LPC, LCPC, LPCC, LMHC
• Social worker	LSW, LISW, CSW, LCSW, MSW, LMSW
Other health care practitioners	
• Doctor of chiropractic (chiropractor)	DC
• Osteopath	DO = diploma in osteopathy (Outside of U.S.: nonphysician practitioner who uses the principles of osteopathy; training may allow use of other credentials)

Note that different countries and localities have different certification, licensing, and registration laws and regulations. This is especially true for mental health professionals.

different from those in the United States; outside of the United States, an awarded DO degree stands for *diploma in osteopathy*, and MOst stands for *master of osteopathy*. Non-US-based DOs also perform osteopathic manipulation (Pollard-Smith & Thomson, 2017); however, they are not physicians, and they are not licensed to practice medicine.

Physicians specialize in a variety of disciplines. Generally, specialties are surgical and nonsurgical. The American College of Surgeons (2022) lists 14 areas of surgical specialization. Orthopaedic (orthopedic) surgeons are most likely to be enlisted to help dancers because they specialize in bones, joints, ligaments, muscles, and tendons.

Nonsurgical specialties are far more numerous, and choosing the right one can be confusing. The nonsurgical physicians who treat dancers are usually primary care physicians with nonsurgical orthopaedic training (and often sports medicine training, too) and physical medicine and rehabilitation physicians (also called physiatrists). When you call for an appointment, ask the office staff if the doctors treat the type of injury for which you need care. The office's web page will be informative, too. It will likely describe what types of doctors are in the office, their educational backgrounds, and what conditions they treat.

Non-MD and Non-DO Medical Practitioners

Several types of medical practitioners do not hold a doctor of medicine (MD) or doctor of osteopathy (DO) degree; in other words, they are not physicians. The following sections describe the ones whom dancers are most likely to access for health care.

Nurse Practitioners

Nurse practitioners are nurses who possess a master's or doctorate degree, and they have specialized clinical training in addition to that required to be a registered nurse. They often work in physicians' offices, hospitals, and urgent care centers—across all medical and surgical specialties—where they increase the capacity of a facility to care for patients. They function as autonomous health care providers, focusing heavily on overall health management, health promotion, health education, and whole-person health care (American Association of Nurse Practitioners, 2022).

Physician Assistants/Associates

Physician assistants (also known as physician associates) practice medicine across the health care spectrum, from primary care to specialty care; they work in all health care settings from primary care clinics to tertiary health care systems. They practice medicine in collaboration with physicians and other members of the health care team, thus increasing access for patients seeking medical care. According to the American Academy of Physician Associates (2022), "PAs (physician associates/physician assistants) are licensed clinicians who practice medicine in every specialty and setting. Trusted, rigorously educated, and trained healthcare professionals, PAs are dedicated to expanding access to care and transforming health and wellness through patient-centered, team-based medical practice" (para. 1).

Podiatrists

Doctors of podiatric medicine—also known as podiatrists (or, in some countries, chiropodists)—are physicians and surgeons for the foot, ankle, and lower leg (American Podiatric Medical Association, 2022). They can undertake nonsurgical approaches to conditions in these areas, such as molding foot orthotics (insoles that correct the anatomical positioning of the feet) and treating corns and ingrown toenails, or they can apply surgical methods when necessary to manage more significant foot and ankle problems. Many podiatrists work with dancers because of the large number of foot and ankle injuries that occur during dance.

Allied Health Professionals

As you can tell from the information in the What Are Allied Health Professionals? sidebar, allied health professionals have important functions in any health care system. It is not practical—or even possible—for medical, surgical, dental, or nursing personnel to provide all health care services. Thus, the practitioners described next are called upon for their specialized roles in delivering excellent, comprehensive care. They are not the only types of allied health professionals, but they represent the ones with whom dancers will most likely engage.

Athletic Trainers

Athletic trainers work under the guidance of or in collaboration with physicians to provide prevention, emergency care, diagnosis, treatment, and rehabilitation of injuries and medical conditions to athletes and other physically active individuals. According to the National Athletic Trainers' Association (2021), "Athletic training is recognized by the American Medical Association (AMA), Health Resources Services Administration (HRSA) and the

What Are Allied Health Professionals?

Dancers typically encounter *allied health professionals* more than any other type of health care provider. Allied health professionals are trained practitioners who provide specific types of health care services and who are not physicians, surgeons, dentists, physician assistants, or nurses. This category of providers includes physical therapists, athletic trainers, massage therapists, and several others. The United States Federal Code defines allied health professionals this way (Legal Information Institute, n.d., 42 U.S. Code § 295p – Definitions. U.S. Code, Title 42, Chapter 6A, Subchapter V, Part G, § 295p. LII):

(5) The term "allied health professional" means a health professional (other than a registered nurse or physician assistant)—

(A) who has received a certificate, an associate's degree, a bachelor's degree, a master's degree, a doctoral degree, or postbaccalaureate training, in a science relating to health care;

(B) who shares in the responsibility for the delivery of health care services or related services, including—

(i) services relating to the identification, evaluation, and prevention of disease and disorders;

(ii) dietary and nutrition services;

(iii) health promotion services;

(iv) rehabilitation services; or

(v) health systems management services; and

(C) who has not received a degree of doctor of medicine, a degree of doctor of osteopathy, a degree of doctor of dentistry or an equivalent degree, a degree of doctor of veterinary medicine or an equivalent degree, a degree of doctor of optometry or an equivalent degree, a degree of doctor of podiatric medicine or an equivalent degree, a degree of bachelor of science in pharmacy or an equivalent degree, a degree of doctor of pharmacy or an equivalent degree, a graduate degree in public health or an equivalent degree, a degree of doctor of chiropractic or an equivalent degree, a graduate degree in health administration or an equivalent degree, a doctoral degree in clinical psychology or an equivalent degree, or a degree in social work or an equivalent degree or a degree in counseling or an equivalent degree.

Department of Health and Human Services (HHS) as an allied health care profession" (para. 1). Athletic trainers have a national certification credential (ATC) as well as state licensing requirements. Athletic therapists are equivalent allied health professionals in Canada and Ireland.

Dietitians

Dietitians provide a variety of advice and consulting about nutrition and meal preparation. Registered dietitians (RD) or registered dietitian nutritionists (RDN) are trained nutrition professionals who

> *advise people on what they should eat in order to achieve healthier lifestyles or a health goal. Some of the job duties that they perform include (but are not limited to): educate others on diet and nutrition, assess a patient's nutritional needs, develop dietetic plans, facilitate group sessions on nutrition and dietetics, provide individual counseling on dietetics and nutrition, help patients in meal planning, collect data, do research, and prepare reports (NutritionEd.org, 2024, para. 4).*

Both the RD and RDN credentials indicate the same training; RD is the more traditional version, and RDN is an updated option (Commission on Dietetic Registration, 2022). Clinical dietitians practice nutritional therapy for medical conditions. Community dietitians focus on education of the public about nutrition, and management dietitians work in food service venues to provide meal planning, menu guidance, and supervision of food preparation operations. In the United States, a registered dietitian (RD or RDN) must also be a licensed dietitian (LD) in states where licensing is required.

Massage Therapists

Massage therapists are licensed providers who are skilled in using manual pressure techniques to treat and restore the body. Massage is a part of integrative medicine that can relieve stress as well as improve pain, function, and circulation (American Massage Therapy Association, 2018). It has positive benefits for muscle tissue (Van Pelt et al., 2021) and for physical and psychological well-being (Espí-López et al., 2020).

Occupational Therapists

Occupational therapists provide therapeutic services that help individuals with injuries, illnesses, or disabilities manage their activities of daily living in the environments where they live and work; it includes working with patients across their life spans. Occupational therapists help adapt a patient's environment to that individual. They are skilled at ensuring that the patient is part of the treatment process (American Occupational Therapy Association, 2022). Occupational therapy assistants may work with occupational therapists in their clinical settings.

Physical Therapists

Physical therapists (called *physiotherapists* or *physios* outside the United States) focus on restoring physical function as they evaluate and treat people with a variety of acute and chronic injuries and illnesses in all age groups. They work in many different settings—including clinics, hospitals, nursing homes, schools, and home health—as therapeutic exercise experts who provide exercise prescriptions, manual therapy techniques, physical function advice, and wellness education (American Physical Therapy Association, 2021). Physical therapy assistants may work with physical therapists in delivering patient care.

Mental Health Professionals

A psychiatrist is a physician who holds a doctor of medicine (MD), doctor of osteopathic medicine (DO in the U.S.), or equivalent degree. Psychiatrists address the diagnosis, treatment, and prevention of mental, emotional, and behavioral health issues, and they are able to assess the psychological and physical aspects of mental health (American Psychiatric Association, 2022). As physicians, psychiatrists can order a wide variety of tests and write prescriptions.

As seen in table 15.1, a variety of specialists exist in psychology, counseling, and social work. They typically specialize in specific age groups or life circumstances of their patients or clients, and they use a variety of tools and techniques to build wellness, healthy behaviors, and emotional resilience (American Psychological Association, 2021). A key factor is the requirement that professionals displaying a Licensed Psychologist credential hold a doctoral degree (PhD or PsyD). Some specialty areas of mental and behavioral health professionals who may interface with dancers include child psychology, sport psychology, industrial and organizational psychology, and other mental and behavioral health practitioners who treat specific conditions such as substance abuse, self-harm, and eating disorders. It is important to remember the axiom *It's okay to not be okay* (National Alliance on Mental Illness, 2022) in reducing the stigma associated with mental health challenges. If you are concerned about your mental health or the mental health of a friend or classmate, please reach out to someone for assistance. You do not need to deal with it on your own. Should the need arise, a number of resources are available in appendix A.

Complementary and Alternative Practitioners

According to the National Center for Complementary and Integrative Health (2021), more than 30 percent of adults and 12 percent of children in the United States utilize health and health care methods that are either not part of mainstream medical practice or that are based on non-Western techniques or philosophies. Dancers may be inclined to consult practitioners in these types of specialties (Haikal et al., 2021; Wang & Russell, 2018). General groupings of these approaches are nutritional, physical, psychological, and combination methods (National Center for Complementary and Integrative Health, 2021). When these methods are used alongside traditional modes of health care, they are termed *complementary care*. When they are used as a substitute for the typical methods used in Western health care, they are termed *alternative practices*. Table 15.2 lists many disciplines that fall under the definition of complementary care. How these practices fit together as part of health care is shown in figure 15.2. Integrative health care involves the careful coordination of conventional and complementary care practices (National Center for Complementary and Integrative Health, 2021).

Acupuncturists assess a patient's syndromes and disharmonies using their diagnostic skills based on principles of traditional Chinese medicine. The basic concept of acupuncture is to use needle insertion at specific places in the body that correlate with anatomical regions or conditions to improve a patient's *qi* (pronounced "chee"). The term *qi* represents a person's life energy or life force; in this way of thinking, *qi* runs through pathways or channels in the body, which are called meridians (Council of Colleges of Acupuncture and Herbal Medicine, n.d.). The technique has been suggested as effective for a variety of conditions; however, pain relief is most verified by research (National Institute for Complementary and Integrative Health, 2016). Because acupuncture is

Table 15.2 Examples of Complementary Health and Health Care Practices

Category of practice	Complementary practices
Nutritional	Herbs
	Vitamins and minerals
	Probiotics
Physical, somatic, and psychological	Tai chi
	Yoga
	Acupuncture
	Massage therapy
	Spinal manipulation
	Osteopathic manipulation
	Art therapy
	Music therapy
	Dance
	Movement therapy
	Mindfulness-based stress reduction
	Qigong
	Hypnotherapy
	Pilates
	Feldenkrais Method
	Alexander Technique
Other	Homeopathy
	Naturopathy
	Reflexology
	Traditional Chinese medicine
	Traditional healers
	Ayurvedic medicine
	Functional medicine

Data from National Center for Complementary and Integrative Health. Available: https://www.nccih.nih.gov/health/complementary-alternative-or-integrative-health-whats-in-a-name.

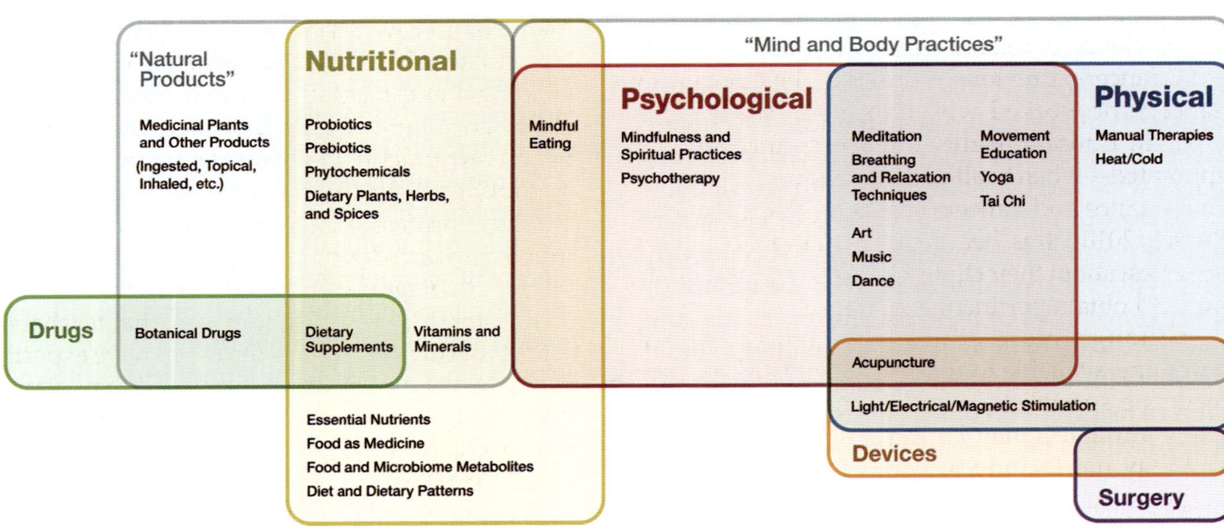

Figure 15.2 Complementary approaches to health care incorporate interfaces between conventional and nonconventional practices. These examples of complementary health approaches fall within the categories of psychological, physical, and nutritional health.

National Center for Complementary and Integrative Health. Available: https://www.nccih.nih.gov/health/complementary-alternative-or-integrative-health-whats-in-a-name.

considered an invasive procedure (since the needles break the skin), treatments should only be applied by qualified, experienced practitioners.

Doctors of chiropractic (chiropractors) are complementary health care providers who treat disorders primarily of the spine, especially malalignment of the vertebrae that can be improved by manipulation. Some chiropractors include conditions beyond the spine (Gliedt et al., 2021). According to the National Board of Chiropractic Examiners (2024), the approach of chiropractors is based on manual techniques that are "natural, nonsurgical, and drugless" (para. 1).

Dance Medicine Specialists

Currently, no standardized or mandatory requirements exist for health care professionals who want to call themselves *dance medicine specialists*, but it is becoming more common for institutions and organizations to offer specialty education related to dance medicine or performing arts medicine, including degrees, certifications, qualifications, and training courses. Because these programs are unregulated and highly varied, clinicians participating in them may or may not obtain real-life experience treating dance related injuries but, at a minimum, should have an interest in or exposure to the nature of dance injuries. Many dance medicine practitioners were (or are) dancers themselves, and this experience is a primary reason they gravitated to this field. Those claiming to specialize in dance medicine should understand dance mechanics, dance training, and the psyche of dancers. They also typically should possess one or more of these characteristics: they have taught dance; lectured about dance injuries, dance science, or related topics; conducted research with dancers; previously provided health care to dancers; or worked with dancers in some other capacity. Dancers readily can sense—and are disappointed—when health care providers do not care about dance and dancers (Lai et al., 2008; Wang & Russell, 2018); thus, health care practitioners should be honest about their clinical background and interests and obtain pertinent experience.

Although more educational pathways are becoming available to those who wish to be dance medicine specialists, obtaining expertise still has many variables, may be introductory or cursory, and may not include methods to correct deficits in dance technique. A skilled health care provider may be adept at diagnosing, correctly treating, and rehabilitating your dance injury, but taking the next step to safely return you to unrestricted dancing may require bigger picture thinking and additional skill sets. Indeed, a full return to dance will be enriched by a multidisciplinary. **collaborative approach** that includes practitioners in the dance teaching and training realms. These individuals are discussed in the next section. In short, not all dance medicine providers can encompass all the skills needed to return an injured dancer to full activity. Dance medicine professionals who are adept at working with dancers demonstrate empathy, know their limits, and readily engage a dancer-patient as a partner in care.

The Role of Professionals Not Licensed in Health Care

Many dancers perceive teachers to be the first-line treatment providers for dance injuries (Air et al, 2014; Russell & Wang, 2018). Although teachers are a valuable resource for dancers, it is important to recognize that they are not licensed health care professionals and do not have any formal training in evaluating and managing dance injuries. Similarly, wellness professionals, professors, strength and conditioning coaches, specialized exercise instructors, and peer dancers have not undergone the rigorous academic and clinical training—nor licensing or registration procedures—necessary to legally practice health care. While it is a natural tendency for these well-intentioned individuals to offer advice based their own experiences with injury, the circumstances and management of each injury are unique to an individual.

Therefore, the appropriate response when approached by a dancer complaining of an injury or pain is to be supportive. Specifically, they should refer a dancer with a suspected injury to a specialized, licensed health care professional while offering emotional and mental encouragement. All advice about an injury should be vetted by a licensed health care practitioner before being implemented. To summarize, instructors, professors, nonlicensed wellness professionals, and anyone else having influence over a dancer (see table 15.3) should never attempt to diagnose or treat dance injuries.

It is important to note, however, that teachers—who know dance students the best—have expertise in dance technique and training, and they play an invaluable supportive role in the rehabilitation of dancers' injuries. Effective teamwork among all stakeholders (dancer, instructors, department leadership, and health care professionals) is important to a dancer's recovery, and it can also be useful in reducing the risk of dance injuries (Bolling et al., 2021; Bolling et al., 2019). Clear and direct communication facilitates focused, reasonable rehabilitation

Table 15.3 **Professionals and Stakeholders Not Licensed to Deliver Health Care**

Artistic staff • Artistic directors • Choreographers • Teachers and instructors • Coaches • Guest artists
Wellness professionals • Strength and conditioning coaches/Personal trainers • Somatic practice instructors • Specialized exercise instructors (Pilates, yoga, Gyrotonics, etc.)
Movement specialists • Kinesiologists • Biomechanists
Others • Human science, exercise science, and biology professors • Peer artists, classmates, friends, and family members who are not medical professionals

goals and helps reduce anxiety in the dancer and the performance production staff. It also reinforces adherence to guidelines and progression in rehabilitation. This integrated approach to athlete health and performance is gaining momentum in the sports literature (Dijkstra et al., 2014; Sporer et al., 2018), and it has direct implications for artistic athletes like dancers, too.

Within this model, the multidisciplinary health care team works synergistically with the coaching (artistic) staff to establish a plan to manage the dancer's health and optimize performance. The **lead practitioner**—who ideally specializes in working with elite performers—is responsible for key clinical decisions related to the dancer's care, but these decisions are made in conjunction with the dancer's and instructors' individual performance goals. This collaborative approach emphasizes the importance of a qualified health care practitioner in the role of a case manager, but it allows autonomy for the staff and dancer to make decisions pertaining to performance and training—as long as they remain within the safety parameters outlined by the clinician.

See the case study in the sidebar for an example of how integrated care can work well.

Knowing When to Pursue Professional Health Care Evaluation

When you are confronted with pain or an injury, there is tremendous value in drawing from the expertise of a knowledgeable health care provider. Pain is one signal that your body uses to alert you to a problem that needs attention; usually, the longer that signal is neglected, the greater the likelihood the problem will worsen. Nevertheless, many dancers avoid seeking care. It is useful to reframe your view of health care as another part of your dance training. For example, consider this question: Would you avoid going to class when your dance teacher wants to help you master a difficult task you have been working toward, such as performing 32 fouettés or perfecting your back shoulder roll? Of course, you wouldn't. Therefore, why would you ignore your body's signals and avoid seeing a physician or other health care professional when they want to help you recover from an injury?

Identifying Signs and Symptoms of Injury

When should a dancer seek out evaluation and treatment for an injury? In chapter 1, *signs* and *symptoms* were introduced as terms that health care practitioners use in reference to evaluating injuries. Signs are characteristics a clinician can see or measure (figure 15.3). Examples of signs include high blood pressure, swelling, a bone deformity that is seen or felt through the skin, and relative looseness of a joint when it is manipulated. Symptoms, on the other hand, are what you feel when something is not quite right; they can be categorized based on severity and how much they affect your ability to participate at full capacity. Examples of symptoms include pain, heart palpitations, blurry vision, and other sensations you feel in your body.

An Integrated Model for Managing a Dancer's Health and Performance

This case study shows clearly how a group of professionals—some licensed health care providers and others not, but all invested in a dancer's well-being and success—work together to create an appropriate plan. The success of this plan relies on skilled health care, effective communication, appropriate accommodations, and well-placed compassion to ensure an injured dancer can continue to dance at as high a level as possible while still respecting the injury process. Notice the integration of various individuals' skills and viewpoints, along with a willingness to embrace modifications for the benefit of the dancer.

A dancer experiences a sharp pain at the back of his ankle that gradually intensifies while jumping during rehearsal. This sensation has been increasing over the past couple of weeks, but now it seems worse. He notifies the teacher that he needs to see the dance department's athletic trainer, someone who specializes in working with performing artists. The teacher reinforces the prudence of this decision, and they dismiss the dancer from rehearsal to seek care.

The athletic trainer performs an initial evaluation and refers the dancer to the department's consulting physician, who also specializes in dance injuries, for X-rays and other imaging to rule out any underlying conditions. The physician diagnoses the injury as Achilles tendinopathy and determines that conservative treatment is appropriate. The dancer follows up with the athletic trainer for manual therapy and rehabilitation exercises.

As part of the treatment, the athletic trainer performs a functional assessment, an evaluation that reveals the dancer forces his turnout due to weakness in the hip; this compensation has contributed to the tendon injury. Moreover, the dancer reports a significant increase in his jumping load recently during rehearsals. The dancer, athletic trainer, teacher, and department chair schedule a meeting to discuss the dancer's treatment plan and goals for the remainder of the semester.

During the meeting, the dancer voices his desire to participate in the fall showcase. It is his senior year, and he hopes to use the video of his performance as an audition piece for professional companies. Collectively, the group decides to keep him in the performance, but transition him to another role that involves less jumping. He also drops an elective technique class to allow time in his schedule to work one-on-one with a Pilates instructor who focuses on exercises and cueing to maximize functional turnout mechanics. The instructor of his remaining technique class advises the dancer to reduce his turnout and decrease the frequency of jumps during center work until his symptoms resolve and the athletic trainer clears him.

Throughout the next three weeks until the fall showcase, the dancer follows the plan precisely while each professional is fully devoted to their role. Progress is made. From a whole-person wellness perspective, the dancer's pain reduces (physical dimension), his strength improves (physical dimension), he attends rehearsals (social dimension), he follows the guidance of the athletic trainer in conjunction with the Pilates instructor and teacher (intellectual dimension), and his emotions are buoyed by the progress (emotional dimension). Overall, he is once again looking forward to staying healthy for the rest of his time in college and to dancing professionally (occupational dimension) as he knows without a doubt that this is what he is destined to do with his life (spiritual dimension).

In this case study, identify all the individuals who participated in some aspect of managing this dancer's care. What were some keys to success? How would breakdowns in communication have affected this situation? Explain the importance of the whole-person wellness approach to success of the dancer in this case (see also chapter 1).

Symptoms are primarily defined as either subclinical or clinical. **Subclinical symptoms** are subtle symptoms that are difficult to report during a clinical evaluation. They may include a difficult-to-describe feeling of pain or a strange pull during a jump. Usually, subclinical symptoms do not limit you from participating; however, you may perceive that they keep you from performing at your optimal level. Therefore, it is valuable to discuss these sensations with a teacher, health care professional, or other trusted individual who can evaluate muscle imbalances, joint looseness, or suboptimal movement patterns. In fact, it may help reduce the chances of an injury.

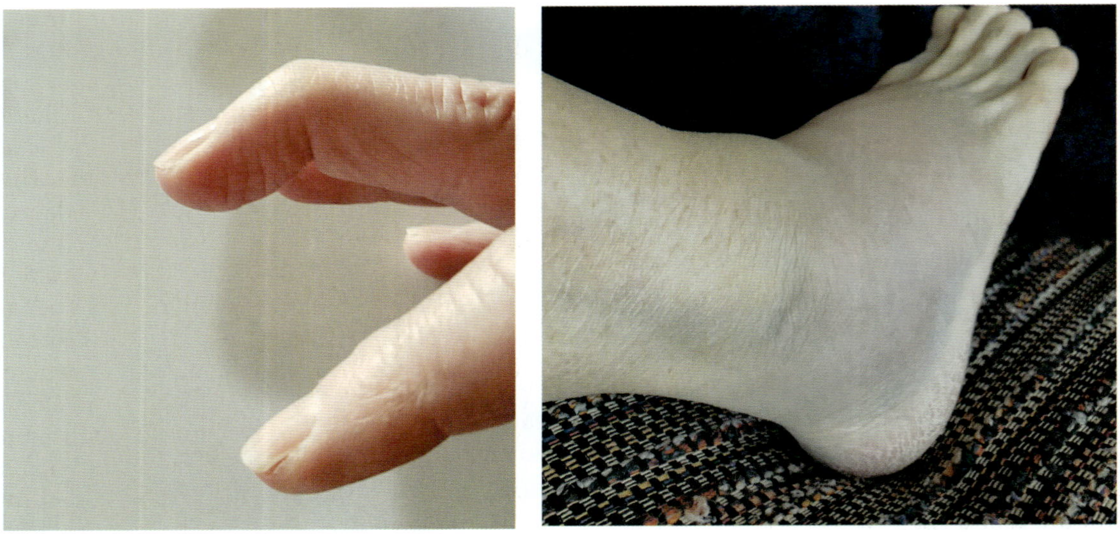

Figure 15.3 Some injuries provide clear signs, or visual clues; others do not. Both of these injuries clearly need attention based on their appearance. However, keep in mind that the absence of an obvious deformity or other outward sign does not mean that an injury is not serious or that it does not need evaluation by a health care professional.

A: Dona Abel; B: Gayanne Grossman

Table 15.4 **Examples of Subclinical and Clinical Symptoms**

Subclinical symptoms	Clinical symptoms (Pain descriptors)
Tightness	Sharp
Pulling	Stabbing
Weakness	Throbbing
Something isn't right	Deep aching
Soreness	Numbness
Wonkiness	Tingling
Imbalance	Shooting

Clinical symptoms, on the other hand, are substantial enough to report to a health care provider; a dancer may purposefully disregard clinical symptoms, but that response is never a good idea. These symptoms provide important information to the clinician as part of an overall diagnostic review. Thus, be sure to describe your symptoms as accurately as possible. Table 15.4 contains examples of subclinical and clinical symptoms.

When mild symptoms arise from lesser injuries such as blisters, cuts, calluses, and minor sprains, you might attempt to self-manage the associated injury. These injuries probably do not warrant evaluation from a health care professional unless red flags develop (as described in the following section). After they heal, consult a teacher, athletic trainer, physical therapist, or other knowledgeable professional to assess for compensatory movement patterns (abnormal activation of muscles[s] to adapt for pain or limitations in joint motion) that could evolve into clinical symptoms. If symptoms continue despite a trial of self-care, you should pursue a health care consultation.

Red Flags of Injury

A **red flag** is a sign or symptom that something may be more serious than it appears, or that an injury is about to progress to a more severe state. If you notice one or more of the following indicators, you should pay attention to it and promptly seek qualified health care advice. These signals should never be ignored, and they should not be self-managed without the guidance of a health care practitioner.

- Persistent or increasing pain
- Pain that disrupts sleep

- Increasing swelling
- Increasing discoloration
- Obvious deformity
- Decreasing function
- Increasing redness (streaking)
- Warm to touch
- Fever or chills
- Numbness
- Tingling

Red Flags of Concussion

While you will find a complete discussion of concussion in dancers in chapter 14, the Concussion Recognition Tool 6 (Echemendia, et al., 2023), or CRT6, pertains to our presentation of red flags. It states that with a head injury,

> *[i]f ANY of the following are reported then the [dancer] should be safely and immediately removed from the [dance activity]. If no qualified medical professional is available, consider transporting by ambulance for urgent medical assessment:*
>
> - *[Dancer] complains of neck pain or tenderness*
> - *Loss of consciousness*
> - *Increasing confusion or deteriorating consciousness state (becoming less responsive, drowsy)*
> - *Severe or increasing headache*
> - *Repeated vomiting*
> - *Increasingly restless, agitative, combative*
> - *Seizure, 'fits,' or convulsion*
> - *Loss of vision or double vision*
> - *Weakness or numbness/tingling in more than one arm or leg*
> - *Visible deformity of the skull*

Adapted from "Concussion Recognition Tool 6," *British Journal of Sports Medicine* 57, no. 11 (2023), 692. doi: 10.1136/bjsports-2023-106851.

The intensity and location of pain are key indicators of what type of injury has occurred and the extent of the tissue damage. The mechanism (cause) of pain also provides important clues. Recall from chapter 10 that *acute injuries* occur suddenly (which is why they are also called traumatic injuries), and they typically result in immediate pain or loss of function, such as when a dancer who lands from a jump and rolls their ankle hears a popping sound accompanied by immediate pain and swelling in the ankle.

In contrast, chronic (overuse) injuries often develop gradually, starting out with mild symptoms that may not seem connected to any specific activity, occurrence, or point in time. Chapter 10 defined *overuse injuries* as a part of *chronic injuries* that can persist for long periods of time when not addressed proactively. One example is a dancer who develops Achilles tendinopathy over the course of several weeks while rehearsing a variation that involves repetitive jumping. It may start out as very manageable, with slight pain, but the desire to keep dancing may override the common sense of seeking care. Again, it is important for you to know that ignoring red flags or pushing through pain may worsen an injury, prolong recovery, and potentially lead to loss of function or even extended time off from dance to allow healing.

Types of Health Care Delivery Settings

University dancers may pursue and receive health care using four basic methods: a student health center, an athletic department clinic, practitioners in the community, and a performing arts medicine clinic (Russell, 2020). These resources are not mutually exclusive, and dancers may use combinations of these settings to pursue care.

The **student health center** is a primary health care clinic dedicated to a university's entire student body. This type of facility is typically staffed by medical doctors, nurse practitioners, physician assistants, and nurses. These professionals are not likely to be trained in or familiar with the specific evaluation of athletes or dancers. Such clinics specialize in preventive care and evaluation of routine primary care issues such as colds, infections, and the varied conditions of a college-aged population.

Athletic department clinics are facilities specializing in sports medicine for collegiate athletes. They are usually staffed by athletic trainers, and often include physical therapists and sports medicine physicians. The clinics excel at treating conventional athletes (e.g., those who play football, volleyball, basketball, soccer, baseball, etc.). They often cannot or will not provide care to dancers because they are busy with their athletes or they are not versed in the specialized knowledge needed to care for dancers' injuries. Occasionally, however, an athletic trainer with a background in dance or who is skilled in dance medicine is available.

Community practitioners are health care providers situated outside of the university setting in the local community around the campus. In the

United States, most frequently they work in **hospital-affiliated outpatient centers** that are overseen by larger hospital institutions or **private practices** that are independently operated rather than paid for or owned by the government or a large company. Some of them may be officially enlisted by the dance department, but in other instances, dancers are on their own to seek care. Depending on your location, qualified dance medicine professionals may or may not be available in your community. Dancers tend to find practitioners by word of mouth (Wang & Russell, 2018). Dance faculty members may maintain a list of providers with whom they have had success in referring their dance students. In the absence of a dedicated on-campus dance medicine clinic, this list is an excellent mechanism of referral because faculty members generally have familiarity with the local community, insights to the health care available in the area, and the ability to develop trusting relationships with medical practitioners.

In a nationalized health care system, dancers may have access to medical practitioners through a country's network where care is provided with no out-of-pocket cost (Air et al., 2014; National Institute of Dance Medicine and Science, 2019). In decentralized health care systems, such as in the United States, dancers may have to arrange payment for whatever services they require either through health insurance or private payment (Wang & Russell, 2018). The extent to which dancers can access specialists will depend on the university's locale and the type of care that is needed.

A dance medicine or **performing arts medicine clinic** located at the university is the ideal setting for a dancer to receive health care. It is a university health care clinic established for the sole purpose of caring for dancers—and perhaps other performing artists—who are also students. The majority of these dance clinics are staffed by athletic trainers, though many are led by physical therapists. Occasionally, community-based physician specialists or physicians from the university's medical center may visit the clinic to provide evaluations, nuanced diagnoses, and other necessary injury management.

Finally, should you have difficulty finding a suitable qualified health care practitioner in your area who understands dance and dancers, you may wish to consider a provider network such as Doctors for Dancers (https://doctorsfordancers.com/). This organization specializes in connecting dancers with qualified dance health practitioners of all types. While focused primarily in the United States, Doctors for Dancers does have some international affiliates and is continually expanding.

Appointment Clinic Versus Walk-In Clinic

When seeking health care, there are several types of facilities you may locate on campus or in the community. It is important to know what the clinic requires of patients and what types of services to expect; for example, you may need to request an appointment to see a practitioner. Most community outpatient facilities (e.g., physicians' offices, physical therapy clinics, orthopaedic or specialty clinics) operate this way.

With the popular increase in on-demand health care, walk-in or no-appointment-needed clinics have become more common. In the university setting, student health centers or athletic department clinics may not require advance appointments; students can walk in at any time during clinic hours and expect same-day care. Another type of **walk-in clinic** is either located inside a retail building (e.g., pharmacy, grocery store, or other convenient location) or is a free-standing structure. This type of clinic is designed to fill the need for quick, uncomplicated treatments for nonemergent illnesses (e.g., headaches, sore throats) and for preventive services (e.g., vaccines, vital sign monitoring). Rarely do these clinics have any advanced medical or imaging equipment. This type of clinic is usually much less expensive than an urgent care or emergency department visit, but it is not appropriate for specialty care or dance-related injuries.

Urgent Care Center Versus Emergency Department

Urgent care centers and **emergency departments** (figure 15.4) also operate on a walk-in basis. Some universities—particularly large urban universities with medical schools—may have on-campus urgent care or emergency departments. Urgent care centers typically only have X-ray capabilities, and they are usually staffed by family medicine physicians or physician assistants who are not trained in dance-related injuries. They frequently have extended hours (weekends and evenings) that receive higher patient volume; this may translate to longer waits to receive care. The usual care they provide includes rudimentary initial assessment of an injury and first aid.

Emergency departments are designed to be an entry point into a hospital for in-patient treatment and life-saving procedures. They are not intended to service minor or nonurgent illness and injury. Patients can walk in or be transported by ambulance. Then, they are triaged (sorted and allocated for treatments) based on the severity of their injury

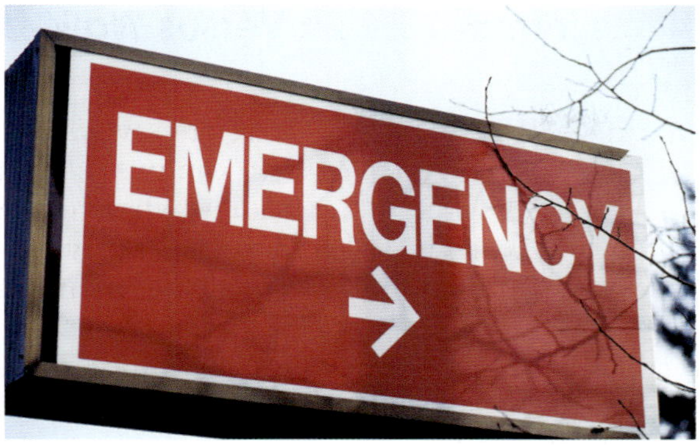

Figure 15.4 Emergency departments are typically expensive, involve long wait times, and lack specialists who understand the nuances of dance-related injuries. These facilities should only be used for life-threatening conditions such as an unstable limb fracture, a severe allergic reaction, a heart attack, or similar situations.

Photodisc

or illness; more serious and life-threatening conditions are expedited to the front of the line. Presenting oneself to an emergency department with a non-life-threatening injury—or an injury that clearly needs advanced medical care—often means a long wait time to see a clinician.

Emergency departments are staffed by a myriad of specialists for emergent situations such as open fractures, penetrating injuries, and head trauma. No specialized dancer-specific or nonemergency care is provided here. For example, even though radiographic imaging capability is available, higher-level imaging such as MRI and CT scans are reserved for true medical emergencies such as strokes. In addition, emergency department fees are very expensive; they cost thousands of U.S. dollars, even for basic treatments. You should avoid using emergency departments for injuries unless an acute (severe and sudden) injury, such as a fracture, dislocation, spine injury, or head trauma, is suspected.

Tips for Successfully Navigating the Health Care System

Although you may be reluctant to seek professional medical care, much can be done to optimize care and facilitate communication. There are huge differences between health care systems across the world. The following are general concepts to help you successfully navigate health care in general. Different mechanisms will vary between countries, regions of countries, and locales. Figure 15.5 provides an example of what you might expect during a health care evaluation.

WWW Visit HK*Propel* to download a copy of figure 15.5.

Navigating Across Multiple Health Care Delivery Systems: A Case Study

A dancer is experiencing ankle pain. She notices it after ramping up rehearsals for a big semester final. After finals, she continues to notice pain in her ankle. She has tried conservative treatment with stretching and icing, but the ankle continues to bother her. First, she goes to the athletic training clinic. The athletic trainer evaluating her is unfamiliar with dance and tells her to brace her ankle. Despite ankle bracing, the dancer continues to have discomfort, so she seeks evaluation at the university's student health center. The nurse practitioner who is staffing the clinic conducts an evaluation and orders an X-ray. The radiologist's reading of the X-ray is normal. The nurse practitioner tells the dancer that the X-ray shows nothing wrong and the ankle should get better on its own.

The dancer becomes a little disconcerted because her ankle continues to bother her. She asks her dance instructor about next steps of pursuing care. The dance instructor recommends a community-based physical therapist who specializes in dance medicine. The dancer receives evaluation and treatment from the physical therapist, who provides resolution of the ankle pain.

The dancer is delighted by the results and asks the physical therapist about a chronic hip pain that has been nagging for many years. The physical therapist refers the dancer to an orthopaedic surgeon who specializes in dance medicine; the surgeon orders an MRI of the hip and finds hip dysplasia (underdeveloped hip joint). Because the dancer is not having severe symptoms, the surgeon recommends ongoing therapies and communicates this with the physical therapist.

In this case study, identify all types of health care professionals and facilities utilized by the dancer. What were their roles? How would utilizing the wrong type of health care facility or medical professional have affected the dancer's care? Explain the importance of working with dance medicine professionals in this case.

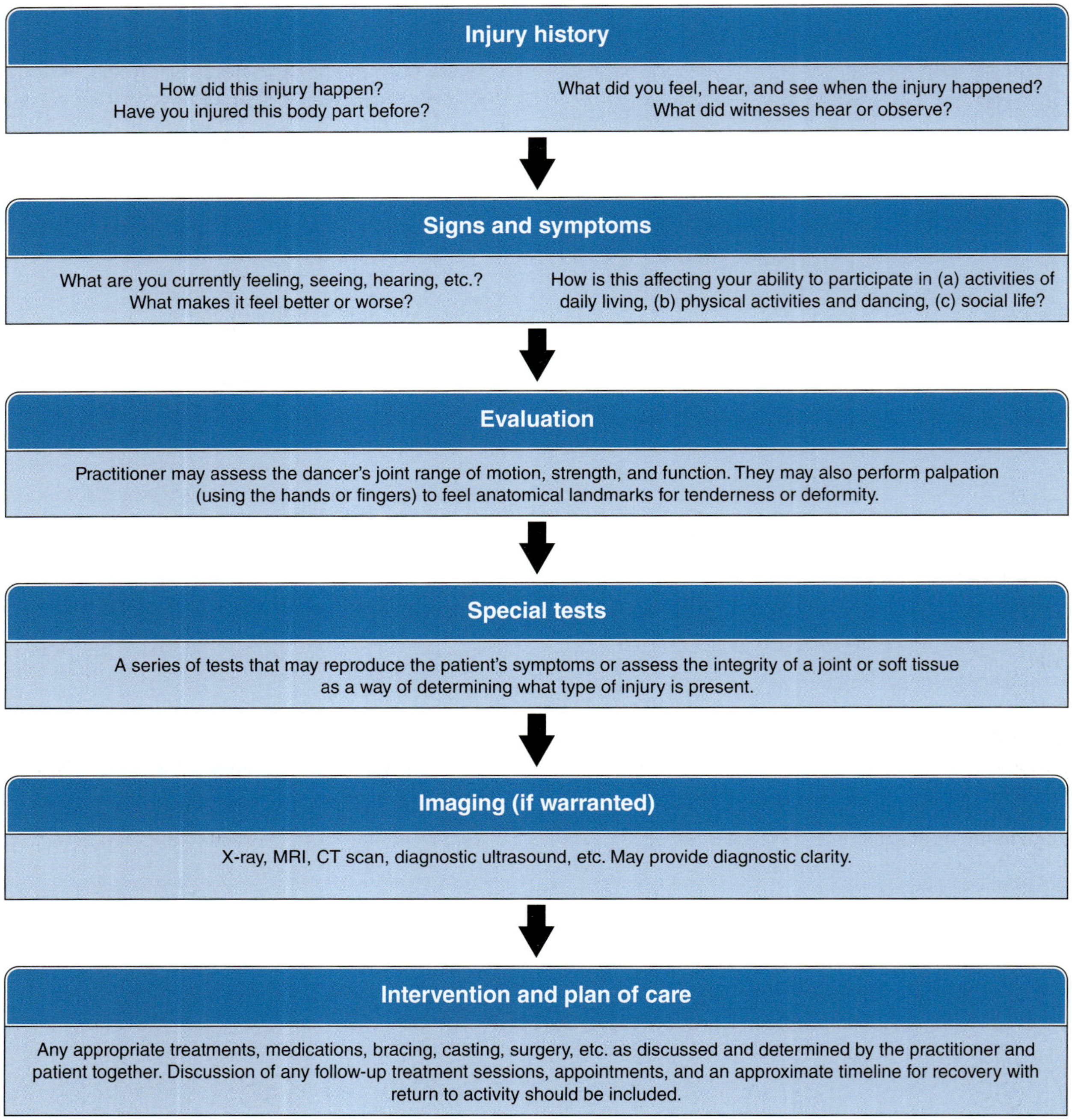

Figure 15.5 The process of evaluating, diagnosing, and establishing a plan of care for a dance injury.

Prior to the visit, you should organize your thoughts. Compile a list of symptoms associated with your clinical concern and a list of questions specific to your injury. These lists will help with clear and succinct communication of concerns to the health care professional. For chronic injuries, it may be helpful to keep a pain diary to document trends, triggers, and treatments that provide the health care professional with insight into what you are experiencing. Table 15.5 shows some sample pain diary questions. You should be prepared to describe the type, location, and intensity of the pain. Numeric and visual pain scales such as those in figures 15.6 and 15.7 are useful and commonly employed tools that a health care professional may use to help gauge the pain intensity associated with your injury (Haefeli & Elfering, 2006). Figure 15.8 shows a common method for a patient to report chronic pain in various parts of the body.

Table 15.5 **Sample Pain Diary**

Date	Pain intensity (Scale 0-10)	Pain description (sharp, throbbing, etc.)	Activities that made pain worse	Activities that made pain better	Medication taken?	Other notes/ observations
1/22	3	Dull	Small jumps in ballet class	Releasing calf with ball before class	Yes; ibuprofen (once per day)	Big test; didn't get much sleep

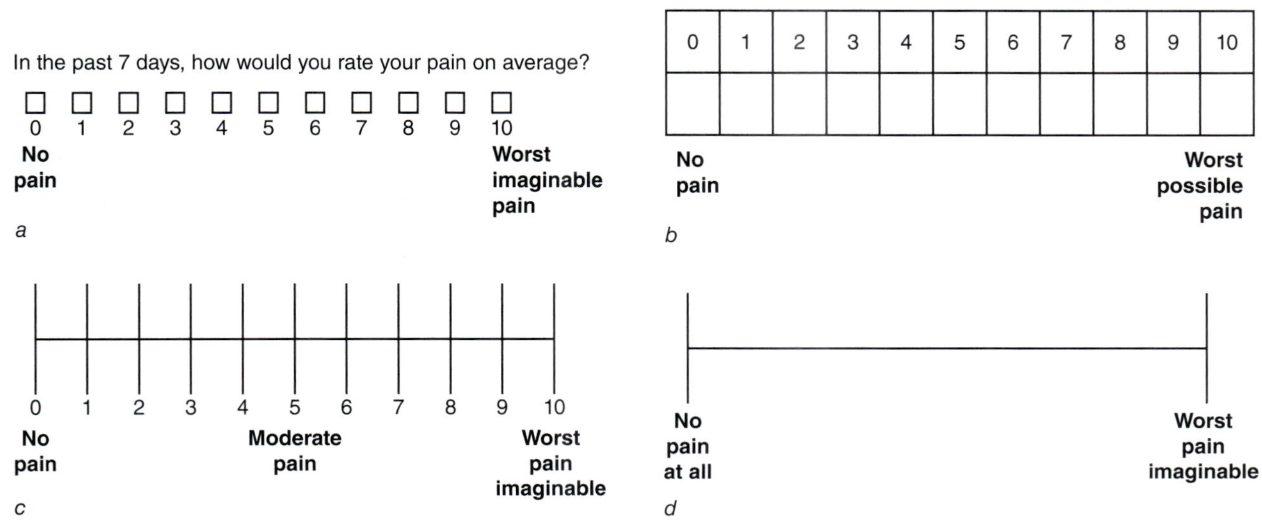

Figure 15.6 Examples of numeric pain rating methods. *(a)* Numeric pain intensity rating scale v1.0 from the Patient-Reported Outcome Measurement Information System (PROMIS). *(b)* and *(c)* Two other commonly used types of graphic rating scales for pain. *(d)* A 100-millimeter visual analogue scale. In this type of scale, a patient makes a vertical slash along the 100-millimeter horizontal line that corresponds to their pain level. The number of millimeters from the left edge to the slash equals their pain score out of 100. Note that the horizontal line must be exactly 100 millimeters long.

A: From "PROMIS Numeric Rating Scale v1.0 - Pain Intensity - 1a," HealthMeasures, (2017), www.healthmeasures.net/index.php?option=com_instruments&view=measure&id=896&Itemid=992.

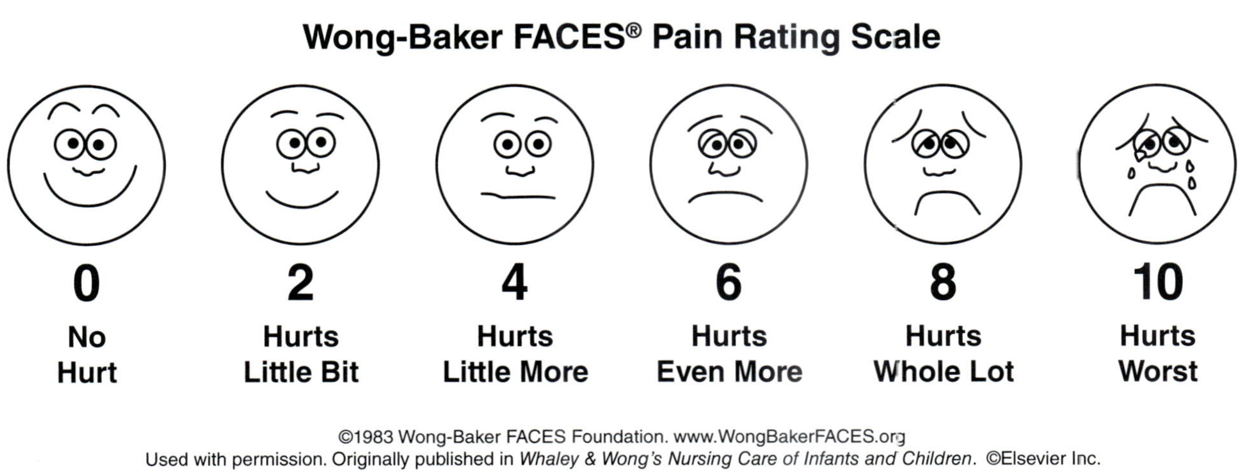

Figure 15.7 Example of a visual pain scale, the Wong-Baker FACES Pain Rating Scale, where a patient circles the face that corresponds to their pain level.

Courtesy Wong-Baker FACES® Foundation

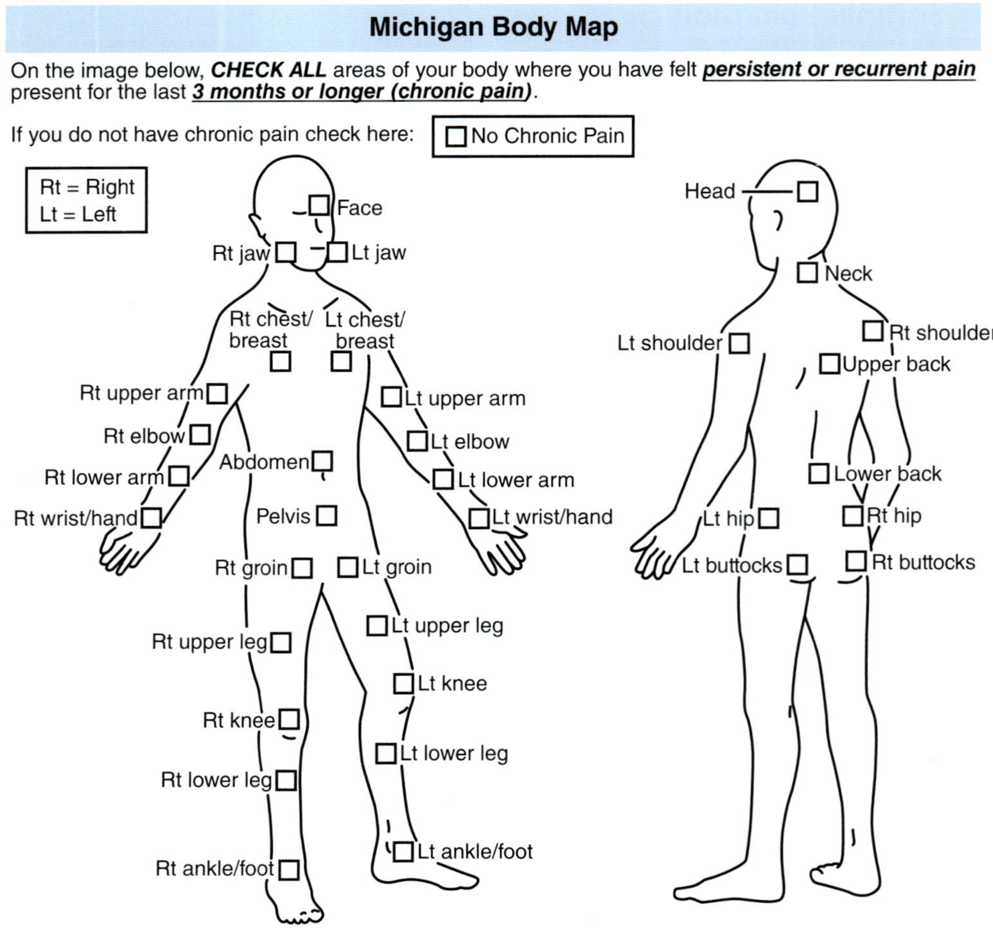

Figure 15.8 The Michigan Body Map is an instrument used to determine where an individual experiences chronic (longer than 3 months) pain.

WWW Go to HK*Propel* to download a pain diary template.

The FACES Scale (figure 15.7) displays a series of human face drawings that become more angst-ridden from left to right, which coincides with an increasing numerical pain scale. This type of scale is used primarily with patients who may have difficulty reporting on a visual analogue or numeric scale, especially children and the elderly. However, this type of pain rating has been reported as valid and reliable for use with adults following orthopaedic surgery (Van Giang et al., 2015), and its appearance is very approachable for use in all types of patients. You can complete any of these common pain scales on your own—including doing so periodically—to track your pain for your own benefit and to help provide your practitioner with an idea of the nature of your pain. As with all topics of patient–clinician dialogue, clear and succinct communication is necessary.

Setting a clear and realistic expectation for the outcome or goal for the medical appointment is also important. While many collegiate dancers do not feel that their clinicians spend enough time with them (Wang & Russell, 2018), most health care practitioners function as part of a system that places them under great pressure to see a given number of patients based on their role. This expectation will likely result in limiting their time with you, even if they would like to spend more time with you. Preparing a list of concerns with specific questions will ensure efficiency; during your health care visit, as much as possible will be accomplished. Depending on the type of health care delivery system, more than one visit may be required. In addition, unless a health care professional is adept at working with dancers, they may give a cursory "All clear" that denies any pathology. While dismissive, this result may at least be a reassuring signal that a significant condition is not present. Be certain to obtain as much information as possible from the practitioner while you have the opportunity.

The other dismissive—and much more frustrating—answer you may receive is the dreaded "Just stop dancing." This advice is poorly conceived, and dancers universally receive it with disdain. The statement is almost always delivered in a condescending manner, and it suggests both a lack of respect for the dancer-patient and an unwillingness to understand the highly physical context of dance. In fact, for some dance injuries, "Stop dancing" is correct advice because to continue would increase the risk of a more serious injury. A stress fracture of the tibia (shin bone) is an example. However, there are more compassionate words with which to deliver the message as well as ways to keep an injured dancer involved in some aspects of dance. Chapter 10 offers more insight into the concept of relative rest as a preferred means to handle such situations. Additionally, whenever a health care visit does not go satisfactorily, a second opinion with a dance medicine specialist should be pursued.

Use of succinct nondance language will likely be required with many health care clinicians. On the other hand, most dance medicine practitioners have previously danced or attended arts functions, and they are familiar with the idiosyncrasies of dance culture (Lai et al., 2008). In these interactions with dance medicine specialists, more time and nuanced evaluation of dance technique may occur. Use of dance language and jargon can readily occur in these dance-specific interactions and evaluations.

If you have had an injured body region imaged with radiology procedures such as X-rays, an MRI (magnetic resonance imaging), or a CT (computed tomography) scan, the images should be brought to whomever you visit for a consultation with a specialist or for a second opinion. Sharing these images allows your providers to review the images themselves rather than rely on the radiologist's report. In today's U.S. health care environment, medical records cannot be sequestered from a patient, so they will be provided for you upon your request. The images are usually copied to a computer disc, and they include the official report of the radiologist who reviewed them. Usually, the disc will include a program that will allow you to view the images on your own computer. Sometimes these records may be available via an online medical records system managed by the medical practice of your provider.

If you visit a dance medicine physician, they may wish to obtain additional imaging to help them make a diagnosis (figure 15.9).

Conclusions and Practical Relevance

Dance-related injuries are common due to the repetitive and physically demanding nature of dance movement. When injuries do occur, proper health care intervention at an appropriate level of care is pivotal to ideal outcomes. Dancers should be aware of clinical signs and symptoms that warrant immediate attention.

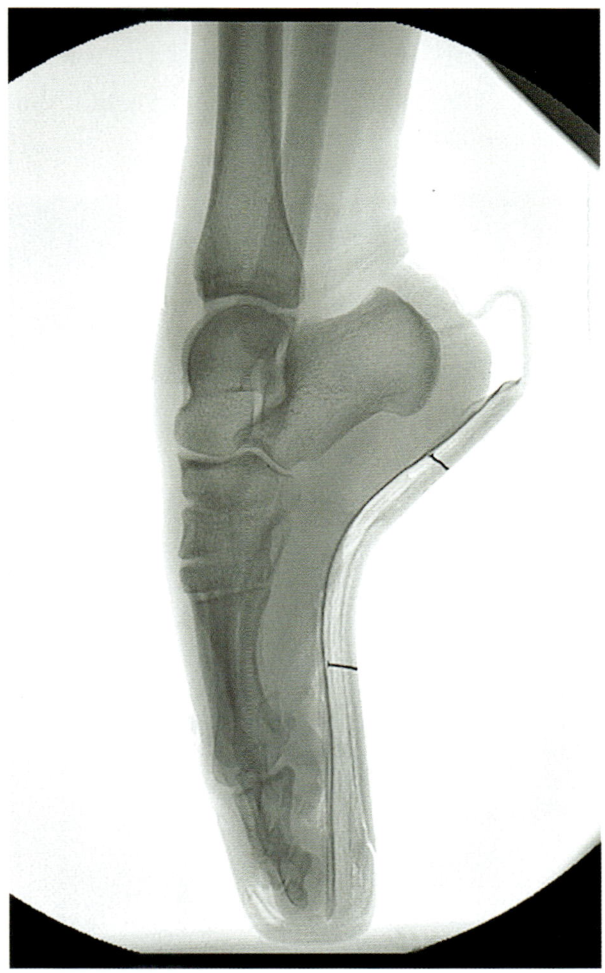

Figure 15.9 Some physicians may order specialized imaging to assess conditions that may be causing a dance injury, such as this X-ray taken while a dancer stands en pointe.

Dr. Jeff Russell

Being able to navigate the health care landscape can help smooth out the experience and optimize care. Healthcare professionals, some of whom are adept at working with dancers, can be found in the setting of student health care, an athletic department clinic, the community around a university, and a performing arts medicine clinic. To optimize health outcomes, adequate communication should occur among medical, allied health, and other health care practitioners; the dance teacher; and the dancer.

Discussion Questions

1. What are the clinical signs and symptoms that warrant immediate attention and timely evaluation by a health care professional?
2. What are the types of facilities dancers may locate on campus or in the community for assessment of their dance-related injury?
3. What is the role of the dance teacher or exercise professional in the management of an injury and in relationship with licensed health care professionals?
4. What are the barriers to adequate and proper health care for dance injuries? Have you encountered any of these barriers? How did you respond? How can such barriers be mitigated?
5. What are some ways you can organize and prepare yourself for attending a medical appointment?

WWW Go to HK*Propel* to access supplemental information and activities connected to chapter content.

16

Navigating Risks and Implementing Best Practices for Success in Dance

Jennifer Deckert, MFA
Margaret Wilson, PhD
Jan Dunn, MS

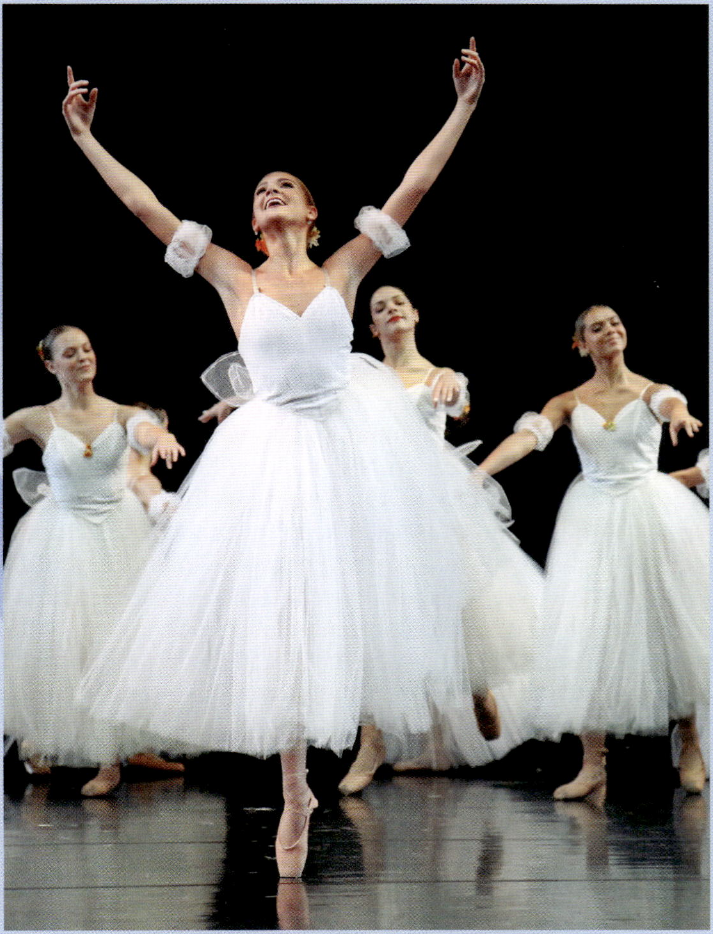

University of South Carolina, Betsy Blackmon Dance Program, Columbia, South Carolina. *Les Sylphides* (2023) reconstructed by Jennifer Deckert after Michel Fokine. Photo: Sadie Whitehead; Dancers: (Foreground) Anna Slade, (Background, L to R) Audrey Rosby, Talbott Carden, Kate Gilchrist.

Key Terms

- advocacy
- emotional risk
- environmental risk
- physical capacity
- raked stage
- safeguarding
- self-care
- sprung floor

As you move forward on your dance wellness journey, this chapter aims to tie up loose ends and send you off with a few reminders. It provides you the opportunity to reflect on what you have studied so far and to consider a variety of principles that are crucial to a successful dance practice. It offers suggestions to fine-tune your wellness, reduce your risk of injury (which includes more than the physical kind), and maximize your performance.

LEARNING OBJECTIVES

After completing this chapter, you will be able to do the following:

- Contextualize the information in the book to help you prepare for success.
- Identify and address environmental and moral safety risks in dance.
- Explain emotional and psychosocial considerations in dance training.
- Create your own identity within a dance environment.
- Describe warm-up and cool-down protocols.
- Implement key concepts to prepare yourself for success as a dancer.
- Advocate for a healthy dance environment.

As a discipline, dance medicine and science endeavors to understand risks for injury and advocate for the best training practices to minimize these risks. The purpose of this book is to provide information on the causes of injury—identifying risk factors, mechanisms, and the physiological and emotional impact that injuries can cause—and help dancers improve and maximize their dance performance. In the previous chapters, you have been introduced to valuable information that will empower you to care for your body, to reduce the risk of injury, and to condition and develop your body and mind for better performance and longevity.

This chapter adds to that discussion by advocating for whole-person wellness—looking at what it takes to balance the physical demands of dance and the artistic goals of the dancer. A dancer's goals and dreams are best achieved by taking control of the care of their whole self. In reality, those goals and dreams can be disrupted by injury—whether it be from an accident or one that develops over time. Injury is an unfortunate reality in physical activity. However, with education and understanding, an injury can be nothing more than a slight detour from the desired path; moreover, it may provide the dancer the time and opportunity to step back, reassess, and gain valuable perspectives while recovering.

Maximizing your **physical capacity** provides a solid foundation for successful training in many modalities, thus expanding your range as a dancer while at the same time increasing your versatility and employability. The field of dance is ever-evolving; physical demands and expressivity look very different today than in generations past; at the same time, genres are blending to make new forms. This constant change is what makes dance so exciting! However, it also means dancers and educators must change along with it. Each generation of artists brings fresh ideas, and fresh ideas bring demands. Examples include asking dancers to be stronger, move more quickly, jump higher, utilize new styles of partnering, and be more adaptive to spaces outside of traditional theater spaces.

The physical body is capable of greatness, but with increased demands, it is more important than ever to look at your training in a holistic way. Training should encompass not only the physical skills but also ways to best fuel the body and support mental wellness. As you navigate this ever-changing field, you must also keep in mind that each new genre, space, and choreographic intention poses a fresh set of physical demands and risks. Each time a new situation is presented, it is imperative that the teacher and dancers recalibrate expectations based on the dancers' capacities and backgrounds as well as prepare the body and mind for new adventures. The following section addresses risks in the dance environment that you may not have evaluated because they are such an integral and embedded aspect of your dance experience.

Environmental Risks

As part of a dance community, you hear and talk about space on a daily basis, using phrases such as *use the space*, *see the space*, *partner with the space*, and *explore the space*. In so many ways the physical space that you inhabit helps to define the movement. However, in a discussion about physical space, it is important not only to see it as a collaborator but also to acknowledge its limitations, namely, **environmental risks**. Where you dance may be consistent from day to day (e.g., in a specific dance studio), or it may change daily while on tour or performing. When assessing and acclimating to a space, there are a variety of factors to consider.

Floors

Dance floors are immeasurably important because they are what support dancers. Figure 16.1 depicts several different types of dance floors. The two primary aspects to consider when assessing the floor are (1) Is it sprung? and (2) What is the surface? Each genre will require a different type of surface. For contemporary and classical dance, a **sprung floor** (built with enough give to absorb some of the daily pounding that dancers experience in the studio) that is made of wood and covered with a vinyl layer for added slip resistance is ideal. Tap dancers may prefer a sprung wood floor without a covering that dampens their characteristic sound. Hip-hop artists often train outdoors on concrete, and certain modern or contemporary performances are danced on irregular, outdoor surfaces.

Research over several decades has shown that a high-quality surface can help reduce shock absorption and reduce risk of injury. The quality of the floor includes the construction of the subfloor and floor as well as the vinyl covering, called *marley* (Hopper & Fong Yan, 2017; Hopper, Allen, et al.,

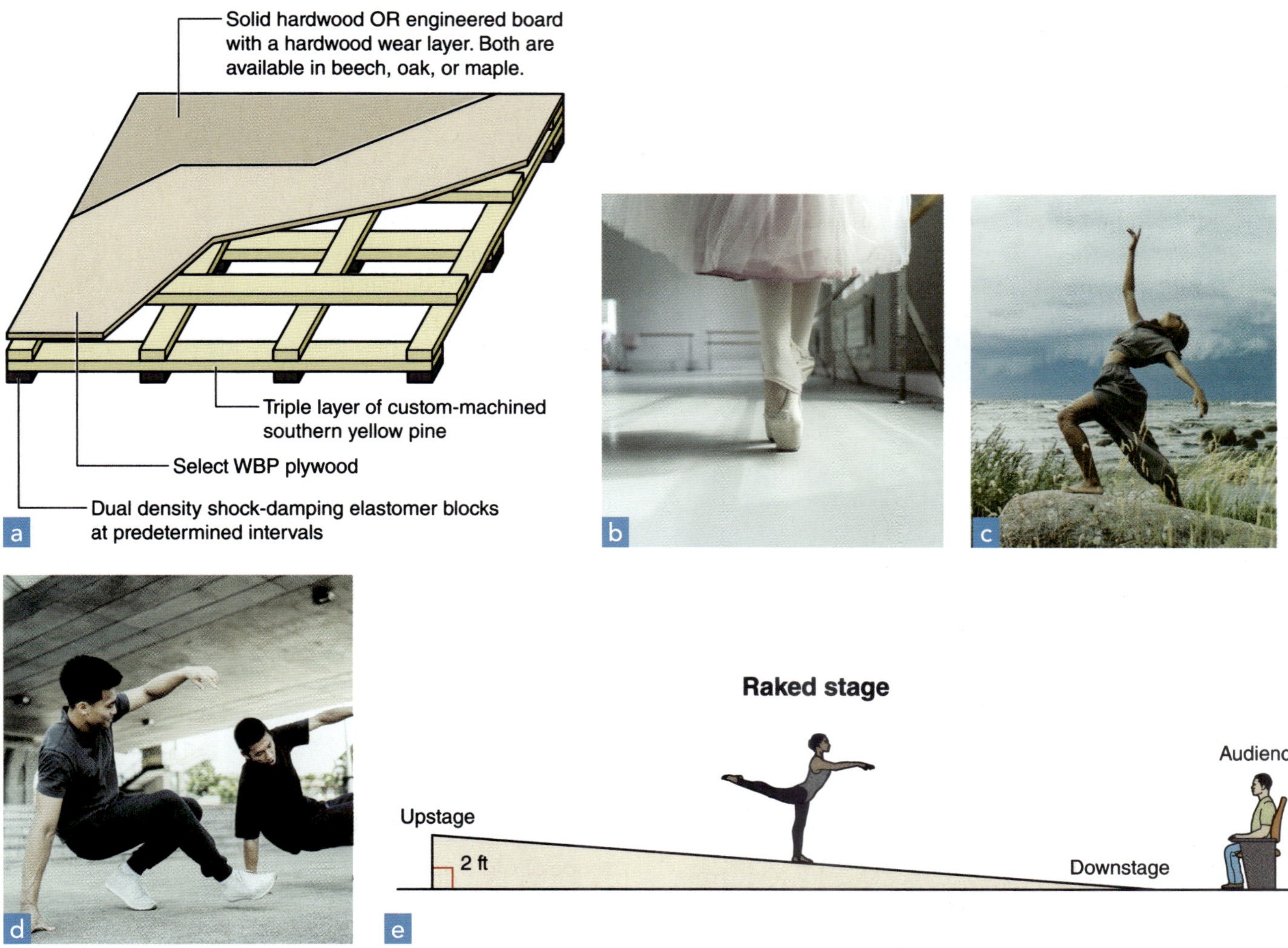

Figure 16.1 Different types of dance floors present different challenges for a dancer. *(a)* Sprung wood floor. *(b)* Floor with vinyl (marley) covering. *(c)* Contemporary dance, especially outdoors, can present many irregular floor types. *(d)* Hip-hop dancers may perform on a number of surfaces, including asphalt or concrete. *(e)* A raked stage.

B: Anastasia Shuraeva on Pexels; C: cottonbro studio on Pexels; D: Allan Mas on Pexels

2014; Hopper, Alderson, et al., 2014; Wanke et al., 2012). Additionally, there are online resources for investigating the importance of a good dance floor. For example, Harlequin Floors, a company that has been working with the dance industry since the 1970s, offers information about the ways that dance flooring can enhance performance and reduce injury (American Harlequin Corporation, 2024).

In addition to floor construction and surface concerns, stages are sometimes *raked* (sloping downward, toward the audience). **Raked stages** present additional concerns for potential risk of injury (Hagins et al., 2007; Felter & Rietveld, 2009). Approximately 20 percent of Broadway and West End productions are performed on a raked stage. Studies have shown that working on this type of surface can double or triple the risk of injury for professional dancers (Pappas & Hagins, 2008; Quin, 2015).

Once you begin to move away from a smooth sprung surface, the injury risk begins to increase because you must absorb more of the impact to your bones and soft tissues that would ordinarily be reduced by the sprung floor. Proper footwear and modified movements (e.g., reduced jumping) can help mitigate these risks; however, working as much as possible on floors that are sprung and have a proper surface provides the best protection. If you do not know about the floor you are dancing on, now is a good time to ask!

Tips for Dancing in Warm Temperatures

- Stay hydrated! Refer to chapter 7 for more information about the importance of proper hydration.
- Certain medications or substances inhibit the sweating mechanism or increase the likelihood of dehydration, thus making a dancer more susceptible to heat stress. Examples include antihistamines and tranquilizers. Alcohol intake also increases the likelihood of heat illness. Cramps related to activity in hot weather are likely, particularly if proper hydration is not maintained.
- Keep in mind that heat stress is not limited to only outdoors in the hot sun. Wherever there is a high air temperature—including indoors—the possibility exists for heat stress. High humidity and lack of air circulation compound the problem.
- Dancers and educators should be aware of the symptoms of heat stress, including headache, fatigue, nausea, faintness, mental confusion or disorientation, clammy skin (for heat exhaustion), and hot and dry skin (for heatstroke, a medical emergency).

Temperature

Have you ever walked into a dance space that is too hot or too cold? Dancers seem to inherently know what temperature is best for their bodies. A studio that is too cold will not allow the body to properly warm up or to stay warm. An overly warm studio is equally undesirable, especially in conditions of high humidity in which the body is unable to cool itself by sweat evaporation as efficiently as it would otherwise. The use of clothing and layers appropriate to the ambient conditions should be supported in environments where the temperature is too cold to retain adequate warmth. In warm or hot environments, proper hydration becomes vital. An ideal temperature for dance should range from 61 to 75 degrees Fahrenheit (16-24 °C) (Quin, 2015).

Safety Protocols and Equipment for Healthy and Clean Spaces

When you are entering a space—whether it be new to you or the one you have danced in for years—make sure you can identify the emergency exits, first aid kit, automated external defibrillator (AED), and any potential hazards. Ensure that the space is clean and free of debris; floors should be swept clean, and equipment for sanitizing touch surfaces should be accessible. All spaces should have safety protocols in place, including actions to take if a dancer becomes injured or has a medical emergency. Finally, proper ventilation is vital. The use of fans, open doors or windows, and proper air filtration systems supports a healthy environment.

While protection from and management of life-threatening attacks and violence in classroom, studio, and performance spaces are outside the scope of this chapter, such occurrences have become all too common. Thus, we recommend that dance educators provide leadership in this area by working with their appropriate institutional administrators and law enforcement officials to formulate action plans in the event of such emergencies. Information about emergency planning presented in chapter 9 will provide a good start.

Know What You Can and Cannot Control

While you may not have control over demanding training and rehearsal schedules or low-quality training or performance facilities, you can control how you prepare your body and take care of it in preparation for a healthy dance career. Warming up, cooling down (see chapter 5), getting adequate rest and proper nutrition (see chapter 7), and maintaining a good balance between strength and flexibility (see chapter 6) will prepare you for all environments and training demands. This book is an excellent resource for understanding how to best prepare your body for performance.

Moral Safety

Another aspect of safety in the dance environment that is not always acknowledged is ethical behavior and moral safety. It considers concerns such as inappropriate or unwanted touch, sexual harassment or abuse, grooming, and gender discrimination. Dance is traditionally hierarchical, with a teacher, choreographer, or director making all of the decisions about how a facility operates. However, today's world has evolved to question such controlling behaviors, especially with minors or populations who may not feel as though they have a voice. The following sections tackle subjects that are important for ensuring your environment is based on consent and respect.

Navigating Physical Touch

From classical partnering and contact improvisation to teacher corrections, physical touch and intimacy have become part of the job when it comes to dance and dance training. However, when considering whole-dancer wellness and well-being, physical contact may not be in the best interest of *every* dancer *all* the time. It can trigger feelings of discomfort or trauma that are important to address prior to moving forward. Asking permission prior to touching another dancer in the room is a great first step, but the field of dance must shift the culture of silence to one of openness and conversation centered on ownership of one's own body.

Dancers often hold the mindset that their body belongs to the art and is therefore at the disposal of the choreographer or instructor in the room. However, questioning this mentality is appropriate, as is normalizing verbal responses such as "I don't feel comfortable trying this lift," "I'm experiencing pain in my left shoulder; I would appreciate if you didn't provide any physical corrections," or even simply "I don't want to be touched today." By opening the dialogue and changing the ways people discuss physical touch and injuries that may limit physical interactions, dance communities begin to establish new levels of trust and build a brave space that honors the whole dancer—body, mind, and soul. Check out the Guidelines for Intimacy Safety in Dance and Theater in appendix B for more information about this topic.

Studio Culture

Dance studios should represent the best places for young students to be—places where they can learn and thrive in a social environment under the supervision of caring and responsible teachers. Vying for parts in recitals and choreography—and even class placements—can provide a healthy level of competition, and students thrive on the opportunity to perform and progress. While this situation is the norm, unfortunately dance studios are not regulated, and dance teacher certification is not required in the United States. Verbal and emotional abuse (often used with the intention—or excuse—

Safeguarding

Some countries have formal guidelines for handling safety concerns (called safeguarding), and these may be applied to dance environments. **Safeguarding** is designed to protect the health and welfare of children, minors, and vulnerable populations. The goal is to ensure the safety and well-being of all participants in dance, recommend proper supervision, and determine adequate teacher-to-student ratios for children. Recommendations are provided for managing security of photography and videography as well as advocating for appropriate touch protocols. In some countries, dance teachers must pass certain criteria (set by the government) to be certified as a safeguarding studio or teacher (Safe in Dance International, 2024) (e.g., www.ukadance.co.uk). In the United States, no agencies or governmental regulations exist for this aspect of dance training. However, dance educators are encouraged to research safeguarding practices and structure their studios along these guidelines regardless of governmental mandates. Educators teaching in a university environment can also find safeguarding measures through their institution to help support a healthy environment.

of challenging the dancer) can trigger trauma in a young dancer. Inadequate supervision, unregulated behavior, expectations for inappropriate dress and choreography, bullying, and lack of tolerance for illness or injury can turn the dance studio into a place of suffering for a dancer. Fortunately, some institutions and **advocacy** organizations around the world are designed to protect the dancer from this type of abuse. See appendix B for more information on creating emotional safety in dance, as well as a list of resource organizations.

Emotional and Psychosocial Considerations

Navigating the physical and ethical safety of a dance environment is just the first step to building and supporting healthy and well dancers. It is important to also reflect on the pressures a dancer experiences from the dance environment itself—often fueling perfectionist tendencies—and the toll this may take on mental health. Chapter 8 provides an in-depth look at psychological wellness and mental health, but there are a few additional factors to consider as they relate to the dance training environment.

Emotional Risks

Dancers are driven by their love of dance and their love of performing; however, alongside this joy and fulfillment, **emotional risk** can also fuel disappointment and frustration. Emotions can exert a powerful effect on training and performance, bringing the dancer up and—sadly—also bringing them down. Exploring ways to find joy and self-fulfillment outside of the studio will bring balance to your practice, as will developing an objective internal voice to understand aspects of dance you struggle with or have not yet attained.

Social Pressures

With its many companies, schools, and programs, dance is a communal activity. All of these dance communities engage groups of dancers in classes, rehearsals, and performances. Within these groups, a wide range of interpersonal dynamics can create a unified and functional ensemble or divide and detract from the goals of the group. Negotiating within these groups can be complicated by competition, stress, or peer pressure. Identifying the ways that you can evaluate your own strengths and preferences, and remove yourself from uncomfortable situations when necessary, will help you develop resilience in these social interactions.

Motivation, Perfectionism, and Burnout

Dance training provides challenges, variety, and opportunities for achievement. However, each dancer must also find their own passion and fulfillment as they maintain their physical practice. Developing physical artistry in dance requires dedication, seeking opportunities for personal growth, and self-motivation. Identifying those elements in dance that test your resolve and bring you success and joy will keep you motivated to work through challenging situations. Thinking about why you dance (for yourself, or for others?), seeing value in what you do, and objectively reflecting on your experiences will help you develop and maintain a healthy mind and body (Mainwaring & Aujla, 2017; Kusner & Schaeffer, 2021). The Dance Well podcast series (Dance Well Podcast, 2024) offers rich content to support these concepts.

Taming Your Inner Dictator

Many dancers are perfectionists; they practice movements over and over to get the timing, line, or quality *just right*; these goals may be physical, technical, or artistic—or all three. The pursuit of the ideal can lead to artistry, or it can lead to frustration. Perfection can be a positive quality when the dancer has high personal standards, self-evaluates, and is not self-critical over mistakes. However, an unhealthy type of perfectionism occurs when the dancer sets unrealistic goals and becomes overly critical when these goals are not achieved. Focusing on a realistic goal and identifying ways in which this goal is strategically achievable is the type of healthy perfectionism that will propel you forward to achieving success (Nordin-Bates, 2014; Nordin-Bates et al., 2017).

Navigating Your Identity Within the Dance Environment

Historically dance has been taught from a position of authority. This has created a culture where dance students look up to their teachers for information, guidance, and expertise. And, as most dance educators were dancers themselves, they are knowledgeable about the field, training expectations, and performance aspirations. Thus, dance classrooms became hallowed spaces where the dancer could gain entrance to a larger world of dance, learning not only dance technique but also expectations for dress, behavior, and protocols.

Within this historical paradigm, dance classrooms and rehearsals were not typically a place for conversation, and dancers were trained to respond only to prompts from the teacher or choreographer. While this protocol created an environment where the dancer's focus was on the material being taught, it did not necessarily allow the dancer to develop agency by asking questions or addressing individual concerns. Dancers would often try to hide injuries or fatigue when they should in fact have communicated such occurrences or requested a modification from the teacher. To avoid this, it is important that dancers also strive to find an identity outside of dance by exploring a holistic sense of self and purpose.

Dance is not only a physical pursuit but also an artistic one. Whereas daily training in technique is an important part of a dancer's success, developing an artistic voice is important as well. Dancers are expected to play roles onstage or express a specific emotion in response to music, but how are these skills developed? You should feel the freedom to consult dance resources to explore your emotions and ideas. This exploration might include character dance, improvisation, reading and writing about dance, or watching performances that expand your understanding of the breadth of dance forms. Dancers can seek stimulus from other sources, such as reading, finding a new hobby, working as a volunteer, or engaging with other social groups to develop self-identity and balance outside of class and training (Kusner & Schaeffer, 2018).

Advocacy

When reflecting on the task of creating a safe space, it can be overwhelming to consider the risks inherent in dance. The first step is understanding that advocacy for safety is multifaceted; moreover, as mentioned previously, one must consider the physical environment as well as the physical and emotional safety of those in the room. Advocating for safe spaces must be a priority for organizations, teachers, and students alike.

As the field develops, the dance community now has the opportunity to support dancers, educators, and artists as they each find their own voice. Teachers must work toward creating teaching and learning environments where dancers are free to ask questions; participate in the artistic process; cultivate agency for their own bodies; and take

Best Practices for Using a Mirror

Sally Radell, MFA, MA, a professor of dance at Emory University, is a leading researcher in the positive and negative effects of working with mirrors in dance training (figure 16.2). She has concluded that mirrors can be very positive as a tool to help dancers learn and as a source of immediate visual feedback; however, they can also be a mechanism for great distraction (Radell et al., 2017; Radell et al., 2020). Beyond a distraction, mirrors can develop a high level of self-consciousness in dancers, may encourage comparison of themselves to others, and may enable disconnection of dancers from their bodies, thus diminishing their proprioception and body awareness. Whereas a mirror can be effective in learning new skills and choreography, once the choreography is learned, rehearsals should be done facing away from a mirror whenever possible, especially because mirrors are not available during performances.

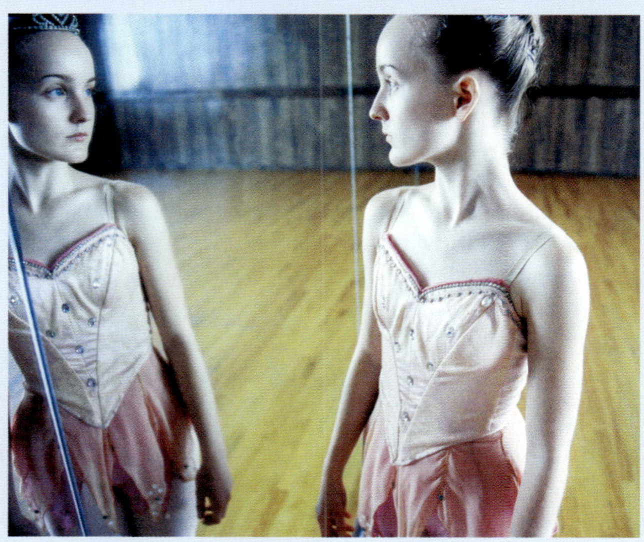

Figure 16.2 While mirrors can be very helpful in dance training, they can also be detrimental.

ownership for their journey as dancers, artists, and creators. This type of environment may look different for every teacher, genre, and location, but the goal should remain the same: to give dancers the space and ability to advocate for their physical and mental well-being.

On the organizational level, administrators must create policies and procedures that are centered on the student experience, clearly outline injury management protocols, and set expectations for proper flooring and temperatures. In addition, organizations are responsible for vetting teachers and others in positions of authority to ensure that they approach their jobs with the safety of the dancers as a priority.

At the classroom level, teachers carry the responsibility of creating an environment where all voices are valid and heard. Through open dialogue and conversations, the studio space must be established as a place where dancers are encouraged to speak, question, and explore. Teachers also must be cognizant of the fact that all dancers come into class with different backgrounds, knowledge, and experiences—including possible trauma. Therefore, each dancer must be treated as an individual rather than with the assumption that all dancers need the same delivery in their training and learning environment.

Finally, what can you—as a dance student—do to advocate for your own safety? Not all dance settings are established in a way that is conducive to healthy and safe dance practices. If you encounter a space that is physically or mentally abusive, that does not support open dialogues, or that presents a physical hazard, it is vital that you withdraw from the situation; then, either seek outside support to work toward productive changes or transfer to a different training program. Dancers have frequently been conditioned to please others and therefore to remain silent in uncomfortable situations. In light of this tendency, self-advocacy is a key skill for all dancers to develop, including working to assess environments that seem unhealthy or dangerous and learning to speak up for their well-being. Ultimately, your health and safety depends on you verbalizing your personal boundaries and demanding a work environment that supports whole-dancer wellness.

How to Best Prepare Yourself for Success

The content of this book may seem overwhelming as you begin to integrate its material into your daily life, but take comfort in knowing that much of your journey is within your control. You should now understand how to (1) engage in outside conditioning, including training your cardiorespiratory system, (2) seek out and implement appropriate stretching and strengthening regimens, (3) explore somatic practices to balance the body and mind, (4) implement optimal nutrition plans that will enhance your performance and overall well-being, and (5) utilize research literature to help support dancer wellness and injury risk reduction.

Warming Up the Body and Mind

It is a dancer's responsibility to prepare their body and mind for class. To maximize the many benefits of this preparation, warming up should be systematic, tailored to your needs and to the class or rehearsal you are preparing for, and helpful in transitioning from previous (nondance) activities, such as arriving from a lecture class in another part of campus or driving in a car to your studio.

In ballet, the first exercises at the barre are often considered to be warm-up activities. Nevertheless, if the dancer is already warm—having moved the joints, dynamically activated the muscles (not by doing static stretches while sitting on the floor), and warmed their body from the inside by raising the heart rate—they will benefit much more from those first pliés. This principle applies to all dance styles and classes.

You are encouraged to create a ritual for yourself in order to take ownership of preparing for class. Having a specific sequence means you can really focus on the intent of the warm-up rather than on simply figuring out something to do. Warm-ups can—and should—be set to music, and you can adjust the movements for the class or rehearsal you are about to enter. Regardless of the exact approach, dedicating time for physical preparation is important.

Mental preparation is equally important. Focusing on your goals for the class or rehearsal, reviewing notes or concepts given in previous sessions, and using mental imagery or visualization to augment your physical practice are all part of preparing your mind for dance. Use this time to set aside worries, concerns, or distractions, and focus on integrating the body and mind by addressing balance or proprioception or by practicing specific breathing techniques to key into the body's responsiveness.

Cooling Down

As beneficial as warming up is, a key element to a dancer's health and injury risk reduction is cooling down. Following the peak combination, the last rehearsal of choreography, or another major dance activity, it is important to bring the body down from the elevated physical, emotional, and mental state required for success in class, rehearsal, or performance. Sadly, it is often the case that no time is allotted for this moment in class; nevertheless, a proper cool-down could be a key to lessening the likelihood of injury, restoring homeostasis in the body, and allowing the body to consolidate its information (Quin, 2015).

Dancers intuitively want to stretch after class. However, sitting down on the floor or lowering the head below the heart in a forward stretch without lowering the heart rate to a near-normal state could be dangerous for some. The reason for this danger is that while the heart and arteries continue to pump blood at a high rate, the veins require the skeletal muscles to assist their return of the blood to the heart. Instead of sitting down or standing, dynamic stretches can gradually decrease in range of motion and intensity (e.g., transitioning from running and jumping to walking and sliding) to lower the heart rate gradually and keep blood from pooling in the lower extremities. Gentle range of motion exercises can continue to mobilize joints, moving fluid throughout the body for muscle relaxation. Stretching is best done when the body is still warm, but the heart rate has decreased, and the body has recovered from physical exertion (Redding & Handman, 2017).

Action Items for Students

1. *Be a purposeful and wise consumer of information.* There is a lot of misinformation about how to be a better, stronger, and more flexible dancer. Just as you have learned not to believe everything you read on the Internet, you must apply this same skepticism to information about your health and well-being. In addition, each body and mind is different; what works for your friend may not work for you. Take the information that works, and discard the rest. You are on a mission to understand what is best for you . . . to explore, to deconstruct, to question, and to develop wisdom.
2. *Incorporate sound science into your dance practice.* As you are vetting sources and information, always try to understand the science behind the recommendation. Then ask, "Is this practice anatomically sound?" and "Is it backed by science?" (Helping you do this is a primary reason for chapter 3 in this book!) If you struggle to answer those questions, you may need to dig a bit deeper to find what you are trying to accomplish. As you approach your dance training with this type of analysis, you may begin to question how a movement is done or the reason behind certain practices. This questioning is the next step in your education. Approach dance with the intention of incorporating your new, healthy knowledge and practice into the classroom and studio.
3. *Work smart with your end goals in mind.* This perspective is incredibly important, especially as you manage and recover from injury or illness. Pushing through pain in one rehearsal or class may result in a longer recovery time or reinjury. This cycle is far too common among dancers, and it often leads to frustration and shortened careers. Always consider the end goal of a full, healthy, and safe recovery; this focus will help to keep things in perspective. For example, maybe taking that extra class or doing large jumps is not the best way to serve your goal. Let that be okay; work smarter, not harder.
4. *Practice self-care.* Dancers are notorious for overtraining, often leading to overuse injuries, disordered eating practices, reduced energy, and burnout. Taking the time to practice **self-care** must be a priority in order to honor the whole-dancer perspective. Enjoy a long lunch with a close friend, get adequate sleep, respect your own limitations and boundaries, read a book, meditate, take a bath, or try other methods of self-care that work for you. Remember that self-care is a necessity; your body and mind help you achieve your goals as a dancer, so caring for them must be a priority.

Considerations for Educators

As an aspiring or well-established educator, it is imperative that you understand the physiological and psychological demands of dance and how to systematically train your students to maximize their wellness under your tutelage. This understanding will yield many benefits for you. Remaining cognizant of the types of injury risks by genre is vital to planning classes and choreography that allows

A Note on Self-Care

The term *self-care* seems to be increasingly present in today's culture, and it can mean anything from a nap to a difficult workout. Keep in mind that self-care is highly personal and should ultimately reduce stress. Since dancers have the tendency to keep pushing themselves, it is important to remember that rest, recovery, and proper nutrition (including hydration) are *all* necessary aspects of self-care. Figure 16.3 offers some ideas for self-care, and there are many others if you put your imagination to work.

Self-care

Self-care should be designed as a pause from the hustle and bustle of your life, something different that you don't get to enjoy often enough. When taking yourself through self-care, silence your phone and put it away. Scrolling through social media is NOT self-care, and neither is binge-watching your streaming service. Eliminate distractions. Be present for yourself. Remember, this is time for YOU and interruptions will reduce self-care's effectiveness.

Pampering
- Have a massage.
- Have a manicure or pedicure.
- Have a bubble bath.
- Take a nap or go to bed early.

Visiting
- Go see a place of natural beauty.
- Stop by a library or bookstore, find a comfortable seat, and sit there reading a book you've not read before.
- Stop by your favorite coffee shop.
- Stop by a boutique and enjoy some window shopping (but don't spend money you don't have).
- Find a place where you can listen to the birds, the ocean waves, the raindrops, the wind, or calming music.
- Drop in to see someone who is special to you.

Roaming and exploring
- Go for a walk or hike.
- Go on a picnic.
- Find a new scent of candle for your home, apartment, or room.
- Find a new blend of tea.
- Find some flowers you can cut for yourself to take home.

Creating
- Make a cup of tea.
- Make a piece of artwork (draw, paint, sculpt, photograph, knit, etc.).
- Write in your journal.
- Plan a book you'd like to write.
- Cook a gourmet meal, an ethnic dish you've been wanting to try, your signature pizza, or your favorite food.
- Make a smoothie, homemade ice cream, or another treat.

Figure 16.3 Several ideas for self-care to help you design your own self-care experiences.

you to consistently train students to maximize their strength and flexibility while nurturing their artistry. Offering options for participation that address other important skills needed for dance and slowly integrating the dancer back into dance create a positive and healthy transition for all involved (Daniels, 2014).

Here are a few other things to consider as you move forward:

1. *Interact with dancers as whole people.* Consider Hettler's six dimensions of wellness (discussed in chapter 1). Work to understand your dancers' perspectives and to support all aspects of their identity.
2. *Be a proper role model.* Acknowledge your own physical limitations with your students by setting your boundaries and modifying movements as needed. Laugh it off when something goes wrong, accept imperfection in the process, fuel your body, take the day off when you are ill, drink lots of water, talk about your hobbies outside of

dance, and take a deep breath when stress starts to creep in. Even if unintended, your actions dictate the energy in the studio. If you want open, healthy, body-aware dancers, you must first find those qualities in yourself.

3. Incorporate sound science into your teaching. Do your research, and build your teaching around practice that is anatomically and physiologically sound.
4. *Always give your best.* Show up, and be present.
5. *Have proper safety protocols and equipment in place.* Have injury action plans, emergency evacuation routes, and first aid kits ready.
6. *Create a physically safe space.* Ensure the floors are sprung and the space is clean.
7. *Create an emotionally safe space.* In other words, create a space in which physical touch is not an assumption but something to ask permission for, and where dancers are expected to speak up when they feel uncomfortable or unsafe.
8. *Work to empower students to take ownership of their learning and well-being.* Provide tools for learning that go beyond watching and repeating. Help them explore their own bodies and capabilities through anatomy lessons, supplemental exercises, resources, and lots of conversation. The best way to empower students is to let them engage in the process; ask them questions that may not have a right answer so that they can exercise their minds. Remove yourself from the position of *power over*, and assume a position of *power with*. By entering the discussion with the students, it gives them the freedom to activate their own sense of wonderment and exploration.
9. *Give the gift of self-care, and model it for your students.* Some days are harder than others. Take care of yourself, but also listen to your students. If they ask for a day to rest or want to have a conversation rather than push themselves physically, it is your opportunity to listen. Sometimes taking a day to learn the tools of visualization, modifications, relaxation, or self-massage is just as valuable as using the time learning how to complete a complex movement.

Conclusions and Practical Relevance

Ultimately, the goal of this book is to advocate for independence and self-empowerment in reducing the risk of dance injuries while at the same time enhancing training and performance for a long and successful career in dance—at every level. Risk is inherent in the field of dance. Thus, the goal should not be to avoid risk. A dancer would never accomplish a fall to the floor, multiple turns, or supported lifts without taking risks. Instead, the goal should be to focus on assessing potential dangers and establishing protocols to mitigate to the extent possible the negative consequences of risk, such as injuries.

Both dancers and teachers should think of risk assessment as you would in swimming. You would not jump into a pool's deep end if you did not already know how to swim, and you would not dive into a lake without knowing its depth and the risk of rocks or other obstructions below the surface. Neither would you, for instance, perform a complex inversion without first knowing how to support yourself. If you are, or plan to become, a teacher, it is important to assess risk and develop solutions for your students. Other examples of risk assessment questions and solutions include *Does the physical space have concrete floors?* Reduce jumps. *Does the dancer lack a fundamental skill necessary to accomplish the task?* Return to basics before adding complexity. Overall, by mindfully approaching new situations, you can maintain confidence, reduce injury risk, and work toward accomplishing the task.

In the unfortunate case of an injury, the teacher and student should find ways to maintain a healthy environment during the rehabilitation process. A healthy environment includes not only physical but also psychological and emotional support, which can be addressed by creating a community of social support and education. Injuries do not last forever; often, dancers who become injured find ways to focus on other capacities or techniques that aid in their return to dance and augment their artistry.

In summary, dancers equally have a responsibility in this process of safety and wellness. Teachers and choreographers can create an open supportive learning space, but dancers must fill it. Throughout this book you have been provided with tools to improve physical and mental health as well as assess and reduce risk. With this information, you now hold the power to succeed—as long as you take personal responsibility for your journey.

Discussion Questions

1. If you have had an injury, what were some things that you learned from this experience? Were there positive outcomes? Did you learn more about your body? If you haven't had an injury, what have you learned from watching fellow dancers deal with an injury?
2. What are some of the risks identified in this chapter that you had not thought about previously? What are the best ways to discuss emotional, occupational, and social risks in a healthy manner?
3. What should you do if you find yourself in a physical environment that you do not feel is safe and how will you approach those in authority over the space to address your concerns?
4. How do you best prepare yourself for success? What are the practices that will help you be successful as a dancer? Can any of these practices apply to success in the other parts of your life, too?

WWW Go to HK*Propel* to access supplemental information and activities connected to chapter content.

Appendix A

International Mental Health Resources

Jo-Anne La Flèche, MPsy, MA; Bonnie Robson, MD, FRCPC; Kathleen McGuire Gaines, BA

As you learned in chapters 8 and 15, mental health is incredibly important for dancers; therefore, it is the first entry in the appendixes of this book. When considering your mental health, remember these two crucial points:

1. When you need help with your mental health, there is no shame in admitting it; and
2. Once you realize you need it, don't hesitate to reach out for help; you can use the resources provided in this appendix.

The resources that follow are intended to assist you in obtaining care for yourself, a fellow dancer, a friend, or a family member. QR codes for several services are provided for quick availability. For readers who are not in the United States, Canada, the United Kingdom, Ireland, or Australia, please locate the similar resources for your country and store them in a readily accessible place *before* they are needed.

TIP: Store these important numbers in your mobile phone with an "A~" in front of them; doing so will put them at the top of your contacts where they are easiest to access (e.g., A~Crisis Text Line; A~National Suicide Prevention Lifeline).

United States

Crisis Text Line
Text HOME to 741 741

National Suicide Prevention Lifeline
Call 988 OR 1-800-273-8255

National Sexual Assault Hotline
1-800-656-4673

The Emily Program Eating Disorder Hotline
1-888-364-5977

Mental Health America
https://mhanational.org

Depression and Bipolar Support
1-800-273-8255

www.dballiance.org

Canada

Crisis Text Line
Text HOME to 686 868

Suicide Prevention Hotline
1-833-456-4566

Canadian Mental Health Association (Mood Disorders and Anxiety)
1-833-456-4566
(in Quebec City: 1-866-277-3553)

www.cmha.ca

National Eating Disorder Information Center
1-866-633-4220

United Kingdom

Crisis Text Line
Text SHOUT to 85258

National Suicide Helpline UK
0800 689 5652

Lifeline (Northern Ireland)
0808 808 8000

Beat Eating Disorders Helpline
0808 801 0677

Ireland

Crisis Text Line
Text HELLO to 50808

Australia

Lifeline Crisis Support Text

Text to 0477 13 11 14

Lifeline Crisis Support Phone

13 11 14

Suicide Call Back Service

1300 659 467

Butterfly Foundation National Helpline (for eating disorders)

1800 33 4673

Other Mental Health Resources

Entertainment Community Fund (formerly The Actor's Fund)—The Dancer's Resource

https://entertainmentcommunity.org/services-and-programs/dancers-resource

Minding the Gap—Mental health resources customized specifically for dancers

www.WeAreMindingTheGap.com

Mental Health First Aid—Training to support people during a mental health crisis (this training is for everyone, not just health care providers)

USA: www.mentalhealthfirstaid.org

International: https://mhfainternational.org

National Alliance on Mental Illness

https://nami.org

1-800-950-6264

Appendix B

Psychological Safety in Dance: Emotions and Intimacy

Emotional Safety in Dance

Misty Lown, ME-PD
Owner and Founder, Misty's Dance Unlimited, LLC

College dance students often teach at their home dance studios or studios near their university and, therefore, regularly interact with children at varying stages of dance training. Thus, it is crucial for you to understand the significance of emotional safety in the dance education atmosphere and how to properly manage it.

Dance is, at its core, about interpersonal connections—among students in a group, within a piece of choreography, between teachers and students, and between dancers and an audience. Achieving these relationships requires a high level of emotional safety—particularly for students as they advance in their training—because dance is, by nature, an activity that requires vulnerability. Bodies are typically clad in leotards and tights; partnering and weight-sharing are a regular part of many genres; emotions allow for storytelling and character building. To fully participate, dancers must become comfortable opening up emotionally.

The Importance of Emotional Safety

Just as educators must keep their students physically safe, they have a responsibility to ensure their emotional safety, too. Young students—some of whom will become professional dance artists, and all of whom will hopefully become conscientious young adults—require an environment where vulnerability is applauded and embraced. They need a place to be their authentic selves and be valued for that authenticity. They need a place to fall (and fail) and have the support to try again and again, strengthening their confidence muscles along with their dance skills.

In that same vein, for some students, emotional safety within the dance studio is an absolute lifeline—a connection beyond the artistic implications. Perhaps their home life isn't stable or their relationships at school are thin. Dance becomes their safety net; it's the place where they can not only be themselves but also be helped in the event that life throws them a curveball. Knowing they have caring grown-ups to confide in and friends to lean on, some students cling to the emotional safety of the studio as their safe haven. These dancers are more willing to open up and thus, to find support. You must properly prepare yourself to be one of those "grown-ups" whenever you have the chance to teach and develop young dancers.

Creating Emotional Safety in Dance

Creating emotional safety in dance starts with educating the educators. It begins with studio owners, program directors, and teachers understanding that their impact goes beyond dance steps and skills. It involves training, such as what is offered through Youth Protection Association for Dance, to define what an emotionally safe space looks like and how to maintain it. For some leaders in dance, it requires a shift in mindset to *put the dancer before the dance*. In other words, the dancer's well-being—physical and emotional—must always be paramount. Of course, a choreographer's creative vision matters, and so does a teacher's curriculum milestone or a studio owner's enrollment goal. However, none of those things should come before the health and wellness of a student.

Feeling emotionally safe in dance is for all who participate. Even the youngest dancers need this assurance, and teachers must realize and act on it. Preschoolers and elementary level students must be allowed to be themselves while they explore their imaginations and feelings as they move through class exercises.

Creating an emotionally safe space for students looks like implementing well-thought, proactive tactics designed to help every dancer feel welcome and supported. Such tactics may include the following:

- Planning a consistent class structure to promote predictability.
- Utilizing "bookends" for each class that include a warm welcome at the beginning and a version of révérence (a dancer's way of saying goodbye and thank you) at the end.
- Offering structured improvisation or freestyle exercises to allow students the freedom to express themselves during a section of class.
- Opening up time for questions during class time, or time for sharing personal reflections.
- Using a smile and warmth in the voice while teaching, in addition to open body language.
- Recognizing the warning signs of possible mental health concerns, and sharing those concerns with the student's parent(s) when needed.

Choreographically, dance educators can encourage student well-being by choosing themes, concepts, costumes, movement, and music that match the dancers' developmental abilities and emotional capacity. For instance, a concept about friendship would be psychologically safe for preteens, while a concept about a love relationship would not. Teachers and choreographers must continually tap into their deep wells of creativity, thinking of the students' well-being first when exploring artistic choices.

Takeaways

As students make progress in their training, there will be more demands on their self-discipline; however, that discipline should not diminish their willingness to be vulnerable. It is a balancing act for which every teacher strives—educating for technique and skill while cultivating a safe space for connections. Emotional safety is necessary for dancers—and dance—to thrive. Great dancing is subjective, but great humans are not. When emotional safety is prioritized, students flourish.

Resources

More Than Just Great Dancing
https://morethanjustgreatdancing.com

Youth Protection Association for Dance
https://ypadnow.com

Nonprofit Education and Advocacy for the Movement Arts
https://neamacares.org

Safe in Dance International
https://safeindance.com

Personal Safety for Dance
https://personalsafetyfordance.com

The Arts Wellbeing Collective
https://artswellbeingcollective.com.au

Mental Health First Aid, from National Council for Mental Wellbeing
www.mentalhealthfirstaid.org/population-focused-modules/youth (youth Mental Health First Aid)

Inner Drive
https://blog.innerdrive.co.uk/sports/10-psychological-safety-tips (ways to support psychological safety)

Dance DATA Project
www.dancedataproject.com/creating-a-safe-dance-environment (college student oriented resources)

National Center on Safe Supportive Learning Environments
https://safesupportivelearning.ed.gov/topic-research/safety/emotional-safety (emotional well-being as related to the school environment)

Boys and Girls Clubs of America
www.bgca.org/news-stories/2023/July/emotional-check-ins-for-kids (ways to support emotional well-being in children)

Guidelines for Intimacy Safety in Dance and Theater

Courtney Abbott, MFA
Freelance intimacy director, actor, and educator

For ages, dance and theater makers have been relying on the talent and courage of individual performers to manifest believable and meaningful moments of physical intimacy, often with no effort to draw a dividing line between what is reality and what is artifice. Consent has rarely been a consideration, let alone a priority. This approach leads to—at worst—deeply damaging abuses of power and—at best—vague storytelling with unpredictable or unrepeatable onstage moments.

Choreographing intimacy work takes the guesswork out of physical storytelling. With guided exercises to practice establishing and honoring one another's boundaries along with a shared language to use around moments of contact, performers can experiment in rehearsal with confidence. The following section includes various topics for you to consider and answers common questions related to the role of intimacy in dance. Whether this aspect of dance is new to you or you are already familiar with it, you are encouraged to explore the resources offered at the end of the section for more information.

What Is Intimacy?

Intimacy is more than just stage kisses. Moments of simulated romance or sex may come to mind at first, but performers may find themselves in intimate contact in partnered dance, in improvisational movement, and even in a devising process. In these situations there is often a disparity in power.

Power Dynamics

Power dynamics are always at play in collaborative work. Teachers and choreographers traditionally have power that their students do not; institutions hold power over those teachers and choreographers; and casting directors, competition judges, and awards committees often exert power over those institutions; the hierarchy goes on and on. Those in positions of greater power must be aware of how those dynamics impact consent.

Consent

Is consent a priority in the space? You can make it one! Get into the habit of checking in with yourself and other dancers about physical touch. Acknowledging your own boundaries and communicating about them gives permission to others to do the same. For example, before rehearsing a partnered dance, one partner may ask the other if the choreography needs any review or revision. Together the two can decide to mark a move, perhaps, or to modify a move, according to both artists' needs. Because of the many power dynamics in artistic spaces, it can be helpful to have an *intimacy professional* facilitate these conversations.

What Does an Intimacy Professional Do?

An intimacy professional assists creative performing artists to craft moments of intimacy that are consensual and repeatable. The intimacy professional will offer artists opportunities to name their boundaries and needs as well as the agency to choose how to address them.

Defining Boundaries Without an Intimacy Professional

There may come a time when you are in a class, or working on a performance piece, or learning choreography in a callback when you discover—to your dismay—that even though your gut, your heart, and your mind tell you there absolutely should be an intimacy professional in the room, there is not an intimacy professional in the room. This scenario may occur when something is happening that crosses your boundaries. For example, the instructor is too hands on for comfort, the dancers you're working with keep pushing to add sexualized emphasis to your piece, the choreographer pairs off couples and teaches a partnered lift that involves one dancer's hand in the other's groin . . . and some part of your brain is thinking . . . um, wait, what about consent?

What can you do in a classroom, rehearsal, or workspace where there is no intimacy professional? You can advocate for consensual practices and define your own boundaries based on your own experiences. You have a right to stand up for yourself. In any context. Period. There is no sacred code that binds you to blindly obey an instructor—especially if a leader is being abusive.

You don't owe anyone access to your body. It's okay to want to change in private. It's okay to not want to perform dance moves that feel uncomfortable to you—both in terms of strength and flexibility and in terms of your comfort with self-touch, with performance of sexuality, or with stereotypically gendered movement.

Your boundaries exist because of your unique experiences, and they are perfect just as they are. When informing someone about a boundary, you are under no obligation to justify that boundary by exposing any details or backstory. If someone asks, you can simply tell them that information is private, or you can check in with them as to why they are asking; maybe all they want is clarity so they can better respect the boundary.

Takeaways

Remember: The dance you can make is unlike anyone else's. Compromising your own boundaries will only serve to suppress your art.

I hope this text has helped you to reflect on the way that consent and intimacy work can contribute positively to your creative spaces. Often, it is urgency—not intentional cruelty—that leads someone to cross a boundary; in their rush to get the result they want, they fail to respect and honor the humans involved. Some of the most important work I do is helping folks to momentarily slow down, take stock, and communicate.

Resources

Intimacy Direction in Dance
www.intimacydirectionindance.com

Moving Body Arts
www.movingbodyarts.com

Theatrical Intimacy Education
www.theatricalintimacyed.com

Intimacy Coordinators of Color
www.intimacycoordinatorsofcolor.com

Momentum Stage, Inc., The Equitable Performing Arts Classroom
www.momentumstage.org/equitable-arts

Appendix C

Screening for Dancer Health

Laura Santos, MS, LAT, ATC

In health care, screening is a tool used to detect increased risk for a condition such as an illness or injury so that an intervention can be applied to limit or prevent harm. Screenings are not predictive. In other words, positive results (results that suggest the presence of a characteristic that needs extra attention) do not foretell for certain that illness or injury will occur. Likewise, negative results (results that suggest the absence of a characteristic that could lead to an illness or injury) do not mean that a condition will not occur. The true value of the positive result of a screening is that it presents an opportunity to connect individuals with resources that can support their health and, in the case of dancers, their performance. Although sometimes overlooked as either inconvenient or intrusive, comprehensive screenings are well worth the time and effort because of their potential to equip students with the skills and knowledge to get the most out of dance training.

Why Implement Dancer Screening?

Recognizing that participation in dance carries inherent risk, medical teams use dancer health screenings to identify challenges to health that can also become barriers to optimal performance. Such challenges include previous history of injury, low energy availability, irregular menstrual patterns, and substance use. Since literature in dance medicine and sports medicine suggests that injury risk is multifactorial, it makes sense to screen for a variety of contributors to that risk. A comprehensive dancer health screening is a combination of various evaluation tools that are tailored to address the unique concerns of the dance population.

Typical Parts of a Dancer Screening Program

When a dancer health screening is implemented at your university or dance company, commonly used components may include the following:

- *Questionnaires* about injury or personal health history, family health history, current activity level, sleep, menstrual history (where applicable), 24-hour food recall, eating attitudes and behaviors, substance use, mood, and more; questionnaires may also screen for concerns such as food insecurity or academic challenges. Such items help inform the concept of whole-person wellness that is woven throughout this book.
- *Anthropometric measurements* such as height, weight, and body composition
- *Vital signs*, including heart rate, temperature, and blood pressure
- *Fitness measurements* such as flexibility, strength, balance, and endurance tests
- *Functional testing* using dance-specific activities that can illuminate deficits or imbalances to be addressed for improved dance performance
- *Equipment fit testing* that identifies how the equipment fits your body, especially footwear evaluation and any specialized wardrobe pieces required for a particular performance

While some types of screening, such as physical fitness tests, might take place in a studio or other open area, it is preferable for other screening activities (e.g., body measurements, interview consultations) to take place in a more private setting so that dancers feel comfortable and so that the discussion may be more fruitful. Health screenings are separate from any skills assessments or placement classes a school or company might conduct, and the results of your individual screenings should be held in confidence between the health care team and you. Sometimes, it may be appropriate for de-identified (all personally identifying information removed), aggregate data to be shared with faculty or used for research purposes; in these instances, the health care team should observe all applicable ethical guidelines and protect your individual identity.

Some health and wellness promotion teams also use screening sessions as an opportunity to gather information about your goals. When reviewing the screening results, you and the team member(s) can collaborate to develop a plan that addresses any potential health or functional challenges while working toward your aims for your dance training. At the bare minimum, you should be made aware of your screening results and provided with appropriate referrals for further evaluation or intervention as needed. Ideally, the health care team will provide all screened students with some level of education about how to reduce injury risk while promoting optimum wellness, health, and resilience.

Takeaways

Screenings incorporated into dance programs can provide very useful reports that guide dancers toward improving their overall health and performance. They can take many forms and gather a wide variety of data. However, the goal of such screenings—and the motivation of the individuals who provide the screenings and use the information they gather—should always be to encourage you toward optimal wellness and to maximize your opportunity to pursue dance in a safe, healthy manner.

Appendix D

Disability Dance and Integrated Dance: Inviting a Radical Re-Visioning

Merry Lynn Morris, PhD, MFA, LMT

Dancers with long-term disabilities represent a dance population that is often overlooked within the dance landscape. When it comes to training precision, reduction of injury risk, injury management methods, and performance opportunities, this population tends to be underserved. Most people who embark on intensive study of dance will experience some form of disability along their preprofessional or professional trajectory. However, people often understand disabilities to be short-term injuries or conditions—be they mental or physical—that will be rehabilitated, returning the dancer to their prior bodily habitus or something very close to it. The gap in understanding is that long-term disability in dance is far more prevalent than discussed and addressed. Many dancers navigate scoliosis, hypermobility conditions, disordered eating or eating disorders, anxiety, permanent age-related changes, and many other mental or physical disabilities. Because of stigma often associated with disability as well as the corresponding expectations of the dance field, dancers tend to conceal these issues, viewing them as a sign of weakness, which potentially leads them to discontinue their dance pursuits.

The Scope of Disability

While some acknowledgment of disabilities occurs in the dance field at large, the scope of disability and its permanence are narrowly conceived. Therefore, training and wellness approaches may also be narrowly conceived. The dance and disability field, as signified by pioneering U.S.-based companies such as Dancing Wheels and AXIS Dance Company, prompts a radical rethinking of traditional approaches to training and artistry, thus allowing an embrace of a much wider breadth of possibilities for dance across a spectrum of bodies (figure D.1).

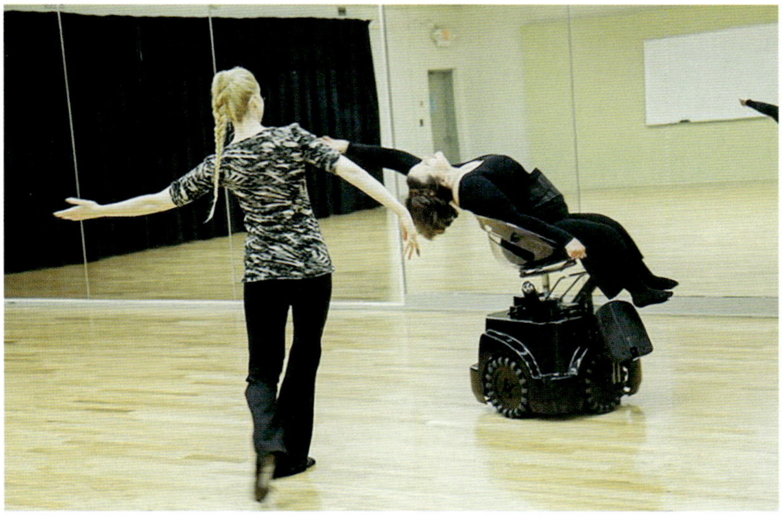

Figure D.1 Marcie Ryan, a professional dancer formerly of the Dancing Wheels company, has an L4-L5 spinal cord injury and typically performs using a manual wheelchair. In this photo, Marcie experiments improvisationally with another dancer, exploring the movement capacities in a prototype power chair that responds to leaning actions of the body through a wearable wireless controller.

University of South Florida College of the Arts

The notion of a dancer with a spinal cord injury, permanent paralysis, amputation, cerebral palsy, spina bifida, intellectual or developmental disability (e.g., autism spectrum disorder), blindness or low vision, or deafness or hard of hearing to be rigorously pursuing dance tends to be excluded from consideration. Other than anecdotal information, little is known about injury patterns, injury prevention, or wellness strategies for dancers with physical, intellectual, developmental, or sensory disabilities.

Questioning Our Current Practice

The dance and disability field invites a questioning of traditional forms of dance practice, including how to address and approach injury. Most dance practice (apart from dance improvisation) is predicated on a body that moves or is expected to move and process information in a prescribed way. This uniform way of moving and processing is frequently mapped onto a room full of bodies, without question.

When a dancer's body does not move in the prescribed way (e.g., due to anatomic restrictions, pain, or injury), what alternatives does that dancer have to adapt the material and yet still feel included in the dance practice (figure D.2)? When a dancer cannot process information in the same way or at the same speed as other dancers in the room, what options are there for that dancer, other than feeling like an outlier—or worse, an outcast—and self-selecting out of dance?

Dance practice and training often assume one bodily norm; therefore, dance is approached in a largely uniform way where students are meant to mirror the exact movement prescription of the teacher and respond to verbal, visual, and tactile cues in specific ways.

However, in an integrated or inclusive setting (figure D.3), the expectations are different in terms of who might be present in the class. Thus, the approach differs. In the integrated or inclusive setting, it is natural to provide alternative techniques when delivering a dance combination, dance cue, or prompt. Space is often made for the dancer to exert agency via multiple choices and help cocreate and collaborate to find solutions to dance goals or concepts. In this setting, bodies with disability are part of the norm; disability, whether short-term or long-term, is viewed as normative rather than as an exception. Adaptation, transposition, experimentation, and creative, collaborative problem solving within a diversity of bodily possibilities are key parts of the training and artistic practice. What if all classes adopted such an approach?

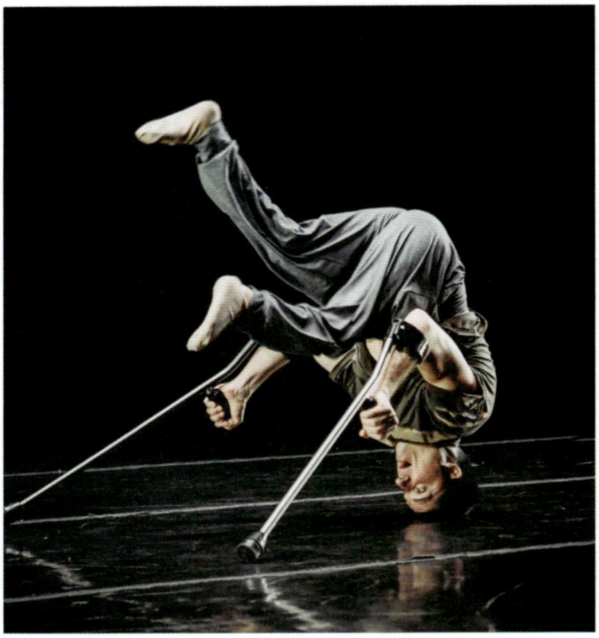

Figure D.2 Luca "LazyLegz" Patuelli is a Canadian breaker who has arthrogryposis and uses his crutches in creative ways to explore innovative movement possibilities.

Tom Kramer

Takeaways

There are several factors on which dancers, dance teachers, choreographers, and health professionals should reflect when taking or teaching class, when treating dancers, or when evaluating dance practice. Ask the following questions of one another, then adopt new approaches to include all dancers.

- What assumptions guide our approach to dance and dancers?
- Who do we think of when we say, "dancer"? Who haven't we considered?
- Who is implicitly left out due to traditional designs and approaches of dance practice?
- Do we know how diverse our students actually are?
- Do students know the true prevalence of the many forms of disability in dance?
- Do students know that disability can be a driver of artistic innovation?

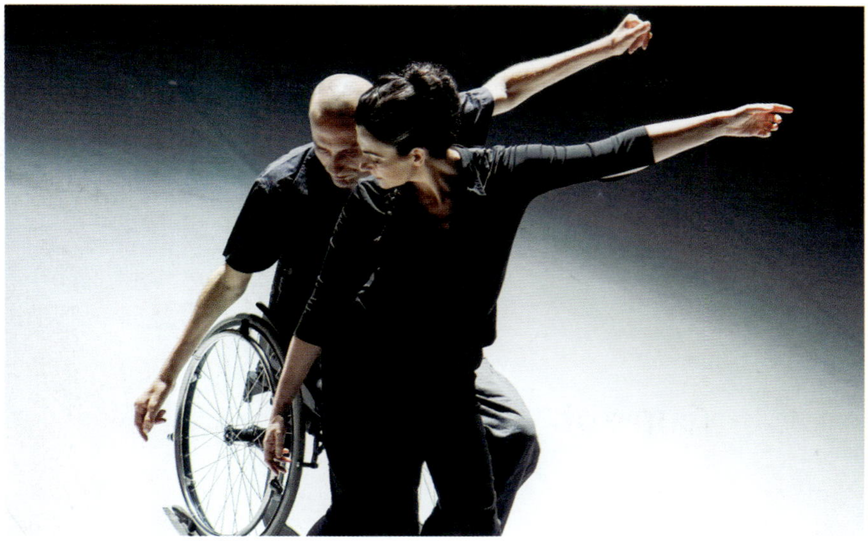

Figure D.3 Israeli dancers Hai Cohen, a wheelchair user with a spinal cord injury, and Tali Wertheim depict physically integrated dance built on contact improvisation methods. They are the comanagers of Israel's Vertigo Power of Balance.
Elad Debi

For Further Reading

Albright, A.C. (2010). *Choreographing difference: The body and identity in contemporary dance*. Wesleyan University Press.

Benjamin, A. (2013). *Making an entrance: Theory and practice for disabled and non-disabled dancers*. Routledge.

Dubon, M., Siegel, R., Smith, J., Tomasic, M. & Morris, M.L. (2021). New directions in dance medicine: Dancers with disabilities, blindness/low vision, and/or deafness/hard of hearing. *Physical Medicine and Rehabilitation Clinics*, 32(1), pp.185-205.

Kuppers, P. (2013). *Disability and contemporary performance: Bodies on the edge*. Routledge.

Wiederholt, E., & Laukkanen, S. (2022). *Breadth of bodies: Discussing disability in dance*. Stance on Dance.

Appendix E

Considerations for Professional Dance

Becoming a professional dancer and then flourishing as one is not an easy undertaking. Nevertheless, it is the dream of many young dancers, including those in college. Navigating this pathway is made easier when you possess specialized insights that illustrate how success is achieved. In this appendix, two health care professionals with decades of experience helping professional dancers thrive offer their insights about the practices that are necessary to excel and how to manage the challenges of touring when you dance for a living.

Life Lessons for Professional Dance From a Health Care Outsider Looking In

Sheyi Ojofeitimi, PT, DPT, OCS, CFMT
Director of Therapy Services, Alvin Ailey American Dance Foundation and Co-Founder, Dance Ready Project

Dancers are incredible beings; indeed, they are unheralded athletes. They pour their heart and soul into their craft, thereby achieving herculean feats with their bodies. I have spent 22 years treating elite preprofessional and professional dancers. I have watched as generations of dancers pursued their dreams; some seemed to reach their goals with ease, while others struggled at every turn. What was the difference between these two groups? What was the secret ingredient? It wasn't the dance elements that most people might expect. In fact, the dancers who "made it" did not always have the best feet, perfect lines, or highest legs; they did, however, use these three essential ingredients: preparation, perspective, and mental flexibility.

The Three Essential Ingredients

1. *Preparation*: This ingredient has less to do with what studio or school you trained at and more to do with *your daily habits* where you are now. How do you prepare your mind and your body for the day ahead? What do you do the night before? What do you do to get ready a few hours or minutes before class, rehearsal, or a performance? Those things that you do consistently will impact your progress. You are probably saying, "My schedule is crazy! I don't have time for anything else!" My response is that if you have time to watch television, then you have time to prepare your body. For example, while watching television, you can roll out and stretch the often-neglected quadriceps, calves, and gluteal muscles. If you binge-watch anything, you can have a whole new amazing body by the time you finish the series!
2. *Perspective*: How do you see yourself? Do you consider yourself an athlete? If not, why not? The truth is that *dancers are athletes*. As a dancer, you should understand and accept this concept. Once you do, you will begin to prioritize health and fitness. The students and professionals I work with who understand it are the ones who have regularly scheduled conditioning before class and rehearsals. They also spend time at the end of the day apologizing to their bodies with acts of self-care such as stretching, rolling out, taking baths, and meditating. Throughout my work with these athletic artists, I noticed that they tended to have fewer injuries and longer careers than those who only danced.
3. *Mental flexibility*: In order to dance better, you often have to *dance less*. For many, that statement does not make any sense, but let me explain: Dance, like any other sport, creates muscle imbalances in the body. Muscle imbalances put you at higher risk of injury.

Doing other activities such as yoga, Pilates, Gyrokinesis, Gyrotonic, and the like helps address and correct these imbalances. The result is a healthier, freer body that translates to better dancing. Where does the mental flexibility come in? It comes with your willingness to try something new—something that will build a part of you besides your dance technique. If you are just hearing this for the first time, I encourage you to try it. Rather than take that third optional dance class for the day, try Pilates or another nondance activity. If you have heard this before and are still struggling to implement it, then this encouragement to invest in your mental flexibility is especially for you.

The Importance of Proper Fuel

Based on my observations of preprofessional and professional dancers over many years, I want to add one more important note to round up my advice to you. It may even be the foundation on which everything else is built. *Feed your cells, not just your stomach.* Your stomach can be full while your cells are still starving. Your cells need the right kind and amount of nutrients to provide you with energy to sustain you physically and mentally. What you consume and when you consume it matters. Remember the word GIGO—garbage in, garbage out. In other words, you get out what you put in. Be intentional about what you put in your body. Chapter 7 is loaded with advice.

Takeaways

Your body is wonderfully made, and it is unique. It is your tool, and it is irreplaceable. Take care of every part of it. Whether or not you intend to pursue dance professionally, these ingredients will serve you well. However, if you are aiming for a professional dance career, they are essential; you cannot succeed without them.

Keys to Success as a Dancer on Tour

Kori L. Kirschner, MS, LAT, ATC, CSCS*D

Dancers have an incredible ability to connect and interact with people while onstage. They have a special relationship with fellow dancers, stagehands, and management as well as with spectators, agents, peers, and everyone in between. As a dancer is sculpted into their artistry from the time they put on their first ballet slipper until they don a 2.5-inch (6 cm) character heel or a jazz shoe, they are engulfed by the world of dance—the wardrobe, the music, the blocking—all of it! Finally, when a dancer commits to touring with a production, everything about this exciting world becomes magnified.

I have worked as an athletic trainer for dancers my entire professional career (over 15 years), with most of it in the touring part of the industry. I have noted the characteristics of successful touring artists, and I am sharing these with you here for your own success. As a dancer, you are educated in many integral components that create discipline, such as critical thinking, perseverance, preparedness, balance, strength, and flexibility. You also have incredible abilities and personality. However, you can prepare for a touring career contract all your life, be at the top of your conservatory class, and still lack the adaptability and boundaries you need to succeed. Without these factors, your career may end before you reach the first city of the tour.

Adaptability to an Ever-Changing Landscape

Adaptability is the quality of being able to adjust to new conditions. As a touring citizen, you will encounter the challenge to be adaptable in varying degrees. Some tour citizens already possess adaptability as a strong character trait, and others find that doing the work to become adaptable creates character-building moments that help them survive life on the road. Both types of individuals have a place. Here are some examples of adaptability on tour:

1. You have been given a schedule for a travel day the night before the company is due to leave. The next day, the departure flight is delayed or cancelled, causing the entire unit to be split between a few different flights that arrive at your destination at all hours of the early morning. Your 4-hour travel day just became a 12-hour travel day, thus

resulting in a so-called day *off* that is not the most restful. You can handle this situation in a couple of ways: You can complain the entire day, have a few too many alcoholic beverages at the airport bar, and stomp up to your touring manager (who has no control over air traffic control or airline management) to give them a piece of your mind after you have posted on social media what an awful day you are having because you will not get your precious rest that you thought you were going to have. Alternatively, you can accept the things you cannot control and adjust accordingly. You can read the book you brought, binge-watch your favorite show on your phone, call a good friend, take a nap, walk around to get in your daily step count, or do a yoga flow for some active recovery while you wait. The second method clearly displays your adaptability.

2. You arrive at your first city on your first professional touring contract. You are responsible for doing your own laundry, grocery shopping, and communicating to your dance captain or the head of wardrobe or props that your costume or prop needs attention. You also need to squeeze in your workout, eat balanced meals, be social, call your loved ones, and be a well-rounded tour citizen. (This same scenario then happens weekly because you travel to a new city every week—or sometimes to two or more cities in a week.) Again, there are two ways one can handle these touring duties: You could have a complete panic attack and emotional meltdown because your mom always did your laundry; fixed your costumes and props; prepared your meals; and organized your dance classes, rehab appointments, and exercise sessions. She also signed you up for your community's summer musical season so you would learn to be social. Alternatively, you can start asking questions to set yourself up for success. Before you leave for tour, you can ask your parents or guardians to teach you how to do your laundry, prep your meals, and communicate with others to obtain assistance. You can also ask another tour citizen for help with these duties. Typically, a touring unit will have a washer and dryer provided by the company for the cast, crew, and staff, so you can sign up for a time slot to do your laundry. If your company has a different arrangement, you may need to do your laundry in the hotel or find a nearby laundromat. For meal prepping, you can learn the unique abilities your fellow tour citizens possess for cooking food at the venue or at the hotel, and you can figure out ways to collaborate for everyone's nutritional benefit. In other words, you can put adaptability in action by choosing this second response.

Adaptability on tour is crucial for longevity in the entertainment environment. Every day, something on the task list will need to be adjusted—from show times and travel days to managing injuries and dark weeks. Understand that adaptability does not give permission to cross over the boundaries of that to which you can reasonably be expected to adapt. Even the most well-rounded, well-adjusted tour citizens must consciously practice balancing adaptability with knowing their boundaries to avoid becoming overextended and overwhelmed. Boundaries are discussed next.

Boundaries That Foster a Wholesome Environment

A boundary is a line that marks the limits of an area; it is a dividing line. A well-rounded tour citizen can successfully interact with many different types of people who have a variety of personalities, and you will encounter many different departments and support staff in a show unit. Establishing healthy boundaries is another crucial component for a long, prosperous, and enjoyable touring experience.

Creating boundaries is not the same as putting in place the emotional fences that provide a sense of safety or defense. Creating these healthy boundaries involves communicating to your fellow tour citizens and community locals that you care for and appreciate them and expressing your desire to be the best tour citizen possible while still protecting your ability to live well on the road. Here are a couple of examples of creating boundaries while on tour:

1. You arrive on tour. On your only day off, the company requests that you drive a vehicle to the airport an hour away to pick up some fellow tour citizens. (You are old enough to be able to drive a company vehicle.) You politely decline the request because you do not feel comfortable driving others in

a company vehicle and you would like a day off work to rest, relax, and recover. You also do not want to put others in potential danger because you are anxious about driving others in the company vehicle. This is a healthy boundary; you know your limits of comfort and stress, and you stay within them.

2. Your roommate invites a couple of friends over, and you are getting very tired. In about 6 hours, you have to be awake and ready for an early-morning public relations event. You can communicate your boundaries in a couple of ways: Before any friends arrive, you discuss room rules with your roommate, and you kindly arrange that the friends should leave no later than an agreed time to permit everyone to get a good night's sleep. Another option is that once the get-together is underway—not realizing the friends would stay so late—you politely communicate to your roommate that you are fading and would like the gathering to move elsewhere so that you can get a good night's sleep and be ready for your morning session.

There are many types of boundaries and varying degrees of implementing them to create a healthy environment on tour. These examples represent only a couple of encounter types you may experience. Overall, you must respect yourself and know your value, including what you can offer to a touring community. Then you must respect and value your fellow tour citizens. Creating healthy boundaries will help build long-lasting friendships and bonds with your touring colleagues.

Takeaways

You can only know what you know, and you can only control what you can control. Communicate to others about areas where you may need assistance, education, or clarity. As a touring citizen, you are living and working as part of an interdependent community. This arrangement may produce a moment (I call it a *human moment*) when someone—even you—makes a mistake or says the wrong thing at the wrong time to the wrong person. It is very important to be adaptable, create healthy boundaries, and communicate appropriately to help minimize those character breaking points. When one of these breaking points does occur, however, it can be an effective learning experience for you and your touring community. Life on tour is very challenging, but it is also adventurous and exhilarating. As you gain experience, you will learn how to find assistance and support while making necessary adjustments.

Appendix F

Artistry and Athletics: The Rigors of College Dance Team

Olivia Placita, BS; assistant coach, dance team, The Ohio State University
Melissa McGhee, BS; head coach, dance team and director, Eugene D. Smith Leadership Institute, The Ohio State University

At many colleges and universities across the United States, there are two types of dance training that seem very different from each other: academic dance for students majoring in dance, and dance team—a genre often associated primarily with sports contests. Collegiate dance teams generate interest from many dancers in traditional academic dance programs. Typically, the dance students who wish to pursue dance team during their college experience come from that background in high school or in their local studio environment. While the two styles of dance training are quite dissimilar, the essences of both have some common bonds that can be appreciated. Moreover, dancers studying in an academic major of dance with an eye on participating for their college dance team should understand the rigors of dance team at the collegiate level in order to maximize their experience and reduce the risk of injury.

The Nature of the Dance Team Environment

The collegiate dance team world has slowly developed from its club sport category at most universities to now being one of the most competitive and rigorous athletic programs among university sports. It continues to gain popularity, and the high-energy choreography of college dance teams is unmistakable (figure F.1). Moreover, dance team is wholly distinct from cheer (cheerleading).

Consistent throughout all college dance team programs are specific standards that must be met. In most situations, college dance teams are seen as ambassadors for their university. While they are easily recognized in front of audiences at many of their school's athletic events, college dance teams

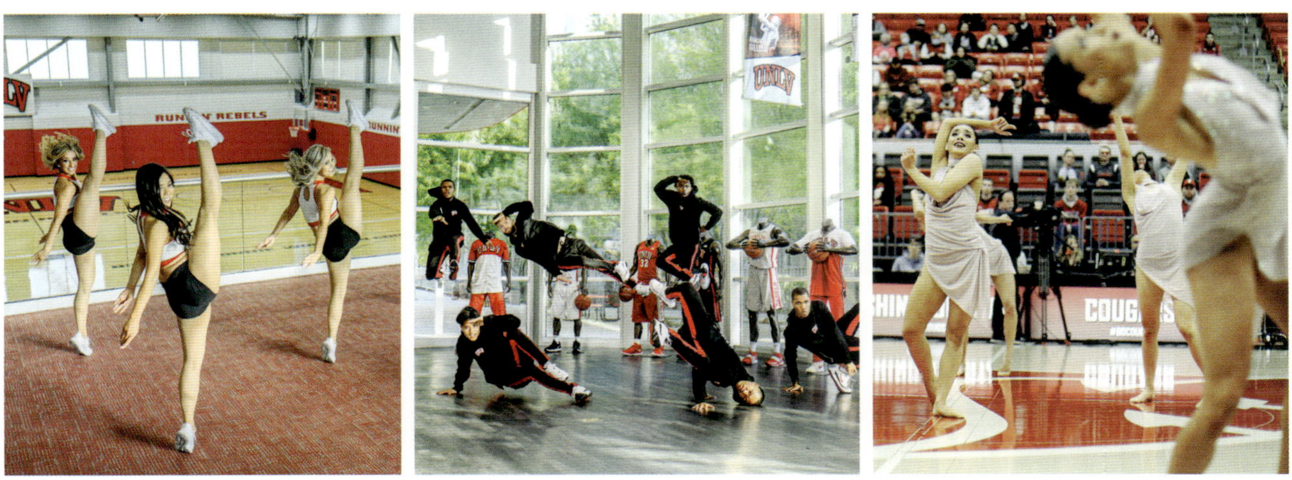

Figure F.1 While there are differences between typical academic dance and dance team, there also are a number of similarities.

A & B: The Rebel Girls + Company. University of Nevada Las Vegas. Photo: Jerry Hughes Photography; C: The Crimson Girls. Washington State University. Photo: Ashley Davis Photo take part in their own rigorous dance training elements that the outside world does not see. Certainly, providing fan spirit activities for sports such as football, basketball, volleyball, hockey, and wrestling is important; however, the heart and soul of most dance team programs is revealed when they are in their own element of dance team competitions.

The pinnacle moment for college dance teams is the national competition. At these events, college programs from across the country travel to one site to contend for awards in categories that include jazz, pom, hip-hop, and game day. Every division at the college dance team national championship is stacked with the best teams in the country. Each of them has trained for 5 to 6 months, building to this one event when they leave every bit of talent, energy, and stamina they have on the dance floor. The combination of artistic expression and athletic power is quite striking.

Preparation for Dance Team Participation

Dance team, like an academic dance program, requires a substantial time commitment. There is a distinction between dance teams focused on success in dance team competitions and those who primarily offer spirit support for their college sports teams. A typical training environment for a competitive dance team is 3 or 4 days a week for 4 hours each day, plus an additional 3 days of physical workouts that include aerobic and anaerobic conditioning and weightlifting. Some universities employ a strength and conditioning coach who has part of their workload assigned to assisting the dancers. Also necessary are specific exercises to develop muscles for the elaborate, dynamic dance performance pieces.

The importance of nutrition, hydration, and recovery cannot be overstated for dance team dancers. Some programs have nutritionists or dietitians who work closely with the dancers to develop appropriate meal plans, especially for the high-intensity physical requirements of the season. The level of challenge to the body is similar to collegiate sports participation, and dance teams' recovery methods are similar, too. These methods may include compression boots and therapeutic cold treatments. While unfortunately not all college dance teams have access to athletic trainers (in spite of the need and benefits of such health care attention), dance team is a rigorous activity for which contemporary measures of reducing the risk of injuries—and proper treatment and rehabilitation regimens for injuries when they do occur—are crucial.

Takeaways

Collegiate dance team participation is increasing in both its following and its participation. Its similarities with traditional academic dance genres, such as ballet, modern, jazz, and others, include creative choreography, passionate dancers, remarkable physicality, and an inscrutable commitment to excellence. As with any dance activity, there is a risk of injury in dance team. However, carefully prescribed training methods and access to specialized health care practitioners will yield many benefits for dance team dancers.

Glossary

accessory navicular—An extra bone that may be found attached to the navicular bone slightly below and forward of the medial ankle at the top of the medial arch; the posterior tibial tendon attaches to it.

Achilles tendon—The largest and strongest tendon in the body, connecting the posterior calf muscles (gastrocnemius and soleus) to the heel bone (calcaneus).

acute injury—Injury that occurs during a sudden, traumatic event and typically results in immediate pain or loss of function.

adenosine triphosphate (ATP)—Important source of energy in the body that drives living cells and actions such as muscle contraction.

advocacy—Promoting the interests of a group or individual.

aerobic—Literally meaning "with air," it refers to the body producing energy with the use of oxygen. It typically involves any exercise that lasts longer than 2 minutes.

aerobic exercise—Describes the oxidative energy system, or refers to physical activity that relies on that system, where oxygen is a component of the energy production processes.

aerobic training—Describes the type of physical activity that is fueled by the production of energy from carbohydrates, amino acids, and fats using physiological processes that incorporate oxygen.

agonist—The muscle (or group of muscles) primarily responsible for creating an action.

allied health professionals—Trained practitioners who provide specific types of health care services and who are not physicians, surgeons, dentists, physician assistants, or nurses. This category of providers includes physical therapists, athletic trainers, massage therapists, and several others.

amenorrhea—The absence of menstruation, often defined as missing one or more menstrual periods. Primary amenorrhea refers to the absence of menstruation in someone who has not had a period by age 15.

anaerobic—Literally meaning "without air," it refers to the body producing energy using processes that do not need oxygen. Describes an energy system, or refers to physical activity that relies on that system, where oxygen is not necessary for completion of the energy production processes.

anaerobic training—Describes the type of physical activity that is fueled by the production of energy using physiological processes that do not incorporate oxygen.

analysis of variance (ANOVA)—An inferential statistical technique that is used to check whether the means of two or more groups are significantly different from one another. ANOVA is used when only one variable is present to calculate the mean, while MANOVA (multivariate ANOVA) is used when two or more than two variables are present.

anatomical snuffbox—Area located at the base of the thumb that is created by the tendons of extensor pollicis longus on one side and the extensor pollicis brevis and abductor pollicis longus on the other.

anorexia nervosa—Clinical eating disorder characterized by voluntary restrictions of food intake, refusing to keep body weight at or above the 85th percentile for height and age, denial of hunger, intense fears of gaining weight, and a distorted body image.

antagonist—The muscle (or group of muscles) responsible for the action that opposes the agonist.

anterior chain system—Muscle groups located at the front of the body.

anterior cruciate ligament (ACL)—Ligament in the knee that attaches the top of the tibia to inside the notch between the two knobs of the bottom of the femur; it functions especially to prevent forward shifting and hyperextension of the knee. It is the primary stabilizer of the knee and is subject to injury when the knee rotates during physical activity.

anterior talofibular ligament (ATFL)—Lateral ligament in the ankle running from the anterior portion of the end of the fibula to the talus. It is the most commonly injured ankle ligament.

anterior tibiofibular ligament—Ligament in the ankle starting at the anterior portion of the tibia and attaching on the lateral fibula that holds the ends of these bones together at the ankle.

antioxidant—A substance (natural or manufactured) that can protect against oxidants such as free radicals. Free radicals have an unpaired electron in their chemical structure that makes them very unstable, reactive, and damaging to cells. Antioxidants can stabilize and neutralize free radicals by donating an electron to a free radical's molecule.

anxiety—Emotional and mental reaction to an anticipated future event or situation that does not exist yet or is unlikely to exist.

aorta—The large artery that carries oxygenated blood away from the heart to the body.

apophysitis—Inflammation occurring at an apophysis (a growth area in a bone where a tendon attaches) that is caused by a tendon pulling on a bone at the tendon's attachment site during repeated contraction of the tendon's muscle.

arthroscopic surgery—Surgery using a slender telescopic instrument that is inserted into a joint.

athlete's foot—Also known as tinea pedis, it is an itchy, scaly foot rash caused by a fungus.

autonomic nervous system—The part of the nervous system that does not require voluntary or conscious input to control bodily functions (e.g., the heart, lungs, and other internal organs are supplied by the autonomic nervous system).

avoidant/restrictive food intake disorder (ARFID)—Avoidance or restriction of certain foods (for reasons other than religious practices) that prevent a person from meeting nutritional or energy needs. ARFID also may be categorized as an eating disorder when its symptoms or unhealthy effects increase.

avulsion—A pulling away of a piece of a bone by tissue attached to it.

basal metabolic rate—The energy needed to keep the body functioning at complete rest, lying still, after a 12-hour fast.

baseline testing—A battery of tests conducted prior to a concussion, usually done before the start of a dance or athletic season. Testing may include a symptom checklist, cognitive tests, balance and coordination assessments, and a visual exam.

body exploitation—Sexualization of the dancing body depicted in a manner that implies sexual readiness (revealing clothing, bodily postures, facial expressions); used to attract customers (dance audience, consumers of pornographic pictures or videos).

body image—Perceptions, attitudes, feelings, and beliefs related to one's body that are based on physical sensations (lived body) and physical appearance (body perceived by others).

bone mineral density—A measure of the amount of minerals (mostly calcium and phosphorous) contained in a certain volume of bone.

bulimia nervosa—Clinical eating disorder characterized by alternating between binging and compensatory behaviors (e.g., excessive training, laxatives), with or without purging.

bunion—Painful swelling of the tissues of the inner portion of the foot along the great toe joint where the toe attaches to the foot, accompanied by hallux valgus.

bunionette—Painful swelling of the tissues of the outer portion of the foot along the fifth toe joint where it attaches to the foot; also called a tailor's bunion.

burnout—Physical, mental, and emotional fatigue caused by chronic stress factors that impair daily functioning.

bursa—Lubricating pad that protects structures in the body that rub against one another, usually during movement.

bursitis—Inflammation and swelling of a bursa that hurts when compressed or pinched by movement.

calcaneofibular ligament (CFL)—Lateral ankle ligament running from the bottom tip of the fibula to the lateral calcaneus.

calcaneus—A bone in the foot known commonly as the heel bone.

cancellous bone—Bone found in the ends of long bones and in the body of short or irregular bones that appears as a lattice of thin bone layers; also called spongy bone.

carbohydrate—A macronutrient supplying energy; found in many forms such as sugars, starches, and fiber.

cardiac output—Amount of blood the heart pumps per minute.

cardiorespiratory fitness—A measure of the ability of the cardiovascular and respiratory systems to work together to supply oxygen to working muscles in response to the stimulus of undertaking physical activity.

catastrophizing—To imagine the worst possible outcome of an action or event: to think about a situation or event as being a catastrophe or having a potentially catastrophic outcome.

central nervous system (CNS)—Body system composed of the brain and spinal cord; it manages body function, movement, sensation, coordination, learning, and behavior.

cerebrospinal fluid—A clear fluid surrounding the brain and spinal cord.

chi-square statistic—Used to determine if observed results are in line with expected results.

chondromalacia patella—Pain and softening of the smooth articular cartilage on the rear of the patella; it is usually caused by the patella not sliding correctly in its groove.

chronic exertional compartment syndrome (CECS)—Painful condition resulting from swelling of muscle tissue within its anatomical enclosure. It produces pressure that interferes with circulation, nerve sensation, and muscle function.

chronic injury—Injury that develops gradually over time and usually occurs from repetitive use of a body area. Also known as *overuse injuries,* they start out as subclinical symptoms, and may not seem connected to any specific activity or point in time.

clinical symptoms—Sensations that are the body's way of signaling an underlying injury or illness and that are felt by the individual; symptoms should not be ignored, and may include sharp, stabbing, throbbing, deep aching, numbness, tingling, and/or shooting pain.

coccydynia—Pain occurring in the coccyx (tailbone) region of the vertebral column.

collaborative approach—Method of medical decisions being made in conjunction with the dance instructor and the dancer that includes the dancer's individual performance goals.

collagen—The most plentiful protein in the body, made of long, tubular, mostly parallel strands. It forms a major portion of connective tissues and skin while providing important support to healthy hair and nails. It also provides a network of support for the cells comprising bone.

concentric contraction—A contraction of a muscle usually resulting in lifting a resistance in a direction opposite to gravity where the muscle shortens while it contracts

concussion—A mild traumatic brain injury caused by forces from an impact to the head or elsewhere on the body that transmits a force to the head and brain.

confidence interval (CI)—A range around a measurement that conveys how precise the measurement is. It is the range of values you expect your true measurement to fall between, within a certain level of confidence (95%, 97%, or 99%).

continence—Ability of an individual to control urination or bowel movements.

contrecoup injury—An injury to the brain that occurs on the opposite side from where the skull was impacted.

contusion—A medical name for a bruise.

core muscles—The muscles of the trunk that form a corsetlike support as a foundation for movement.

core stability—Ability of the trunk musculature to control the position and rigidity of the trunk; it is important in creating a solid foundation for movements of the extremities.

correlation coefficient (r)—Describes the size and direction of a relationship between two variables. Coefficients range from 1.0 to –1.0. A positive correlation means that as one variable increases, so does the other. A negative correlation means that as one variable increases, the other decreases. The farther a coefficient is from 0, the stronger the relationship is between the two variables. Note that correlation does not establish a cause-and-effect relationship (see Schober et al., 2018).

coup injury—An injury to the brain that occurs at the point where the skull was impacted.

cranium—The bony portion of the skull that surrounds the brain.

creep—Tendency of a tissue to first deform to a certain length and then, over time, to continue to slowly lengthen when under a constant stress.

cross-training—The action or practice of engaging in two or more sports or types of exercise to improve fitness or performance in one's main sport. In a dance context, refers to the use of non-dance physical training to improve a dancer's overall fitness level and consequently improve their ability to engage in dance activity that requires a high physiological demand.

cryotherapy—The use of cold (e.g., ice, cold pack, frozen peas) to provide treatment to an injury.

cuboid syndrome—Abnormal movement of the cuboid bone related to changes in the joint mechanics of the lateral midfoot and, possibly, torn ligaments that hold the cuboid in place.

deep extensor compartment—Area in the forearm containing the adductor pollicis longus, extensor pollicis longus, extensor pollicis brevis, extensor indicis, and supinator muscles.

deep flexor compartment—Area in the forearm containing the flexor digitorum profundus, flexor pollicis longus, and pronator quadratus muscles.

deltoid ligament—Strong, triangular shaped group of ligaments on the inner aspect of the ankle that connects the tip of the tibia to the medial surface of the foot bones below the ankle.

depression—Clinical mood disorder manifested by low mood; loss of interest in activities; significant changes in weight, appetite, or sleeping habits; feeling agitated or without energy; impaired concentration and decision-making abilities; feelings of worthlessness; toxic guilt; or thoughts about death or suicide, with or without a plan.

dislocation—When the bones of a joint slide apart and do not return to their normal position without manipulation.

disordered eating—A spectrum between normal eating and an eating disorder that may include symptoms and behaviors of eating disorders but at a lesser frequency or lower level of severity. Includes behaviors and beliefs that prevent one's consumption of the nutritional ingredients required for energy needs and optimal dance performance. Disordered eating may include restrictive eating, compulsive eating, or irregular or inflexible eating patterns.

distress—Negative stress that hampers one's physical, emotional and mental well-being, as well as one's ability to deal appropriately with a challenging situation.

dorsiflexion—Movement at the ankle joint such that the foot moves upward, or toward the leg, as seen in a plié movement. (Dancers often call this flexing the foot, though really it is flexion of the ankle and this terminology is much less common than dorsiflexion.)

dysmenorrhea—The medical term for painful menstrual periods. Primary dysmenorrhea is caused by uterine contractions; secondary dysmenorrhea is related to other pain-inducing conditions such as endometriosis or pelvic inflammatory disease.

eating disorder—Clinically diagnosed eating disturbance that has damaging effects on global wellness, most often associated with body image concerns and distortions.

eccentric contraction—A contraction of a muscle that usually results in lowering a resistance in the direction of gravity where the muscle lengthens in a controlled way while it contacts.

edema—A medical name for swelling.

elastic deformation—A temporary change in length caused by a tension force, with restoration to the original length after the tension force is removed.

elasticity—The ability of tissues to return to their original length following stretching.

emergency action plan (EAP)—A living document that outlines steps to be undertaken should an emergency arise.

emergency department—An entry point to a hospital for in-patient treatment and life-saving procedures. These facilities should only be used for severe conditions such as an unstable limb fracture, a severe allergic reaction, a heart attack, or similar situations.

emotional risk—Any aspect of one's environment that may cause emotional trauma.

empirical rule—In statistics, the 68–95–99.7 rule, also known as the empirical rule, is a shorthand used to remember the percentage of values that lie within an interval estimate in a normal distribution: 68%, 95%, and 99.7% of the values lie within one, two, and three standard deviations of the mean, respectively.

endurance (muscular endurance)—The ability of a muscle to resist fatigue while contracting or to contract repeatedly without fatiguing.

energy availability—The energy available to the body for all metabolic processes after considering exercise energy expenditure. It is estimated by subtracting exercise energy expenditure from total energy intake; the remaining energy is presented in kilocalories (kcal) per kilogram (kg) of fat-free mass. An energy availability of 45 kcal per kg fat-free mass per day is recommended. Energy availability below this number is considered suboptimal, and low energy availability is less than 30 kcal per kg fat-free mass per day. Low energy availability can not only impair physical performance but can also provoke many medical complications, including insufficient peak bone mass and menstrual dysfunction.

environmental risk—Any aspect of one's physical surroundings that may cause physical injury.

eustress—Positive form of stress; it is energizing, and it may help a person heighten performance and overcome obstacles.

eversion—Turning the sole of the foot outward, away from the inside of the ankle and foot (in dance terms: *winging*).

evidence-based practice—The integration of the best available research evidence with clinical expertise and patient measurements, which allows for the application of research to the real world.

extensibility—Capacity of a tissue to stretch.

extrinsic motivation—The desire to succeed related to factors that are external to you, such as a desire to please a choreographer, director, teacher, or parent.

fascia—Thin sheet or wrapping of connective tissue that encapsulates every organ, blood vessel, bone, nerve fiber, and muscle fiber as well as groups or bundles of these structures.

fast-twitch (type II) muscle fiber—A fast-contracting muscle fiber that has a high capacity for short-term anaerobic work.

fat—A macronutrient of many different structures that supplies energy; also needed by the human body for insulation and as an energy reserve.

fat-free mass—Body weight minus fat mass. Fat-free mass consists of bone, muscle, vital organs, and extracellular fluid. While sometimes used interchangeably, lean body mass is a different mass as it also typically includes essential fat.

fiber—A type of complex carbohydrate that is not absorbed or digested by the body.

fibularis—An anatomical term for three muscles contained in the lower leg that have attachments to the fibula: fibularis longus, fibularis brevis, and fibularis tertius; an equivalent term to peroneus.

first aid—Early care provided for an acute injury or illness.

first responder—Professional who provides care at the scene of an emergency, such as a police officer, firefighter, emergency medical technician, or paramedic (titles vary internationally).

flexibility—A measure of how far a joint is able to move through its range of motion; often seen as how far the limb moves from its standard anatomical position.

form closure—Creation of stability in a joint by close congruity of the surfaces of the bones that form the joint; seen especially in the sacroiliac joints.

fracture—Any disruption of bone that occurs from overuse or an acute injury.

gender disparity—Unfair social treatment based on gender, generally in favor of men.

genotype—The genetic constitution of an individual organism.

gluteals—Also known as the glutes, a group of three muscles (gluteus maximus, gluteus medius, and gluteus minimus) that make up the buttock area. Often the term refers only to the largest of the group, the gluteus maximus, which constitutes the bulk of the area.

glycemic index (GI)—An indicator that allows ranking of foods based on their overall effect on blood sugar levels. The carbohydrate in low-GI foods or meals is released into the bloodstream more slowly than that from high-GI foods or meals.

glycolytic energy system—Metabolic process that breaks down glucose into pyruvate and allows resynthesis of two ATP molecules.

Golgi tendon organs—Sensory receptors in muscle tendon that sense changes in muscle tension.

growth plate—The portion of skeletally immature bone where bone growth occurs.

hallux valgus—Abnormal deviation of the big toe away from the midline of the body or toward the other toes of the foot; it is often associated with wearing shoes that are ill-fitting for the forefoot.

hamstrings—The three muscles of the posterior thigh.

healing environment—Positive circumstances that support healing; includes internal, interpersonal, behavioral, and external domains.

health—Generally defined as the absence of disease.

hematoma—A pooling or collection of blood in a localized area of the body after an injury. In the context of head injuries, it refers to a collection of blood in or around the brain.

hemorrhage—Bleeding. In the context of head injuries, it refers to bleeding in or around the brain.

high ankle sprain—Ankle injury with a rotational force that spreads the tibia and fibula at the ankle joint and injures the anterior tibiofibular ligament and the fibrous connection between the tibia and fibula.

hip external rotators—A group of six muscles that lie posterior to each hip joint and that are responsible for externally rotating (turning out) the hip and lower extremity.

holistic—A view of an entity based on considering the complete system of that entity. The word is derived from the Greek word *hólos*, which means "whole." In the context of wellness, holistic is synonymous with whole-person.

hospital-affiliated outpatient center—A medical facility designed for procedures, treatment, or other services that do not require an overnight stay at a hospital; such centers are overseen by a local hospital institution.

hypermobility—Increased range of motion (ROM) of joints or joint laxity. It may occur normally in children or adolescents or as the result of a disease (e.g., Marfan's Syndrome or Ehlers-Danlos Syndromes).

hypertonic—Fluid with a greater number of dissolved particles than body fluids.

hypertrophy—The increase in size of skeletal muscle resulting from the increased size of individual muscle fibers.

hypothesis—A statement that predicts the result of a quantitative research project. For example, "Participating in a six-week leg strengthening program will improve jump height in dancers." Usually, a hypothesis states a possible answer to a research question.

hypotonic—Fluid with fewer dissolved particles than body fluids.

iliac crest—The top edge of the broad, winglike portion (the ilium) of each half of the pelvis.

iliotibial band (ITB)—Fibrous thickening from the tensor fasciae latae muscle that extends from the iliac crest down the lateral part of the thigh to the lateral part of the fibula just below the knee. It provides stability to the knee and assists with flexion and extension of the knee.

immediate responder—The first helper on the scene of an emergency; they may or may not have formal emergency care training.

impingement—Compression of a tendon or bursa between two bones or the impact of two bones coming together.

in vivo—In the living body.

incidence—A measure of new episodes of an injury or illness that occur within a population during a certain amount of time.

incontinence—Inability of an individual to control urination or bowel movements.

injury—An occurrence that causes damage to tissue in the body from either overuse or a traumatic event.

integrated health care—Care provided by a coordinated care team of providers devoted to addressing the whole-person needs of patients.

intensity—How hard the body is working during exercise.

interosseous membrane—Strong, fibrous tissue that runs between two bones along their length; in the lower extremity, it connects the tibia and fibula.

intra-abdominal pressure (IAP)—The pressure inside the abdominal cavity, which is increased by bearing down as in a bowel movement, especially when holding the breath; it is also increased by contraction of the core musculature.

intrinsic motivation—The desire to succeed related to an internal drive, such as the pure joy of movement rather than external thoughts of being good or bad at dance.

inversion—Turning the sole of the foot inward, toward the inside of the ankle and foot (in dance terms: *sickling*). This is the most common mechanism by which an ankle sprain occurs.

isotonic—Fluid having a similar composition to body fluids.

joint capsule—A ligamentous sheath that surrounds a joint.

labrum—A ring of elastic-like cartilage that runs around the perimeter of the glenoid fossa in the shoulder and provides added stability to the humerus as it moves.

lactate threshold—Denotes the intensity of exercise when an abrupt increase occurs in lactate accumulation in blood and muscle.

laxity—A state of looseness around a joint because structures surrounding the joint are loose, torn, or weak.

lead practitioner—Health care professional who specializes in working with elite performers and is responsible as the health care team leader for key clinical decisions related to a dancer's care.

ligament—Fibrous band of soft tissue that is made mostly of collagen and connects two bones.

Lisfranc sprain—An injury to the ligaments that support the Lisfranc joints of the midfoot; this can be a very troublesome injury and must not be missed or ignored.

lumbopelvic—A region of the body incorporating the L4-L5 and L5-S1 (L = lumbar; S = sacral) spinal segments, the right and left sacroiliac joints, the pubic symphysis, and the right and left hips.

macronutrients—Nutrients needed by humans in large amounts; measured in grams that can supply daily energy; types include carbohydrate, protein, fat, and alcohol.

Mann-Whitney U test—A statistical test used to compare whether a difference exists in the dependent variable for two independent groups.

mean—Also called the average, the mean is the sum of all measurements in the dataset divided by the number of measurements.

mechanism of injury (MOI)—The manner in which a physical injury occurs, typically described in terms of forces (e.g., sickling of the ankle causing a lateral sprain or excessive valgus force at the knee landing a jump).

medial collateral ligament (MCL)—Ligament running along the medial (inner) portion of the knee that stabilizes the knee joint.

median—The middle number in a dataset sorted from lowest number to highest, or vice versa.

menarche—The occurrence of a female's first menstrual period.

meninges—Three protective layers of connective tissue that cover the brain, nerves, and skull.

meniscus—Fibrous piece of cartilage within a joint; in the lower extremity, two are located in the knee; the plural is *menisci*.

mental imagery—Mental representation of objects, ideas, or situations stored in one's memory or imagination.

metatarsals—The five bones located in the middle portion of the foot. Metatarsal 1 is on the great toe side, and metatarsal 5 is on the pinky toe side.

micronutrients—Nutrients needed by humans in small amounts; vitamins and minerals.

mindfulness—The practice of a nonjudgmental and moment-to-moment awareness toward one's experience (bodily feelings, emotions, thoughts, or activities).

mode—The number that is repeated most often in a dataset.

motor control—The process of initiating, directing, and grading purposeful voluntary movement.

motor neuron—A nerve that carries a signal from the central nervous system to a location in the body that causes an action, such as a muscle contraction, at that location.

muscle fascicle—A group of muscle fibers contained in a covering of perimysium.

muscle fiber—A group of myofibrils contained in a covering of endomysium.

muscle spindle—Sensory receptor in skeletal muscle that senses changes in muscle length and rate of lengthening.

muscular endurance—The ability to maintain muscular force over a prolonged period of time.

myocardium—The anatomical name for the heart muscle; *my-* means "muscle," and *cardi-* means "heart."

myofascial trigger point—Hyperirritable spot in a muscle, usually caused by overuse or stress, and often found within a taut band of skeletal muscle. These spots are painful on compression, and they can cause pain to be referred to other locations nearby.

myofibril—A portion of a muscle fiber that contains the myofilaments actin and myosin.

myotatic reflex—A reflex that causes a muscle to contract in response to the muscle being stretched; it is also called the stretch reflex. The reflex is moderated by the spinal cord rather than by the brain.

net protein balance—The difference between protein synthesis (making new protein) and protein breakdown (also called degradation). If net protein balance is positive, then protein synthesis is greater than protein breakdown; if net protein balance is negative, protein breakdown is greater than protein synthesis.

neuroma—Benign mass or thickening of a nerve.

odds ratio—A statistical test used to quantify how strong the association is between two sets of observations.

open access—A type of journal article publishing in which a fee is paid to a journal, usually by an article's authors or the authors' institution, to cover the costs of publishing the article. This system allows anyone in the world to freely access the article without a subscription to the journal where the article is published.

overload principle—Challenging the body beyond its normal limits in order to achieve physical gains.

oxidative energy system—Complex sequence of metabolic processes that allows the full oxidation of glucose and resynthesis of 32 ATP molecules.

oxygen uptake—The rate at which oxygen is consumed and delivered to working tissues via the cardiorespiratory system; symbolized by $\dot{V}O_2$ with the units milliliters of oxygen (O_2) per kilogram of body weight per minute.

parasympathetic nervous system—Subdivision of the autonomic nervous system that regulates the body's functions outside of voluntary control and leading to decreased arousal.

patellar subluxation—Occurs when the patella (kneecap) slides out of its groove on the femur.

patella—Relatively flat, triangular, movable bone that forms the anterior point of the knee and protects the front of the knee joint. Its posterior ridge fits into a groove on the front of the femur.

peer review—A process by which experts in the field (i.e., peers of the authors of an article) review an article for proper methods, accuracy of results, and importance of conclusions to determine if the article is acceptable for publication.

pelvic floor—The structures that enclose the bottom of the pelvis to help support the lower abdominal contents such as the intestines, rectum, bladder, and reproductive organs.

pelvic floor muscles—The layers of muscle that enclose and support the opening at the bottom of the pelvis.

pelvic ring—The circular formation created by the two pelvic halves connected anteriorly at the pubic symphysis and posteriorly by the sacrum of the vertebral column.

perfectionistic concerns—Excessive worries about making mistakes and a rigid quest for the absence of flaws.

performance anxiety—Generally known as stage fright, an anxiety disorder associated with the stress of performing, especially in front of an audience.

performing arts medicine clinic—A health care clinic, often based in a university, that is established for the sole purpose of caring for dancers (and perhaps other performing artists). If housed at a university, the patients are typically the university's dance students.

periodization—The planned manipulation of exercise training variables including load, sets, repetitions (reps), exercise duration, intensity, and scheduled periods of rest versus training to reach targeted goals.

personal identity—The sense of being unique according to personal attributes, life experiences, and role identities (e.g., dancer, daughter, son, friend).

personal protective equipment (PPE) —Physical barriers to prevent infection of a responder while giving care.

phalanges—Small bones of the toes and fingers; the singular form is *phalanx*.

phosphagen energy system—Metabolic process that breaks down phosphocreatine to allow resynthesis of one ATP molecule.

physical capacity—The ability of a person to accomplish a physical task.

phytonutrients—A broad name for a variety of compounds of plant origin; they are most abundant and concentrated in colorful plants. There are thousands of phytonutrients, and they include polyphenols and antioxidants.

plantar fascia—Fan-shaped bundle of fibrous connective tissue on the bottom of the foot. It is intricately intertwined with the muscles of the foot, and it has connective, supportive, and shock-absorbing functions.

plantar fasciitis—Inflammation of the plantar fascia in the sole of the foot that causes pain in the heel or arch.

plantar flexion—Movement of the foot in a downward direction at the ankle (pointing the foot), as seen in rising to relevé or continuing to the toes en pointe.

plantar plate—Ligaments that support the undersides of the metatarsophalangeal joints in the toes.

plastic deformation—A permanent change in length or form of a structure that is caused by a constant force application.

plyometrics—A form of exercise that uses fast, powerful movements to improve a person's speed and power during functional tasks.

polyphenol—Naturally occurring compounds abundant in plants. They include flavonoids (found in plants such as broccoli, celery, and citrus fruits) and phenolic acids (found in plants such as strawberries, coffee, and vinegar).

positive adaptation—Process of the body becoming accustomed to exercise.

postconcussive syndrome or **persistent postconcussion symptoms**—Currently defined as concussion symptoms that continue beyond 4 weeks from the initial injury; these terms continue to be debated in concussion research.

posterior chain system—Muscle groups located in the rear of the body.

posterior talofibular ligament (PTFL)—Ligament that runs from the rear lower part of the fibula to the rear of the talus

posterior tilt of the pelvis—Tipping the pelvis backward.

postprandial—After food intake.

post-traumatic stress disorder (PTSD)—A set of stress reactions (such as flashbacks, nightmares, and panic attacks) following a traumatic event.

power-based culture—A competitive culture dominated by one individual or a minority of individuals who set rules, values, and practices as well as make important decisions that influence the whole organization.

power—The ability of a muscle to exert force quickly; explosiveness.

prevalence—The percentage of a population that experiences an injury or illness or has a specific characteristic at a given point in time.

prevention—Keeping a problem from happening by creating prophylaxis or safeguards to completely avoid it.

primary sources—Researchers' original sources for which they have used the scientific method to examine and describe phenomenon, test a hypothesis, explain results, or make some inferences from their observations.

private practices—Independently operated medical facilities, not paid for or owned by the government or a larger company such as a hospital.

probability value (P value)—A number that indicates whether or not a statistically significant difference exists between or among the tested variables.

pronation—Rolling in of the ankle and foot that positions the weight along the inside border of the foot such that the arch becomes lower than typical. Often associated with flatfeet.

prone—Lying on the front of the body.

proprioception—Perception or awareness of the position and movement of the body and its segments.

protein—An essential macronutrient that is made up of amino acids. Protein has many roles in the body, including maintaining body tissues.

psychosocial factors—Personal characteristics and family and social relationships that may influence global well-being (e.g., the ability to withstand high levels of pain, toxic competitiveness, invalidating comparisons, intensive physical training, emotional setbacks and losses, adverse childhood experiences (ACE), current traumatic events, family problems, lack of social skills, and/or social isolation.

pubic bone—A bar of bone on the pelvis that can be felt just above the genitals. The pubic bones of the two pelvic halves join in the front at that location.

pubic symphysis dysfunction—Pain or instability created at the junction where the two pelvic halves meet anteriorly (at the pubic symphysis).

Q angle—The angle formed between the line of the quadriceps muscles and the patella tendon; it is also known as the quadriceps angle. A typical Q angle is 12 degrees for men and 17 degrees for women.

quadriceps—The four muscles located on the front of the thigh.

qualitative research—Research that explores ideas or phenomena and that focuses on questions about experiences, feelings, opinions, culture, and social or emotional health.

quantitative research—Research that involves collecting and interpreting numerical data.

raked stage—Performance surface in which the back of the stage is raised higher than the front of the stage.

randomized controlled trial—Type of research where researchers study the effects of an intervention by randomly assigning participants to groups. At least one group takes part in the intervention, and one group does not take part in any intervention.

rating of perceived exertion (RPE)—A scale to measure the level of exertion a person feels during physical activity.

reciprocal inhibition—When muscles on one side of the joint relax to accommodate contraction on the other side of the joint.

red flags—Clinical signs and symptoms that warrant immediate medical attention; examples are increasing pain, increasing swelling, increasing discoloration, obvious deformity, decreasing function, inability to bear weight.

rehabilitation phases—General structure or framework for research-based injury rehabilitation; utilizes protected motion, controlled motion, and return to function phases to promote optimal healing and reduce risk of reinjury.

relative energy deficiency in sport (REDs)—A complex and potentially serious physiological condition caused by insufficient intake of energy via food; it compromises the body's ability to sustain itself.

relative rest—A strategic reduction or alteration in dance activities to allow symptom resolution and injury healing without requiring a dancer to be completely removed from dance; this is normally arranged between a health care practitioner and a dancer, and often includes the dancer's teacher(s), as well.

repetitive overuse injury—Injury that occurs from repeated movements or sustained postures of daily activities (e.g., using a computer, household chores, dance) that lead to musculoskeletal pain and dysfunction.

resting metabolic rate—The energy the body needs to sustain essential processes such as heartbeat, breathing, core temperature at complete rest, and lying still in a quiet environment.

restorative sleep—The period of sleep when your body's energy demand decreases so your body and mind can be repaired and restored, essentially resetting you for another day of activity.

reversibility principle—Training adaptations are lost when exercise training ceases.

risk reduction—Decreasing the likelihood of an injury, disease, or health-related condition by altering one or more risk factors.

rotator cuff—A group of four muscles (subscapularis, supraspinatus, infraspinatus, and teres minor) that originate on the scapula and attach around the rounded portion of the upper humerus; they control rotational movements of the shoulder joint.

sacroiliac—The junction between the sacrum and the ilium of a pelvic bone; also refers to a slightly immovable joint between the sacrum and a pelvic bone, with one on each side of the sacrum.

sacrum—The block of bone made of five fused vertebrae that is located near the bottom of the spine. The pelvic halves attach to the spine on either side of the sacrum.

safeguarding—Formal guidelines for handling safety concerns; they are meant to protect an individual from harm.

scapula—Colloquially known as a shoulder blade, an irregular, somewhat flat bone located on the posterior shoulder. The plural is *scapulae.*

scapular depression—Sliding the scapulae (shoulder blades) downward, as in lowering the shoulders after shrugging.

scapular dyskinesis—A condition in which the scapula's position is altered while at rest or during movement because of poorly functioning muscles; symptoms are created by the resulting faulty range of motion.

secondary sources—The compilation of information gathered from primary sources.

self-care—Actions that increase a person's whole-person wellness, especially a purposeful intention to counteract stressors in one's life.

self-compassion—Unconditional kindness and comfort toward self and others as part of one's human condition.

self-directed abuse—Neglect of personal needs and normalization of discomfort, pain, and injury.

self-esteem—Overall sense of personal value based on feelings of personal efficacy, self-worth, and personal dignity where one acts according to human values.

self-fulfilling prophecies—Predictions that become true due to the attitudes or behaviors of the one who believes them.

self-talk—Statements or verbalizations (positive or negative) regarding oneself. These statements may be explicit and audible to an outside observer, or they may be covert, inner dialogue.

sensory neuron—A nerve that carries a signal from a location in the body to the central nervous system to provide information about the body's status.

sesamoids—Two small bones under the ball of the foot that are embedded in the tendons of the flexor hallucis brevis muscle. They act as pulleys that increase the mechanical advantage of the tendons in flexing the great toe.

shin splints—Inflammation of the tibial and toe extensor muscles along their attachments on the tibia that is caused by repeated microtrauma (as in running or jumping).

shoulder instability—Looseness of the shoulder's ball-and-socket joint that causes problems with shoulder mechanics and may lead to pain and injury.

signs—Identifying markers of an illness, injury, or health-related condition that can be observed (usually by a clinician during an evaluation).

sit (or sitz) bones—Anatomically called the ischial tuberosities, they are the two protrusions of bone from the pelvis located in the buttocks area on which one sits.

skull fracture—A break in any of the bones surrounding the head.

slow-twitch (type I) muscle fiber—A slow-contracting muscle fiber that has a high capacity for long-term aerobic work.

specificity principle—Improvement in a particular physiological characteristic of the body is incurred by placing a training demand on the body that is related to developing that physiological characteristic.

sphincter—A circular opening from the inside of the body to the outside; the size of the opening and the exit of substances through it are usually controlled by a circular muscle around the opening.

spinal extension—Bending the trunk upward and backward when returning from spinal flexion, or bending the trunk backward from standing straight up. The latter is also called *spinal hyperextension.*

spinal flexion (spinal forward flexion)—Bending the trunk forward.

spinal hyperextension—Bending the trunk backward from a position of standing straight up.

spinal lateral flexion—Bending the trunk toward one side. Right lateral flexion is bending toward the right, and left lateral flexion is bending toward the left.

spinal rotation—Turning the trunk toward one side while keeping the hips relatively stationary. Right rotation is turning toward the right, and left rotation is turning toward the left.

spondylolisthesis—An injury that usually occurs at the level of lumbar vertebra 4 or 5; a fracture occurs in the pars interarticularis portion of the vertebra, resulting in part of the vertebra slipping forward.

spondylolysis—An injury that usually occurs at the level of lumbar vertebra 4 or 5; the pars interarticularis portion of the vertebra has a stress fracture defect. Unlike spondylolisthesis, this injury is not fractured through the bone, so part of the vertebra does not slip forward.

sprain—Disruption of ligamentous tissue, usually due to trauma that stretches (grade I), partially tears (grade II), or fully tears (grade III) a ligament.

sprung floor—A type of dance floor construction that absorbs shock. Sprung floors are built with wooden battens arranged in a crossing pattern under the floor. Foam or rubber feet are often added beneath the floor surface.

standard deviation (SD)—How much the values within a group of numbers differ from the mean of those numbers. A SD closer to 0 indicates that the values in the dataset are close to the mean, while a SD farther from 0 indicates that the values are spread out over a wider range.

standard precautions—Accepted strategies designed to decrease the risk of infection.

statistics—A set of mathematical tests used to infer information about a population.

stoicism—A pattern of enduring and not revealing physical or emotional pain or hardship.

strain—Disruption of muscles or tendons, usually due to trauma that stretches (grade I), partially tears (grade II), or fully tears (grade III) a muscle or tendon.

strength—The ability of a muscle to produce enough tension to overcome resistance.

stress—Instinctive and global body response to a perceived threat to one's well-being in the face of a challenging situation; may be positive (eustress) or negative (distress).

stress fracture—Area in a bone where repeated stress creates pain and (possibly) a tiny hairline fracture.

stretch-shortening cycle—Eccentric (lengthening) contraction of a muscle immediately followed by concentric (shortening) contraction of the same muscle.

stretch tolerance—The experience of decreasing discomfort at the end range of a stretch.

stroke volume—Amount of blood the heart pumps per beat.

student health center—A primary health care clinic dedicated to a university's entire student body. Such clinics specialize in preventive care and evaluation of routine primary care issues such as colds, infections, and the varied conditions of a college-aged population.

study design—The set of methods used to answer a research question.

subclinical symptoms—Subtle symptoms, not recognizable in a clinical evaluation and possibly not limiting a dancer's participation, but that may be perceived as affecting the dancer's ability to perform at their optimal level.

subconcussive impacts—Repetitive, symptomless head impacts that can build up over time, leading to changes in the brain or causing a concussion to occur from a lower-than-expected force.

subluxation—When the bones of a joint slide apart and spontaneously return to their normal position.

subsymptom threshold aerobic exercise training—Light aerobic exercise performed during concussion recovery that is at an intensity that does not increase symptoms.

superficial extensor compartment—Area in the forearm containing the brachioradialis, extensor carpi radialis brevis, extensor carpi radialis longus, extensor digitorum, extensor digiti minimi, extensor carpi ulnaris, and anconeus muscles.

superficial flexor compartment—Area in the forearm containing the pronator teres, the flexor carpi radialis longus, the palmaris longus, the flexor carpi ulnaris, and the flexor digitorum superficialis muscles, all of which originate from the medial epicondyle.

supination—Rolling out of the ankle and foot that positions the weight along the outside border of the foot such that the arch becomes higher than typical. Often associated with high-arched feet.

supine—Lying on one's back.

supine tabletop position—A position of a leg when lying on the back such that the hip and knee are at approximately 90-degree angles. Thus, the thigh is perpendicular to the floor, and the lower leg is parallel to the floor.

sympathetic nervous system—Subdivision of the autonomic nervous system that regulates the body's functions outside of voluntary control and leading to increased arousal.

symptoms—What someone with an illness, injury, or health-related condition feels and can report.

synovial sheath—Tubular lubricating sleeve that surrounds tendons in locations where a tendon is subject to irritation, such as passing through a tunnel or around a bone.

synovium—The inside lining of a joint or a tunnel-like structure through which a tendon passes; it provides lubrication to the joint or to the tendon to allow smooth motion.

systematic review—A standardized method to extract, compile, analyze, and review information from the existing research literature about a specific research question.

talus—Tarsal bone at the top of the foot that bears the weight of the body and is part of the ankle joint.

tendinitis—Inflammation in a tendon.

tendinopathy—Painful condition of a tendon commonly associated with overuse injury.

tendinosis—Condition of degeneration in a tendon.

tendon—A cord of strong, fibrous connective tissue, made mostly of collagen, that attaches a muscle to a bone.

tenosynovitis—Condition of inflammation of a tendon and its surrounding synovial sheath.

tensor fasciae latae (TFL)—Muscle that arises from the anterior part of the iliac crest on the pelvis and travels to its insertion at the iliotibial band (ITB) about one-third of the way down the lateral thigh.

thixotropy—Phenomenon in which the viscosity of a substance decreases under an applied stress, such as pressure.

thoracic cavity—The space contained inside the ribs and sternum (breastbone). The heart, lungs, thymus gland, esophagus, and trachea, along with the diaphragm and several other muscles, are located here.

thorax/thoracic—The chest part of the trunk where the ribs are located. *Thoracic* is the adjective form of *thorax*.

tidal volume—Amount of air a person inhales per breath.

transversus abdominis (TA)—A corsetlike muscle of the abdomen with fibers that run parallel to the floor when standing. It is an important muscle for controlling abdominal pressure; therefore, it is also essential for assisting with breath control.

traumatic brain injury (TBI)—A disturbance of brain function due to an external force.

traumatic injury—Injury caused by a sudden external force to the body, such as a blow from a blunt object, a collision with another person, a fall, or an unexpected physical load; it usually requires immediate treatment.

triangular fibrocartilage complex (TFCC)—A load-bearing arrangement of structures between two bones in the wrist and the ulna of the forearm; it acts as a stabilizer for the ulnar aspect of the wrist.

tryptophan—An essential amino acid required for normal growth in humans; it has a role in the creation of various proteins involved in energy metabolism as well as the sleep cycle.

t-test—A type of inferential statistic used to determine whether a significant difference exists between the means of two groups of data. It is also called *Student's t-test.*

urgent care center—Medical facility with extended hours, but that have limited imaging and treatment capabilities; their services include rudimentary initial assessment of an injury and first aid.

valgus—Direction of an anatomical structure away from the midline of the body, such as hallux valgus in the great toe.

varus—Direction of an anatomical structure toward the midline of the body, such as genu varus in the knee.

vascular—Referring to the blood vessels.

vertebra—A single bone of the vertebral column (spine); the plural is *vertebrae.*

vestibular and ocular rehabilitation—A type of therapy targeted at the balance and visual systems that helps to address symptoms of concussion like dizziness, balance, coordination, and vision issues.

virtuosity—A high level of technical skill in the practice of a fine art.

viscosity—A tissue's resistance to deformation under an applied stress.

walk-in clinic—Medical facility typically located inside a retail building or in a free-standing structure; designed to fill the need for quick, uncomplicated treatments for nonemergent illnesses and for preventive services.

wellness—Having an optimal level of each of several characteristics necessary for a person to live. This book incorporates a six-dimensional view of wellness.

whiplash—An injury that results from the neck being forcibly bent backward, sideways, or forward; a whiplash movement can cause a concussion.

z-score (z value)—A standardized score that allows comparison of numbers in relationship to the mean and standard deviation. In calculating z-scores of a group of numbers, the mean of the numbers is a z-score of 0. One standard deviation away from the mean—in either a positive or negative direction from 0—is a z-score of ±1.00. Two standard deviations away from the mean is a z-score of ±2.00, and three standard deviations away from the mean is a z-score of ±3.00.

References

Foreword

Solomon, R. & Solomon, J. (2023). *Dance Medicine & Science Bibliography* (9th ed.). International Association for Dance Medicine & Science.

Chapter 1

Allen, N., Nevill, A.M., Brooks, J.H.M., Koutedakis, Y., & Wyon, M.A. (2013). The effect of a comprehensive injury audit program on injury incidence in ballet: A 3-year prospective study. *Clinical Journal of Sport Medicine, 23*(5), 373-378. https://doi.org/10.1097/JSM.0b013e3182887f32

Allen, N., Ribbans, W.J., Nevill, A.M., & Wyon, M.A. (2014). Musculoskeletal injuries in dance: A systematic review. *International Journal of Physical Medicine & Rehabilitation, 3*(1), 1000252. https://doi.org/10.4172/2329-9096.1000252

Ammer, C. (2003). *The American Heritage Dictionary of Idioms.* https://idioms.thefreedictionary.com/an+ounce+of+prevention+is+worth+a+-pound+of+cure

Anand Prakash, A. (2017). Medical attention seeking dance injuries: systematic review of case reports. *The Physician and Sportsmedicine, 45*(1), 64-74. https://doi.org/10.1080/00913847.2017.1270700

Bekker, S., & Clark, A.M. (2016). Bringing complexity to sports injury prevention research: From simplification to explanation. *British Journal of Sports Medicine, 50*(24), 1489-1490. https://doi.org/10.1136/bjsports-2016-096457

Biernacki, J.L., Stracciolini, A., Fraser, J. Micheli, L., & Sugimoto, D. (2018). Risk factors for lower-extremity injuries in female ballet dancers. *Clinical Journal of Sport Medicine, 31*(2), e64-e79. https://doi.org/10.1097/jsm.0000000000000707

Bittencourt, N.F.N., Meeuwisse, W.H., Mendonça, L.D., Nettel-Aguirre, A., Ocarino, J.M., & Fonseca, S.T. (2016). Complex systems approach for sports injuries: Moving from risk factor identification to injury pattern recognition—Narrative review and new concept. *British Journal of Sports Medicine, 50*(21), 1309-1314. https://doi.org/10.1136/bjsports-2015-095850

Bolling, C., van Mechelen, W., Pasman, H.R., & Verhagen, E. (2018) Context matters: Revisiting the first step of the 'sequence of prevention' of sports injuries. *Sports Medicine, 48*(10), 2227-2234. https://doi.org/10.1007/s40279-018-0953-x

Bolling, C., Barboza, S.D., van Mechelen, W., & Pasman, H.R. (2019). How elite athletes, coaches, and physiotherapists perceive a sports injury. *Translational Sports Medicine, 2*, 17-23. https://doi.org/10.1002/tsm2.53

Bolling, C., Mellette, J., Pasman, H.R., Van Mechelen, W., & Verhagen, E. (2019). From the safety net to the injury prevention web: Applying systems thinking to unravel injury prevention challenges and opportunities in Cirque du Soleil. *BMJ Open Sport and Exercise Medicine, 5*(1), e000492. https://doi.org/10.1136/bmjsem-2018-000492

Bolling, C., van Rijn, R.M., Pasman, H.R., van Mechelen, W., & Stubbe, J.H. (2021). In your shoes: A qualitative study on the perspectives of professional dancers and staff regarding dance injury and its prevention. *Translational Sports Medicine, 4*, 386-394. https://doi.org/10.1002/tsm2.226

Bronner, S., Ojofeitimi, S., & Rose, D. (2003). Injuries in a modern dance company. *American Journal of Sports Medicine, 31*(3), 365-373. https://doi.org/10.1177/03635465030310030701

Bronner, S., & Wood, L. (2017). Impact of touring, performance schedule, and definitions on 1-year injury rates in a modern dance company. *Journal of Sports Sciences, 35*(21), 2093-2104. https://doi.org/10.1080/02640414.2016.1255772

Çevik, C., Cigĕrci, Y., Kılıç, İ., & Uyar, S. (2020). Relationship between smartphone addiction and meaning and purpose of life in students of health sciences. *Perspectives in Psychiatric Care, 56*(3), 705-711. https://doi.org/10.1111/ppc.12485

Clarsen, B., Myklebust, G., & Bahr, R. (2013). Development and validation of a new method for the registration of overuse injuries in sports injury epidemiology: The Oslo Sports Trauma Research Centre (OSTRC) Overuse Injury Questionnaire. *British Journal of Sports Medicine, 47*(8), 495-502. https://doi.org/10.1136/bjsports-2012-091524

Clarsen, B., Rønsen, O., Myklebust, G., Flørenes, T. W., & Bahr, R. (2014). The Oslo Sports Trauma Research Center questionnaire on health problems: a new approach to prospective monitoring of illness and injury in elite athletes. *British Journal of Sports Medicine, 48*(9), 754-760. https://doi.org/10.1136/bjsports-2012-092087

Ekstrand, J., Lundqvist, D., Davison, M., D'Hooghe, M., & Pensgaard, A.M. (2019). Communication quality between the medical team and the head coach/manager is associated with injury burden and player availability in elite football clubs. *British Journal of Sports Medicine, 53*(5), 304-308 https://doi.org/10.1136/bjsports-2018-099411

Ekstrand, J., Lundqvist, D., Lagerbäck, L., Vouillamoz, M., Papadimitiou, N., & Karlsson, J. (2018). Is there a correlation between coaches' leadership styles and injuries in elite football teams? A study of 36 elite teams in 17 countries. *British Journal of Sports Medicine. 52*(8), 527-531. https://doi.org/10.1136/bjsports-2017-098001

Finch, C. (2006). A new framework for research leading to sports injury prevention. *Journal of Science and Medicine in Sport, 9,* 3-9. https://doi.org/10.1016/j.jsams.2006.02.009

Finch, C.F., & Donaldson, A. (2010). A sports setting matrix for understanding the implementation context for community sport. *British Journal of Sports Medicine, 44*(13), 973-978. https://doi.org/10.1136/bjsm.2008.056069

Fuller, M., Moyle, G.M., Hunt, A.P., & Minett, G.M. (2020). Injuries during transition periods across the year in pre-professional and professional ballet and contemporary dancers: A systematic review and meta-analysis. *Physical Therapy in Sport. 44,* 14-23. https://doi.org/10.1016/j.ptsp.2020.03.010

Hincapié, C.A., Morton, E.J., & Cassidy, J.D. (2008). Musculoskeletal injuries and pain in dancers: A systematic review. *Archives of Physical Medicine and Rehabilitation, 89*(9), 1819-1829. https://doi.org/10.1016/j.apmr.2008.02.020

Hulme, A., Thompson, J., Nielsen, R.O., Read, G.J.M., & Salmon, P.M. (2018). Towards a complex systems approach in sports injury research: Simulating running-related injury development with agent-based modelling. *British Journal of Sports Medicine, 53*(9), 560-569. https://doi.org/10.1136/bjsports-2017-098871

Jacobs, C.L., Hincapié, C.A., & Cassidy, J.D. (2012). Musculoskeletal injuries and pain in dancers: A systematic review update. *Journal of Dance Medicine & Science, 16*(2), 74-84.

Johnson, J.A. (1986). *New dimensions in wellness: A context for living.* Slack.

Kenny, S.J., Palacios-Derflingher, L., Whittaker, J.L., & Emery, C.A. (2017). The influence of injury definition on injury burden in pre-professional ballet and contemporary dancers. *Journal of Orthopaedic & Sports Physical Therapy, 89*(9), 1819-1829. https://doi.org/10.2519/jospt.2018.7542

Kenny, S.J., Whittaker, J.L., & Emery, C.A. (2016). Risk factors for musculoskeletal injury in pre-professional dancers: A systematic review. *British Journal of Sports Medicine. 50*(16), 997-1003. https://doi.org/10.1136/bjsports-2015-095121

King, J., Roberts, C., Hard, S., & Ardern, C.L. (2018). Want to improve return to sport outcomes following injury? Empower, engage, provide feedback and be transparent: 4 habits! *British Journal Sports Medicine, 53*(9), 526-527. https://doi.org/10.1136/bjsports-2018-099109

Laws, H. (2005). *Fit to Dance 2: Report of the second national inquiry into dancers' health and injury in the UK.* One Dance UK.

Lee, L., Reid, D., Cadwell, J., & Palmer, P. (2017). Injury incidence, dance exposure and the use of the Movement Competency Screen (MCS) to identify variables associated with injury in full-time pre-professional dancers. *International Journal of Sports Physical Therapy, 12*(3), 352-370.

Liederbach, M., Dilgen, F.E., & Rose, D.J. (2008). Incidence of anterior cruciate ligament injuries among elite ballet and modern dancers: A 5-year prospective study. *American Journal of Sports Medicine, 36*(9), 1779-1788. https://doi.org/10.1177/0363546508323644

Liederbach, M., Hagins, M., Gamboa, J.M., & Welsh, T.M. (2012). Assessing and reporting dancer capacities, risk factors, and injuries: Recommendations from the IADMS Standard Measures Consensus Initiative. *Journal of Dance Medicine & Science, 16*(4), 139-153.

McEwen, K., & Young, K. (2011). Ballet and pain: Reflections on a risk-dance culture. *Qualitative*

Research in Sport, Exercise and Health. 3, 152-173. https://doi.org/10.1080/2159676X.2011.572181

McGlashan, A.J., & Finch, C.F. (2010). The extent to which behavioural and social sciences theories and models are used in sport injury prevention research. *Sports Medicine, 40*(10), 841-858. https://doi.org/10.2165/11534960-000000000-00000

National Wellness Institute (NWI). (n.d.). *Six Dimensions of Wellness: National Wellness Institute.* https://members.nationalwellness.org/page/Six_Dimensions

O'Brien, J., Donaldson, A., & Finch, C.F. (2016). It will take more than an existing exercise programme to prevent injury. *British Journal of Sports Medicine, 50*(5), 264-265. https://doi.org/10.1136/bjsports-2015-094841

Ojofeitimi, S. & Bronner, S. (2011). Injuries in a modern dance company effect of comprehensive management on injury incidence and cost. *Journal of Dance Medicine & Science, 15*(3), 116-122. https://doi.org/10.1177/1089313X1101500304

Roberts, T.A., Daniels, E.A., Weaver, J.M., & Zanovitch, L.S. (2022). "Intermission!" A short-term social media fast reduces self-objectification among pre-teen and teen dancers. *Body Image, 43*, 125–133. https://doi.org/10.1016/j.bodyim.2022.08.015

Russell, J.A. (2013). Preventing dance injuries: Current perspectives. *Open Access Journal of Sports Medicine, 4,* 199-210. https://doi.org/10.2147/OAJSM.S36529

Smith, T.O., Davies, L., De Medici, A., Hakim, A., Haddad, F., & MacGregor, A. (2016). Prevalence and profile of musculoskeletal injuries in ballet dancers: A systematic review and meta-analysis. *Physical Therapy in Sport, 19*, 50-56. https://doi.org/10.1016/j.ptsp.2015.12.007

Swarbrick, M. (2006). A wellness approach. *Psychiatric Rehabilitation Journal, 29*(4), 311-314. https://doi.org/10.2975/29.2006.311.314

Unsworth, D.A., Russell, J.A., & Martiny, A.C. (2014). Presence of Staphylococcus aureus on university dance studio floors and barres: a preliminary investigation. *Journal of Dance Medicine & Science, 18*(3), 115–120. https://doi.org/10.12678/1089-313X.18.3.115

van Mechelen, W., Hlobil, H., & Kemper, H. C. (1992). Incidence, severity, aetiology and prevention of sports injuries. A review of concepts. *Sports Medicine, 14*(2), 82–99. https://doi.org/10.2165/00007256-199214020-00002

van Seters, C., van Rijn, R.M., van Middelkoop, M., & Stubbe, J.H. (2020). Risk factors for lower-extremity injuries among contemporary dance students. *Clinical Journal of Sport Medicine. 30*(1), 60-66. https://doi.org/10.1097/JSM.0000000000000533

Vera, A.M., Barrera, B.D., Peterson, L.E., Yetter, T.R., Dong, D., Delgado, D.A., McCulloch, P. C., Varner, K.E., & Harris, J.D. (2020). An injury prevention program for professional ballet: A randomized controlled investigation. *Orthopaedic Journal of Sports Medicine, 8*(7). https://doi.org/10.1177/2325967120937643

Vriend, I., Coehoorn, I., & Verhagen, E. (2015). Implementation of an app-based neuromuscular training programme to prevent ankle sprains: a process evaluation using the RE-AIM Framework. *British Journal of Sports Medicine, 49*(7), 484–488. https://doi.org/10.1136/bjsports-2013-092896

Vriend, I., Gouttebarge, V., van Mechelen, W., & Verhagen, E. A. L. M. (2016). Neuromuscular training is effective to prevent ankle sprains in a sporting population: a meta-analysis translating evidence into optimal prevention strategies. *Journal of ISAKOS: Joint Disorders & Orthopaedic Sports Medicine, 1*(4), 202–213. https://doi.org/10.1136/jisakos-2016-000062

World Health Organization (WHO). (1946, July 22). Constitution of the World Health Organization. https://apps.who.int/gb/bd/PDF/bd47/EN/constitution-en.pdf?ua=1

Chapter 2

Adam, M.U., Brassington, G.S., Steiner, H., & Matheson, G.O. (2004). Psychological factors associated with performance-limiting injuries in professional ballet dancers. *Journal of Dance Medicine & Science, 8*(2), 43-46.

Akehurst, S. & Oliver, E.J. (2014). Obsessive passion: A dependency associated with injury-related risky behaviour in dancers. *Journal of Sports Sciences, 32*(3), 259-267. https://doi.org/10.1080/02640414.2013.823223

Alimena, S., Air, M.E., Gribbin, C., & Manejias, E. (2016). Utilization of routine primary care services among dancers. *Journal of Dance Medicine & Science, 20*(3), 95-102. https://doi.org/10.12678/1089-313X.20.3.95

Allen, N., Nevill, A., Brooks, J., Koutedakis, Y., & Wyon, M. (2012). Ballet injuries: Injury incidence and severity over 1 year. *Journal of Orthopaedic & Sports Physical Therapy, 42*(9), 781-A781. https://doi.org/10.2519/jospt.2012.3893

Anderson, R., & Hanrahan, S.J. (2008). Dancing in pain: Pain appraisal and coping in dancers. *Journal of Dance Medicine & Science, 12*(1), 9-16.

Andhare, N., Yeole, U., & Tannu, M. (2018). Effect of intrinsic muscle training on balance in Bharatanatyam dancers: Randomized control trial. *International Journal of Science and Healthcare Research, 3*(4), 208-212.

Andrzejewski, C.E., Wilson, A.M., & Henry, D. J. (2013). Considering motivation, goals, and mastery orientation in dance technique. *Research in Dance Education, 14*(2), 162-175. https://doi.org/10.1080/14647893.2012.733364

Arbinaga, F. (2018). Self-reported perceptions of sleep quality and resilience among dance students. *Perceptual and Motor Skills, 125*(2), 351-368. https://doi.org/10.1177/0031512518757352

Armstrong, R. (2019). Dance screening practices in dance companies, dance schools and university dance programmes: An international survey of current practices. *Journal of Clinical Case Reports.* https://doi.org/10.33118/oaj.clin.2019.01.007

Armstrong, R., & Greig, D.M. (2018). The Beighton score as a predictor of Brighton criteria in sport and dance. *Physical Therapy in Sport, 32*, 145-154. https://doi.org/10.1016/j.ptsp.2018.04.016

Aujla, I., & Farrer, R. (2015). The role of psychological factors in the career of the independent dancer. *Frontiers in Psychology, 6*(1688). https://doi.org/10.3389/fpsyg.2015.01688

Azzi, M.S. (1996). Multicultural Tango: the impact and the contribution of the Italian immigration to the Tango in Argentina. *International Journal of Musicology*, 437-453.

Bahr, R., & Krosshaug, T. (2005). Understanding injury mechanisms: A key component of preventing injuries in sport. *British Journal of Sports Medicine, 39*(6), 324-329. https://doi.org/10.1136/bjsm.2005.018341

Banio, A. (2016). Influence of rehabilitation on health of ballroom dancers after sports injuries. *Central European Journal of Sport Sciences and Medicine, 14*, 63-71. https://doi.org/10.18276/cej.2016.2-07

Bejjani, F.J., Halpern, N., Pio, A., Dominguez, R., Voloshin, A., & Frankel, V.H. (1988). Musculoskeletal demands on flamenco dancers: A clinical and biomechanical study. *Foot & Ankle, 8*(5), 254-263. https://doi.org/10.1177/107110078800800505

Berglund, C.L., Philips, L.E., & Ojofeitimi, S. (2006). Flexor hallucis longus tendinitis among dancers. *Orthopaedic Physical Therapy Practice, 18*(3), 26.

Biernacki, J.L., Stracciolini, A., Fraser, J., J. Micheli, L., & Sugimoto, D. (2021). Risk factors for lower-extremity injuries in female ballet dancers: A systematic review. *Clinical Journal of Sport Medicine, 31*(2), e64-e79. https://doi.org/doi:10.1097/JSM.0000000000000707

Bowerman, E., Whatman, C., Harris, N., Bradshaw, E., & Karin, J. (2014). Are maturation, growth and lower extremity alignment associated with overuse injury in elite adolescent ballet dancers? *Physical Therapy in Sport, 15*(4), 234-241. https://doi.org/10.1016/j.ptsp.2013.12.014

Bria, S., Bianco, M., Galvani, C., Palmieri, V., Zeppilli, P., & Faina, M. (2011). Physiological characteristics of elite sport-dancers. *J Sports Med Phys Fitness, 51*(2), 194-203.

Bronner, S., & Bauer, N.G. (2018). Risk factors for musculoskeletal injury in elite pre-professional modern dancers: A prospective cohort prognostic study. *Physical Therapy in Sport, 31*, 42-51. https://doi.org/10.1016/j.ptsp.2018.01.008

Bronner, S., Codman, E., Hash-Campbell, D., & Ojofeitimi, S. (2016). Differences in preseason aerobic fitness screening in professional and pre-professional modern dancers. *Journal of Dance Medicine & Science, 20*(1), 11-22. https://doi.org/10.12678/1089-313X.20.1.11

Bronner, S., & Wood, L. (2017). Impact of touring, performance schedule, and definitions on 1-year injury rates in a modern dance company. *Journal of Sports Sciences, 35*(21), 2093-2104. https://doi.org/10.1080/02640414.2016.1255772

Byhring, S., & Bø, K. (2002). Musculoskeletal injuries in the Norwegian National Ballet: A prospective cohort study. *Scandinavian Journal of Medicine & Science in Sports, 12*(6), 365-370.

Cahalan, R., Bargary, N., & O'Sullivan, K. (2018). Pain and injury in elite adolescent Irish dancers: A cross-sectional study. *Journal of Dance Medicine & Science, 22*(2), 91-99. https://doi.org/10.12678/1089-313X.22.2.91

Cahalan, R., Bargary, N., & O'Sullivan, K. (2019). Dance exposure, general health, sleep and injury in elite adolescent Irish dancers: A prospective study. *Physical Therapy in Sport*, *40*, 153-159. https://doi.org/10.1016/j.ptsp.2019.09.008

Cahalan, R., O'Sullivan, P., Purtill, H., Bargary, N., Ni Bhriain, O., & O'Sullivan, K. (2016). Inability to perform because of pain/injury in elite adult Irish dance: A prospective investigation of contributing factors. *Scandinavian Journal of Medicine & Science in Sports*, *26*(6), 694-702. https://doi.org/10.1111/sms.12492

Cahalan, R., Purtill, H., O'Sullivan, P., & O'Sullivan, K. (2015). A cross-sectional study of elite adult Irish dancers: Biopsychosocial traits, pain, and injury. *Journal of Dance Medicine & Science*, *19*(1), 31-43. https://doi.org/10.12678/1089-313X.19.1.31

Campbell, R.S., Lehr, M.E., Livingston, A., McCurdy, M., & Ware, J.K. (2019). Intrinsic modifiable risk factors in ballet dancers: Applying evidence based practice principles to enhance clinical applications. *Physical Therapy in Sport*, *38*, 106-114. https://doi.org/10.1016/j.ptsp.2019.04.022

Campoy, F.A., Coelho, L.R., Bastos, F.N., Netto Júnior, J., Vanderlei, L.C., Monteiro, H.L., Padovani, C.R., & Pastre, C.M. (2011). Investigation of risk factors and characteristics of dance injuries. *Clinical Journal of Sport Medicine*, *21*(6), 493-498. https://doi.org/10.1097/JSM.0b013e318230f858

Castillo-López, J.M., Munuera-Martínez, P.V., Algaba-Guisado, C., Reina-Bueno, M., Salti-Pozo, N., & Vargas-Macías, A. (2016). Pathologic disorders of the foot in professional female flamenco dancers. *Journal of the American Podiatric Medical Association*, *106*(1), 54-59. https://doi.org/10.7547/14-111

Castillo-López, J.M., Vargas-Macías, A., Domínguez-Maldonado, G., Lafuente-Sotillos, G., Ramos-Ortega, J., Palomo-Toucedo, I.C., Reina-Bueno, M., & Munuera-Martínez, P.V. (2014). Metatarsal pain and plantar hyperkeratosis in the forefeet of female professional flamenco dancers. *Medical Problems of Performing Artists*, *29*(4), 193-197.

Challis, J., Cahalan, R., Jakeman, P., NiBhriain, O., Cronin, L., & Reeves, S. (2020). Dietary intake, body composition, and nutrition knowledge of Irish dancers. *Journal of Dance Medicine & Science*, *24*(3), 105-112. https://doi.org/10.12678/1089-313X.24.3.105

Chandan, S., Tamaria, S., Gaur, D., Chadha, C., & Sharma, P. (2018). Cross-sectional study of foot posture index, navicular drop and arch index in Kathak dancers. *International Journal of Research and Review*, *5*(6), 157-164. https://doi.org/10.4444/ijrr.1002/627

Chatterjea, A. (1996). Training in Indian classical dance: A case study. *Asian Theatre Journal*, *13*(1), 68-91. https://doi.org/10.2307/1124303

Costa, M.S.S., Ferreira, A.S., Orsini, M., Silva, E.B., & Felicio, L.R. (2016). Characteristics and prevalence of musculoskeletal injury in professional and non-professional ballet dancers. *Brazilian Journal of Physical Therapy*, *20*(2), 166-175. https://doi.org/10.1590/bjpt-rbf.2014.0142

Cuellar-Moreno, M. (2016). Flamenco dance. Characteristics, resources and reflections on its evolution. *Cogent Arts & Humanities*, *3*(1), 1260825. https://doi.org/10.1080/23311983.2016.1260825

Dang, Y., Koutedakis, Y., & Wyon, M. (2020). Fit to Dance survey: Elements of lifestyle and injury incidence in Chinese dancers. *Medical Problems in Performing Artists*, *35*(1), 10-18. https://doi.org/10.21091/mppa.2020.1002

DeMann, L.E., Jr. (1997). Sacroiliac dysfunction in dancers with low back pain. *Manual Therapy*, *2*(1), 2-10. https://doi.org/10.1054/math.1997.0280

Doyle-Lucas, A.F., Akers, J.D., & Davy, B.M. (2010). Energetic efficiency, menstrual irregularity, and bone mineral density in elite professional female ballet dancers. *Journal of Dance Medicine & Science*, *14*(4), 146-154.

Eberman, L., Miletic, A., Kostic, R., & Miletic, D. (2011). Pain prevalence among competitive international dancers. *International Journal of Athletic Therapy and Training*, *16*(1), 13-16. https://doi.org/10.1123/ijatt.16.1.13

Ekegren, C.L., Quested, R., & Brodrick, A. (2014). Injuries in pre-professional ballet dancers: Incidence, characteristics and consequences. *Journal of Science and Medicine in Sport*, *17*(3), 271-275. https://doi.org/10.1016/j.jsams.2013.07.013

Ellison, J., & Partridge, J.A. (2012). Relationships between shame-coping, fear of failure, and perfectionism in college athletes. *Journal of Sport Behavior*, *35*(1), 19-39.

Emery, L.L. (1981). Review of *Jazz Dance* by M. Stearns & J. Stearns. *Dance Research Journal, 13*(2), 33-34. https://doi.org/10.2307/1478408

Fong Yan, A., Hiller, C., Smith, R., & Vanwanseele, B. (2011). Effect of footwear on dancers: A systematic review. *Journal of Dance Medicine & Science, 15*(2), 86-92.

Fong Yan, A., Hiller, C., Sinclair, P.J., & Smith, R.M. (2014). Kinematic analysis of sautés in barefoot and shod conditions. *Journal of Dance Medicine & Science, 18*(4), 149-158. https://doi.org/10.12678/1089-313X.18.4.149

Forczek, W., Baena-Chicón, I., & Vargas-Macías, A. (2017). Movement concepts approach in studies on flamenco dancing: A systematic review. *European Journal of Sport Science, 17*(9), 1161-1176. https://doi.org/10.1080/17461391.2017.1359680

Fuller, C.W., Ekstrand, J., Junge, A., Andersen, T.E., Bahr, R., Dvorak, J., Hägglund, M., McCrory, P., & Meeuwisse, W.H. (2006). Consensus statement on injury definitions and data collection procedures in studies of football (soccer) injuries. *Scandinavian Journal of Medicine & Science in Sports, 16*(2), 83-92. https://doi.org/10.1111/j.1600-0838.2006.00528.x

Fuller, M., Moyle, G.M., Hunt, A.P., & Minett, G.M. (2020). Injuries during transition periods across the year in pre-professional and professional ballet and contemporary dancers: A systematic review and meta-analysis. *Physical Therapy in Sport, 44*, 14-23. https://doi.org/10.1016/j.ptsp.2020.03.010

Grčić, V., Miletić, A., & Kuzmanić, B. (2015). Construction of tests for evaluating the level of hip hop performance. *Research in Physical Education, Sport & Health*, 4(1), 57-60.

Guarino, L., & Oliver, W. (2014). *Jazz dance: A history of the Roots and branches*. University Press of Florida.

Hackney, M.E., Kantorovich, S., & Earhart, G.M. (2007). A study on the effects of Argentine tango as a form of partnered dance for those with Parkinson disease and the healthy elderly. *American Journal of Dance Therapy, 29*(2), 109-127.

Hill, C.V. (2014). *Tap dancing America: A cultural history*. Oxford University Press.

Hanna, K., Hanley, A., Huddy, A., McDonald, M., & Willer, F. (2017). Physical activity participation and nutrition and physical activity knowledge in university dance students. *Medical Problems of Performing Artists, 32*(1), 1-7. https://doi.org/10.21091/mppa.2017.1001

Harrison, C., & Ruddock-Hudson, M. (2017). Perceptions of pain, injury, and transition-retirement: The experiences of professional dancers. *Journal of Dance Medicine & Science, 21*(2), 43-52. https://doi.org/10.12678/1089-313X.21.2.43

Herbert, R.D., de Noronha, M., & Kamper, S.J. (2011). Stretching to prevent or reduce muscle soreness after exercise. The Cochrane Database of Systematic Reviews, (7), CD004577. https://doi.org/10.1002/14651858.CD004577.pub3

Higginbotham, O., & Cahalan, R. (2020). The collegiate Irish dancer's experience of injury: A qualitative study. *Medical Problems of Performing Artists, 35*(1), 1-9. https://doi.org/10.21091/mppa.2020.1001

Hincapié, C.A., & Cassidy, J.D. (2010). Disordered eating, menstrual disturbances, and low bone mineral density in dancers: A systematic review. *Archives of Physical Medicine and Rehabilitation, 91*(11), 1777-1789.E1. https://doi.org/10.1016/j.apmr.2010.07.230

Homans, J. (2013). *Apollo's angels: A history of ballet*. Granta Books.

Hubbard, K.W. (2008). Valuing cultural context and style: Strategies for teaching traditional jazz dance from the inside out. *Journal of Dance Education, 8*(4), 110-116. https://doi.org/10.1080/15290824.2008.10387371

Icon Collective, LLC. (2024). *Hip hop history: From streets to the mainstream*. https://www.iconcollective.edu/hip-hop-history

International Dance Federation. (n.d.). Retrieved July 27, 2021, from www.idfdance.com/eng/pages/index

International Olympic Committee. (2020). *Breaking*. https://olympics.com/en/news/breaking-break-dancing-rules-format-moves

Jacobs, C. L., Hincapié, C.A., & Cassidy, J.D. (2012). Musculoskeletal injuries and pain in dancers: A systematic review update. *Journal of Dance Medicine & Science, 16*(2), 74-84.

James, A. S., & Lazarczuk, S.L. (2019). Epidemiology of injuries in West End performers. *Journal of Dance Medicine & Science, 23*(4), 139-144. https://doi.org/10.12678/1089-313X.23.4.139

Jeffries, A.C., Wallace, L., Coutts, A.J., Cohen, A.M., McCall, A., & Impellizzeri, F.M. (2020). Injury, illness, and training load in a professional contemporary dance company: A prospective study.

Journal of Athletic Training, *55*(9), 967-976. https://doi.org/10.4085/1062-6050-477-19

Kalyva, S., Yannakoulia, M., Koutsouba, M., & Venetsanou, F. (2021). Disturbed eating attitudes, social physique anxiety, and perceived pressure for thin body in professional dancers. *Research in Dance Education*, 1-12. https://doi.org/10.1080/14647893.2021.1940124

Kauther, M.D., Wedemeyer, C., Kauther, K.M., Weidle, P.A., Wegner, A., & von Knoch, M. (2009). Das "Headspin Hole" bei Breakdancern—Medizinische Erstbeschreibung eines häufigen Uberlastungsschadens [Breakdancer's "Headspin Hole"—first description of a common overuse syndrome]. *Sportverletzung Sportschaden*, *23*(1), 52–53. https://doi.org/10.1055/s-0028-1109219

Kenny, S.J., Palacios-Derflingher, L., Shi, Q., Whittaker, J.L., & Emery, C.A. (2019). Association between previous injury and risk factors for future injury in preprofessional ballet and contemporary dancers. *Clinical Journal of Sport Medicine*, *29*(3). https//doi.org/ 10.1097/JSM.0000000000000513

Kenny, S.J., Whittaker, J.L., & Emery, C.A. (2016). Risk factors for musculoskeletal injury in preprofessional dancers: A systematic review. *British Journal of Sports Medicine*, *50*(16), 997. https://doi.org/10.1136/bjsports-2015-095121

Kim, S. & Kim, J. (2007). Mood after various brief exercise and sport modes: Aerobics, hip-hop dancing, ice skating, and body conditioning. *Perceptual and Motor Skills*, *104*(3 Pt 2), 1265-1270. https://doi.org/10.2466/pms.104.4.1265-1270

Klockare, E., Gustafsson, H., & Nordin-Bates, S.M. (2011). An interpretative phenomenological analysis of how professional dance teachers implement psychological skills training in practice. *Research in Dance Education*, *12*(3), 277-293. https://doi.org/10.1080/14647893.2011.614332

Knight, C.J., Berrow, S.R., & Harwood, C.G. (2017). Parenting in sport. *Current Opinion in Psychology*, *16*, 93-97. https://doi.org/10.1016/j.copsyc.2017.03.011

Knight, K.L. (2008). Editorial. More precise classification of orthopaedic injury types and treatment will improve patient care. *Journal of Athletic Training*, *43*(2), 117-118. https://doi.org/10.4085/1062-6050-43.2.117

Kopytko, T. (2011). Cultural dance: Arangetram classical dance graduation Indian style. *DANZ Quarterly: New Zealand Dance* (25 Spring), 6-7.

Korczynski, M., Nguyen, A., & Snyder, T. (2020). The "Cone-Head" sign: Magnetic resonance image findings of the "Headspin Hole," An overuse injury found in breakdancers. *Radiology Case Reports*, *15*(5), 489-491. https://doi.org/10.1016/j.radcr.2020.01.038

Koutedakis, Y. (2000). "Burnout" in dance: The physiological viewpoint. *Journal of Dance Medicine & Science*, *4*(4), 122-127.

Krosshaug, T., Andersen, T.E., Olsen, O.E., Myklebust, G., & Bahr, R. (2005). Research approaches to describe the mechanisms of injuries in sport: Limitations and possibilities. *British Journal of Sports Medicine*, *39*(6), 330-339. https://doi.org/10.1136/bjsm.2005.018358

Lakes, R. (2005). The messages behind the methods: The authoritarian pedagogical legacy in western concert dance technique training and rehearsals. *Arts Education Policy Review*, *106*(5), 3-20.

Lalli, G. (2004). A North Indian classical dance form: Lucknow Kathak. *Visual Anthropology*, *17*(1), 19-43. https://doi.org/10.1080/08949460490273997

Leanderson, C., Leanderson, J., Wykman, A., Strender, L.-E., Johansson, S.-E., & Sundquist, K. (2011). Musculoskeletal injuries in young ballet dancers. *Knee Surgery, Sports Traumatology, Arthroscopy*, *19*(9), 1531-1535. https://doi.org/10.1007/s00167-011-1445-9

Lee, L., Reid, D., Cadwell, J., & Palmer, P. (2017). Injury incidence, dance exposure and the use of the Movement Competency Screen (MCS) to identify variables associated with injury in full-time pre-professional dancers. *International Journal of Sports Physical Therapy*, *12*(3), 352-370.

Liederbach, M., Hagins, M., Gamboa, J.M., & Welsh, T.M. (2012). Assessing and reporting dancer capacities, risk factors, and injuries: Recommendations from the IADMS Standard Measures Consensus Initiative. *Journal of Dance Medicine & Science*, *16*(4), 139-153.

Logue, D.M., Madigan, S.M., Melin, A., Delahunt, E., Heinen, M., Donnell, S.-J.M., & Corish, C.A. (2020). Low energy availability in athletes 2020: An updated narrative review of prevalence, risk, within-day energy balance, knowledge, and impact on sports performance. *Nutrients*, *12*(3), 835. https://doi.org/10.3390/nu12030835

Mainwaring, L.M., & Finney, C. (2017). Psychological risk factors and outcomes of dance injury: A systematic review. *Journal of Dance Medicine & Science, 21*(3), 87-96. https://doi.org/10.12678/1089-313X.21.3.87

Mainwaring, L.M., Krasnow, D., & Kerr, G. (2001). And the dance goes on: Psychological impact of injury. *Journal of Dance Medicine & Science, 5*(4), 105-115.

Malkogeorgos, A., Mavrovouniotis, F., Zaggelidis, G., & Ciucurel, C. (2011). Common dance related musculoskeletal injuries. *Journal of Physical Education and Sport, 11*(3), 259-266.

Malliou, P., Rokka, S., Beneka, A., Mavridis, G., & Godolias, G. (2007). Reducing risk of injury due to warm up and cool down in dance aerobic instructors. *Journal of Back and Musculoskeletal Rehabilitation, 20*(1), 29-35. https://doi.org/10.3233/BMR-2007-20105

Masal, S. & Borkar, P. (2021). Epidemiology of musculoskeletal injuries in Indian classical dancers: A systematic review. *International Journal of Physical Education, Sports and Health, 8*(3), 310-319.

Mayers, L., Bronner, S., Agraharasamakulam, S., & Ojofeitimi, S. (2010). Lower extremity kinetics in tap dance. *Journal of Dance Medicine & Science, 14*(1), 3-10.

Mayers, L., Judelson, D., & Bronner, S. (2003). The prevalence of injury among tap dancers. *Journal of Dance Medicine & Science, 7*(4), 121-125.

McCabe, T., Wyon, M., Ambegaonkar, J., & Redding, E. (2013). A bibliographic review of medicine and science research in DanceSport. *Medical Problems of Performing Artists, 28*, 70-79. https://doi.org/10.21091/mppa.2013.2013

McEwen, K., & Young, K. (2011). Ballet and pain: Reflections on a risk-dance culture. *Qualitative Research in Sport, Exercise and Health*, 3(2), 152-173. https://doi.org/10.1080/2159676X.2011.572181

McGuinness, D., & Doody, C. (2006). The injuries of competitive Irish dancers. *Journal of Dance Medicine & Science, 10*(1-2), 35-39.

Mickeviciene, D. (2004). Ritual dance as a form of worship: A case of Bharata Nāṭyam. *Acta Orientalia Vilnensia*, 5, 228-241. https://doi.org/10.15388/aov.2004.18247

Miletic, D., Miletic, A., & Milavic, B. (2015). Age-related progressive increase of lower back pain among male dance sport competitors. *Journal of Back and Musculoskeletal Rehabilitation, 28*(3), 551-560. https://doi.org/10.3233/bmr-140555

Miller, K.E., & Hoffman, J.H. (2009). Mental well-being and sport-related identities in college students. *Sociology in Sport Journal, 26*(2), 335-356. https://doi.org/10.1123/ssj.26.2.335

Ministry of Culture, Government of India. (n.d.). *Dance.* Retrieved July 28, 2021, from www.indiaculture.nic.in/dance

Moita, J.P., Nunes, A., Esteves, J., Oliveira, R., & Xarez, L. (2017). The relationship between muscular strength and dance injuries: A systematic review. *Medical Problems of Performing Artists, 32*(1), 40-50. https://doi.org/10.21091/mppa.2017.1002

Murgia, C. (2013). Overuse, tissue fatigue, and injuries. *Journal of Dance Medicine & Science, 17*(3), 92-100. https://doi.org/10.12678/1089-313X.17.3.92

Nair, S.P., Kotian, S., Hiller, C., & Mullerpatan, R. (2018). Survey of musculoskeletal disorders among Indian dancers in Mumbai and Mangalore. *Journal of Dance Medicine & Science, 22*(2), 67-74. https://doi.org/10.12678/1089-313x.22.2.67

National Dance Council of America. (2021). *History.* https://www.ndca.org/pages/ndca_history/Default.asp

Netting, L.D. (1998). Lyrical jazz dance defined. *Journal of Physical Education, Recreation & Dance, 69*(5), 7-8. https://doi.org/10.1080/07303084.1998.10605544

Noh, Y.E., Morris, T., & Andersen, M.B. (2005). Psychosocial factors and ballet injuries. *International Journal of Sport and Exercise Psychology, 3*(1), 79-90. https://doi.org/10.1080/1612197X.2005.9671759

Novosel, B., Sekulic, D., Peric, M., Kondric, M., & Zaletel, P. (2019). Injury occurrence and return to dance in professional ballet: Prospective analysis of specific correlates. *International Journal of Environmental Research and Public Health, 16*(5), 765. https://doi.org/10.3390/ijerph16050765

Ojofeitimi, S., & Bronner, S. (2011). Injuries in a modern dance company effect of comprehensive management on injury incidence and cost. *Journal of Dance Medicine & Science, 15*(3), 116-122.

Ojofeitimi, S., Bronner, S., & Woo, H. (2012). Injury incidence in hip hop dance. *Scandinavian Journal of Medicine and Science Sports, 22*(3), 347-355. https://doi.org/10.1111/j.1600-0838.2010.01173.x

One Dance UK. (2011). *Industry standards: Working to ensure high standards for dancers' health, well-being and performance*. https://www.onedanceuk.org/programmes/industry-standards

Padham, M., & Aujla, I. (2014). The relationship between passion and the psychological well-being of professional dancers. *Journal of Dance Medicine & Science, 18*(1), 37-44. https://doi.org/10.12678/1089-313X.18.1.37

Pandya, A. (2014). Role of Nattuvanar in Bharatanatyam. *Naad-Nartan Journal of Dance & Music, 2*(2), 89-91.

Panhale, V.P., Walankar, P.P., & Sridhar, A. (2020). Analysis of postural risk and pain assessment in Bharatanatyam dancers. *Indian Journal of Occupational and Environmental Medicine, 24*(2), 66-71. https://doi.org/10.4103/ijoem.IJOEM_190_19

Patterson, E.L., Smith, R.E., Everett, J.J., & Ptacek, J.T. (1998). Psychosocial factors as predictors of ballet injuries: Interactive effects of life stress and social support. *Journal of Sport Behavior, 21*(1), 101-112.

Paul, J., & Kapoor, S. (1998). Dance related injuries among Bharatanatyam dancers. *Indian Anthropologist, 28*(2), 21-33. www.jstor.org/stable/41932561

Pettersen, S.D., Aslaksen, P.M., & Pettersen, S.A. (2020). Pain processing in elite and high-level athletes compared to non-athletes. *Frontiers in Psychology, 11*, 1908. https://doi.org/10.3389/fpsyg.2020.01908

Pollard-Smith, T., & Thomson, O.P. (2017). Professional ballet dancers' experience of injury and osteopathic treatment in the UK: A qualitative study. *Journal of Bodywork and Movement Therapies, 21*(1), 148-156. https://doi.org/10.1016/j.jbmt.2016.06.009

Premelč, J., Vučković, G., James, N., & Dimitriou, L. (2019). A retrospective investigation on age and gender differences of injuries in DanceSport. *International Journal of Environmental Research and Public Health, 16*(21). https://doi.org/10.3390/ijerph16214164

Quested, E., & Duda, J.L. (2009). Perceptions of the motivational climate, need satisfaction, and indices of well-and ill-being among hip hop dancers. *Journal of Dance Medicine & Science, 13*(1), 10-19.

Quinn, M., Miltenberger, R., James, T., & Abreu, A. (2017). An evaluation of auditory feedback for students of dance: Effects of giving and receiving feedback. *Behavioral Interventions, 32*(4), 370-378. https://doi.org/10.1002/bin.1492

Raja, S.N., Carr, D.B., Cohen, M., Finnerup, N.B., Flor, H., Gibson, S., Keefe, F.J., Mogil, J.S., Ringkamp, M., Sluka, K.A., Song, X.-J., Stevens, B , Sullivan, M.D., Tutelman, P.R., Ushida, T., & Vader, K. (2020). The revised International Association for the Study of Pain definition of pain: Concepts, challenges, and compromises. *PAIN, 161*(9), 1976-1982.

Ramkumar, P.N., Farber, J., Arnouk, J., Varner, K.E., & Mcculloch, P. (2016). Injuries in a professional ballet dance company: A 10-year retrospective study. *Journal of Dance Medicine & Science, 20*(1), 30-37. https://doi.org/10.12678/1089-313X.20.1.30

Reynolds, M., Kerchief, B., & Boyce, D. (2013). A descriptive study on injury prevalence among female ballet, jazz, and modern dancers. *Journal of Women's Health Physical Therapy, 37*(2), 83-90. https://doi.org/10.1097/JWH.0b013e31829da683

Riding McCabe, T., Ambegaonkar, J.P., Redding, E., & Wyon, M. (2014). Fit to dance survey: A comparison with dancesport injuries. *Medical Problems of Performing Artists, 29*(2), 102-110. https://doi.org/10.21091/mppa.2014.2021

Rip, B., Fortin, S., & Vallerand, R.J. (2006). The relationship between passion and injury in dance students. *Journal of Dance Medicine & Science, 10*(1-2), 14-20.

Rizzoli, R., Bischoff-Ferrari, H., Dawson-Hughes, B., & Weaver, C. (2014). Nutrition and bone health in women after the menopause. *Women's Health, 10*(6), 599-608. https://doi.org/10.2217/WHE.14.40

Rocha, P., McClelland, J., Sparrow, T., & Morris, M.E. (2017). The biomechanics and motor control of tap dancing. *Journal of Dance Medicine & Science, 21*(3), 123-129. https://doi.org/10.12678/1089-313X.21.3.123

Royo, A.L.Y. (2010). Indian classical dance: A sacred art? *Journal of Hindu Studies, 3*(1), 114-123. https://doi.org/10.1093/jhs/hiq008.

Russell, J.A. (2013). Preventing dance injuries: Current perspectives. *Open Access Journal of Sports Medicine, 4*, 199-210. https://doi.org/10.2147/oajsm.S36529

Sanders, D.J., Walker, A.J., Prior, K.E., Poyssick, A.N., & Arent, S.M. (2021). Training demands and physiological profile of cross-disciplined collegiate female dancers. *Journal of Strength & Con-*

ditioning Research, 35(8). https://doi.org/10.1519/JSC.0000000000003107

Sekulic, D., Prus, D., Zevrnja, A., Peric, M., & Zaletel, P. (2020). Predicting injury status in adolescent dancers involved in different dance styles: A prospective study. *Children, 7*(12), 297. https://doi.org/10.3390/children7120297

Shaw, J.W., Springham, M., Brown, D.D., Mattiussi, A.M., Pedlar, C.R., & Tallent, J. (2020). The validity of the session rating of perceived exertion method for measuring internal training load in professional classical ballet dancers. *Frontiers in Physiology, 11*, 480. https://doi.org/10.3389/fphys.2020.00480

Shen Yun Performing Arts. (n.d.). *7 Differences between ballet and classical Chinese dance*. www.shenyunperformingarts.org

Simon, J., Hall, E., & Docherty, C. (2014). Prevalence of chronic ankle instability and associated symptoms in university dance majors: An exploratory study. *Journal of Dance Medicine & Science, 18*(4), 178-184. https://doi.org/10.12678/1089-313X.18.4.178

Simpson, N.S., Gibbs, E.L., & Matheson, G.O. (2017). Optimizing sleep to maximize performance: Implications and recommendations for elite athletes. *Scandinavian Journal of Medicine & Science in Sports, 27*(3), 266-274. https://doi.org/10.1111/sms.12703

Soares Campoy, F.A., Raquel de Oliveira Coelho, L., Bastos, F.N., Júnior, J.N., Marques Vanderlei, L.C., Luiz Monteiro, H., Padovani C.B., & Pastre C.M. (2011). Investigation of risk factors and characteristics of dance injuries. *Clinical Journal of Sport Medicine, 21*(6), 493-498. https://doi.org/10.1097/JSM.0b013e318230f858

Southwick, H., & Crupi, M. (2017). A screening program for the young dancer: Perspectives on what and why to include in a screen. In R. Solomon, J. Solomon, & L.J. Micheli (Eds.), *Prevention of Injuries in the Young Dancer* (pp. 43-62). Springer International. https://doi.org/10.1007/978-3-319-55047-3_3

Steinberg, N., Siev-Ner, I., Peleg, S., Dar, G., Masharawi, Y., Zeev, A., & Hershkovitz, I. (2011). Injury patterns in young, non-professional dancers. *Journal of Sports Sciences, 29*(1), 47-54. https://doi.org/10.1080/02640414.2010.521167

Steinberg, N., Siev-Ner, I., Peleg, S., Dar, G., Masharawi, Y., Zeev, A., & Hershkovitz, I. (2012). Extrinsic and intrinsic risk factors associated with injuries in young dancers aged 8-16 years. *Journal of Sports Sciences, 30*(5), 485-495. https://doi.org/10.1080/02640414.2011.647705

Surgenor, B.R., Redding, E., & Cahalan, R. (2020). Periodization, training load prescription and monitoring. In R. Cahalan (Ed.), *Complete Irish dancer: Optimization of health and performance in Irish dancers* (pp. 117-134). Nova Sports.

Tajet-Foxell, B., & Rose, F.D. (1995). Pain and pain tolerance in professional ballet dancers. *British Journal of Sports Medicine, 29*(1), 31-34. https://doi.org/10.1136/bjsm.29.1.31

Tjukov, O., Engeroff, T., Vogt, L., Banzer, W., & Niederer, D. (2020). Injury profile of hip-hop dancers. *Journal of Dance Medicine & Science, 24*(2), 66-72. https://doi.org/10.12678/1089-313X.24.2.66

Toney-Butler, T.J., & Varacallo, M. (2021). Motor vehicle collisions. In *StatPearls*. StatPearls.

Toyoda, E. (2012). Acculturation through a leisure activity: The Argentine Tango in Japan. *Asian Journal of Latin American Studies 25*(2), 1-26.

Ursej, E., Sekulic, D., Prus, D., Gabrilo, G., & Zaletel, P. (2019). Investigating the prevalence and predictors of injury occurrence in competitive hip hop dancers: Prospective analysis. *International Journal of Environmental Research and Public Health, 16*(17), 3214. https://doi.org/10.3390/ijerph16173214

USA Dance. (n.d.). *DanceSport*. https://usadance.org/page/WhatisDanceSport

Vaczi, M., Tekus, E., Atlasz, T., Cselko, A., Pinter, G., Balatincz, D., Kaj, M., & Wilhelm, M. (2016). Ballroom dancing is more intensive for the female partners due to their unique hold technique. *Physiology International, 103*(3), 392-401. https://doi.org/10.1556/2060.103.2016.3.11

Vaganova, A. (1969). *Basic principles of classical ballet: Russian ballet technique*. Dover.

van Rijn, R.M., & Stubbe, J.H. (2021). Generalized joint hypermobility and injuries: A prospective cohort study of 185 pre-professional contemporary dancers. *Journal of Clinical Medicine, 10*(5), 1007. https://doi.org/10.3390/jcm10051007

van Seters, C., van Rijn, R.M., van Middelkoop, M., & Stubbe, J.H. (2020). Risk factors for lower-extremity injuries among contemporary dance students. *Clinical Journal of Sport Medicine, 30*(1), 60-66. https://doi.org/10.1097/JSM.0000000000000533

van Winden, D., van Rijn, R.M., Savelsbergh, G., Oudejans, R., & Stubbe, J. H. (2020). Limited coping skills, young age, and high BMI are risk factors for injuries in contemporary dance: A 1-year prospective study. *Frontiers in Psychology, 11*, 1452. https://doi.org/10.3389/fpsyg.2020.01452

van Winden, D.P.A.M., van Rijn, R.M., Richardson, A., Savelsbergh, G.J.P., Oudejans, R.R.D., & Stubbe, J.H. (2019). Detailed injury epidemiology in contemporary dance: A 1-year prospective study of 134 students. *BMJ Open Sport & Exercise Medicine, 5*(1), e000453. https://doi.org/10.1136/bmjsem-2018-000453

Vargas-Macías, A., Baena-Chicón, I., Gorwa, J., Michnik, R.A., Nowakowska-Lipiec, K., Gómez-Lozano, S., & Forczek-Karkosz, W. (2021). Biomechanical effects of flamenco footwork. *Journal of Human Kinetics, 80*, 19-27. https://doi-org /10.2478/hukin-2021-0086

Vassallo, A.J., Trevor, B.L., Mota, L., Pappas, E., & Hiller, C.E. (2019). Injury rates and characteristics in recreational, elite student and professional dancers: A systematic review. *Journal of Sports Sciences, 37*(10), 1113-1122. https://doi.org/10.1080/02640414.2018.1544538

Wang, K. (1985). *The history of Chinese dance*. China Books & Periodicals.

Wang, T.J., & Russell, J.A. (2018). A tenuous pas de deux: Examining university dancers' access to and satisfaction with healthcare delivery. *Medical Problems of Performing Artists, 33*(2), 111–117. https://doi.org/10.21091/mppa.2018.2018

Wanke, E.M., Mill, H., Wanke, A., Davenport, J., Koch, F., & Groneberg, D.A. (2012). Dance floors as injury risk: Analysis and evaluation of acute injuries caused by dance floors in professional dance with regard to preventative aspects. *Medical Problems of Performing Artists, 27*(3), 137-142. https://doi.org/10.21091/mppa.2012.3025

Wanke, E.M., Arendt, M., Mill, H., & Groneberg, D.A. (2013). Occupational accidents in professional dance with focus on gender differences. *Journal of Occupational Medicine and Toxicology, 8*(1), 35. https://doi.org/10.1186/1745-6673-8-35

Wanke, E.M., Arendt, M., Mill, H., Koch, F., Wanke, A., & Groneberg, D.A. (2014). Traumatic injuries in revue dancers. *Journal of Dance Medicine & Science, 18*(1), 22-28. https://doi.org/10.12678/1089-313X.18.1.22

Wanke, E.M., Kunath, E.K., Koch, F., Davenport, J., Weisser, B., Groneberg, D.A., Mache, S., Endres, E., & Vitzthum, K. (2012). Survey of health problems in musical theater students: A pilot study. *Medical Problems of Performing Artists, 27*(4), 205–211.

Witkoś, J., & Hartman-Petrycka, M. (2021). Implications of Argentine Tango for health promotion, physical well-being as well as emotional, personal and social life on a group of women who dance. *International Journal of Environmental Research and Public Health, 18*(11), 5894. https://doi.org/10.3390/ijerph18115894

World Dance Council. (2023). *Welcome to the World Dance Council*. https://www.wdcdance.com/

World DanceSport Federation. (2022). History. https://www.worlddancesport.org/WDSF/History

World DanceSport Federation. (2024a). WDSF members. https://www.worlddancesport.org/Member

World DanceSport Federation. (2024b). Within world sports. https://www.worlddancesport.org/About/Olympic

Chapter 3

Abergel, R.E., Tuesta, E., & Jarvis, D.N. (2021). The effects of acute physical fatigue on sauté jump biomechanics in dancers. *Journal of Sports Sciences, 39*(9), 1021-1029. https://doi.org/10.1080/02640414.2020.1854425

Allen, N. (2019). *Injury Prevention and Management for Dancers*. Crowood Press.

Altbach, P.G., & de Wit, H. (2018). Too much academic research is being published. *University World News*. www.universityworldnews.com/post.php?story=20180905095203579

Blakeslee, S. (2004). The CRAAP Test. *LOEX Quarterly, 31*(3), 6-7.

Bulkley, D., & Jarvis, D. N. (2023). Dancers exhibit decreases in postural control after fatigue. *Sports Biomechanics*, 1–12. Online ahead of print. https://doi.org/10.1080/14763141.2023.2212643

Clippinger, K. (2023). *Dance Anatomy and Kinesiology* (3rd ed.). Human Kinetics.

Du Prel, J.B., Hommel, G., Röhrig, B., & Blettner, M. (2009). Confidence interval or p-value?: Part 4 of a series on evaluation of scientific publications.

Deutsches Ärzteblatt International, 106(19), 335-339. https://doi.org/10.3238/arztebl.2009.0335

Haas, J.G. (2018). *Dance Anatomy* (2nd ed.). Human Kinetics.

Jeffries, A. C., Wallace, L., Coutts, A. J., Cohen, A. M., McCall, A., & Impellizzeri, F. M. (2020). Injury, illness, and training load in a professional contemporary dance company: A prospective study. *Journal of Athletic Training, 55*(9), 967–976. https://doi.org/10.4085/1062-6050-477-19

Robin, K. & Morton, J. (2019). *Dancing Longer, Dancing Stronger* (2nd ed.). Princeton Book Company.

McLeod, S.A. (2019). Z-score: Definition, calculation and interpretation. Simply Psychology. www.simplypsychology.org/z-score.html

Novosel, B., Sekulic, D., Peric, M., Kondric, M., & Zalatel, P. (2019). Injury occurrence and return to dance in professional ballet: prospective analysis of specific correlates. *International Journal of Environmental Research and Public Health, 16*(765), 1-11.

Pollard-Smith, T., & Thomson, O.P. (2017). Professional ballet dancers' experience of injury and osteopathic treatment in the UK: A qualitative study. *Journal of Bodywork and Movement Therapies, 21*(1), 148-156. https://doi.org/10.1016/j.jbmt.2016.06.009

Quin, S., Rafferty, S., Tomlinson, C. (2015). *Safe Dance Practice.* Human Kinetics.

Schober, P., Boer, C., & Schwarte, L.A. (2018). Correlation coefficients: Appropriate use and interpretation. *Anesthesia and Analgesia, 126*(5), 1763-1768. https://doi.org/10.1213/ANE.0000000000002864

Simmel, L (2014). *Dance Medicine in Practice: Anatomy, Injury Prevention, Training.* Routledge.

Szumilias, M. (2010). Explaining odds ratios. *Journal of the Canadian Academy of Child and Adolescent Psychiatry, 19*(3): 227-229.

Chapter 4

Beck, S., Redding, E., & Wyon, M.A. (2015). Methodological considerations for documenting the energy demand of dance activity: A review. *Frontiers in Psychology, 6*, 568. https://doi.org/10.3389/fpsyg.2015.00568

Blanksby, B.A., & Reidy, P.W. (1988). Heart rate and estimated energy expenditure during ballroom dancing. *British Journal of Sports Medicine, 22*, 57-60. https://doi.org/10.1136/bjsm.22.2.57

Borg, G.A. (1982). Psychophysical bases of perceived exertion. *Medicine & Science in Sports & Exercise, 14*, 377-381.

Bronner, S., & Wood, L. (2017). Impact of touring, performance schedule, and definitions on 1-year injury rates in a modern dance company. *Journal of Sports Sciences, 35*(21), 2093-2104. https://doi.org/10.1080/02640414.2016.1255772

Cohen, J.L., Segal, K.R., & McArdle, W.D. (1982). Heart rate response to ballet stage performance. *The Physician & Sportsmedicine, 10*(11), 120-122; 125-130; 133.

Cizek, E., Kelly, P., Kress, K., & Mattfeldt-Beman, M. (2016). Factors affecting healthful eating among touring popular musicians and singers. *Medical Problems of Performing Artists, 31*(2), 63-68. https://doi.org/10.21091/mppa.2016.2013

Hopper, L.S., Allen, N., Wyon, M., Alderson, J.A., Elliott, B.C., & Ackland, T.R. (2014). Dance floor mechanical properties and dancer injuries in a touring professional ballet company. *Journal of Science and Medicine in Sport, 17*(1), 29-33. https://doi.org/10.1016/j.jsams.2013.04.013

Hopper, L.S., Wheeler, T.J., Webster, J.M., Allen, N., Roberts, J.R., & Fleming, P.R. (2014). Dancer perceptions of the force reduction of dance floors used by a professional touring ballet company. *Journal of Dance Medicine & Science, 18*(3), 121-130. https://doi.org/10.12678/1089-313X.18.3.121

Jeffries, A.C., Wallace, L., & Coutts, A.J. (2017). Quantifying training loads in contemporary dance. *International Journal of Sports Physiology and Performance, 12*(6), 796-802.

Jones, A.M., & Carter, H. (2000). The effect of endurance training on parameters of aerobic fitness. *Sports Medicine, 29*(6), 373-386.

Kenney, L.W., Wilmore, J.H., & Costill, D.L. (2021). *Physiology of sport and exercise* (8th ed.). Human Kinetics.

Liiv, H., Jurimae, T., Klonova, A., & Cicchella, A. (2013). Performance and recovery: Stress profiles in professional ballroom dancers. *Medical Problems of Performing Artists, 28*(2), 65-69.

McArdle, W.D., Katch, F.L., & Katch, V.L. (2023). *Exercise Physiology: Nutrition, Energy and Human Performance* (9th ed.). Lippincott, Williams & Wilkins.

Needham-Beck, S., Wyon, M.A., & Redding, E. (2019). The relationship between performance competence and cardiorespiratory fitness in contemporary dance. *Medical Problems of Performing Artists, 34*(2), 79-84.

Redding, E., Weller, P., Ehrenberg, S., Irvine, S., Quin, E., Rafferty, S., Wyon, M., & Cox, C. (2009). The development of a high intensity dance performance fitness test. *Journal of Dance Medicine & Science, 13*(1), 3-9.

Redding, E., & Wyon, M. (2003). Strengths and weaknesses of current methods for evaluating the aerobic power of dancers. *Journal of Dance Medicine & Science, 7*(1), 10-16.

Schantz, P.G., & Astrand, P.O. (1984). Physiological characteristics of classical ballet. *Medicine and Science in Sports and Exercise, 16*(5), 472-476.

Shaw, J.W., Springham. M., Brown, D.D., Mattiussi, A.M., Pedlar, C.R., & Tallent, J. (2020). The validity of the session rating of perceived exertion method for measuring internal training load in professional classical ballet dancers. *Frontiers in Physiology, 11,* 480. https://doi.org/10.3389/fphys.2020.00480

Stephens, N., & Wyon, M.A. (2020). Physiological characteristics of musical theatre performers and the effect on cardiorespiratory demand whilst singing and dancing. *Medical Problems of Performing Artists, 35*(1), 54-58.

Surgenor, B., & Wyon, M.A. (2019). Measuring training load in dance: The construct validity of session-RPE. *Medical Problems of Performing Artists, 34*(1), 1-5. https://doi.org/10.21091/mppa.2019.1002

Twitchett, E.A., Koutedakis, Y., & Wyon, M.A. (2009). Physiological fitness and professional classical ballet performance: A brief review. *Journal of Strength and Conditioning Research, 23*(9), 2732–2740. https://doi.org/10.1519/JSC.0b013e3181bc1749

Twitchett, E., Angioi, M., Koutedakis, Y., & Wyon, M. (2009). Video analysis of classical ballet performance. *Journal of Dance Medicine & Science, 13*(4), 124-128.

Twitchett, E., Nevill, A., Angioi, M., Koutedakis, Y., & Wyon, M. (2011). Development, validity, and reliability of a ballet-specific aerobic fitness test. *Journal of Dance Medicine & Science, 15*(3), 123-127.

World DanceSport Federation. (2023). *WDSF Breaking Rules and Regulations Manual* (version 6). https://dancesport.app.box.com/s/fowfqyiedh1z3vryqa0a963acptv1vhv

Wyon, M., Redding, E., Abt, G., Head, A., & Sharp, N.C.C. (2003). Development, reliability, and validity of a multistage dance specific aerobic fitness test (DAFT). *Journal of Dance Medicine & Science, 7*(3), 80-84.

Wyon, M.A., Abt, G., Redding, E., Head, A., & Sharp, N.C.C. (2004). Oxygen uptake during modern dance class, rehearsal, and performance. *Journal of Strength and Conditioning Research, 18*(3), 646.

Wyon, M. (2006). Testing an aesthetic athlete: Contemporary dance and classical ballet dancers. In E.M. Winter, A.M. Jones, R.C.R. Davison, P.D. Bromley, & T. Mercer (Eds.), *Sport and exercise physiology testing guidelines: Volume II—Exercise and clinical testing: The British Association of Sport and Exercise Sciences Guide*. Routledge.

Wyon, M.A., Deighan, M.A., Nevill, A.M., Doherty, M., Morrison, S.L., Allen, N., Jobson, S.J., & George, S. (2007). The cardiorespiratory, anthropometric, and performance characteristics of an international/national touring ballet company. *Journal of Strength and Conditioning Research, 21*(2), 389-393. https://doi.org/10.1519/R-19405.1

Wyon, M.A., Twitchett, E., Angioi, M., Clarke, F., Metsios, G., & Koutedakis, Y. (2011). Time motion and video analysis of classical ballet and contemporary dance performance. *International Journal of Sports Medicine, 32*(11), 851–855. https://doi.org/10.1055/s-0031-1279718

Wyon, M.A., Allen, N., Cloak, R., Beck, S., Davies, P., & Clarke, F. (2016). Assessment of maximum aerobic capacity and anaerobic threshold of elite ballet dancers. *Medical Problems of Performing Artists, 31*(3), 145-150. https://doi.org/10.21091/mppa.2016.3027

Wyon, M.A., Harris, J., Adams, F., Cloak, R., Clarke, F., & Bryant, J. (2018). Cardiorespiratory profile and performance demands of elite hip-hop dancers: Breaking and new style. *Medical Problems of Performing Artists, 33*(3), 198-204.

Chapter 5

Asmussen, E., & Mazin, B. (1978). Recuperation after muscular fatigue by "diverting activities." *European Journal of Applied Physiology and Occupational Physiology, 38*(1), 1-7. https://doi.org/10.1007/BF00436747

Brumitt, J., & Cuddeford, T. (2015). Current concepts of muscle and tendon adaptation to strength and conditioning. *International Journal of Sports Physical Therapy, 10*(6), 748–759.

Clark J.E. (2016). The impact of duration on effectiveness of exercise, the implication for periodization of training and goal setting for individuals who are overfat, a meta-analysis. *Biology of Sport, 33*(4), 309-333. https://doi.org/10.5604/20831862.1212974

Farmer, C., & Brouner, J. (2021). Perceptions of strength training in dance. *Journal of Dance Medicine & Science, 25*(3), 160-168. https://doi.org/10.12678/1089-313X.091521a

Fletcher, R.A., & Ebert, A. (1978). *Every Body is Beautiful.* Lippincott Williams & Wilkins.

Friedman, P., & Eisen, G. (2005). *The Pilates Method of Physical and Mental Conditioning.* Viking Studio.

Haas, J. (2017). *Dance Anatomy* (2nd ed.). Human Kinetics.

Hackney, A.C., Kallman, A.L., & Ağgön, E. (2019). Female sex hormones and the recovery from exercise: Menstrual cycle phase affects responses. *Biomedical Human Kinetics, 11*(1), 87-89. https://doi.org/0.2478/bhk-2019-0011

Hamilton, W.G., Hamilton, L.H., Marshall, P., & Molnar, M. (1992). A profile of the musculoskeletal characteristics of elite professional ballet dancers. *American Journal of Sports Medicine, 20*(3), 267–273. https://doi.org/10.1177/036354659202000306

Hong, A.R., & Kim, S.W. (2018). Effects of Resistance Exercise on Bone Health. *Endocrinology and Metabolism, 33*(4), 435–444. https://doi.org/10.3803/EnM.2018.33.4.435

Jones, C.M., Griffiths, P.C., & Mellalieu, S.D. (2017). Training load and fatigue marker associations with injury and illness: A systematic review of longitudinal studies. *Sports Medicine, 47*(5), 943-974. https://doi.org/10.1007/s40279-016-0619-5

Kenney, W.L., Wilmore, J.H., & Costill, D.L. (2022). *Physiology of Sport and Exercise* (8th ed.). Human Kinetics.

Kent, A., Camner, J., & Camner, C. (1984). *The Dancers' Body Book.* HarperCollins.

Lansky, C.P. (2020). Tiler Peck's Top 10 Tips for Training at Home. *Pointe Magazine.* https://pointemagazine.com/tiler-peck-instagram-classes

Liederbach, M., Schanfein, L., & Kremenic, I.J. (2013). What is known about the effect of fatigue on injury occurrence among dancers? *Journal of Dance Medicine & Science, 17*(3), 101-108. https://doi.org/10.12678/1089-313x.17.3.101

Marks, A. (2017). Target your dancers' weak spots with New York City Ballet's hot new tools. *Dance Magazine.* https://dance-teacher.com/target-weak-spots-for-dancers

McArdle W., Katch, F.I. & Katch, V.L. (2023). *Exercise Physiology: Nutrition, Energy, and Human Performance* (9th ed.). Lippincott Williams & Wilkins.

Nicholas J.A. (1975). Risk factors, sports medicine and the orthopedic system: an overview. *Journal of Sports Medicine, 3*(5), 243–259. https://doi.org/10.1177/036354657500300507

Pilates, J.H., & Miller, W.J. (1945). *Return to Life Through Contrology.* Ravenio Books.

Romero-Moraleda, B., Coso, J.D., Gutiérrez-Hellín, J., Ruiz-Moreno, C., Grgic, J., & Lara, B. (2019). The influence of the menstrual cycle on muscle strength and power performance. *Journal of Human Kinetics, 68*, 123-133. https://doi.org/10.2478/hukin-2019-0061

Sands, W.A., Wurth, J.J., & Hewit, J.K. (2012). *The National Strength and Conditioning Association's (NSCA) Basics of Strength and Conditioning Manual.* www.nsca.com/contentassets/116c55d64e1343d2b264e05aaf158a91/basics_of_strength_and_conditioning_manual.pdf

Storm, J.M., Wolman, R., Bakker, E., & Wyon, M.A. (2018). The relationship between range of motion and injuries in adolescent dancers and sportspersons: A systematic review. *Frontiers in Psychology, 9*, 287. https://doi.org/10.3389/fpsyg.2018.00287

Thomas, M.H., & Burns, S.P. (2016). Increasing lean mass and strength: A comparison of high frequency strength training to lower frequency strength training. *International Journal of Exercise Science, 9*(2), 159-167.

Thompson, C. (2020). Diaphragmatic breathing. *Dance Teacher, 42*(4), 52-53.

Teitz, C.C. (1986). First aid, immediate care, and rehabilitation of knee and ankle injuries in dancers and athletes. In C.G. Shell (Ed.), *The Dancer as Athlete.* Human Kinetics.

Vitale, K.C., Owens, R., Hopkins, S.R., & Malhotra, A. (2019). Sleep hygiene for optimizing recovery in athletes: Review and recommendations. *International Journal of Sports Medicine, 40*(8), 535-543. https://doi.org/10.1055/a-0905-3103

Wyon, M.A., & Koutedakis, Y. (2013) Muscular fatigue considerations for dance. *Journal of Dance Medicine & Science, 17*(2), 63-69.

Chapter 6

Apostolopoulos, N. (2010). microStretching-A practical approach for recovery and regeneration. *New Studies in Athletics, 25,* 81-97

Apostolopoulos, N., Metsios, G.S., Flouris, A.D., Koutedakis, Y., & Wyon, M.A. (2015). The relevance of stretch intensity and position: A systematic review. *Frontiers in Psychology, 6,* 1128. https://doi.org/10.3389/fpsyg.2015.01128

Behara, B. & Jacobson, B.H. (2017). Acute effects of deep tissue foam rolling and dynamic stretching on muscular strength, power, and flexibility in Division I linemen. *Journal of Strength and Conditioning Research, 31*(4), 888-892. https://doi.org/10.1519/JSC.0000000000001051

Blackmon, A. & Faulkner, E. (2019). *Bending without breaking—implications of hypermobility in dancers.* Dance/USA Task Force on Dancer Health. https://danceusa.s3.us-east-2.amazonaws.com/page_uploads/Bending%20Without%20Breaking%20PDF.pdf

Blackmon, A.M. & Kirollos, A. (2020). *Postpartum guidelines for dancers.* Dance/USA Task Force on Dancer Health. https://danceusa.s3.us-east-2.amazonaws.com/page_uploads/Post-Partum%20Guidelines%20for%20Dancers%20Jan%202020.pdf

Capobianco, R.A., Mazzo, M.M., & Enoka, R.M. (2019). Self-massage prior to stretching improves flexibility in young and middle-aged adults. *Journal of Sports Sciences, 37*(13), 1543-1550. https://doi.org/10.1080/02640414.2019.1576253

Clippinger, K.S. (2024). *Dance Anatomy and Kinesiology* (3rd ed.). Human Kinetics.

Day, H., Koutedakis, Y., & Wyon, M.A. (2011). Hypermobility and dance: A review. *International Journal of Sports Medicine, 32,* 485-489. https://doi.org/10.1055/s-0031-1273690

Eby, S., & Alfano, A. (2012). Physical modalities in sports medicine. In F.G. O'Connor, D.J. Casa, B.A. Davis, P. St. Pierre, R.E. Sallis, & R.P. Wilder (Eds.), *ACSM's Sports Medicine: A Comprehensive Review* (pp. 484-492). Wolters Kluwer Health.

Fagnani, F., Giombini, A., DiCesare, A., Pigozzi, F., & DiSalvo, V. (2006). The effects of a whole-body vibration program on muscle performance and flexibility in female athletes. *American Journal of Physical Medicine & Rehabilitation, 85*(12), 956-962. https://doi.org/10.1097/01.phm.0000247652.94486.92

Fox, S.I., & Rompolski, K. (2022). *Human physiology* (16th ed.). McGraw Hill.

Herzog, W. (2019). The problem with skeletal muscle series elasticity. *BMC Biomedical Engineering, 1*(28), 1-14. https://doi.org/10.1186/s42490-019-0031-y

Hindle, K.B., Whitcomb, T.J., Briggs, W.O., & Hong, J. (2012). Proprioceptive neuromuscular facilitation (PNF): Its mechanisms and effects on range of motion and muscular function. *Journal of Human Kinetics, 31,* 105-113. https://doi.org/10.2478/v10078-012-0011-y

Holt, L.E., Pelham, T.W., & Holt, J. (2008). *Flexibility: a concise guide to conditioning, performance enhancement, injury prevention, and rehabilitation.* Humana Press.

Hotta, K., Behnke, B.J., Arjmandi, B., Ghosh, P., Chen, B., Brooks, R., Maraj, J.J., Elam, M.L., Mahar, P., Kurien, D., Churchill, A., Spulveda, J.L., Kabolowsky, M.B., Christou, D.D., & Muller-Delp, J.M. (2018). Daily muscle stretching enhances blood flow, endothelial function, capillarity, vascular volume and connectivity in aged skeletal muscle. *Journal of Physiology, 596*(10), 1903-1917. https://doi.org/10.1113/JP275459

Kandel, E.R., Schwartz, J.H., Jessell, T.M., Siegelbaum, S.A., & Hudspeth, A.J. (Eds.). (2013). *Principles of neural science* (5th ed.). McGraw-Hill.

Knierim, J. (2020). *Neuroscience online.* McGovern Medical School at UTHealth. https://nba.uth.tmc.edu/neuroscience/m/s3/chapter02.html

Knight, I., McCormack, M., & Bird, H. (2012). *Managing joint hypermobility—A guide for dance teachers. (info sheet #7).* South West Music School. https://cpdfordanceteachers.files.wordpress.com/2012/09/managing-joint-hypermobily-syndrome-a-guide-for-teachers.pdf

Kozai, A., & Surgenor, B. (2017). *The importance of a good warm-up: Are you warm enough to start dancing?* International Association for Dance Medicine and Science. https://iadms.org/media/5788/iadms-resource-paper-the-importance-of-a-good-warm-up.pdf

Kruse, N.T. & Scheuermann, B.W. (2017). Cardiovascular responses to skeletal muscle stretching:

"Stretching" the truth or a new exercise paradigm for cardiovascular medicine? *Sports Medicine, 47*(12), 2507-2520. https://doi.org/10.1007/s40279-017-0768-1

Lakie, M., & Campbell, K.S. (2019). Muscle thixotropy—Where are we now? *Journal of Applied Physiology, 126*, 1790-1799. https://doi.org/10.1152/japplphysiol.00788.2018

Lauersen, J.B., Bertelsen, D.M., & Andersen, L.B. (2014). The effectiveness of exercise interventions to prevent sports injuries: a systematic review and meta-analysis of randomised controlled trials. *British Journal of Sports Medicine, 48*(11), 871-877.

Liguori, G., & American College of Sports Medicine (ACSM). (2020). *ACSM's guidelines for exercise testing and prescription*. Lippincott Williams & Wilkins.

Lima, C.D., Wong, L.E., Wong, M.A., Levya, W.D., Pinto, R.S., Cadore, E.L., & Ruas, C.V. (2016). Acute effects of static vs. ballistic stretching on strength and muscular fatigue between ballet dancers and resistance trained women. *Journal of Strength and Conditioning Research, 30*(11), 3220-3227. https://doi.org/10.1519/JSC.0000000000001606

Lima, C.D., Ruas, C.V., Behm, D.G., & Brown, L.E. (2019). Acute effects of stretching on flexibility and performance: A narrative review. *Journal of Science in Sport and Exercise, 1*(1), 29-37. https://doi.org/10.1007/s42978-019-0011-x

Lis, A., de Castro, C., & Nordin, M. (2012). Biomechanics of tendons and ligaments. In M. Nordin & V.H. Frankel (Eds.), *Basic biomechanics of the musculoskeletal system* (4th ed., pp. 102-127). Lippincott Williams & Wilkins.

Manejias, E. (2020). *Pregnancy in dance*. Dance/USA Task Force on Dancer Health. https://danceusa.s3.us-east-2.amazonaws.com/page_uploads/Pregnancy%20&%20Dance%20Jan%202020.pdf

McCormack, M., Briggs, J., Hakim, A., & Grahame, R. (2004). Joint laxity and the benign joint hypermobility syndrome in student and professional ballet dancers. *Journal of Rheumatology, 31*(1), 173-178.

Monteiro, E.R., Vigotsky, A.D., da Silva Novaes, J., & Škarabot, J. (2018). Acute effects of different anterior thigh self-massage on hip range-of-motion in trained men. *International Journal of Sports Physical Therapy, 13*(1), 104-113. https://doi.org/10.26603/ijspt20180104

Oxford University Press. (2023). Flexible. *Oxford English dictionary*. www.oed.com/search/dictionary/?scope=Entries&q=flexible

Osawa, Y., & Oguma, Y. (2013). Effects of vibration on flexibility: A meta-analysis. *Journal of Musculoskeletal and Neuronal Interactions, 13*(4), 442-453.

Petrofsky, J.S., Laymon, M., & Lee, H. (2013). Effect of heat and cold on tendon flexibility and force to flex the human knee. *Medical Science Monitor, 19*, 661-667. https://doi.org/10.12659/MSM.889145

Rumian, A.P., Wallace, A.L., & Birch, H.L. (2007). Tendons and ligaments are anatomically distinct but overlap in molecular and morphological features—A comparative study in an ovine model. *Journal of Orthopaedic Research, 25*(4), 458-464.

Sands, W.A., McNeal, J.R., Stone, M.H., Russell, E.M., & Jemni, M. (2006). Flexibility enhancement with vibration: Acute and long-term. *Medicine and Science in Sports & Exercise, 38*(4), 720-725. https://doi.org/10.1249/01.mss.0000210204.10200.dc

Shinno, H., Kurose, S., Yamanaka, Y., Higurashi, K., Fukushima, Y., Tsutsumi, H., & Kimura, Y. (2017). Evaluation of a static stretching intervention on vascular endothelial function and arterial stiffness. *European Journal of Sports Science, 17*(5), 586-592. https://doi.org/10.1080/17461391.2017.1284267

Shrier, I., & Gossal, K. (2000). Myths and truths of stretching: Individualized recommendations for healthy muscles. *The Physician and Sportsmedicine, 28*(8), 57-63. https://doi.org/10.3810/psm.2000.08.1159

Simmel, L. (2014). *Dance medicine in practice* (J. Michael & L. Simmel, Trans.). Routledge.

Škarabot, J., Beardsley, C., & Štirn, I. (2015). Comparing the effects of self-myofascial release with static stretching on ankle range-of-motion in adolescent athletes. *International Journal of Sports Physical Therapy, 10*(2), 203-212.

Small, K., Naughton, L., & Matthews, M. (2008). A systematic review into the efficacy of static stretching as part of a warm-up for the prevention of exercise-related injury. *Research in Sports Medicine, 16*(3), 213-231.

Waldhelm, A., Gacek, M., Davis, H., Saia, C., & Kirby, B. (2019). Acute effects of neural gliding on athletic performance. *International Journal of Sports Physical Therapy, 14*(4), 603-612. https://doi.org/10.26603/ijspt20190603

Weerapong, P., Hume, P.A., & Kong, G.S. (2005). The mechanisms of massage and effects on performance, muscle recovery and injury prevention. *Sports Medicine, 35*(3), 235-256. https://doi.org/10.2165/00007256-200535030-00004

Wilke, J., Macchi, V., DeCaro, R., & Stecco, C. (2019). Fascia thickness, aging and flexibility: Is there an association? *Journal of Anatomy, 235*(1), 43-49. https://doi.org/10.1111/joa.12902

Wilke, J., Niederer, D., Vogt, L., & Banzer, W. (2016). Remote effects of lower limb stretching: Preliminary evidence for myofascial connectivity? *Journal of Sports Sciences, 34*(22), 2145-2148. https://doi.org/10.1080/02640414.2016.1179776

Wilke, J., Vogt, L., Niederer, D., & Banzer, W. (2017). Is remote stretching based on myofascial chains as effective as local exercise? A Randomized-controlled trial. *Journal of Sports Sciences, 35*(20), 2021–2027. https://doi.org/10.1080/02640414.2016.1251606

Woods, K., Bishop, P., & Jones, E. (2007). Warm-up and stretching in the prevention of muscular injury. *Sports Medicine, 37*(12), 1089-1099. https://doi.org/10.2165/00007256-200737120-00006

Wyon, M. (2010). Stretching for dance. *IADMS Bulletin for Teachers, 2*(1), 9-12. https://iadms.org/media/2940/iadms-bulletin-vol2n1.pdf

Zugel, M., Maganaris, C.N., Wilke, J., Jurkat-Rott, K., Klingler, W., Wearing, S.C., Findley, T., Barbe, M.F., Steinacker, J.M., Vleeming, A., Bloch, W., Schleip, R., & Hodges, P.W. (2018). Fascial tissue research in sports medicine: From molecules to tissue adaptation, injury and diagnostics: Consensus statement. *British Journal of Sports Medicine, 52*(23), 1497. https://doi.org/10.1136/bjsports-2018-099308

Chapter 7

Academy of Nutrition and Dietetics, Dietitians of Canada, and American College of Sports Medicine. (2016). Nutrition and athletic performance. *Medicine & Science in Sports & Exercise 48*(3), 543-568. doi: 10.1249/MSS.0000000000000852

Afaghi, A., O'Connor, H., & Chow, C.M. (2007). High-glycemic-index carbohydrate meals shorten sleep onset. *American Journal of Clinical Nutrition, 85*(2), 426-430. https://doi.org/10.1093/ajcn/85.2.426

Ambegaonkar, J.P., & Brown, A.F. (2021). Nutrition periodization in dancers. *Physical Medicine and Rehabilitation Clinics of North America, 32*(1), 65-73. https://doi.org/10.1016/j.pmr.2020.09.001

Baker L. B. (2017). Sweating rate and sweat sodium concentration in athletes: a review of methodology and intra/interindividual variability. *Sports Medicine, 47*(Suppl 1), 111–128. https://doi.org/10.1007/s40279-017-0691-5

Benson, J.E., Geiger, C.J., Eiserman, P.A., & Wardlaw, G.M. (1989). Relationship between nutrient intake, body mass index, menstrual function, and ballet injury. *Journal of the American Dietetic Association, 89*(1), 58-63.

Binks, H., Vincent, G.E., Gupta, C., Irwin, C., & Khalesi, S. (2020). Effects of diet on sleep: A narrative review. *Nutrients, 12*(4), 1-18. https://doi.org/10.3390/nu12040936

Bravo, R., Matito, S., Cubero, J., Paredes, S.D., Franco, L., Rivero, M., Rodríguez, A.B., & Barriga, C. (2013). Tryptophan-enriched cereal intake improves nocturnal sleep, melatonin, serotonin, and total antioxidant capacity levels and mood in elderly humans. *Age, 35*(4), 1277-1285. https://doi.org/10.1007/s11357-012-9419-5

Brown, A.F., Welsh, T., Panton, L.B., Moffatt, R., & Ormsbee, M. J. (2020). Higher-protein intake improves body composition index in female collegiate dancers. *Applied Physiology, Nutrition, and Metabolism, 45*(5), 547–554.

Brown, D.D. (2018). Nutritional considerations for the vegetarian and vegan dancer. *Journal of Dance Medicine & Science, 22*(1), 44-53.

Brown, M.A., Howatson, G., Quin, E., Redding, E., & Stevenson, E.J. (2017). Energy intake and energy expenditure of preprofessional female contemporary dancers. *PLoS ONE, 12*(2), 1-13. https://doi.org/10.1371/journal.pone.0171998

Brown, M.A., Stevenson, E.J., & Howatson, G. (2018). Whey protein hydrolysate supplementation accelerates recovery from exercise-induced muscle damage in females. *Applied Physiology, Nutrition, and Metabolism, 43*(4), 324-330.

Brown, M.A., Stevenson, E.J., & Howatson, G. (2019). Montmorency tart cherry (Prunus cerasus L.) supplementation accelerates recovery from exercise-induced muscle damage in females. *European Journal of Sport Science, 2, 19*(1), 95-102.

Bulka, C.M., Davis, M.A., Karagas, M.R., Ahsan, H., & Argos, M. (2017). The unintended consequences of a gluten-free diet. *Epidemiology, 28*(3), e24-e25. https://doi.org/10.1097/EDE.0000000000000640

Camaschella, C. (2019). Iron deficiency. *Blood, 133*(1), 30-39. https://doi.org/10.1182/blood-2018-05-815944

Carbone, J.W., McClung, J.P., & Pasiakos, S.M. (2012). Skeletal muscle responses to negative energy balance: Effects of dietary protein. *Advances in Nutrition, 3*(2), 119-126. https://doi.org/10.3945/an.111.001792

Chadwick, R. (2004). Nutrigenomics, individualism and public health. *Proceedings of the Nutrition Society, 63*(1), 161-166. https://doi.org/10.1079/pns2003329

Challis, J., Cahalan, R., Jakeman, P., Nibhriain, O., Cronin, L., & Reeves, S. (2020). Dietary intake, body composition and nutrition knowledge of Irish dancers. *Journal of Dance Medicine & Science, 24*(3), 105-112.

Close, G.L., Baar, K., Sale, C., & Bermon, S. (2019). Nutrition for the prevention and treatment of injuries in track and field athletes. *International Journal of Sport Nutrition and Exercise Metabolism, 29*(2), 189-197. https://doi.org/10.1123/ijsnem.2018-0290

Coso, J.D., Estevez, E., Baquero, R.A., & Mora-Rodriguez, R. (2008). Anaerobic performance when rehydrating with water or commercially available sports drinks during prolonged exercise in the heat. *Applied Physiology, Nutrition, and Metabolism, 33*(2), 290-298.

Craig, W.J., Mangels, A.R., Fresán, U., Marsh, K., Miles, F.L., Saunders, A.V., Haddad, E.H., Heskey, C.E., Johnston, P., Larson-Meyer, E. and Orlich, M. (2021). The safe and effective use of plant-based diets with guidelines for health professionals. *Nutrients, 13*(11), 4144. https://doi.org/10.3390/nu13114144

Dressler, P., Gehring, D., Zdzieblik, D., Oesser, S., Gollhofer, A., & König, D. (2018). Improvement of functional ankle properties following supplementation with specific collagen peptides in athletes with chronic ankle instability. *Journal of Sports Science and Medicine, 17*(2), 298-304. https://doi.org/10.1016/j.jbmt.2018.09.037

FAO, IFAD, UNICEF, WFP & WHO. (2022). The State of Food Security and Nutrition in the World 2022. Repurposing food and agricultural policies to make healthy diets more affordable. Rome, FAO. https://doi.org/10.4060/cc0639en

Frankenfield, D. (2006). Energy expenditure and protein requirements after traumatic injury. *Nutrition in Clinical Practice, 21*(5), 430-437. https://doi.org/10.1177/0115426506021005430

Frusztajer, N.T., Dhuper, S., Warren, M.P., Brooks-Gunn, J., & Fox, R.P. (1990). Nutrition and the incidence of stress fractures in ballet dancers. *American Journal of Clinical Nutrition, 51*(August), 779-783.

Gupta, L., Morgan, K., & Gilchrist, S. (2017). Does elite sport degrade sleep quality? A systematic review. *Sports Medicine, 47*(7), 1317-1333. https://doi.org/10.1007/s40279-016-0650-6

Harris, J.A., & Benedict, F.G. (1918). A biometric study of human basal metabolism. *Proceedings of the National Academy of Sciences of the United States of America, 4*(12), 370-373. https://doi.org/10.1073/pnas.4.12.370

Harvard University T.H. Chan School of Public Health. (2023). The nutrition source: Antioxidants. www.hsph.harvard.edu/nutritionsource/antioxidants

Howatson, G., Bell, P.G., Tallent, J., Middleton, B., McHugh, M.P., & Ellis, J. (2012). Effect of tart cherry juice (Prunus cerasus) on melatonin levels and enhanced sleep quality. *European Journal of Nutrition, 51*(8), 909-916. https://doi.org/10.1007/s00394-011-0263-7

Jagim, A.R., Camic, C.L., Kisiolek, J., Luedke, J., Erickson, J., Jones, M.T., & Oliver, J.M. (2018). Accuracy of resting metabolic rate prediction equations in athletes. *Journal of Strength & Conditioning Research, 32*(7), 1875-1881.

Jeukendrup, A.E. (2017). Periodized nutrition for athletes. *Sports Medicine, 47*(Suppl 1), 51-63. https://doi.org/10.1007/s40279-017-0694-2

Jones, L.C., Cleary, M.A., Lopez, R.M., Zuri, R.E., & Lopez, R. (2008). Active dehydration impairs upper and lower body anerobic power. *Journal of Strength and Conditioning Research, 22*(2), 455-463.

Keay, N., Overseas, A.D., & Francis, G. (2020). Indicators and correlates of low energy availability in male and female dancers. *BMJ Open Sport and Exercise Medicine, 6*(1). https://doi.org/10.1136/bmjsem-2020-000906

Lakićević N. (2019). The effects of alcohol consumption on recovery following resistance exercise: A systematic review. *Journal of Functional Morphology and Kinesiology*, *4*(3), 41. https://doi.org/10.3390/jfmk4030041

Lerner, B.A., Green, P.H.R., & Lebwohl, B. (2019). Going against the grains: Gluten-free diets in patients without celiac disease—Worthwhile or not? *Digestive Diseases and Sciences*, *64*(7), 1740-1747. https://doi.org/10.1007/s10620-019-05663-x

Lis, D.M., Stellingwerff, T., Shing, C.M., Ahuja, K.D.K., & Fell, J.W. (2015). Exploring the popularity, experiences, and beliefs surrounding gluten-free diets in nonceliac athletes. *International Journal of Sport Nutrition and Exercise Metabolism*, *25*(1), 37-45. https://doi.org/10.1123/ijsnem.2013-0247

McArdle, W.D., Katch, F.I., & Katch, V.L. (2015). Body composition, energy balance, and weight control. *Exercise Physiology: Nutrition, Energy, and Human Performance.* (8th ed., pp. 727-833). Wolters Kluwer.

Mettler, S., Mitchell, N., & Tipton, K.D. (2010). Increased protein intake reduces lean body mass loss during weight loss in athletes. *Medicine and Science in Sports and Exercise*, *42*(326), 326-337. https://doi.org/10.1249/MSS.0b013e3181b2ef8e

Mountjoy, M., Sundgot-Borgen, J., Burke, L., Carter, S., Constantini, N., Lebrun, C., Meyer, N., Sherman, R., Steffen, K., Budgett, R., & Ljungqvist, A. (2014). The IOC consensus statement: Beyond the female athlete triad—Relative energy deficiency in sport (RED-S). *British Journal of Sports Medicine*, *48*(7), 491–497. https://doi.org/10.1136/bjsports-2014-093502

Mountjoy, M., Ackerman, K.E., Bailey, D.M., Burke, L.M., Constantini, N., Hackney, A.C., Heikura, I.A., Melin, A., Pensgaard, A.M., Stellingwerff, T., Sundgot-Borgen, J.K., Torstveit, M.K., Jacobsen, A.U., Verhagen, E., Budgett, R., Engebretsen, L., & Erdener, U. (2023). 2023 International Olympic Committee's (IOC) consensus statement on Relative Energy Deficiency in Sport (REDs). *British Journal of Sports Medicine*, *57*(17), 1073–1097. https://doi.org/10.1136/bjsports-2023-106994

Niland, B., & Cash, B.D. (2018). Health benefits and adverse effects of a gluten-free diet in non-celiac disease patients. *Gastroenterology & Hepatology*, *14*(2), 82-91.

O'Brien, C.P., & Lyons, F. (2000). Alcohol and the athlete. *Sports Medicine 2*, *29*(5), 295-300.

Owens, D.J., Twist, C., Cobley, J.N., Howatson, G., & Close, G.L. (2019). Exercise-induced muscle damage: What is it, what causes it and what are the nutritional solutions? *European Journal of Sport Science*, *19*(1), 71-85. https://doi.org/10.1080/17461391.2018.1505957

Phillips, S.M. (2004). Protein requirements and supplementation in strength sports. *Nutrition*, *20*(7-8), 689-695. https://doi.org/10.1016/j.nut.2004.04.009

Ramkumar, P.N., Farber, J., Arnouk, J., Varner, K.E., & Mcculloch, P.C. (2016). Injuries in a professional ballet dance company: A 10-year retrospective study. *Journal of Dance Medicine & Science*, *20*(1), 30-37. https://doi.org/10.12678/1089-313X.20.1.30

Rodriguez, N.N.R., Di Marco, N., Langley, S., & DiMarco, N.M. (2009). American College of Sports Medicine, American Dietetic Association, and Dietitians of Canada joint position statement: Nutrition and athletic performance. *Medicine and Science in Sports and Exercise*, *41*(3), 709-731. https://doi.org/10.1249/MSS.0b013e31819further0eb86

Schaal, K., Tafflet, M., Nassif, H., Thibault, V., Pichard, C., Alcotte, M., Guillet, T., El Helou, N., Berthelot, G., Simon, S., & Toussaint, J.F. (2011). Psychological balance in high level athletes: Fender-based differences and sport-specific patterns. *PloS One*, *6*(5), e19007. http://doi.org/10.1371/journal.pone.0019007

Shaw, G., Lee-Barthel, A., Ross, M.L.R., Wang, B., & Baar, K. (2017). Vitamin C-enriched gelatin supplementation before intermittent activity augments collagen synthesis. *American Journal of Clinical Nutrition*, *105*(1), 136-143. https://doi.org/10.3945/ajcn.116.138594

Singh, P., Arora, A., Strand, T.A., Leffler, D.A., Catassi, C., Green, P.H., Kelly, C.P, Ahuja, V., & Makharia, G.K. (2018). Global prevalence of celiac disease: Systematic review and meta-analysis. *Clinical Gastroenterology and Hepatology*, *16*(6), 823-836.e2 https://doi.org/10.1016/j.cgh.2017.06.037

Smith-Ryan, A.E., Hirsch, K.R., Saylor, H.E., Gould, L.M., & Blue, M.N.M. (2020). Nutritional considerations and strategies to facilitate injury recovery and rehabilitation. *Journal of Athletic Training*, *55*(9), 918-930. https://doi.org/10.4085/1062-6050-550-19

Sousa, M., Carvalho, P., Moreira, P., & Teixeira, V. (2013). Nutrition and nutritional issues for dancers. *Medical Problems of Performing Artists*, *28*(3), 119-123.

Spiro, A., & Buttriss, J. (2014). Vitamin D: an overview of vitamin D status and intake in Europe. *Nutrition Bulletin*, *39*(4), 322-350.

Thomas, D.T., Erdman, K.A., & Burke, L.M. (2016). Nutrition and athletic performance. *Medicine and Science in Sports and Exercise, 48*(3), 543-568.

Tipton, K.D. (2015). Nutritional support for exercise-induced injuries. *Sports Medicine, 45*(1), 93-104. https://doi.org/10.1007/s40279-015-0398-4

Vella, L.D., & Cameron-Smith, D. (2010). Alcohol, athletic performance and recovery. *Nutrients*, 2(8), 781-789. https://doi.org/10.3390/nu2080781

Vitale, K., & Getzin, A. (2019). Nutrition and supplement update for the endurance athlete: Review and recommendations. *Nutrients, 11*(6), 1-20. https://doi.org/10.3390/nu11061289

van Vliet, S., Burd, N.A., & van Loon, L.J. (2015). The skeletal muscle anabolic response to plant-versus animal-based protein consumption. *Journal of Nutrition, 145*(9), 1981–1991. https://doi.org/10.3945/jn.114.204305

Walsh, N.P., Halson, S.L., Sargent, C., Roach, G.D., Nédélec, M., Gupta, L., Leeder, J., Fullagar, H.H., Coutts, A.J., Edwards, B.J., Pullinger, S.A., Robertson, C.M., Burniston, J.G., Lastella, M., Le Meur, Y., Hausswirth, C., Bender, A.M., Grandner, M.A., & Samuels, C.H. (2021). Sleep and the athlete: Narrative review and 2021 expert consensus recommendations. *British Journal of Sports Medicine, 55*(7), 356-368. https://doi.org/10.1136/bjsports-2020-102025

Watson, A.M. (2017). Sleep and athletic performance. *Current Sports Medicine Reports, 16*(6), 413-418. https://doi.org/10.1249/JSR.0000000000000418

Wolman, R., Wyon, M.A., Koutedakis, Y., Nevill, A.M., Eastell, R., & Allen, N. (2013). Vitamin D status in professional ballet dancers: Winter vs. summer. *Journal of Science and Medicine in Sport, 16*(5), 388-391. https://doi.org/10.1016/j.jsams.2012.12.010

Wyon, M.A., Wolman, R., Kolokythas, N., Sheriff, K., Galloway, S., & Mattiussi, A. (2018). Effect of vitamin D supplementation in elite adolescent dancers on muscle function and injury incidence: A randomised double-blind study. *International Journal of Sports Physiology and Performance, 14*(1), 55-59.

Chapter 8

Aalami, M., Jafarnejad, F., & ModarresGharavi, M. (2016). The effects of progressive muscular relaxation and breathing control technique on blood pressure during pregnancy. *Iranian Journal of Nursing and Midwifery Research, 21*(3), 331-336.

Akehurst, S., & Oliver, E.J. (2014). Obsessive passion: A dependency associated with injury- related risky behaviour in dancers. *Journal of Sports Sciences, 32*(3), 259-267.

Alexias, G., & Dimitropoulou, E. (2011). The body as a tool: Professional classical ballet dancers' embodiment. *Research in Dance Education, 12* (2), 87-104.

American Psychiatric Association. (2022). *Diagnostic and statistical manual of mental disorders* (5th ed.). American Psychiatric Association.

Angyal, C. (2021). *Turning pointe: How a new generation of dancers is saving ballet from itself.* Bold Type.

Anxiety and Depression Association of America (ADAA) (2021). Anxiety disorders: facts and statistics. https://adaa.org/understanding-anxiety/facts-statistics

Araújo, A., Gaines, K., Goonan, B., & Skvarla, L. (2021). *Case study in mental health of dancers and impacts of a preventative mental health program.* [Unpublished data]. Minding the Gap and Point Park University.

Arcelus, J., Witcomb, G.L., & Mitchell, A. (2014). Prevalence of eating disorders amongst dancers: A systemic review and meta-analysis. *European Eating Disorders Review, 22*(2), 92-101.

Australian Institute of Health and Welfare. (2023). Mental health: Prevalence and impact of mental illness. www.aihw.gov.au/mental-health/overview/prevalence-and-impact-of-mental-illness

Batson, G., & Wilson, M. (2017). Rest and Recovery. In M.V. Wilmerding, & D. Krasnow, (Eds.), *Dancer Wellness* (pp.84-92). Human Kinetics.

Brackenridge, C.H, Bishopp, D., Moussall, S., & Tapp, J. (2008). The characteristics of sexual abuse in sport: A multidimensional scaling analysis of events described in media reports. *International Journal of Sport and Exercise Psychology, 6*(4), 385-406.

Canadian Mental Health Association. (2022). Fast facts about mental health and mental illness. https://cmha.ca/fast-facts-about-mental-illness

Cena, H., Barthels, F., Cuzzolaro, M., Bratman, S., BrytekMatera, A, Dunn, T., Varga, M., Missbach, B. & Donini, L.M. (2018). Definition and diagnostic criteria for orthorexia nervosa: A narrative review of the literature. *Eating and Weight Disorders – Studies on Anorexia, Bulimia and Obesity, 24*(2),209-246. https://doi.org/10.1007/s40519-018-0606-y

Dance Data Project. (2021). Global ballet leadership report. www.dancedataproject.com/wp-content/uploads/2021/12/2020-2021-Global-Ballet-Leadership-Report.pdf

Dehdari, T., Heidarnia, A., Ramezankhani, A., Sadeghian, S., & Ghofranipour, F. (2009). Effects of progressive muscular relaxation training on quality of life in anxious patients after coronary artery bypass graft surgery. *Indian Journal of Medical Research, 129*(5), 603-608.

DeWolfe, C.E.J., Scott, D., & Seaman, K.A. (2021). Embrace the challenge: Acknowledging a challenge following negative self-talk improves performance. *Journal of Applied Sport Psychology, 33*(5), 527-540.

Elliott, I.A. (2017). A self-regulation model of sexual grooming. *Trauma, Violence & Abuse, 18*(1), 83-97. https://doi.org/10.1177/1524838015591573

Forcier, M.F. (2017). Code of silence: A call to action to address and prevent abuse in dance communities. *The Dance Current*, https://thedancecurrent.com/article/code-silence

Fortin, S., Trudel, S., & Rail, G. (2009). Incorporation paradoxale des normes esthétiques et de santé chez les danseurs contemporains. [Paradoxical incorporation of aesthetic and health standards among contemporary dancers.] In S. Fortin (Dir.), *Danse et Santé, du Corps Intime au Corps Social. [Dance and Health, from the Intimate Body to the Social Body.]* (pp. 9-45). Presses De l'Université du Québec.

Garcia-Dantas, A., Amado Alonso, D, Sánchez-Miguel, P.A., & del Río Sánchez, C. (2018). Factors dancers associate with their body dissatisfaction. *Body Image, 25*, 40-47.

Green, J. (2001). Socially constructed bodies in American dance classrooms. *Research in Dance Education, 2* (2), 155-173.

Hardy, J. (2006) Speaking clearly: A critical review of the self-talk literature. *Psychology of Sport and Exercise, 7*(1), 81-97.

Hobden, R. (2009). La prévention des problèmes de santé dans les écoles et compagnies de danse. [Prevention of health problems in schools and dance companies.] In S. Fortin (Dir.), *Danse et Santé, du Corps Intime au Corps Social [Dance and Health, from the Intimate Body to the Social Body.]*(pp. 215- 224). Presses de l'Université du Québec.

Jackson, J. (2005). My dance and the ideal body: Looking at the ballet practice from the inside out. *Research in Dance Education, 6* (1), 25-40.

Kabat-Zinn, J. (2016). *Wherever you go, there you are: Mindfulness meditation in everyday life* (10th ed.). Little Brown Book Group.

Karin, J., Haggard, P., & Christensen, J. (2017). Mental training. In M.V. Wilmerding & D. Krasnow (Eds.), *Dancer wellness* (pp. 57-69). Human Kinetics.

Keah, N., Overseas, A., & Francis, G. (2020). Indicators and correlates of low energy availability in male and female dancers. *BMJ Open Sport & Exercise Medicine, 6 (1)*, 1-7.

Kelly, D. (2012). *Ballerina: Sex, scandal and suffering beyond the symbol of perfection.* Greystone Books.

Kenny, D.T. (2011). *The psychology of music performance anxiety.* Oxford University Press.

Krasnow, D., & Wilmerding, M.V. (2015) (Eds.). *Motor learning and control for dance.* Human Kinetics.

Kveton-Bohnert, L.A. (2017). *The voices of classical ballet dancers: Alleviating maladaptive perfectionism through resilience, mindful learning and self-compassion* [Qualitative study from semi-structured interviews]. Proquest Dissertations: Saybrook University.

La Flèche, J. (2014, November 19). Live interview with Ms. Irma Sandrey. New York, NY.

La Flèche, J. (2018). The silence after the applause: Dealing with post-performance depression. *The Dance Current.* https://thedancecurrent.com/article/silence-after-applause

La Flèche, J. (2019). Big little secrets: Understanding abuse and trauma in dance, part II. https://thedancecurrent.com/article/big-little-secrets-part-ii

La Flèche, J. (2020). Big little secrets: Understanding abuse and trauma in dance, part I. *The Dance Current*, January/February:52-53.

Lakes, R. (2005). The messages behind the methods: The authoritarian pedagogical legacy in western concert dance technique training and rehearsals. *Arts Education Policy Review, 106*(5), 3-16.

Lee, C. (1999). *Ballet in western culture, a history of its origins and evolution.* Allyn & Bacon.

Mainwaring, L., & Aujla, I. (2017). Psychological wellness. In M.V. Wilmerding & D. Krasnow (Eds.), *Dancer wellness* (pp.71-82). Human Kinetics.

Mainwaring, L., & Finney, C. (2017). Psychological risk factors and outcomes of dance injury. A systematic review. *Journal of Dance Medicine & Science, 21* (3), 87-96.

Mainwaring, L., & Krasnow, D. (2010). Teaching the dance class: Strategies to enhance skill acquisition, mastery and positive self-image. *Journal of Dance Education, 10*(1), 14- 21.

Martha Graham Reflects on Her Art and a Life in Dance. (1985, March 31). *The New York Times*. p. H1. www.nytimes.com/1985/03/31/arts/martha-graham-reflects-on-her-art-and-a-life-in-dance.html

McEwen, K., & Young, K. (2011). Ballet and pain: Reflections on a risk-dance culture. *Qualitative Research in Sport, Exercise and Health, 3*(2), 152-173.

McGuire, K. (2016, October 31). Tackling depression. *Dance Magazine*. www.dancemagazine.com/tackling-depression-2307044490.html

McManus, S, Bebbington P, Jenkins R, & Brugha, T. (Eds.). (2016). *Mental health and wellbeing in England: Adult psychiatric morbidity survey 2014*. Leeds: NHS Digital. https://assets.publishing.service.gov.uk/government/uploads/system/uploads/attachment_data/file/556596/apms-2014-full-rpt.pdf

Moola, F., & Krahn, A. (2018). A dance with many secrets: The experience of emotional harm from the perspective of past professional female dancers in Canada. *Journal of Aggression, Maltreatment & Trauma, 27* (3), 256-274

Mountjoy, M., Brackenridge, C., Arrington, M., Blauwet, C., Carska-Sheppard, A., Fasting, K., Kirby, S., Leahy, T., Marks, S., Martin, K., Starr, K., Tiivas, A., & Budgett, R. (2016). International Olympic Committee consensus statement: harassment and abuse (non-accidental violence) in sport. *British Journal of Sports Medicine, 50*(17), 1019–1029. https://doi.org/10.1136/bjsports-2016-096121

Mruk, C.J. (2013). *Self-esteem and positive psychology: Research, theory and practice* (4th ed.). Springer.

Nasio. J.D. (2007). *Mon corps et ses images.* [*My body and its images.*] Éditions Payot.

National Alliance on Mental Illness. (2021). Mental health by the numbers. www.nami.org/mhstats

Neff, K.D., & Knox, M.C. (2017). Self-compassion. In V. Zeigler-Hill & T.K. Shackelford (Eds.), *Encyclopedia of personality and individual differences* (pp.1-8). Springer International.

Nordin-Bates, S.M. (2020) Striving for perfection or for creativity? A dancer's dilemma. *Journal of Dance Education, 20*(1), 23-24.

Nordin-Bates, S. (2023). *Essentials of dance psychology.* Human Kinetics.

Oliver, W. (2005). Reading the ballerina's body: Susan Bordo sheds light on Anastasia Volochkova and Heidi Guenther. *Dance Research Journal, 37*(2), 38-54.

Oliver, W. (2008). Body image in the dance class. *Journal of Physical Education, Recreation & Dance, 79*(5), 18-41.

Papalia, D., & Martorell, G. (2021). *Experience human development* (14th ed). McGraw-Hill.

Papaefstathiou, M., Rhind, D., & Brackenridge, C. (2013). Child protection in ballet: Experiences and views of teachers, administrators and ballet students. *Child Abuse Review, 22*, 127-141.

Parent, S. & Fortier, K. (2018). Comprehensive overview of the problem of violence against athletes in sport. *Journal of Sport & Social Issues, 42*(4), 227-246.

Pickard, A. (2012). Schooling the dancer: The evolution of an identity as a ballet dancer. *Research in Dance Education, 13*(1), 25-46.

Pickard, A. (2013). Ballet body belief: Perceptions of an ideal ballet body from young ballet dancers. *Research in Dance Education, 14*(1), 3-19.

Pollatou, E., Bakali, N., Theodorakis, Y., & Goudas, M. (2010). Body image in female professional and amateur dancers. *Research in Dance Education, 11*(2), 131-137.

Price, B.R., & Pettijohn, T.F. (2006). The effect of ballet dance attire on body and self-perception of female dancers. *Social Behavior and Personality, 34*(8), 991-98.

Quin, E., Rafferty, S., & Tomlinson, C. (2015). *Safe dance practice*. Human Kinetics.

Radell, S.A., Keneman, M.L., Mandradjieff, M.P., Adame, D.D., & Cole, S.P. (2017). Comparison study of body image satisfaction between beginning- and advanced-level female ballet students. *Journal of Dance Medicine & Science, 21* (4), 135-143.

Radell, S.A., Mandradjieff, M.P., Adame, D.D,. & Cole, S.P. (2020). Impact of mirrors on body image of beginning modern and ballet students. *Journal of Dance Medicine & Science, 24* (3), 126-134.

Reardon CL, Hainline B, Aron CM, Baron D, Baum AL, Bindra A, Budgett R, Campriani N, Castaldelli-Maia JM, Currie A, Derevensky JL, Glick ID, Gorczynski P, Gouttebarge V, Grandner MA, Han DH, McDuff D, Mountjoy M, Polat A…Engebretsen L. Mental health in elite athletes: International Olympic Committee consensus statement. (2019). *British Journal of Sports Medicine, 53*, 667-699.

Rip, B., Fortin S., & Vallerand, R.J. (2006). The relationship between passion and injury in dance students. *Journal of Dance Medicine & Science, 10*, 14-20.

Ritenburg, H.M. (2010). Frozen landscapes: A Foucauldian genealogy of the ideal ballet dancers' body. *Research in Dance Education, 11*(1), 71-85.

Saigal, M. (2021). Language matters: Shifting how we speak about food and bodies to prevent eating disorders and promote dancer health. Performing Arts Medicine Association Annual Symposium, June 24, 2021.

Smith-Theodore, D. (2021). The language of eating disorders from a psychological perspective . . . Are we helping or harming? Performing Arts Medicine Association Annual Symposium, June 27, 2021.

Steiger, H., & Thaler, L. (2016). Eating disorders, gene–environment interactions and the epigenome: Roles of stress exposures and nutritional status. *Physiology & Behavior, 162*, 181-185. https://doi.org/10.1016/j.physbeh.2016.01.041

Sterne, S., & Patsalidou, C. (2017). Bone health. In M.V. Wilmerding & D. Krasnow (Eds.), *Dancer wellness* (pp. 113-127). Human Kinetics.

Stirling, A.E., & Kerr, G. (2013). The perceived effects of elite athletes' experiences of emotional abuse in the coach-athlete relationship. *International Journal of Sport and Exercise Psychology, 11*(1), 87-100.

Stop Street Harassment. (2018). *The facts behind the #Me Too movement: A national study on sexual harassment & assault*. Stop Street Harassment. www.stopstreetharassment.org/wp-content/uploads/2018/01/Full-Report-2018-National-Study-on-Sexual-Harassment-and-Assault.pdf

Taylor, J., & Estanol, E. (2015). *Dance psychology for artistic and performance excellence*. Human Kinetics.

Thompson, P., & Jaque, S.V. (2016). Visiting the muse: Creativity, coping, and PTSD in talented dancers and athletes. *American Journal of Play, 8*(3), 363-378.

Troxel, W.M., Rodriguez, A., Seelam, R., Dong, L., Perez, L.G., Tucker, J.S., Siconolfi, D., & D'Amico, E.J. (2022). A latent class approach to understanding longitudinal sleep health and the association with alcohol and cannabis use during late adolescence and emerging adulthood. *Addictive Behaviors, 134*, 107417. https://doi.org/10.1016/j.addbeh.2022.107417

U.S. Department of Veterans Affairs. (2020). PTSD: National Center for PTSD. What is PTSD? www.ptsd.va.gov/understand/what/index.asp

van Winden, D., van Rijn, R.M., Savelsbergh, G.J.P., Oudejans, R.R.D., & Stubbe, J.H. (2020a). Characteristics and extent of mental health issues in contemporary dance students. *Medical Problems of Performing Artists, 35* (3),121-129.

van Winden, D., van Rijn, R.M., Savelsbergh, G.J.P., Oudejans, R.R.D., & Stubbe, J.H. (2020b). Limited coping skills, young age, and high BMI are risk factors for injuries in contemporary dance: A 1-year prospective study. *Frontiers in Psychology, 11*:1452.

van Zelst, L., Clabaugh, A., & Morling, B. (2004). Dancers' body esteem, fitness esteem and self-esteem in three contexts. *Journal of Dance Education, 4* (2), 48-57.

Victorino, R.C. (2020). The Eisenhower Matrix: Prioritize your time on what matters most. https://slab.com/blog/eisenhower-matrix

Wingenroth, L. (2018, June). #DancersToo: Is the dance world finally ready to address sexual harassment? *Dance Magazine*, pp. 31-33.

Zhao, L., Wu, H., Zhou, X., Wang, Q., Zhu, W., & Chen, J. (2012). Effects of progressive muscular relaxation training on anxiety, depression and quality of life of endometriosis patients under gonadotrophin-releasing hormone agonist therapy. *European Journal of Obstetrics, Gynecology, and Reproductive Biology, 162*(2), 211-215. https://doi.org/10.1016/j.ejogrb.2012.02.029

Chapter 9

Andersen, J.C., Courson, R.W., Kleiner, D.M., & McLoda, T.A. (2002). National Athletic Trainers' Association position statement: Emergency planning in athletics. *Journal of Athletic Training, 37*(1), 99-104.

Ashkenazi, I., & Hunt, R. C. (2019). You're it-you've got to save someone: Immediate responders, not bystanders. *Frontiers in Public Health, 7*, 361. https://doi.org/10.3389/fpubh.2019.00361

Centers for Disease Control and Prevention. (2019). *Standard precautions for all patient care*. CDC. www.cdc.gov/infectioncontrol/basics/standard-precautions.html

Fouad A.F., Abbott P.V., Tsilingaridis G., Cohenca N., Lauridsen E., Bourguignon C., O'Connell A., Flores M.T., Day P.F., Hicks L., Andreasen J.O., Cehreli Z.C., Harlamb S., Kahler B., Oginni A., Semper M., & Levin L. (2020). International Association of Dental Traumatology guidelines for the management of traumatic dental injuries: 2. Avulsion of permanent teeth. *Dental Traumatology. 36*(4):331-342. https://doi.org/10.1111/edt.12573

Hernandez, B.L.M., & Strickland, G. (2005). School health and safety: Standards for dance education and dance in physical education. *Journal of Physical Education, Recreation & Dance, 76*(4), 20-25.

Integrated Community Solutions. (2023). What is ICSAVE? https://icsave.org

Jamshaid, S., Banhidy, N., Ghedia, R., & Seymour, K. (2023). Where should epistaxis education be focused? A comparative study between the public and healthcare workers on knowledge of first aid management methods of epistaxis. *Journal of Laryngology and Otology, 137*(4), 408–412. https://doi.org/10.1017/S0022215122001098

Kleinknecht v. Gettysburg College, 989 F2d 1360 (3rd Cir 1993). https://law.resource.org/pub/us/case/reporter/F2/989/989.F2d.1360.92-7160.html

Mitchell, K.B., Gugerty, L., & Muth, E. (2008). Effects of brief training on use of automated external defibrillators by people without medical expertise. *Human Factors, 50*(2), 301-310. https://doi.org/10.1518/001872008X250746

National Wellness Institute (NWI). (n.d.). *Six Dimensions of Wellness: National Wellness Institute.* https://nationalwellness.org/resources/six-dimensions-of-wellness

Oliver, G.J., Walter, D.P., & Redmond, A.D. (2017). Prehospital deaths from trauma: Are injuries survivable and do bystanders help? *Injury 48*(5), 985-991. https://doi.org/10.1016/j.injury.2017.02.026.

Pelto, H.F., & Drezner, J.A. (2020). Design and implementation of an emergency action plan for sudden cardiac arrest in sport. *Journal of Cardiovascular Translational Research, 13*(3), 331-338. https://doi.org/10.1007/s12265-020-09988-1

Potter, B.W., & Martin, R.D. (2009). Testing the emergency action plan in athletics. *International Journal of Athletic Therapy & Training, 14*(6), 29-32.

Singletary, E.M., Zideman, D.A., Bendall, J.C., Berry, D.A., Borra, V., Carlson, J.N., Cassan, P., Chang, W.-T., Charlton, N.P., Djärv, T., Douma, M.J., Epstein, J.L., Hood, N.A., Markenson, D.S., Meyran, D., Orkin, A., Sakamoto, T., Swain, J.M., Woodin, J.A., . . . Lee, C.-C. (2020). 2020 International consensus on first aid science with treatment recommendations. *Resuscitation, 156,* A240-A282. https://doi.org/10.1016/j.resuscitation.2020.09.016

Vassallo, A.J., Hiller, C., Stamatakis, E., & Pappas, E. (2017). Epidemiology of dance-related injuries presenting to emergency departments in the United States, 2000-2013. *Medical Problems of Performing Artists, 32*(3), 170-175. https://doi.org/10.21091/mppa.2017.3028

Weir J.D. (1997). Effective management of epistaxis in athletes. *Journal of Athletic Training, 32*(3), 254–255.

World Health Organization. (2007). Standard precautions in healthcare. In WHO, *Aide-memoire: Epidemic and pandemic alert and response.* World Health Organization. www.who.int/csr/resources/publications/EPR_AM2_E7.pdf

Chapter 10

Alexander, J., Richards, J., Attah, O., Cheema, S., Snook, J., Wisdell, C., May, K., & Selfe, J. (2018). Delayed effects of a 20-min crushed ice application on knee joint position sense assessed by a functional task during a re-warming period. *Gait & Posture, 62,* 173-178. https://doi.org/10.1016/j.gaitpost.2018.03.015

Anderson, R., Hanrahan, S.J., (2008). Dancing in pain: Pain appraisal and coping in dancers. *Journal of Dance Medicine & Science, 12*(1), 9-16.

Beahrs, T.R., Reagan, J., Bettin, C.C., Grear, B.J., Murphy, G.A., & Richardson, D.R. (2019). Smoking effects in foot and ankle surgery: An evidence-based review. *Foot & Ankle International, 40*(10), 12261232. https://doi.org.proxy.library.ohio.edu/10.1177/1071100719867942

Bleakley, C.M., Glasgow, P., & MacAuley, D.C. (2012). PRICE needs updating, should we call the POLICE?. *British Journal of Sports Medicine, 46*(4), 220-221. https://doi.org/10.1136/bjsports-2011-090297

Bleakley, C.M., McDonough, S.M., MacAuley, D.C., & Bjordal, J. (2006). Cryotherapy for acute ankle sprains: A andomized controlled study of two different icing protocols. *British Journal of Sports Medicine, 40*(8), 700-705. https://doi.org/10.1136/bjsm.2006.025932

Brukner P., & Khan, K. (2018). *Clinical Sports Medicine* (5th ed.). McGraw Hill Education.

Dubois, B., & Esculier, J. F. (2020). Soft-tissue injuries simply need PEACE and LOVE. *British Journal of Sports Medicine, 54*(2), 72-73. https://doi.org/10.1136/bjsports-2019-101253

DuBose, J., MacAllister, L., Hadi, K., & Sakallaris, B. (2018). Exploring the concept of healing spaces. *HERD, 11*(1), 43–56. https://doi.org/10.1177/1937586716680567

Herrera, E., Sandoval, M.C., Camargo, D.M., & Salvini, T.F. (2010). Motor and sensory nerve conduction are affected differently by ice pack, ice massage, and cold water immersion. *Physical Therapy, 90*(4), 581-591. https://doi.org/10.2522/ptj.20090131

Jung, M.K., Callaci, J.J., Lauing, K.L., Otis, J.S., Radek, K.A., Jones, M.K., & Kovacs, E.J. (2011). Alcohol exposure and mechanisms of tissue injury and repair. *Alcoholism, Clinical and Experimental Research, 35*(3), 392–399. https://doi.org/10.1111/j.1530-0277.2010.01356.x

Lyrtzis, C., Natsis, K., Papadopoulos, C., Noussios, G., & Papathanasiou, E. (2011). Efficacy of paracetamol versus diclofenac for Grade II ankle sprains. *Foot & Ankle International, 32*(6), 571–575. https://doi.org/10.3113/FAI.2011.0571

Macedo, C.S., Alonso, C.S., Liporaci, R.F., Vieira, F., & Guirro, R.R. (2014). Cold water immersion of the ankle decreases neuromuscular response of lower limb after inversion movement. *Brazilian Journal of Physical Therapy, 18*(1), 93-97. https://doi.org/10.1590/s1413-35552012005000132

Malanga, G.A., Yan, N., & Stark, J. (2015). Mechanisms and efficacy of heat and cold therapies for musculoskeletal injury. *Postgraduate Medicine, 127*(1), 57-65. https://doi.org/10.1080/00325481.2015.992719

Mitchell, A.C., & Thain, P.K. (2011). The effect of intermittent ice application on dynamic postural control. *Journal of Strength and Conditioning Research, 25*, S62-S63. https://doi.org/10.1097/01.JSC.0000395678.91938.67

Mirkin, G., & Hoffman, M. (1978). *The Sports Medicine Book.* Little, Brown and Company.

Pollitt, E.E., & Hutt, K. (2021). Viewing injury in dancers from a psychological perspective - A literature review. *Journal of Dance Medicine & Science, 25*(2), 75-79. https://doi.org/10.12678/1089-313X.061521a

Potts, J.C., & Irrgang, J.J. (2001). Principles of rehabilitation of lower extremity injuries in dancers. *Journal of Dance Medicine and Science, 5*(2), 51-61.

Rickman, A.M., Ambegaonkar, J.P., & Cortes, N. (2012). Core stability: Implications for dance injuries. *Medical Problems of Performing Artists, 27*(3), 159-164. https://doi.org/10.21091/mppa.2012.3028

Russell, J.A. (2013). Preventing dance injuries: Current perspectives. *Open Access Journal of Sports Medicine, 4*, 199-210. https://doi-org /10.2147/OAJSM.S36529

Sabo, M. (2013). Physical therapy rehabilitation strategies for dancers: A qualitative study. *Journal of Dance Medicine & Science, 17*(1), 11-17. https://doi.org/10.12678/1089-313x.17.1.11

Stein, C.J., Gleason, C.N., Pepin, M.J., Kinney, S.A., Southwick, H.L., Park, E.R., & Stracciolini, A. (2016). Cigarette smoking among dancers of different ages and levels of training. *Journal of Dance Medicine & Science, 20*(4), 174-180. https://doi.org/10.12678/1089-313x.20.4.174

Stovitz, S. D., & Johnson, R. J. (2003). NSAIDs and musculoskeletal treatment: what is the clinical evidence?. *The Physician and Sportsmedicine, 31*(1), 35–52. https://doi.org /10.3810/psm.2003.01.160

Wang, Y., Li, S., Zhang, Y., Chen, Y., Yan, F., Han, L., & Ma, Y. (2021). Heat and cold therapy reduce pain in patients with delayed onset muscle soreness: A systematic review and meta-analysis of 32 randomized controlled trials. *Physical Therapy in Sport, 48*, 177-187. https://doi.org/10.1016/j.ptsp.2021.01.004

Chapter 11

Albisetti, W., Perugia, D., De Bartolomeo, O., Tagliabue, L., Camerucci, E., & Calori, G.M. (2010). Stress fractures of the base of the metatarsal bones in young trainee ballet dancers. *International Orthopaedics, 34*(1), 51–55. https://doi.org/10.1007/s00264-009-0784-3

Bronner, S. (2021). Injury characteristics in pre-professional modern dancers: Prospective study of differences due to sex, training year, and external causal mechanisms. *Journal of Dance Medicine & Science, 25*(2), 117-130. https://doi.org/10.12678/1089-313X.061521g

Campbell, R., Lehr, M., Livingston, A., McCurdy, M., & Ware, J. K. (2019). Intrinsic modifiable risk factors in ballet dancers: Applying evidence based practice principles to enhance clinical applications.

Physical Therapy in Sport, 28, 206-114. https://doi.org/10.1016/j.ptsp.2019.04.022

Dalley, A. F. & Agur A. M. R. (2023). *Moore's Clinically Oriented Anatomy.* (9th ed.). Wolters Kluwer.

Daneshmandia, H., Sakib, F., Shahheidaric, S., & Khoorid, A. (2011). Lower extremity malalignment and its linear relation with Q angle in female athletes. *Procedia – Social and Behavioral Sciences, 15*, 3349–3354.

Durall, C.J. (2011). Examination and treatment of cuboid syndrome: A literature review. *Sports Health, 3*(6), 514-519. https://doi.org/10.1177/1941738111405965

Ekegren, C., Quested, R., & Brodrick, A. (2014). Injuries in pre-professional ballet dancers: Incidence, characteristics and consequences. *Journal of Science and Medicine in Sport, 17*, 271-275. https://doi.org/10.1016/j.jsams.2013.07.013

Hamilton, W.G. (1982). Sprained ankles in ballet dancers. *Foot & Ankle, 3*(2), 99-102. https://doi.org/10.1177/107110078200300208

Kadel, N. (2014) Foot and ankle problems in dancers. *Physical Medicine and Rehabilitation Clinics of North America, 25*(4), 829-44. https://doi.org/10.1016/j.pmr.2014.06.003

Kadel, N., & Donaldson-Fletcher, E. (2004). Lisfranc fracture-dislocation in a male ballet dancer during take-off of a jump: A case report. *Journal of Dance Medicine & Science, 8*(2), 56-58.

Kalbouneh, H., Alajoulin, O., Alsalem, M., Humoud, N., Shawaqfeh, J., Alkhoujah, M., Abu-Hassan, H., Mahafza, W., & Badran, D. (2017). Incidence and anatomical variations of accessory navicular bone in patients with foot pain: A retrospective radiographic analysis. *Clinical Anatomy, 30*(4), 436-444. https://doi.org/10.1002/ca.22876

Kelikian, A.S., & Sarrafian, S.K. (2011). *Sarrafian's Anatomy of the Foot and Ankle: Descriptive, Topographic, Functional.* (3rd ed.). Lippincott Williams & Wilkins.

Liederbach, M., Dilgen, F. E., & Rose, D. J. (2008). Incidence of anterior cruciate ligament injuries among elite ballet and modern dancers: a 5-year prospective study. *American Journal of Sports Medicine, 36*(9), 1779–1788. https://doi.org/10.1177/0363546508323644

Lin, C., Lee, I., Liao, J., Wu, H., & Su, F. (2011). Comparison of postural stability between injured and uninjured ballet dancers. *American Journal of Sports Medicine, 39*(6),1324-1331.

Mahieu, N., Witvrouw, E., Stevens, V., Tiggelen, D., & Roget P. (2006). Intrinsic risk factors for the development of Achilles tendon overuse injury: A prospective study. *American Journal of Sports Medicine, 34*(2), 226-235.

Nwawka, O.K., Hayashi, D., Diaz, L.E., Goud, A.R., Arndt, W.F., 3rd, Roemer, F.W., Malguria, N., & Guermazi, A. (2013). Sesamoids and accessory ossicles of the foot: anatomical variability and related pathology. *Insights into Imaging, 4*(5), 581–593. https://doi.org/10.1007/s13244-013-0277-1

O'Kane, J.W., & Kadel, N. (2008). Anterior impingement syndrome in dancers. *Current Reviews in Musculoskeletal Medicine.* 1, 12-16. https://doi.org/10.1007/s12178-007-9001-4

O'Loughlin, P.F., Hodgkins, C.W., & Kennedy, J.G. (2008). Ankle sprains and instability in dancers. *Clinics in Sports Medicine, 27*(2), 247-262. https://doi.org/10.1016/j.csm.2007.12.006

Peng, H.-T., Chen, W.C., Kernozek, T.W., Kim, K., & Song, C.-Y. (2015). Influences of patellofemoral pain and fatigue in female dancers during ballet jump-landing. *International Journal of Sports Medicine*, 36(9), 747-753. https://doi.org/10.1055/s-0035-1547220

Prakash, A.A. (2017). Medical attention seeking dance injuries: Systematic review of case reports. *The Physician and Sportsmedicine, 45*(1), 64-74. https://doi.org/10.1080/00913847.2017.1270700

Ramkumar, P.N., Farber, J., Arnouk, J., Varner, K.E., & Mcculloch, P.C. (2016). Injuries in a professional ballet dance company: A 10-year retrospective study. *Journal of Dance Medicine & Science, 20*(1), 30–37. https://doi.org/10.12678/1089-313X.20.1.30

Russell, J.A. (2010). Acute ankle sprain in dancers. *Journal of Dance Medicine & Science.* 14(3), 89-96.

Russell, J.A., Kruse, D.W., Koutedakis, Y., McEwan, I.M., & Wyon, M.A. (2010). Pathoanatomy of posterior ankle impingement in ballet dancers. *Clinical Anatomy, 23*(6), 613–621. https://doi.org/10.1002/ca.20991

Steib S., Zech A., Hentschke C., & Pfeifer, K. (2013). Fatigue-induced alterations of static and dynamic postural control in athletes with a history of ankle sprain. *Journal of Athletic Training*, 48(2), 203-8.

Sueki, D., & Brechter, J. (2010). *Orthopedic Rehabilitation Clinical Advisor.* Mosby Elsevier.

Waterman, B.R., Belmont, P.J., Cameron, K.L., Svoboda, S J., Alitz, C.J., & Owens, B.D. (2011). Risk factors for syndesmotic and medial ankle sprain: Role of sex, sport, and level of competition. *American Journal of Sports Medicine*, *39*(5), 992-998. https://doi.org/10.1177/0363546510391462

Chapter 12

Armstrong, A., & Hubbard, M.C. (2018). *AAOS essentials of musculoskeletal care*. Jones & Bartlett Learning.

Aroori, S., & Spence, R.A. (2008). Carpal tunnel syndrome. *The Ulster Medical Journal*, *77*(1), 6-17.

Beighton, P., Solomon, L., & Soskolne, C.L. (1973). Articular mobility in an African population. *Annals of the Rheumatic Diseases*, *32*(5), 413–418. https://doi.org/10.1136/ard.32.5.413

Brenner, J.S., Council on Sports Medicine and Fitness. (2016). Sports specialization and intensive training in young athletes. *Pediatrics, 138*, e20162148. https://doi.org/10.1542/peds.2016-2148

Burkhart, S.S., Morgan, C.D., & Kibler, W.B. (2003). The disabled throwing shoulder: Spectrum of pathology. Part I: Pathoanatomy and biomechanics. *Arthroscopy, 19*(4), 404-420. https://doi.org/10.1053/jars.2003.50128

Burn, M.B., McCulloch, P.C., Lintner, D.M., Liberman, S.R., & Harris, J.D. (2016). Prevalence of scapular dyskinesis in overhead and nonoverhead athletes: a systematic review. *Orthopaedic Journal of Sports Medicine*, *4*(2), 2325967115627608. https://doi.org/10.1177/2325967115627608

Casadei, K., & Kiel, J. (2023). Triangular Fibrocartilage Complex. In *StatPearls*. StatPearls Publishing.

Coogan, S.M., Hansen-Honeycutt, J., Fauntroy, V., & Ambegaonkar, J.P. (2021). Upper-body strength endurance and power norms in healthy collegiate dancers: A 10-year prospective study. *Journal of Strength & Conditioning Research, 35*(6), 1599-1603.

https://doi.org/10.1519/JSC.0000000000004016

Crosbie, J., Kilbreath, S.L., Hollmann, L., & York, S. (2008). Scapulohumeral rhythm and associated spinal motion. *Clinical Biomechanics*, *23*(2), 184-192. https://doi.org/10.1016/j.clinbiomech.2007.09.012

DeFroda, S.F. (2018). Skier's or gamekeeper's thumb. In Eltorai, A.E.M., Eberson, C. P., & Daniels, A.H., (Eds.). *Essential Orthopedic Review.* (pp. 89-90). Springer.

de Villeneuve Bargemon, J.B., Jaloux, C., Viaud-Ambrosino, S., & Kachouh, N. (2021). A jersey finger diagnostic trap: Rupture of the flexor digitorum profundus tendon and the flexor digitorum superficialis tendon. *Trauma Case Reports, 34*, 100476. https://doi.org/10.1016/j.tcr.2021.100476

Englert, C., Zellner, J., Koller, M., Nerlich, M., & Lenich, A. (2013). Elbow dislocations: A review ranging from soft tissue injuries to complex elbow fracture dislocations. *Advances in Orthopedics, 2013*, 951397. https://doi-org./10.1155/2013/951397

Fares, M.Y., Boufadel, P., Daher, M., Koa, J., Khanna, A., & Abboud, J.A. (2023). Anterior shoulder instability and open procedures: History, indications, and clinical outcomes. *Clinics in Orthopedic Surgery, 15*(4), 521–533. https://doi.org/10.4055/cios23018

Head, L., Gencarelli, J.R., Allen, M., & Boyd, K.U. (2015). Wrist ganglion treatment: Systematic review and meta-analysis. *Journal of Hand Surgery, 40*(3), 546-53.e8. https://doi.org/10.1016/j.jhsa.2014.12.014

Henderson G, (2021, December 10). It's time to rethink hyperspecialization for young dancers. *Dance Teacher.* https://dance-teacher.com/its-time-to-rethink-hyperspecialization-for-young-dancers

Kibler, W.B., & Sciascia, A.D. (2017). *Disorders of the Scapula and Their Role In Shoulder Injury.* Springer International.

Leanderson, C., Leanderson, J., Wykman, A., Strender, L.E., Johansson, S.E., & Sundquist, K. (2011). Musculoskeletal injuries in young ballet dancers. *Knee Surgery, Sports Traumatology, Arthroscopy, 19*(9), 1531-1535. https://doi.org/10.1007/s00167-011-1445-9

Leddy, J.P., & Packer, J.W. (1977). Avulsion of the profundus tendon insertion in athletes. *Journal of Hand Surgery, 2*(1), 66-69. https://doi.org/10.1016/s0363-5023(77)80012-9

Ojofeitimi, S., Bronner, S., & Woo, H. (2012). Injury incidence in hip hop dance. *Scandinavian Journal of Medicine & Science in Sports, 22*(3), 347-355. https://doi.org/10.1111/j.1600-0838.2010.01173.x

Paine, R., & Voight, M.L. (2013). The role of the scapula. *International Journal of Sports Physical Therapy, 8*(5), 617-629.

Panagiotopoulos, A.C., & Crowther, I.M. (2019). Scapular dyskinesia, the forgotten culprit of shoulder pain and how to rehabilitate. *SICOT-J, 5*, 29. https://doi.org/10.1051/sicotj/2019029

Popkin, C.A., Bayomy, A.F., & Ahmad, C.S. (2019). Early sport specialization. *Journal of the American Academy of Orthopaedic Surgeons, 27*(22), e995-e1000. https://doi.org/10.5435/JAAOS-D-18-00187

Saccomanno, M. F., Fodale, M., Capasso, L., Cazzato, G., & Milano, G. (2014). Generalized joint laxity and multidirectional instability of the shoulder. *Joints, 1*(4), 171–179. https://doi.org/10.11138/jts/2013.1.4.171

Schaeffer, M. (2022, September 25). Can dance cues drive scapular dyskinesia? Flyspace Physical Therapy. https://www.flyspacephysicaltherapy.nyc/post/can-dance-cues-drive-scapular-dyskinesia

Schroeder, N.S., & Goldfarb, C.A. (2015). Thumb ulnar collateral and radial collateral ligament injuries. *Clinics in Sports Medicine, 34*(1), 117-126. https://doi.org/10.1016/j.csm.2014.09.004

Sides, S.N., Ambegaonkar, J.P., & Caswell, S.V. (2009). High incidence of shoulder injuries in collegiate modern dance students. *International Journal of Athletic Therapy and Training, 14*(4), 43-46.

Smith, P.J., Gerrie, B.J., Varner, K.E., McCulloch, P.C., Lintner, D.M., & Harris, J.D. (2015). Incidence and prevalence of musculoskeletal injury in ballet: a systematic review. *Orthopaedic Journal of Sports Medicine, 3*(7), 2325967115592621. https://doi.org/10.1177/2325967115592621

Tsiouti, N., & Wyon, M. (2021). Injury occurrence in break dance: An online cross-sectional cohort study of breakers. *Journal of Dance Medicine & Science, 25*(1), 2-8. https://doi.org/10.12678/1089-313X.031521a

Wanke, E.M., Arendt, M., Mill, H., Koch, F., Wanke, A., & Groneberg, D.A. (2014). Traumatic injuries in revue dancers. *Journal of Dance Medicine & Science, 18*(1), 22-28. https://doi.org/10.12678/1089-313X.18.1.22

Wanke, E.M., Mill, H., Arendt, M., Wanke, A., Koch, F., & Groneberg, D.A. (2014). Occupational accidents in professional dancers with regard to different professional dance styles. *Work, 49*(4), 597–606. https://doi.org/10.3233/WOR-131736

Wipperman, J., & Goerl, K. (2016). Carpal tunnel syndrome: Diagnosis and management. *American Family Physician, 94*(12), 993-999.

Wu, Y.T., Chen, S.R., Li, T.Y., Ho, T.Y., Shen, Y.P., Tsai, C.K., & Chen, L.C. (2019). Nerve hydrodissection for carpal tunnel syndrome: A prospective, randomized, double-blind, controlled trial. *Muscle & Nerve, 59*(2), 174-180. https://doi.org/10.1002/mus.26358

Chapter 13

Bowling, A. (1989). Injuries to dancers: Prevalence, treatment, and perceptions of causes. *British Medical Journal, 298*(6675), 731-734.

Champion, L.M., & Chatfield, S.J. (2008). Measurement of turnout in dance research: A critical review. *Journal of Dance Medicine & Science, 12*(4), 121-135.

Charbonnier, C., Kolo, F.C., Duthon, V.B., Magnenat-Thalmann, N., Becker, C.D., Hoffmeyer, P., & Menetrey, J. (2011). Assessment of congruence and impingement of the hip joint in professional ballet dancers: A motion capture study. *American Journal of Sports Medicine, 39*(3), 557-566. https://doi.org/10.1177/0363546510386002

Coplan, J.A. (2002). Ballet dancer's turnout and its relationship to self-reported injury. *Journal of Orthopaedic and Sports Physical Therapy, 32*(11), 579-584. http://doi.org/10.2519/jospt.2002.32.11.579

D'Hemecourt, P., & Luke, A. (2012). Sport-specific biomechanics of spinal injuries in aesthetic athletes (dancers, gymnasts, and figure skaters). *Clinics in Sports Medicine, 31*(3), 397-408.

De Mattos Lourenco, T.R., Matsuoka, P.K., Baracat, E.C., & Haddad, J.M. (2018). Urinary incontinence in female athletes: A systematic review. *International Urogynecology Journal, 29*(12), 1757-1763. https://doi.org/10.1007/s00192-018-3629-z

Deslandes, M., Guillin, R., Cardinal, E., Hobden, R., & Bureau, N.J. (2008). The snapping iliopsoas tendon: New mechanisms using dynamic sonography. *American Journal of Roentgenology, 190*(3), 576-581. https://doi.org/10.2214/AJR.07.2375

Dumoulin, C., Cacciari, L.P., & Hay-Smith, E.J.C. (2018). Pelvic floor muscle training versus no treatment, or inactive control treatments, for urinary incontinence in women. *Cochrane Database of Systematic Reviews, 10*, CD005654. https://doi.org/10.1002/14651858.CD005654.pub4

Duthon, V.B., Charbonnier, C., Kolo, F.C., Magnenat-Thalmann, N., Becker, C.D., Bouvet, C., Coppens, E., Hoffmeyer, P., & Menetrey, J. (2013). Correlation of clinical and magnetic resonance imaging findings in hips of elite female ballet dancers. *Arthroscopy, 29*(3), 411–419. https://doi.org/10.1016/j.arthro.2012.10.012

Eickmeyer, S.M. (2017). Anatomy and physiology of the pelvic floor. *Physical Medicine and Rehabilitation Clinics of North America, 28*(3), 455-460. https://doi.org/10.1016/j.pmr.2017.03.003

Elattar, O., Choi, H.-R., Dills, V.D., & Busconi, B. (2016). Groin injuries (athletic pubalgia) and return to play. *Sports Health, 8*(4), 313-323. https://doi.org/10.1177/1941738116653711

Emery, S., Cook, J., Ferrar, K., & Mayes, S. (2021). Deep hip external rotator muscle size in ballet dancers compared to non-dancing athletes, and associations to pain. *Physical Therapy in Sport, 51*, 58-64. https://doi.org/10.1016/j.ptsp.2021.06.010

Emery, S., Cook, J., Ferris, A.R., Smith, P., & Mayes, S. (2019). Hip flexor muscle size in ballet dancers compared to athletes, and relationship to hip pain. *Physical Therapy in Sport, 38*, 146-151. https://doi.org/10.1016/j.ptsp.2019.05.003

Frank, C., Kobesova, A., & Kolar, P. (2013). Dynamic neuromuscular stabilization & sports rehabilitation. *International Journal of Sports Physical Therapy, 8*(1), 62-73.

Gelabert, R. (1986). Dancers' spinal syndromes. *Journal of Orthopaedic and Sports Physical Therapy, 7*(4), 180-191. https://doi.org/10.2519/jospt.1986.7.4.180

Gildea, J.E., Hides, J.A., & Hodges, P.W. (2013). Size and symmetry of trunk muscles in ballet dancers with and without low back pain. *Journal of Orthopaedic and Sports Physical Therapy, 43*(8), 525-533. https://doi.org/10.2519/jospt.2013.4523

Grierson, M. (2019). Management of the dancer's spine. In L. Elson (Ed.), *Performing Arts Medicine* (pp. 89-95). Elsevier.

Griffin, D.R., Dickenson, E.J., O'Donnell, J., Agricola, R., Awan, T., Beck, M., Clohisy, J.C., Dijkstra, H.P., Falvey, E., Gimpel, M., Hinman, R.S., Hölmich, P., Kassarjian, A., Martin, H.D., Martin, R., Mather, R.C., Philippon, M.J., Reiman, M.P., Takla, A., Thorborg, K., … Bennell, K.L. (2016). The Warwick Agreement on femoroacetabular impingement syndrome (FAI syndrome): an international consensus statement. *British Journal of Sports Medicine, 50*(19), 1169–1176. https://doi.org/10.1136/bjsports-2016-096743

Hamilton, W.G., Hamilton, L.H., Marshall, P., & Molnar, M. (1992). A profile of the musculoskeletal characteristics of elite professional ballet dancers. *American Journal of Sports Medicine, 20*(3), 267-273.

Harris, J.D., Gerrie, B.J., Varner, K.E., Lintner, D.M., & McCulloch, P.C. (2016). Radiographic prevalence of dysplasia, cam, and pincer deformities in elite ballet. *American Journal of Sports Medicine, 44*(1), 20-27. https://doi.org/10.1177/0363546515601996

Haylen, B.T., de Ridder, D., Freeman, R.M., Swift, S.E., Berghmans, B., Lee, J., Monga, A., Petri, E., Rizk, D.E., Sand, P.K., & Schaer, G.N. (2010). An International Urogynecological Association (IUGA)/International Continence Society (ICS) joint report on the terminology for female pelvic floor dysfunction. *International Urogynecology Journal, 21*(1), 5-26. https://doi.org/10.1007/s00192-009-0976-9

Hodges, P.W., Eriksson, A.E.M., Shirley, D., & Gandevia, S.C. (2005). Intra-abdominal pressure increases stiffness of the lumbar spine. *Journal of Biomechanics, 38*(9), 1873-1880. https://doi.org/10.1016/j.jbiomech.2004.08.016

Jenkins, J.B., Wyon, M., & Nevill, A. (2013). Can turnout measurements be used to predict physiotherapist-reported injury rates in dancers? *Medical Problems of Performing Artists, 28*(4), 230-235.

Kadel, N.J., Teitz, C.C., & Kronmal, R.A. (1992). Stress fractures in ballet dancers. *American Journal of Sports Medicine, 20*(4), 445-449. https://doi.org/10.1177/036354659202000414

Keim, H.A., & Kirkaldy-Willis, W.H. (1980). Low back pain. *Clinical Symposia, 32*(6), 1-35.

Kemp, J.L., Risberg, M.A., Mosler, A., Harris-Hayes, M., Serner, A., Moksnes, H., Bloom, N., Crossley, K.M., Gojanovic, B., Hunt, M.A., Ishøi, L., Mathieu, N., Mayes, S., Scholes, M.J., Gimpel, M., Friedman, D., Ageberg, E., Agricola, R., Casartelli, N.C., Diamond, L.E., … Bizzini, M. (2020). Physiotherapist-led treatment for young to middle-aged active adults with hip-related pain: consensus recommendations from the International Hip-related Pain Research Network, Zurich 2018. *British Journal of Sports Medicine, 54*(9), 504–511. https://doi.org/10.1136/bjsports-2019-101458

Khan, K., Brown, J., Way, S., Vass, N., Crichton, K., Alexander, R., Baxter, A., Butler, M., & Wark, J. (1995). Overuse injuries in classical ballet. *Sports Medicine, 19*(5), 341–357. https://doi.org/10.2165/00007256-199519050-00004

Khan, K., Roberts, P., Nattrass, C., Bennell, K., Mayes, S., Way, S., Brown, J., McMeeken, J., & Wark, J. (1997). Hip and ankle range of motion in elite classical ballet dancers and controls. *Clinical Journal of Sport Medicine, 7*(3), 174–179. https://doi.org/10.1097/00042752-199707000-00004

Kocjan, J., Adamek, M., Gzik-Zroska, B., Czyżewski, D., & Rydel, M. (2017). Network of breathing. Multifunctional role of the diaphragm: A review. *Advances in Respiratory Medicine, 85*(4), 224-232. https://doi.org/10.5603/ARM.2017.0037

Krasnow, D., Wilmerding, M.V., Stecyk, S., Wyon, M., & Koutedakis, Y. (2011). Biomechanical research in dance: A literature review. *Medical Problems of Performing Artists, 26*(1), 3-23.

Lewis, C.L., Laudicina, N.M., Khuu, A., & Loverro, K.L. (2017). The human pelvis: Variation in structure and function during gait. *Anatomical Record, 300*(4), 633-642. https://doi.org/10.1002/ar.23552

Lirette, L.S., Chaiban, G., Tolba, R., & Eissa, H. (2014). Coccydynia: An overview of the anatomy, etiology, and treatment of coccyx pain. *Ochsner Journal, 14*(1), 84-87.

Longhino, V., Bonora, C., & Sansone, V. (2011). The management of sacral stress fractures: Current concepts. *Clinical Cases in Mineral and Bone Metabolism, 8*(3), 19-23.

Mayes, S., Ferris, A.R., Smith, P., Garnham, A., & Cook, J. (2016a). Atraumatic tears of the ligamentum teres are more frequent in professional ballet dancers than a sporting population. *Skeletal Radiology, 45*(7), 959-967. https://doi.org/10.1007/s00256-016-2379-6

Mayes, S., Ferris, A.R., Smith, P., Garnham, A., & Cook, J. (2016b). Professional ballet dancers have a similar prevalence of articular cartilage defects compared to age- and sex-matched non-dancing athletes. *Clinical Rheumatology, 35*(12), 3037-3043. https://doi.org/10.1007/s10067-016-3389-4

Mayes, S., Ferris, A.R., Smith, P., Garnham, A., & Cook, J. (2016c). Similar prevalence of acetabular labral tear in professional ballet dancers and sporting participants. *Clinical Journal of Sport Medicine, 26*(4), 307-313. https://doi.org/10.1097/jsm.0000000000000257

Mayes, S., Ferris, A.R., Smith, P., Garnham, A., & Cook, J. (2017). Bony morphology of the hip in professional ballet dancers compared to athletes. *European Radiology, 27*(7), 3042-3049. https://doi.org/10.1007/s00330-016-4667-x

Mayes, S., Ferris, A.R., Smith, P., & Cook, J. (2018). Obturator externus was larger, while obturator internus size was similar in ballet dancers compared to nondancing athletes. *Physical Therapy in Sport, 33*, 1-6. https://doi.org/10.1016/j.ptsp.2018.06.001

Mayes, S., Ferris, A.R., Smith, P., & Cook, J. (2020). Hip joint effusion-synovitis is associated with hip pain and sports/recreation function in female professional ballet dancers. *Clinical Journal of Sport Medicine, 30*(4), 341-347. https://doi.org/10.1097/JSM.0000000000000595

Mayes, S., Smith, P., Stuart, D., & Cook, J. (2021). Joint hypermobility does not increase the risk of developing hip pain, cartilage defects, or retirement in professional ballet dancers over 5 years. *Clinical Journal of Sport Medicine, 31*(6), e342-e346. https://doi.org/10.1097/jsm.0000000000000862

Mayes, S., Smith, P., Stuart, D., Semciw, A., & Cook, J. (2021). Hip joint cartilage defects in professional ballet dancers: A 5-year longitudinal study. *Clinical Journal of Sport Medicine, 31*(6), e335-e341. https://doi.org/10.1097/jsm.0000000000000818

McMillan, R.M., Mayes, S., Cook, J., Semciw, A.I., Plass, L.M., & Pizzari, T. (2023). Gluteal muscle size and quality in professional ballet dancers compared to non-dancing athletes. *Journal of Dance Medicine & Science, 27*(3), 119–129. https://doi.org/10.1177/1089313X231177161

Meister, M.R., Sutcliffe, S., Ghetti, C., Chu, C.M., Spitznagle, T., Warren, D.K., & Lowder, J.L. (2019). Development of a standardized, reproducible screening examination for assessment of pelvic floor myofascial pain. *American Journal of Obstetrics and Gynecology, 220*(3), 255.e1-255.e9. https://doi.org/10.1016/j.ajog.2018.11.1106

Milanesi, R., & Caregnato, R.C.A. (2016). Intra-abdominal pressure: An integrative review. *Einstein, 14*(3), 423-430. https://doi.org/10.1590/S1679-45082016RW3088

Mitchell, R.J., Gerrie, B.J., McCulloch, P.C., Murphy, A.J., Varner, K.E., Lintner, D.M., & Harris, J.D. (2016). Radiographic evidence of hip microinstability in elite ballet. *Arthroscopy, 32*(6), 1038-1044.e1. https://doi.org/10.1016/j.arthro.2015.12.049

Negus, V., Hopper, D., & Briffa, N.K. (2005). Associations between turnout and lower extremity injuries in classical ballet dancers. *Journal of Ortho-*

paedic and Sports Physical Therapy, 35(5), 307-318. https://doi.org/10.2519/jospt.2005.35.5.307

Pires, T., Pires, P., Moreira, H., & Viana, R. (2020). Prevalence of urinary incontinence in high-impact sport athletes: A systematic review and meta-analysis. *Journal of Human Kinetics, 73*, 279-288. https://doi.org/10.2478/hukin-2020-0008

Prather, H., Dugan, S., Fitzgerald, C., & Hunt, D. (2009). Review of anatomy, evaluation, and treatment of musculoskeletal pelvic floor pain in women. *PM & R, 1*(4), 346-358. https://doi.org/10.1016/j.pmrj.2009.01.003

Quaghebeur, J., Petros, P., Wyndaele, J.J., & De Wachter, S. (2021). The innervation of the bladder, the pelvic floor, and emotion: A review. *Autonomic Neuroscience: Basic & Clinical, 235*, 102868. https://doi.org/10.1016/j.autneu.2021.102868

Quanbeck, A.E., Russell, J.A., Handley, S.C., & Quanbeck, D.S. (2017). Kinematic analysis of hip and knee rotation and other contributors to ballet turnout. *Journal of Sports Sciences, 35*(4), 331-338. https://doi.org/10.1080/02640414.2016.1164335

Reid, D.C., Burnham, R.S., Saboe, L.A., & Kushner, S.F. (1987). Lower extremity flexibility patterns in classical ballet dancers and their correlation to lateral hip and knee injuries. *American Journal of Sports Medicine, 15*(4), 347-352.

Smith, T.O., de Medici, A., Oduoza, U., Hakim, A., Paton, B., Retter, G., Haddad, F.S., & Macgregor, A. (2017). National survey to evaluate musuloskeletal health in retired professional ballet dancers in the United Kingdom. *Physical Therapy in Sport, 23*, 82–85. https://doi.org/10.1016/j.ptsp.2016.07.009

Sorrigueta-Hernández, A., Padilla-Fernandez, B.-Y., Marquez-Sanchez, M.-T., Flores-Fraile, M.-C., Flores-Fraile, J., Moreno-Pascual, C., Lorenzo-Gomez, A., Garcia-Cenador, M.-B., & Lorenzo-Gomez, M.-F. (2020). Benefits of physiotherapy on urinary incontinence in high-performance female athletes. Meta-analysis. *Journal of Clinical Medicine, 9*(10), 3240. https://doi.org/10.3390/jcm9103240

Stokes, I.A., Gardner-Morse, M.G., & Henry, S.M. (2010). Intra-abdominal pressure and abdominal wall muscular function: Spinal unloading mechanism. *Clinical Biomechanics, 25*(9), 859-866. https://doi.org/10.1016/j.clinbiomech.2010.06.018

Sutton-Traina, K., Smith, J.A., Jarvis, D.N., Lee, S.P., & Kulig, K. (2015). Exploring active and passive contributors to turnout in dancers and non-dancers. *Medical Problems of Performing Artists, 30*(2), 78-83. https://doi.org/10.21091/mppa.2015.2013

Swain, C.T.V., Bradshaw, E.J., Ekegren, C L., & Whyte, D.G. (2019). The epidemiology of low back pain and injury in dance: A systematic review. *Journal of Orthopaedic and Sports Physical Therapy, 49*(4), 239-252. https://doi.org/10.2519/jospt.2019.8609

Talasz, H., Kremser, C., Kofler, M., Kalchschmid, E., Lechleitner, M., & Rudisch, A. (2011). Phase-locked parallel movement of diaphragm and pelvic floor during breathing and coughing-A dynamic MRI investigation in healthy females. *International Urogynecology Journal, 22*(1), 61-68. https://doi.org/10.1007/s00192-010-1240-z

Teitz, C.C., & Kilcoyne, R.F. (1998). Premature osteoarthrosis in professional dancers. *Clinical Journal of Sport Medicine, 8*(4), 255-259.

Teixeira, R.V., Colla, C., Sbruzzi, G., Mallmann, A., & Paiva, L.L. (2018). Prevalence of urinary incontinence in female athletes: A systematic review with meta-analysis. *International Urogynecology Journal, 29*(12), 1717-1725. https://doi.org/10.1007/s00192-018-3651-1

van Arkel, R.J., Amis, A.A., Cobb, J.P., & Jeffers, J.R. (2015). The capsular ligaments provide more hip rotational restraint than the acetabular labrum and the ligamentum teres: An experimental study. *Bone & Joint Journal, 97-B*(4), 484-491. https://doi.org/10.1302/0301-620X.97B4.34638

van Dijk, C.N., Lim, L.S., Poortman, A., Strubbe, E.H., & Marti, R.K. (1995). Degenerative joint disease in female ballet dancers. *American Journal of Sports Medicine, 23*(3), 295-300.

Vassallo, A.J. (2017). *Safe Dance Report IV: Investigating Injuries in Australia's Professional Dancers*. Australian Dance Council. https://ausdance.org.au/?ACT=73&file=2404

Washington, I., Mayes, S., Ganderton, C., & Pizzari, T. (2016). Differentials in turnout among professional classical ballet dancers. *Medical Problems of Performing Artists, 31*(3), 160-165. https://doi.org/10.21091/mppa.2016.3029

Waxenbaum, J.A., Reddy, V., Williams, C., & Futterman, B. (2022). Anatomy, back, lumbar vertebrae. In *StatPearls*. StatPearls Publishing.

Winder, B., Lindegren, K., & Blackmon, A. (2023). Prevalence of urinary incontinence and other pelvic floor-related symptoms in female professional dancers. *Journal of Dance Medicine & Science, 27*(1), 50–55. https://doi.org/10.1177/1089313X231176629

Chapter 14

Abrahams, S., Fie, S.M., Patricios, J., Posthumus, M., & September, A.V. (2014). Risk factors for sports concussion: An evidence-based systematic review. *British Journal of Sports Medicine, 48*(2), 9197. https://doi.org/10.1136/bjsports-2013-092734

Albano, M., Alpini, D.C., & Carbone, G.V. (2014). Whiplash and sport. In D.C. Alpini, G. Brugnoni, & A. Cesarani (Eds.), *Whiplash injuries: Diagnosis and treatment* (pp. 127-137). Springer Milan. https://doi.org/10.1007/978-88-470-5486-8_13

Aromatario, M., Torsello, A., D'Errico, S., Bertozzi, G., Sessa, F., Cipolloni, L., & Baldari, B. (2021). Traumatic epidural and subdural hematoma: Epidemiology, outcome, and dating. *Medicina, 57*(2), 125. https://doi.org/10.3390/medicina57020125

Asplund, C.A., O'Connor, F.G., & Noakes, T.D. (2011). Exercise-associated collapse: An evidence-based review and primer for clinicians. *British Journal of Sports Medicine, 45*(14), 1157-1162. https://doi.org/10.1136/bjsports-2011-090378

Boyette, J., Pemberton, J., & Bonilla-Velez, J. (2015). Management of orbital fractures: Challenges and solutions. *Clinical Ophthalmology*, 2127. https://doi.org/10.2147/OPTH.S80463

Buckley, T.A., Baugh, C.M., Meehan, W.P., & DiFabio, M.S. (2017). Concussion management plan compliance: A study of NCAA Power 5 conference schools. *Orthopaedic Journal of Sports Medicine, 5*(4), 2325967117702606. https://doi.org/10.1177/2325967117702606

Cho, C.H., Song, K.S., Min, B.W., Lee, S.M., Chang, H.W., & Eum, D.S. (2009). Musculoskeletal injuries in break-dancers. *Injury, 40*(11), 1207-1211. https://doi.org/10.1016/j.injury.2009.05.019

Custer, A., Sufrinko, A., Elbin, R.J., Covassin, T., Collins, M., & Kontos, A. (2016). High baseline postconcussion symptom scores and concussion outcomes in athletes. *Journal of Athletic Training, 51*(2), 136-141. https://doi.org/10.4085/1062-6050-51.2.12

DeMatteo, C.A., Randall, S., Lin, C.-Y.A., & Claridge, E. A. (2019). What comes first: Return to school or return to activity for youth after concussion? Maybe we don't have to choose. *Frontiers in Neurology, 10*, 792. https://doi.org/10.3389/fneur.2019.00792

Domene, P.A., Stanley, M., & Skamagki, G. (2018). Injury surveillance of nonprofessional salsa dance. *Journal of Physical Activity and Health, 15*(10), 774-780.

Drew, L.B., & Drew, W.E. (2004). The contrecoup-coup phenomenon: A new understanding of the mechanism of closed head injury. *Neurocritical Care, 1*(3), 385-390. https://doi.org/10.1385/NCC:1:3:385

Echemendia, R.J., Ahmed, O.H., Bailey, C.M., Bruce, J.M., Burma, J.S., Davis, G.A., Gioia, G., Howell, D.R., Fuller, G.W., Master, C.L., van Ierssel, J., Pardini, J., Schneider, K.J., Walton, S.R., Zemek, R., Patricios, J.S. (2023) The Concussion Recognition Tool 6 (CRT6). *British Journal of Sports Medicine, 57*(11),692-694.

Echemendia, R.J., Brett, B.L., Broglio, S., Davis, G.A., Giza, C.C., Guskiewicz, K.M., Harmon, K.G., Herring, S., Howell, D.R., Master, C.L., Valovich McLeod, T.C., McCrea, M., Naidu, D., Patricios, J., Putukian, M., Walton, S.R., Schneider, K.J., Burma, J.S., Bruce, J.M. (2023) Introducing the Sport Concussion Assessment Tool 6 (SCAT6). *British Journal of Sports Medicine, 57*(11), 619-621.

Ellis, M.J., Leddy, J., & Willer, B. (2016). Multi-disciplinary management of athletes with post-concussion syndrome: An evolving pathophysiological approach. *Frontiers in Neurology, 7*, 136. https://doi.org/10.3389/fneur.2016.00136

Haines, D.E. (2015). *Neuroanatomy in clinical context: An atlas of structures, sections, systems, and syndromes* (9th edition). Wolters Kluwer Health.

Harmon, K.G., Clugston, J.R., Dec, K., Hainline, B., Herring, S.A., Kane, S., Kontos, A.P., Leddy, J.J., McCrea, M.A., Poddar, S.K., Putukian, M., Wilson, J.C., & Roberts, W.O. (2019). American Medical Society for Sports Medicine position statement on concussion in sport. *Clinical Journal of Sport Medicine, 29*(2), 87-100. https://doi.org/10.1097/JSM.0000000000000720

Hynes, L.M., & Dickey, J.P. (2006). Is there a relationship between whiplash-associated disorders and concussion in hockey? A preliminary study. *Brain Injury, 20*(2), 179-188. https://doi.org/10.1080/02699050500443707

Iverson, G.L., Gardner, A.J., Terry, D.P., Ponsford, J.L., Sills, A.K., Broshek, D.K., & Solomon, G.S. (2017). Predictors of clinical recovery from concussion: A systematic review. *British Journal of Sports Medicine, 51*(12), 941-948. https://doi.org/10.1136/bjsports-2017-097729

Kauther, M.D., Wedemeyer, C., Wegner, A., Kauther, K.M., & von Knoch, M. (2009). Breakdance injuries and overuse syndromes in amateurs and professionals. *The American Journal of Sports Medicine, 37*(4), 797-802. https://doi.org/10.1177/0363546508328120

Khellaf, A., Khan, D.Z., & Helmy, A. (2019). Recent advances in traumatic brain injury. *Journal of Neurology, 266*(11), 2878-2889. https://doi.org/10.1007/s00415-019-09541-4

Kish, R.L., & Koutures, C.G. (2016). The invisible injury: Supporting the recovery of dancers with concussions. *Journal of Physical Education, Recreation & Dance, 87*(8), 27-33. https://doi.org/10.1080/07303084.2016.1216482

Grove, J.R., Main, L.C., Sharp, L. (2013). Stressors, recovery processes, and manifestations of training distress in dance. *Journal of Dance Medicine and Science, 87*(8),70-78.

Kroshus, E., Cameron, K.L., Coatsworth, J.D., D'Lauro, C., Kim, E., Lee, K., Register-Mihalik, J.K., Milroy, J.J., Roetert, E.P., Schmidt, J.D., Silverman, R.D., Warmath, D., Wayment, H.A., & Hainline, B. (2020). Improving concussion education: Consensus from the NCAA-Department of Defense Mind Matters Research & Education Grand Challenge. *British Journal of Sports Medicine, 54*(22), 1314-1320. https://doi.org/10.1136/bjsports-2020-102185

Kroshus, E., & Chrisman, S.P.D. (2019). A new game plan for concussion education. *Health Education & Behavior, 46*(6), 916-921. https://doi.org/10.1177/1090198119859414

Leddy, J., Baker, J.G., Haider, M.N., Hinds, A., & Willer, B. (2017). A physiological approach to prolonged recovery from sport-related concussion. *Journal of Athletic Training, 52*(3), 299-308. https://doi.org/10.4085/1062-6050-51.11.08

Leddy, J.J., Burma, J.S., Toomey, C.M., Hayden, A., Davis, G.A., Babl, F.E., Gagnon, I., Giza, C.C., Kurowski, B.G., Silverberg, N.D., Willer, B., Ronksley, P.E., Schneider, K.J. (2023) Rest and exercise early after sport-related concussion: A systematic review and meta-analysis. *British Journal of Sports Medicine*, 57(12), 762-770.

Leddy, J.J., Haider, M.N., Ellis, M.J., Mannix, R., Darling, S.R., Freitas, M.S., Suffoletto, H. N., Leiter, J., Cordingley, D.M., & Willer, B. (2019). Early subthreshold aerobic exercise for sport-related concussion: A randomized clinical trial. *JAMA Pediatrics, 173*(4), 319-325. https://doi.org/10.1001/jamapediatrics.2018.4397

Lee, J.Y., Lin, L., & Tan, A. (2020). Prevalence of pole dance injuries from a global online survey. *The Journal of Sports Medicine and Physical Fitness, 60*(2), 270-275. https://doi.org/10.23736/S0022-4707.19.09957-2

Lin, K., & Wroten, M. (2022). Ranchos Los Amigos. In *StatPearls*. StatPearls. 2024 Jan. www.ncbi.nlm.nih.gov/books/NBK448151

Maron, B.J., Haas, T.S., Murphy, C.J., Ahluwalia, A., & Rutten-Ramos, S. (2014). Incidence and causes of sudden death in U.S. college athletes. *Journal of the American College of Cardiology, 63*(16), 1636-1643. https://doi.org/10.1016/j.jacc.2014.01.041

McAllister, T., & McCrea, M. (2017). Long-term cognitive and neuropsychiatric consequences of repetitive concussion and head-impact exposure. *Journal of Athletic Training, 52*(3), 309-317. https://doi.org/10.4085/1062-6050-52.1.14

McCrory, P., Meeuwisse, W., Dvorak, J., Aubry, M., Bailes, J., Broglio, S., Cantu, R.C., Cassidy, D., Echemendia, R.J., Castellani, R.J., Davis, G.A., Ellenbogen, R., Emery, C., Engebretsen, L., Feddermann-Demont, N., Giza, C.C., Guskiewicz, K.M., Herring, S., Iverson, G. L., . . . Vos, P.E. (2017). Consensus statement on concussion in sport—The 5th international conference on concussion in sport held in Berlin, October 2016. *British Journal of Sports Medicine, 51*(11), 838-847. https://doi.org/10.1136/bjsports-2017-097699

McIntyre, L., & Campo, M. (2017). Descriptive values for dancers on baseline concussion tools. *Journal of Athletic Training, 52*(11), 1035-1040. https://doi.org/10.4085/1062-6050-52.10.14

McIntyre, L., & Liederbach, M. (2016). Concussion knowledge and behaviors in a sample of the dance community. *Journal of Dance Medicine & Science, 20*(2), 79-88. https://doi.org/10.12678/1089-313X.20.2.79

McPherson, A.L., Nagai, T., Webster, K.E., & Hewett, T.E. (2019). Musculoskeletal injury risk after sport-related concussion: A systematic review and meta-analysis. *The American Journal of Sports Medicine, 47*(7), 1754-1762. https://doi.org/10.1177/0363546518785901

Mortazavi, M.M., Denning, M., Yalcin, B., Shoja, M.M., Loukas, M., & Tubbs, R.S. (2013). The intracranial bridging veins: A comprehensive review of their history, anatomy, histology, pathology, and neurosurgical implications. *Child's Nervous*

System, 29(7), 1073-1078. https://doi.org/10.1007/s00381-013-2054-3

Natali, A.L., Reddy, V., & Leo, J.T. (2020). Neuroanatomy, middle meningeal arteries. In *StatPearls*. StatPearls. www.ncbi.nlm.nih.gov/books/NBK519545

Patricios, J.S., Schneider, K.J., Dvorak, J., Ahmed, O.H., Blauwet, C., Cantu, R.C., Davis, G.A., Echemendia, R.J., Makdissi, M., McNamee, M., Broglio, S., Emery, C.A., Feddermann-Demont, N., Fuller, G.W., Giza, C.C., Guskiewicz, K.M., Hainline, B., Iverson, G.L., Kutcher, J.S., Leddy, J.J., … Meeuwisse, W. (2023). Consensus statement on concussion in sport: the 6th International Conference on Concussion in Sport—Amsterdam, October 2022. *British Journal of Sports Medicine, 57*(11), 695–711. https://doi.org /10.1136/bjsports-2023-106898

Patricios, J.S., Davis, G.A., Ahmed, O.H., Blauwet, C., Schneider, G.M., Purcell, L.K., Echemendia, R.J., Fremont, P., Fuller, G.W., Herring, S.A., Harmon, K.G., Loosemore. M., Makdissi, M., O'Halloran, P., Putukian, M., Turner, M., Webborn, N., Yeates, K.O., van Ierssel, J., Schneider, K.J. (2023) Introducing the Sport Concussion Office Assessment Tool 6 (SCOAT6). *British Journal of Sports Medicine, 57*(11), 648-650.

Prisk, V.R., & Hamilton, W.G. (2008). Stress fracture of the first rib in weight-trained dancers. *American Journal of Sports Medicine, 36*(12), 2444-2447. https://doi.org/10.1177/0363546508326710

Purcell, L.K., Davis, G.A., & Gioia, G.A. (2019). What factors must be considered in 'return to school' following concussion and what strategies or accommodations should be followed? A systematic review. *British Journal of Sports Medicine, 53*(4), 250-250. https://doi.org/10.1136/bjsports-2017-097853

Rebbeck, T., Evans, K., & Elliott, J.M. (2019). Concussion in combination with whiplash-associated disorder may be missed in primary care: Key recommendations for assessment and management. *Journal of Orthopaedic and Sports Physical Therapy, 49*(11), 819-828. https://doi.org/10.2519/jospt.2019.8946

Russell, J.A., McIntyre, L., Stewart, L., & Wang, T. (2021). Concussions in dancers and other performing artists. *Physical Medicine and Rehabilitation Clinics of North America, 32*(1), 155-168. https://doi.org/10.1016/j.pmr.2020.09.007

Scorza, K.A., & Cole, W. (2019). Current concepts in concussion: Initial evaluation and management. *American Family Physician, 99*(7), 426-434.

Silverberg, N.D., Iaccarino, M.A., Panenka, W.J., Iverson, G.L., McCulloch, K.L., Dams-O'Connor, K., Reed, N., & McCrea, M. (2020). American Congress of Rehabilitation Medicine Brain Injury Interdisciplinary Special Interest Group Mild TBI Task Force. Management of concussion and mild traumatic brain injury: A synthesis of practice guidelines. *Archives of Physical Medicine and Rehabilitation, 101*(2), 382-393.

Stein, C., Kinney, S., McCrystal, T., Carew, E., Bottino, N., Meehan, W., & Micheli, L. (2014). Dance-related concussion: A case series. *Journal of Dance Medicine and Science, 18*(2), 53-61.

Stemper, B.D., Shah, A.S., Harezlak, J., Rowson, S., Mihalik, J.P., Duma, S.M., Riggen, L.D., Brooks, A., Cameron, K.L., Campbell, D., DiFiori, J.P., Giza, C.C., Guskiewicz, K.M., Jackson, J., McGinty, G.T., Svoboda, S.J., McAllister, T.W., Broglio, S.P., McCrea, M., & the CARE Consortium Investigators. (2019). Comparison of head impact exposure between concussed football athletes and matched controls: Evidence for a possible second mechanism of sport-related concussion. *Annals of Biomedical Engineering, 47*(10), 2057-2072. https://doi.org/10.1007/s10439-018-02136-6

Tsiouti, N., & Wyon, M. (2021). Injury occurrence in break dance: An online cross-sectional cohort study of breakers. *Journal of Dance Medicine & Science, 25*(1), 2-8. https://doi.org/10.12678/1089-313X.031521a

Van de Graaff, K.M, Rhees, R.W., & Palmer, S.L. (2013). Central nervous system. In Van de Graaff, K.M, Rhees, R.W., & Palmer, S.L. *Schaum's Outline of Human Anatomy and Physiology*, (4th ed., pp. 162–181). McGraw-Hill Education.

Waltzman, D., & Sarmiento, K. (2019). What the research says about concussion risk factors and prevention strategies for youth sports: A scoping review of six commonly played sports. *Journal of Safety Research, 68*, 157-172. https://doi.org/10.1016/j.jsr.2018.11.005

Warmath, D., & Winterstein, A.P. (2019). Reporting skill: The missing ingredient in concussion reporting intention assessment. *Sports Health, 11*(5), 416-424. https://doi.org/10.1177/1941738119856609

Yau, R.K., Golightly, Y.M., Richardson, D.B., Runfola, C.D., Waller, A.E., & Marshall, S.W. (2017). Potential predictors of injury among pre-professional ballet and contemporary dancers. *Journal of Dance Medicine & Science, 21*(2), 53-63.

Chapter 15

Air, M.E., Grierson, M.J., Davenport, K.L., & Krabak, B.J. (2014). Dissecting the doctor-dancer relationship: Health care decision making among American collegiate dancers. *PM & R: the Journal of Injury, Function, and Rehabilitation, 6*(3), 241-24. https://doi.org/10.1016/j.pmrj.2013.09.001

American Academy of Physician Associates. (2022). *What is a PA?* AAPA. www.aapa.org/what-is-a-pa

American Association of Nurse Practitioners. (2022). *What's a nurse practitioner?* AANP. www.aanp.org/about/all-about-nps/whats-a-nurse-practitioner

American College of Surgeons. (2022). *Education: What are the surgical specialties?* ACS. www.facs.org/for-medical-professionals/education/online-guide-to-choosing-a-surgical-residency/guide-to-choosing-a-surgical-residency-for-medical-students/faqs/specialties

American Massage Therapy Association. (2018). *Massage therapy in integrative care & pain management.* American Massage Therapy Association.

American Occupational Therapy Association. (2022). *Become an OT/OTA: About occupational therapy.* AOTA, www.aota.org/career/become-an-ot-ota/about-the-profession

American Physical Therapy Association. (2021). *Choose physical therapy.* APTA. www.choosept.com

American Podiatric Medical Association. (2022). *What is a podiatrist?* APMA. www.apma.org/podiatristsFAQ

American Psychiatric Association. (2022). *What is psychiatry?* American Psychiatric Association. https://psychiatry.org/patients-families/what-is-psychiatry

American Psychological Association. (2021). *APA-approved standards and guidelines.* APA. www.apa.org/about/policy/approved-guidelines

Bolling, C., Mellette, J., Pasman, H.R., Van Mechelen, W., & Verhagen, E. (2019). From the safety net to the injury prevention web: Applying systems thinking to unravel injury prevention challenges and opportunities in Cirque du Soleil. *BMJ Open Sport and Exercise Medicine, 5*(1), 1-9. https://doi.org/10.1136/bmjsem-2018-000492

Bolling, C., van Rijn, R.M., Pasman, H R., van Mechelen, W., & Stubbe, J.H. (2021). In your shoes: A qualitative study on the perspectives of professional dancers and staff regarding dance injury and its prevention. *Translational Sports Medicine, 4,* 386-394 https://doi.org/10.1002/tsm2.226

Commission on Dietetic Registration. (2022). *Registered dietitian (RD) or registered dietitian nutritionist (RDN) certification.* CDR. www.cdrnet.org/certifications/registered-dietitian-rd-certification

Council of Colleges of Acupuncture and Herbal Medicine. (n.d.). *Learn about acupuncture medicine.* CCAHM. www.ccahm.org/ccaom/Learn_about_AOM.asp

Dijkstra H.P., Pollock N., Chakraverty R., & Alonso J.M. (2014). Managing the health of the elite athlete: A new integrated performance health management and coaching model. *British Journal of Sports Medicine, 48*(7), 523-531. https://doi.org/10.1136/bjsports-2013-093222

Echemendia R.J., Ahmed O.H., Bailey C.M., Bruce J.M., Burma J.S., Davis G.A., Gioia G., Howell D.R., Fuller G.W., Master C.L., van Ierssel J., Pardini J., Schneider K.J., Walton S.R., Zemek R., Patricios J.S. (2023). Concussion recognition tool 6. *British Journal of Sports Medicine, 57*(11), 692. https://10.1136/bjsports-2023-106851

Espí-López, G.V., Serra-Añó, P., Cuenca-Martínez, F., Suso-Martí, L., & Inglés, M. (2020). Comparison between classic and light touch massage on psychological and physical functional variables in athletes: A randomized pilot trial. *International Journal of Therapeutic Massage & Bodywork, 13*(3), 30-37.

Gliedt, J.A., Perle, S.M., Puhl, A.A., Daehler, S., Schneider, M.J., & Stevans, J. (2021). Evaluation of United States chiropractic professional subgroups: A survey of randomly sampled chiropractors. *BMC Health Services Research, 21*(1), 1049. https://doi.org/10.1186/s12913-021-07081-0

Haefeli, M., & Elfering, A. (2006). Pain assessment. *European Spine Journal, 15*(Suppl 1), S17-S24. https://doi.org/10.1007/s00586-005-1044-x

Haikal, L., Boissonnault, È., Boudier-Revéret, M., & Dagher, J.H. (2021). Dancers' perceptions of accessibility and quality of the relationship with healthcare professionals in Quebec. *Medical Problems of Performing Artists, 36*(4), 245-262. https://doi.org/10.21091/mppa.2021.4028

HealthMeasures. (2017). *PROMIS numeric rating xcale v1.0 - Pain intensity - 1a.* Health Measures. www.

healthmeasures.net/index.php?option=com_instruments&view=measure&id=896&Itemid=992

Lai, R.Y., Krasnow, D., & Thomas, M. (2008). Communication between medical practitioners and dancers. *Journal of Dance Medicine & Science, 12*(2), 47-53

Legal Information Institute. (n.d.). 42 U.S. Code § 295p – Definitions. U.S. Code, Title 42, Chapter 6A, Subchapter V, Part G, § 295p. LII. www.law.cornell.edu/uscode/text/42/295p

National Alliance on Mental Illness. (2022). *Personal Stories: It's Okay to Not be Okay.* NAMI. www.nami.org/Personal-Stories/It-s-Okay-Not-to-Be-Okay

National Athletic Trainers' Association. (2021). Athletic training: What is athletic training? NATA. www.nata.org/about/athletic-training

National Board of Chiropractic Examiners. (2024). *Chiropractic care.* NBCE. www.nbce.org/about-nbce/chiropractic-care

National Center for Complementary and Integrative Health. (2021). *Complementary, alternative, or integrative health: What's in a name?* NIH. www.nccih.nih.gov/health/complementary-alternative-or-integrative-health-whats-in-a-name

National Center for Complementary and Integrative Health. (2016). *Acupuncture: In Depth.* NIH. www.nccih.nih.gov/health/acupuncture-in-depth

National Institute of Dance Medicine and Science. (2019). *Healthcare.* NIDMS. www.nidms.co.uk/healthcare

NutritionEd.org. (2024). What is a registered dietitian nutritionist? www.nutritioned.org/what-is-a-registered-dietitian-nutritionist/

Pollard-Smith, T., & Thomson, O.P. (2017). Professional ballet dancers' experience of injury and osteopathic treatment in the UK: A qualitative study. *Journal of Bodywork and Movement Therapies, 21*(1), 148-156. https://doi.org/10.1016/j.jbmt.2016.06.009

Rinonapoli, G., Graziani, M., Ceccarini, P., Razzano, C., Manfreda, F., & Caraffa, A. (2020). Epidemiology of injuries connected with dance: A critical review on epidemiology. *Medicinski Glasnik, 17*(2), 256-264. https://doi.org/10.17392/1201-20

Russell, J.A. (2013). Preventing dance injuries: Current perspectives. *Open Access Journal of Sports Medicine, 4*, 199-210. https://doi.org/10.2147/OAJSM.S36529

Russell, J.A. (2020). Clinical care of performing arts students in the university setting: A successful model with wide potential. In S.H. Lee, M.L. Morris, & S.V. Nicosia (Eds.), *Perspectives in performing arts medicine practice* (pp. 395-418). Springer. https://doi.org/10.1007/978-3-030-37480-8_25

Thomas, H., & Tarr, J. (2009). Dancers' perceptions of pain and injury: Positive and negative effects. *Journal of Dance Medicine & Science, 13*(2), 51-59.

Sporer, B.C., & Windt, J. (2018). Integrated performance support: Facilitating effective and collaborative performance teams. *British Journal of Sports Medicine, 52*(16),1014-1015. https://doi.org/10.1136/bjsports-2017-097646

Van Giang, N., Chiu, H.Y., Thai, D.H., Kuo, S.Y., & Tsai, P.S. (2015). Validity, sensitivity, and responsiveness of the 11-face faces pain scale to postoperative pain in adult orthopedic surgery patients. *Pain Management Nursing, 16*(5), 678–684. https://doi.org/10.1016/j.pmn.2015.02.002

Van Pelt, D.W., Lawrence, M.M., Miller, B F., Butterfield, T.A., & Dupont-Versteegden, E.E. (2021). Massage as a mechanotherapy for skeletal muscle. *Exercise and Sport Sciences Reviews, 49*(2), 107–114. https://doi.org/10.1249/JES.0000000000000244

Weigert, B. (2005). Does prior training affect risk of injury in university dance programs? *Medical Problems of Performing Artists, 20*(3), 115-118. https://doi.org/10.21091/mppa.2005.3023

Wang, T.J., & Russell, J.A. (2018). A tenuous pas de deux: Examining university dancers' access to and satisfaction with healthcare delivery. *Medical Problems of Performing Artists, 33*(2), 111-117. https://doi.org/10.21091/mppa.2018.2018

Chapter 16

American Harlequin Corporation. (2024). *Dance.* https://us.harlequinfloors.com/en/markets/dance/

Dance Well Podcast. (2024). *360 Degrees of Health and Wellness for Dancers.* www.dancewellpodcast.com/

Daniels, K. (2014). Technique class participation options for injured dancers. *International Association for Dance Medicine & Science resource paper for dancers and teachers.* IADMS. https://iadms.org/media/5787/iadms-resource-paper-technique-class-participation-for-injured-dancers.pdf

Felter, A.A., & Rietveld, A.B. (2009). Relation between dance floors and dance injuries. *Medical Problems of Performing Artists, 24*(1), 47.

Hagins, M., Pappas, E., Kremenic, I., Orishimo, K.F., & Rundle, A. (2007). The effect of an inclined landing surface on biomechanical variables during a jumping task. *Clinical Biomechanics, 22*(9), 1030-1036. https://doi.org/10.1016/j.clinbiomech.2007.07.012

Hopper L., & Fong Yan, A. (2016). The dance environment. In M.V. Wilmerding & D.H. Krasnow (Eds.), *Dancer wellness* (pp. 4-12). Human Kinetics.

Hopper, L.S., Allen, N., Wyon, M., Alderson, J.A., Elliott, B.C., & Ackland, T.R. (2014). Dance floor mechanical properties and dancer injuries in a touring professional ballet company. *Journal of Science and Medicine in Sport, 17*(1), 29-33. https://doi.org/10.1016/j.jsams.2013.04.013

Hopper, L.S., Alderson, J.A., Elliott, B.C., Ackland, T.R., & Fleming, P.R. (2014). Do dance floor force reduction and static stiffness represent dynamic floor stiffness during dance landings? *Procedia Engineering, 72*, 931-936. https://doi.org/10.1016/j.proeng.2014.06

Kusner, E. & Shaeffer, M. (Hosts). (2018, Sep. 26). A dancer's identity (No. 14) [Audio podcast episode with guest Dr. Elizabeth Morray]. In *DanceWell*. Wav Records. www.dancewellpodcast.com/news/2018/9/26/episode-14-a-dancers-identity.

Kusner, E. & Shaeffer, M. (Hosts). (2021, Oct. 2). Resilience. (No. 90) [Audio podcast episode with guest Michelle Dwarka]. In *DanceWell*. Wav Records. www.dancewellpodcast.com/news/2021/10/2/episode-90-resilience

Mainwaring, L., Aujla, I. (2017). Psychological wellness. In M.V. Wilmerding & D.H. Krasnow (Eds.), *Dancer wellness* (pp. 71-81), Human Kinetics.

Nordin-Bates, S.M. (2014). Perfectionism. *International Association for Dance Medicine & Science resource paper for dancers and teachers*. IADMS. https://iadms.org/media/5910/iadms-resource-paper-perfectionism.pdf

Nordin-Bates, S.M , Raedeke, T.D., & Madigan, D.J. (2017). Perfectionism, burnout, and motivation in dance: A replication and test of the 2 × 2 model of perfectionism. *Journal of Dance Medicine & Science, 21*(3), 115-122. https://doi.org/10.12678/1089-313X.21.3.115

Pappas, E., & Hagins, M. (2008). The effects of "raked" stages on standing posture in dancers. *Journal of Dance Medicine & Science, 12*(2), 54-58.

Quin, E., Rafferty, S., & Tomlinson, C. (2015). *Safe dance practice*. Human Kinetics.

Radell, S.A., Keneman, M.L., Mandradjieff, M.P., Adame, D.D., & Cole, S.P. (2017). Comparison study of body image satisfaction between beginning-and advanced-level female ballet students. *Journal of Dance Medicine & Science, 21*(4), 135-143. https://doi.org/10.12678/1089-313X.21.4.135

Radell, S.A., Mandradjieff, M.P., Adame, D.D., & Cole, S.P. (2020). Impact of mirrors on body image of beginning modern and ballet students. *Journal of Dance Medicine & Science, 24* (3), 126-134. https://doi.org/10.12678/1089-313X.24.3.126

Redding, E., & Handman, P.G. (2017). Cross training and conditioning. In M.V. Wilmerding & D.H. Krasnow (Eds.), *Dancer Wellness* (pp. 37-53). Human Kinetics.

Safe in Dance International. (2024). *Optimising performance. Minimising injury. Enhancing dance*. www.safeindance.com/

Wanke, E.M., Mill, H., Wanke, A., Davenport, J., Koch, F., & Groneberg, D.A. (2012). Dance floors as injury risk: analysis and evaluation of acute injuries caused by dance floors in professional dance with regard to preventative aspects. *Medical Problems of Performing Artists, 27*(3), 137-142. https://doi.org/10.21091/mppa.2012.3025

Index

Note: The italicized *f* and *t* following page numbers refer to figures and tables, respectively.

D

Q

R

S

About the Editor

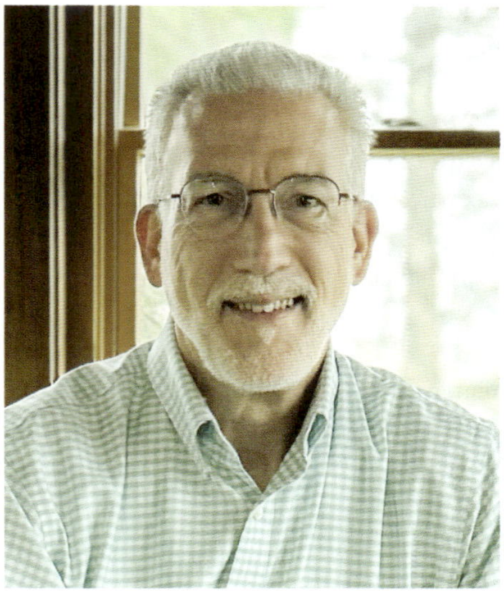

Ruth Russell

Jeffrey A. Russell, PhD, ATC, is an associate professor of athletic training and the director of Science and Health in Artistic Performance (SHAPe) at Ohio University, where he studies artists in dance, music, theater, circus, film and television, and marching band. His PhD in dance medicine and science is from the University of Wolverhampton in England. He has served on the boards of the International Association for Dance Medicine & Science and the Performing Arts Medicine Association. He is a founding board member of The Bridge Dance Project, the founder of the International Task Force on Head Impacts and Trauma in Stunts, and an ambassador and research advisor for the Australian Stunts Organisation. His international research group focuses primarily on concussions in film and television stunt performers as well as health care access for dancers in the commercial industry and on university dance teams. Other research from his lab includes magnetic resonance imaging (MRI) of the ankle in ballet dancers and the use of dance socks to reduce forces on dancers' feet. He has published and spoken extensively on a variety of topics in performing arts medicine. Dr. Russell and his wife, Ruth, live in Athens, Ohio.

About the Contributors

Courtney Abbott, MFA, (she/they) has been an intimacy director since 2018. Prior to this work, they taught consent and bystander intervention to the United States Armed Forces. She holds certificates in mental health first aid (National Council for Behavioral Health), nonviolent communication (NYCNVC), and narrative therapy technique (Evanston Family Therapy Center) and studied trauma healing with The Global Gratitude Alliance and with Gender Reconciliation International. Recent collaborations include Steppenwolf Theatre, Chicago Shakespeare Theater, Northwestern University, Redtwist Theatre, and About Face Theatre. They are a proud alum of Northwestern (bachelor's degree in theater, 2004) and Ohio University (master's degree in acting, 2021).

Jatin P. Ambegaonkar, PhD, ATC, OT, CSCS, FIADMS, is associate dean for research and professor of athletic training in the School of Kinesiology in the College of Education and Human Development at George Mason University in Virginia. He is the founding codirector of George Mason University's Sports Medicine Assessment Research and Testing Laboratory. Dr. Ambegaonkar is the editor in chief of the *Journal of Dance Medicine & Science*, serves on the editorial board of the *Journal of Athletic Training*, and peer reviews for over 25 professional journals. He has served on the board of directors for the International Association for Dance Medicine & Science and chaired the association's research committee. Dr. Ambegaonkar has published over 80 articles and given over 150 professional presentations. Professionally, Dr. Ambegaonkar is certified as an athletic trainer, strength and conditioning specialist, and occupational therapist.

Amanda (Mandy) Blackmon, PT, DPT, OCS, CMTPT, received her doctor of physical therapy (DPT) degree from Emory University in 2005. Dr. Blackmon is a board-certified specialist in orthopaedic physical therapy with 18 years of clinical experience treating patients with musculoskeletal conditions. She specializes in treating performing artists and dancers, and she is the head physical therapist for Atlanta Ballet. Mandy owns a private practice in Atlanta and is a managing partner for Atlanta Dance Medicine, with multiple locations in the Atlanta area. Dr. Blackmon is adjunct faculty in the DPT program at Mercer University in Atlanta, Georgia. Mandy is also an instructor for Myopain Seminars in the Janet Travell dry needling training program. She is involved in multiple performing arts medicine organizations, including the performing arts special interest group for the American Physical Therapy Association, the Dance/USA Task Force on Dancer Health, the Performing Arts Medicine Association, and is on the board of the International Association for Dance Medicine & Science.

Linda Bluestein, MD, is a former ballet dancer, board-certified anesthesiologist, integrative pain medicine physician, and assistant professor at the Medical College of Wisconsin, Central Wisconsin. She has extensive experience treating individuals with complex hypermobility disorders, educating and coaching dancers and studio owners, and conducting research on hypermobile dancers. Dr. Bluestein completed her anesthesiology residency at the Mayo Graduate School of Medicine after receiving her medical degree from the University of California–Los Angeles School of Medicine. She founded and hosts the podcast *Bendy Bodies With the Hypermobility MD*, is widely published, and has given numerous national and international presentations. As a leading specialist in connective tissue disorders, Dr. Bluestein worked with the nonprofit Chronic Pain Partners to create the first online continuing medical education program about Ehlers-Danlos Syndromes. Dr. Bluestein's website is www.hypermobilitymd.com.

Caroline Bolling, PT, PhD, is a sports physiotherapist and postdoctoral researcher at the Amsterdam Collaboration on Health & Safety in Sports, IOC Research Center, Amsterdam UMC, in the Netherlands. Her publications focus on injury prevention, complexity, and qualitative research. She is also a teacher at the Master Sports Physiotherapy Hogeschool in Utrecht, Netherlands. For her master's degree in public health at UFMG in Belo Horizonte, Brazil, she studied injuries and health of professional dancers. Her PhD highlighted the athlete's and artist's voice in injury prevention research, and it was nominated for a *British Journal of Sports Medicine* PhD award. She was physiotherapist of the

Brazilian national gymnastics team and Minas Tenis Clube, and she was head therapist of Cirque du Soleil (*Quidam*, *Corteo*, *Paramour*, and CDS at sea, *Kooza*).

Ann F. Brown, PhD, CISSN, FIADMS, is an associate professor, associate dean for graduate studies, and director of the Human Performance Laboratory at the University of Idaho. Her research focuses primarily on the influence of exercise, nutrition, and supplementation on body composition, the menstrual cycle, and the overall health among females of all ages. More specifically, Brown focuses on lifestyle interventions centered around optimizing female physiology. Dr. Brown's background in dance is a featured aspect of her research, with which she contributes to the growing body of literature in dance science and nutrition. She is a member and fellow of the International Association for Dance Medicine & Science and serves on the editorial board for its journal, *Journal of Dance Medicine & Science.* Additionally, she is a member of the National Strength and Conditioning Association, for whom she has contributed textbook chapters (*NSCA's Guide to Sport and Exercise Nutrition, Second Edition*). She is a member of the International Society for Sport Nutrition and has contributed textbook chapters to the third edition of *Nutritional Sciences: From Fundamentals to Food.*

Kevin M. Brown, MeEd, ATC, is the director of sports medicine for KORT Physical Therapy. He is the athletic trainer for the Louisville Ballet, Actors Theatre of Louisville, and The Vision Dance Center. Kevin serves on the National Athletic Trainers' Association Council on Practice Advancement performing arts committee and is president of the Performing Arts Athletic Trainers' Society. He is a member of the International Association for Dance Medicine & Science, the Performing Arts Medicine Association, the Dance/USA Task Force on Dancer Health, and the Select Medical dance medicine advisory board.

Meghan A. Brown, PhD, FHEA, SENR, is a senior lecturer in sport and exercise nutrition at Leeds Beckett University, and she contributes to undergraduate and postgraduate provision as well as research activity in the Carnegie School of Sport. Meghan has provided nutrition support to a variety of athletes across different levels as a registered sport and exercise nutritionist. She has many research interests, but she focuses mainly on nutrition and exercise metabolism—specifically nutritional interventions to promote recovery in female dancers, which was the focus of her PhD at Northumbria University. Meghan has worked closely with dancers, and she has a special interest in energy availability and the specific requirements of female athletes.

Róisín Cahalan, PhD, PT, is a chartered physiotherapist, academic, and researcher, and works as an Associate Professor in Physiotherapy at the University of Limerick, Ireland. She also is the world's leading authority on pain and injury in Irish dancing. She is a qualified Irish dancing teacher and adjudicator and former professional dancer; she performed the female lead role with *Riverdance: The Show* and toured with the production for over 8 years. Her PhD and postdoctoral work focus on injury screening and prevention in Irish dancing as well as collegiate contemporary dancing. She is the editor and main author of the book *Complete Irish Dancer: Optimization of Health and Performance in Irish Dancers*, and she was nominated for an International Association for Dance Medicine & Science Dance Educator Award in 2020.

Jasmine D. Challis, RD, MRes, is an accredited nutritionist and dietitian on the UK Sport and Exercise Nutrition Register, focusing on dance. She has worked across the dance field for over 30 years, giving talks, running workshops, and providing one-on-one sessions for dancers and dance students. She is coauthor of the *International Association for Dance Medicine & Science (IADMS) Nutrition Resource Paper* as well as the nutrition chapters in a number of dancer health books. Her book *Nutrition for Dance and Performance* was published by Routledge in 2023. She is on the board of The Bridge Dance Project. She has presented at the International Association for Dance Medicine & Science annual conference regularly. She completed a master's degree in sport and exercise science (with distinction) in 2018; her research project was with Irish dancers.

Debra A. Crookshanks, BSc, PT, is an Australian trained and registered clinical physiotherapist working exclusively in the dance medicine space in Australia. She is the author of *The Safe Dance 3 Report*, commissioned by the Australia Council/Ausdance, has written and presented syllabuses for the anatomy and dance medicine components of university and tertiary education–based programs, and teaches and mentors graduate and postgraduate dance students in dance medicine and science. She received an award from the Australian Physiotherapy Association for services in dance, and she has served as a board member of the International Association for Dance Medicine & Science.

Kathleen L. Davenport, MD, is the director of physiatry at the Hospital for Special Surgery Florida. She serves as president (2023–2025) on the board of directors for the International Association for Dance Medicine & Science and is the company physician for Miami City Ballet. She is the editor for the *Physical Medicine and Rehabilitation Clinics of North America* Dance Medicine issue, published in 2021. She has published numerous articles in both scientific journals and popular media. She lectures regularly at national and international conferences to advance wellness in athletes and dancers.

Jennifer Deckert, MFA, is an associate professor of dance at the University of South Carolina in Columbia, South Carolina, where she serves as the director of dance and associate chair of the department of theatre and dance. She has been an active member of the International Association for Dance Medicine & Science for the past 19 years and has served on their board of directors and dance educators' committee. Her research interests include dynamic alignment, the effects of fatigue, and the integration of wellness-based training into the classroom and university environment. Jennifer holds a master of fine arts degree from the University of Utah.

Diane Diefenderfer is an associate professor of teaching in the dance department of the University of California, Irvine, where she teaches ballet technique and directs the Pilates program for dancer wellness. Diane enjoyed a 20-year career in dance as a soloist with the Frankfurt, Eglevsky, and Los Angeles Ballet companies. She encountered the Pilates Method in 1978 while rehabilitating from an injury, subsequently practicing Pilates as a supplement to her dance training and instructor apprenticeship. A second-generation Pilates teacher, she holds the honorable distinction of being awarded a master teacher certification from legendary teacher and mentor Ron Fletcher, a disciple of Joseph and Clara Pilates. Diane is a nationally certified Pilates teacher (NCPT), is a regular presenter for Pilates Method Alliance conferences, is on the faculty of Pilates Anytime, and is a contributing author to *Women's Health and Wellness Across the Lifespan* from Lippincott Williams & Wilkins.

Amanda M. Donahue, MS, ATC, is the athletic trainer for the Palladino School of Dance & School of the Arts at Dean College in Franklin, Massachusetts. She completed her bachelor's degree in athletic training from Northeastern University and her master's degree in kinesiology from the University of Illinois at Urbana-Champaign. Her first exposure to working with professional dancers was during her internship for the Radio City Rockettes athletic training staff as an undergraduate student. She has also had the opportunity to provide per diem athletic training services for the Boston Ballet. She has been a member of the National Athletic Trainers' Association (NATA) since 2010, and she has served as the chair of NATA's Council of Practice Advancement performing arts committee. She has also written articles specific to performing arts for *NATA News* and the NATA blog. She has been a member of the International Association for Dance Medicine & Science for the past 8 years, and she has presented at their annual conference both in the United States and internationally multiple times. She also has served as the External Organization Liaison for the Performing Arts Athletic Trainers' Society and is one of the society's founding members. In addition, she was interviewed by and provided exercises for *Dance Magazine*, discussing preparation for inversions and floor work in dance.

Jan Dunn, MS, is a dance educator and dance medicine specialist, Pilates rehabilitation specialist, Franklin Method educator, and former university dance instructor. She is currently cochair of The Bridge Dance Project. She is on the U.S. advisory board of Safe in Dance International and is the dance wellness editor for 4Dancers.org. She was one of the founders of the International Association for Dance Medicine & Science, serving 21 years as president, as executive director, and on the board of directors. She founded and served as chair of the National Dance Association's committee on dance medicine and science, and she was organizer and cochair of the 2004 International Dance Medicine Conference in Taiwan. She founded Denver Dance Medicine Associates as well as the wellness programs of several universities. Her degrees are in dance and exercise science, specializing in dance science.

Lauren Elson, MD, is the director of dance medicine for Spaulding Rehabilitation at Harvard Medical School. She is a former professional dancer and dance instructor and a current performer. She is board certified in physical medicine and rehabilitation and in sports medicine. She is on the board of directors of the International Association for Dance Medicine & Science and is the chair of the freelance dancer committee on the Dance/USA task force for dance health. She has lectured nationally and internationally on dance medicine and edited the textbook *Performing Arts Medicine.*

Gary Galbraith, MFA, is a professor of dance and artistic director of dance at Case Western Reserve University. Prior to his university appointment, he was a principal dancer with the Martha Graham Dance Company, for which he danced most of the major male roles. He is also the founder and director of the Dancer Wellness Project, in which he has consulted with professional dance companies and universities around the world. Along with being the chair of the injury surveillance committee for Dance/USA's task force on dancer health, he has been a longtime member of the International Association for Dance Medicine & Science as well as the Performing Arts Medicine Association.

Gayanne Grossman, PT, EdM, BFA, FIADMS, is a dancer, educator, author, physical therapist for dancers, and researcher. She served on the board of directors of the International Association for Dance Medicine & Science (IADMS) for 14 years and currently serves on the Board of The Bridge Dance Project. Gayanne is adjunct faculty for the Peabody Institute, Johns Hopkins University, where she teaches kinesiology. She is the author of the textbook *Dance Science: Anatomy, Movement Analysis, Conditioning* and the editor in chief of the *IADMS Bulletin for Dancers and Teachers*. She published original peer-reviewed research, most notably on turnout measurement, and wrote the hip chapter for the American Physical Therapy Association's monograph on dance medicine. Gayanne has lectured worldwide on dance medicine and science.

Jacqui Greene Haas, MA, AT Ret., is a retired performing arts athletic trainer who served as the on-site performing arts medicine supervisor and athletic trainer for Mercy Health at Cincinnati Ballet for almost 30 years. She is a former professional ballet dancer, and she has a bachelor's degree in dance from the University of South Florida; her athletic training education is from the University of Cincinnati, and her master's degree is from Northern Kentucky University. Jacqui is proud to be the author of two editions of the Human Kinetics publication *Dance Anatomy*, and she currently teaches dance physiology, Pilates, foundations, and ballet at Northern Kentucky University's School of the Arts. She is a member of the National Athletic Trainers' Association, the International Association for Dance Medicine & Science, and the Bridge Dance Project.

Melody Hrubes, MD, a physician at Rothman Orthopaedic in New York City, is board certified in physical medicine and rehabilitation as well as sports medicine. She currently serves as the medical director for the Radio City Rockettes, medical lead for the Team USA Olympic breaking team, and team physician coordinator for the U.S. Soccer Federation U17 women's national team. Dr. Hrubes has worked with multiple dance and theater companies and is president-elect of the Performing Arts Medicine Association. She also serves on the board of directors of the American Medical Society for Sports Medicine and is a fellow of the American College of Sports Medicine.

Danielle N. Jarvis, PhD, ATC, is a professor of kinesiology at California State University, Northridge, where she teaches course work in biomechanics, dance science, and evidence-based practice. She is the director of LEAAP (Laboratory for Evaluating Athletic & Aesthetic Performance), where she conducts biomechanics research addressing questions related to movement coordination during skilled athletic activities. She received a bachelor of science degree in athletic training and exercise science with a minor in dance from Ithaca College; a master of science degree in kinesiology (with an emphasis in dance) from California State University, Northridge; and a PhD in biokinesiology (with an emphasis in biomechanics) from the University of Southern California. She is certified as an athletic trainer by the National Athletic Trainers' Association and is an active member of the International Association for Dance Medicine & Science.

Nancy J. Kadel, MD, is a foot and ankle orthopaedic surgeon specializing in the diagnosis and treatment of musculoskeletal foot and ankle injuries and the care of dancers. She sees patients at the Seattle Clinic for Performing Artists/Sound Spine and Joint Physicians. Dr. Kadel is past president of the International Association for Dance Medicine & Science and past president of the Performing Arts Medicine Association. She has authored articles on many topics, including stress fractures in ballet dancers, foot and ankle issues in dancers, and biomechanics of the midfoot ligaments en pointe. Previously, Dr. Kadel was associate professor of orthopaedics at the University of Washington and at the University of California, San Francisco. She received Top Doc awards in California and Washington. Dr. Kadel is a consulting orthopaedist for several Seattle area dance companies.

Steven J. Karageanes, DO, FAOASM, is a physician of sports medicine and performing arts medicine in Novi, Michigan. He is a founding member of

Athletes and the Arts, is on the board of directors of the American Association of Orthopedic Medicine, is president of Nonprofit Education and Advocacy for the Movement Artists, and is on the advisory board of The Bridge Dance Project. He serves on the editorial board of *Clinical Journal of Sports Medicine* and was editor of the textbook *Principles of Manual Sports Medicine*. He is a past president of the American Osteopathic Academy of Sports Medicine.

Lynnette Khoo-Summers, PT, DPT, is an associate professor in the physical therapy program and department of orthopaedics at Washington University School of Medicine. She received her undergraduate degree in public relations and dance from Colorado State University. She received her master's degree in physical therapy and then her clinical doctorate from Washington University School of Medicine. Her expertise is in the movement system impairment theory, and she uses this concept for injury prevention and rehabilitation of all musculoskeletal and orthopaedic conditions. She was a coauthor for two chapters in the second volume for *Movement System Impairment Theory*. Her specialty is treating all performing artists in the faculty practice clinic as well as providing performance day coverage at theaters in St. Louis. She is codirector, with Dr. Devyani Hunt, of the Medical Program for Performing Artists at Washington University School of Medicine. She is a member of the American Physical Therapy Association and is part of their performing arts special interest group. She is also a member of the International Association for Dance Medicine & Science and the Performing Arts Medicine Association.

Kori L. Kirschner, MS, LAT, ATC, CSCS*D, is an athletic trainer, certified strength and conditioning specialist, and Manager of Ship Operations for Performing Arts Athletic Training and Physical Therapy with Next Level Physiotherapy and Performance in Orlando, Florida. She is a trailblazing athletic trainer who has taken her skills and adventurous spirit across six continents to support the health and wellness of performing athletes. She was one of the first athletic trainers to establish preventive health maintenance programs at Walt Disney World and later at Feld Entertainment Inc. She has provided health care to the Radio City Rockettes on tour and in New York as well as to Cirque du Soleil's *La Nouba* in Orlando, Florida. She is a member of the National Athletic Trainers' Association and the National Strength and Conditioning Association. Kori has given many conference presentations, mentored athletic training students, and given interviews around the world regarding her work creating athletic training programs for touring performing artists.

Robin Kish, MS, MFA, is an associate professor in dance at Chapman University. Robin blends her background in dance and science creating innovative educational programs supporting the development of safe and effective dance training programs. She has presented research and developed education lectures for the Performing Arts Medicine Association, International Association for Dance Medicine & Science, and National Dance Education Organization. She is a founding board member of The Bridge Dance Project. She coauthored *The Embodied Dancer: A Guide to Optimal Performance* and the second edition of *Dancing Longer, Dancing Stronger: A Dancer's Guide to Improving Technique and Preventing Injury*. A former modern dancer and a product of the private studio and competition environment, she is passionate about bringing dancer wellness and safe teaching practices to the industry.

Jo-Anne La Flèche, MPsy, MA, is a clinical and performance psychologist with a master's degree in dance. She works as resident psychologist at L'École Supérieure de Ballet du Québec in Montréal, where she teaches performance psychology and psycho-pedagogy as well as providing counseling to students. She gives workshops and lectures on performance psychology and dancer mental health in Canada, the United States, and Europe. She has written several articles and informational papers and is a psychology consultant for *Dance Magazine* and *Dance Teacher* magazine. She gives dance therapy workshops on self-esteem and embodiment to dancers and nondancers. La Flèche is a member of the Performing Arts Medicine Association and takes part in working groups on dancer health: Personal Safety for Dance, The Bridge Dance Project, the International Association for Dance Medicine & Science mental health advisory group, and the Dance/USA task force on dancer health. She is a board member and past president (2021-2022) of Healthy Dancer Canada.

Monica Lorenzo, MS, ATC, is the founder of the first athletic training program in the National Basketball Association (NBA) with New York Knicks Entertainment. She currently serves as head athletic trainer in this role as well as director of health, wellness, and physical education of the Trevor Day School in New York City. She received her bachelor of science degree in athletic training from the State University of New York (SUNY) Stony Brook University in 2008 and her master's degree in rehabilitative science and corrective exercise from California University of Pennsylvania in 2010. Monica is the founder of Pro Athletic Solutions LLC, which contracts athletic trainers providing care to NBA and pro sport entertainment teams. Monica has served as an athletic trainer for the *Radio City Christmas Spectacular* and Cirque Du Soleil. Through her second company, ROMO Fit Inc., Monica provides athletic training care, including strength and conditioning for performing artists. Monica is passionate about education for performing artists, and she lectures at national dance conventions and university performance departments on injury prevention methods for the performing artist.

Misty Lown, ME-PD, is the founder of More Than Just Great Dancing, a licensed dance studio affiliation program that reaches over 100,000 dance students each week. She is also the former owner of Youth Protection Association for Dance and owner and founder of Misty's Dance Unlimited, which has been named one of the Top 50 Studios in the Nation by *Dance Spirit* magazine. She has been recognized as Teacher of the Year by Eclipse, named Outstanding Businesswoman of the Year by the YWCA, and awarded the Pope John XXIII Award for Distinguished Service by Viterbo University. Misty has authored over 100 industry articles and blogs. She is the author of *One Small Yes* and is currently a PhD candidate at Concordia University in Chicago.

Susan Mayes, PhD, AM, is the Australian Ballet's director of artistic health and has been their principal physiotherapist since 1997. Mayes also consults for national and international professional sports. Mayes was appointed an adjunct research fellow at La Trobe University following completion of her PhD in 2017 on hip joint health in professional ballet dancers, and she received La Trobe University's Distinguished Alumni Award in 2018. She leads a dance research partnership between Australian Ballet and La Trobe University and has been invited to speak at international conferences and lectures throughout Australia and Europe. Mayes was awarded an Order of Australia in 2020 for her role in injury prevention and improving outcomes for ballet dancers.

Melissa McGhee, BS, is the head coach of The Ohio State University dance team. Before stepping into the head coach role, she was also a member of the dance team, where she gained knowledge and qualifications to establish herself as head coach. Within the previous 5 years, she has led the team to win nine national championships in the NCAA Division IA pom, jazz, and game day divisions at the Universal Dance Association college national championships.

Kathleen McGuire Gaines, BA, is a former ballet dancer, a mental health advocate, and the founder of Minding the Gap, a social good company that seeks to see mental health regarded with the same seriousness in dance as physical health. She and her collaborators work directly with dance institutions to deliver mental health skills programs and design protocols to support dancers and dance teaching artists. Her research on the mental health of dancers has been presented at the International Association for Dance Medicine & Science conference and the Performing Arts Medical Association symposium. Kathleen is also a certified mental health first aid instructor and a contributing writer to *Dance Magazine*.

Lauren McIntyre, ATC, has been an athletic trainer at the Harkness Center for Dance Injuries at NYU Langone Health since 2010. Over the course of her career, Lauren has worked with thousands of dancers and performers to rehabilitate injury and optimize performance. Lauren's research focuses on dance injury epidemiology and concussions in dance. Her work is published in the *Journal of Athletic Training* and *Physical Medicine & Rehabilitation Clinics of North America*, among other publications. She presents regularly on injury surveillance and dance concussion and has been the lead or coauthor of presentations at 15 national and international conferences.

Merry Lynn Morris, PhD, MFA, LMT, is a dance educator, researcher, and choreographer who has worked within academia for 25 years. She teaches dance science courses for undergraduate dance students and spearheads the certificate program in dance medicine and science at University of South Florida. Dr. Morris is a licensed manual therapist and worked in the alternative medicine sector for 15 years. She is also active in the dance and disability community at local, regional, national, and international levels through teaching, research, leadership, and activism. She has earned five U.S. patents, and her research scholarship appears in such journals as *Medical Problems of Performing Artists*, *Journal of*

Technology and Innovation, *Research in Dance Education*, *Medical Science Educator*, and *Physical Medicine and Rehabilitation*. Morris coedited the book *Perspectives in Performing Arts Medicine Practice: A Multidisciplinary Approach*. She is an active member of the International Association for Dance Medicine & Science.

Carina Nasrallah, MS, ATC, LAT, CISSN, PAM-C, is a certified and licensed athletic trainer for Houston Methodist Hospital and serves as head athletic trainer for the Houston Ballet. She has a bachelor of arts in dance from Belhaven University and a master of science in athletic training from Shenandoah University, where she also completed a graduate certificate in performing arts medicine. She is an active member of the International Association for Dance Medicine & Science and the Performing Arts Athletic Trainers' Society, and is a certified sports nutritionist from the International Society for Sports Nutrition. She has served as adjunct faculty at Shenandoah University and Virginia Commonwealth University (VCU), and she has presented nationally and internationally on cross-training for dancers, health care for collegiate and professional dancers, and the management of performing arts injuries.

Sarah Needham-Beck, PhD, is a research fellow in exercise physiology and program coordinator of the master's degree in dance science at the University of Chichester, United Kingdom. Sarah conducts research both with personnel working in physically demanding occupations and with student and professional dancers. Sarah received both her PhD (2017) and master's degree (2010) in dance science from Trinity Laban Conservatoire of Music and Dance, where her research focused on cardiorespiratory fitness in contemporary dance training and performance. She has published original research in journals, including the *Journal of Strength and Conditioning Research*, *Medical Problems of Performing Artists*, and *Frontiers in Psychology: Performance Science*. Sarah is a long-standing member of the International Association for Dance Medicine & Science (IADMS), where she formerly served as chair of the student and promotion committees and currently serves on the IADMS board as a director-at-large.

Katherine Nicole Krizo, MS, LAT, ATC, began ballroom dancing during her undergraduate education at The Ohio State University (OSU). As a member of DanceSport at OSU, she competed and placed in many collegiate and amateur competitions around the United States in all four styles, rising through the levels. Some of her most noteworthy titles include 2019 National Collegiate DanceSport Champion in Championship Smooth and Pre-Championship Latin with partner Anthony English and 2020 WDSF World Smooth Championship Semifinalist with partner Jonathan Wolfgram. While completing her master's degree in athletic training at Indiana University (IU), she conducted research on injuries in ballroom dancers and was the graduate assistant athletic trainer for the IU ballet department. Following that, she returned to OSU to complete an athletic training internship with the men's gymnastics and fencing teams. Currently she is a performing arts athletic trainer at the University of North Carolina School of the Arts.

Sheyi Ojofeitimi, PT, DPT, OCS, CFMT, is director of therapy services and health and safety advisor for the Alvin Ailey American Dance Foundation and co-founder of the Dance Ready Project. A licensed physical therapist for 22 years, she oversees the care of Alvin Ailey Dance Foundation's staff and dancers (both professional and preprofessional). She has worked with several Broadway and off-Broadway shows, including *Wicked*, *Once On This Island*, *Avenue Q*, *The Book of Mormon*, and *Freestyle Love Supreme*. For 10 years, she served as senior research associate at the Analysis of Dance and Movement (ADAM) Center, a biomechanics laboratory conducting research on movement and injury patterns in dancers. She is author on 17 peer-reviewed journal articles, including two examining the effect of comprehensive management on injury incidence and cost in a modern dance company and another measuring the extreme kinematics in selected hip-hop dance sequences. She holds a doctoral degree in physical therapy, specializing in dance medicine and biomechanics. She teaches injury prevention and performance enhancement workshops to underserved dancers in the U.S., Africa, and the Caribbean. She also serves as a peer reviewer for the *Journal of Dance Medicine & Science*.

Olivia Placita, BS, was a seven-time national championship member of The Ohio State University dance team from 2019 through 2022. She graduated with a degree in health promotion, nutrition, and exercise science from The Ohio State University in May of 2022. Following graduation, Olivia stepped into the assistant coaching position for The Ohio State University dance team.

Emma Redding, PhD, FIADMS, is the director of the Victorian College of the Arts at University of Melbourne, Australia. Prior to this position, she was a professor of performance science at Trinity Laban Conservatoire of Music and Dance in London, England. Emma is a trained dancer and holds a PhD in applied biological sciences. At Trinity Laban she co-wrote the world's first master's degree in dance science, and she is cofounder of the UK National Institute for Dance Medicine and Science. Emma is a fellow and past president of the International Association for Dance Medicine & Science and serves as associate editor for the *Journal of Dance Medicine & Science*. In 2022, Emma was awarded as a member of the Most Excellent Order of the British Empire (MBE) for her services to dance.

Bonnie E. Robson, MD, FRCPC, is a retired psychiatrist who since 1983 has specialized in performance arts medicine. Until 2013, she consulted athletes and artists at Pivot Sport Medicine and was an assistant professor in the faculty of medicine at University of Toronto. She was a consultant for the National Ballet School of Canada and Quinte Ballet School and is currently a consultant for Ballet Jorgen. She has presented at national and international conferences. She was published in juried and public journals such as *Medical Problems of Performing Artists* and *Journal of Dance Medicine & Science* and served on their editorial boards. She has served on the board of the Performing Arts Medicine Association (PAMA) and of NETWORK Schools. She was honored by the latter with a lifetime achievement award and by PAMA with the Bill Dawson Award. She was a member of the Dance/USA task force on dancer health and serves on the membership committee of Healthy Dancer Canada, from which she received their lifetime achievement award in 2022. She currently is a member of Personal Safety for Dance and is a past member of the board of The Bridge Dance Project and the International Association for Dance Medicine & Science mental health working group.

Laura Santos, MS, LAT, ATC, served for nearly two decades as the lead athletic trainer and associate director for health services at the University of North Carolina School of the Arts, a public performing arts conservatory. She now provides clinical and outreach services on a freelance basis with the goal of enhancing health and performance for dancers at all levels. She has presented performing arts medicine content at regional, national, and international conferences, including the Winston-Salem Dance Medicine (WiSDM) Conference [formerly City of Arts and Innovation Dance Medicine (CAIDM) Conference], the National Athletic Trainers' Association (NATA) Clinical Symposia, and the International Association for Dance Medicine & Science (IADMS) Annual Meeting. In 2014, she was recognized by the NC Athletic Trainers' Association as Emerging Practices Athletic Trainer of the Year.

Rose Schmieg, DHSc, PT, ATC, CISSN, CSCS, is the founding director of the Shenandoah University Division of Athletic Training. She has directed a master's degree program in athletic training as well as graduate certificate programs in performing arts medicine (PAM) and performing arts health and fitness (PAHF). The PAM and PAHF graduate certificates are uniquely interprofessional, and they are the first of their kind in the United States. Dr. Schmieg led the development of the Shenandoah Performing Arts Rehabilitation Center, an on-campus clinic. In this center, Dr. Schmieg performs wellness screening, orthopaedic assessment, injury management, and research on conservatory students. Dr. Schmieg is a physical therapist and athletic trainer. She is certified in manual therapy, sports nutrition, and strength and conditioning. She is a member of the Performing Arts Medicine Association and the International Association for Dance Medicine & Science. Dr. Schmieg is currently serving as the Shenandoah University interim dean of the School of Health Professions.

Meg Schneider, MS, ATC, is a certified athletic trainer with years of experience in the performing arts setting. Meg has been the assistant athletic trainer for the Radio City Rockettes in New York City since 2004. In 2013, she joined the Chicago Bulls Entertainment team, where she created and implemented their first-ever athletic training program. Meg has consistently donated her time to medical conferences and National Athletic Trainers' Association (NATA) committees. She was the NATA performing arts representative for 4 years after serving several years on the committee. Meg is a founding member of the Performing Arts Athletic Training Society, and she serves as board treasurer. Most recently, she has served on the medical board for iAct, helping with the Darfur refugee soccer teams. Her greatest accomplishment is being mom to her sons, Benjamin and William.

Selina Shah, MD, FACP, FAMSSM, is a board-certified sports medicine and internal medicine physician in private practice in Walnut Creek, California. She is the company physician for several dance companies in the San Francisco Bay Area. She is the team physician for USA Artistic Swimming and also a physician for USA Gymnastics, USA Weightlifting, and USA Figure Skating. She provides coverage for Broadway shows and Cirque du Soleil. She is past treasurer and board member for the International Association for Dance Medicine & Science. She is a past board member for The Bridge Dance Project and serves on the executive committee for the Dance/USA Task Force on Dancer Health. She has lectured nationally and internationally on various dance medicine topics. She has published papers in medical journals and books, including criteria on determining readiness for pointe and her original research on demographics and dance injuries in modern dance and other injury case reports.

Kelli Sharp, DPT, is an associate professor and the chair of the department of dance in the Claire Trevor School of the Arts at University of California, Irvine (UCI). Sharp serves as the director of the Medical Humanities Center and is a vice chair for research in physical medicine and rehabilitation at the UCI Medical Center. Her lab at UCI takes a multidisciplinary approach, integrating the application of clinical neuroscience to the study of dance, while conversely using dance as a therapeutic tool in the rehabilitation of human disease/injury. The first theme of her research program is movement science, which applies principles from biomechanics, motor learning, and neural plasticity to enhance injury prevention, motor control, and physical performance. The second theme of Sharp's research program is using movement therapies to treat individuals with neurological disorders (e.g., using dance training to help rehabilitate individuals with brain injuries).

Nefeli Tsiouti, PT, MA, MSc, is a physiotherapist and sports massage therapist at HealthAlign Medical & Health Centre in Cyprus. She works as a dance scientist, researcher, and educator of Project Breakalign, an international hip-hop research project she founded in 2013. She is a scientific collaborator at the European University Cyprus School of Medicine, and she received the Sports Therapist of the Year award in 2018 from the Federation of Holistic Therapists. Nefeli has been appointed as a judge for the local qualifiers of the Olympic Games 2024 in breaking. She is an author of breaking-related science works published in the *Journal of Dance Medicine & Science* and other journals and books. She has devoted her work to pioneering breaking science to give back to the community of hip-hop.

Desiree A. Unsworth, PT, DPT, is a licensed physical therapist and Pilates instructor who specializes in treating dancers and performing artists. Desiree graduated with her doctor of physical therapy degree from Northwestern University in 2018, where she was named an Edelsberg Scholar. Post-graduation, Desiree worked at Westside Dance Physical Therapy treating New York City Ballet dancers, School of American Ballet students, and Broadway performers. Her past company and show coverage include Alvin Ailey American Dance Theater, Joffrey Ballet, Hubbard Street Dance Chicago, *West Side Story* (2021 film), and Berkeley Repertory Theatre. She is a member of the International Association for Dance Medicine & Science and the American Physical Therapy Association, has presented research at their conferences, and is published in the *Journal of Dance Medicine & Science*.

Tina J. Wang, MD, is a board-certified physical medicine and rehabilitation physician specializing in fascia and performing arts medicine. Dr. Wang practices a unique blend of osteopathic medicine, integrative medicine, and regenerative medicine at her private practice, Tupelo Pointe, where she treats performing artists with hypermobility. Dr. Wang is also an assistant professor for University of California, Riverside (UCR) and Loma Linda University School of Medicine. One of Dr. Wang's areas of academic interest is in the emerging field of fascia. She is a fascia researcher and her clinical research focuses on hypermobility spectrum disorders and Ehlers-Danlos syndromes.

Margaret Wilson, PhD, is a professor emerita in the department of theater and dance at the University of Wyoming (UW). Along with Jennifer Deckert, she cofounded the first undergraduate bachelor's program in dance science and the vertical dance program at UW. Her research focuses on balance, vertical dance, and applications of dance science in teaching. Her work has been published in the *Journal of Dance Medicine & Science* and biomechanics journals. She has served on the International Association for Dance Medicine & Science (IADMS) board of directors, the IADMS dance educators' committee, and the Dance Science and Somatics Educators organization. She was a UW Presidential Research Scholar in 2020, and was awarded a Wyoming Governor's Arts Award in 2022 and the IADMS Dance Educators Award in 2023.

Brooke Winder, DPT, is a licensed physical therapist and board-certified specialist in orthopaedic physical therapy. She is an associate professor and coordinator of the dance science degree program at California State University, Long Beach, where she teaches courses in dance injury risk management, anatomy, wellness, Pilates, and conditioning for dancers. Dr. Winder also specializes clinically in the management of pelvic floor dysfunction in dancers and other artistic athletes. She performs research and lectures nationally and internationally to both the health care and performing arts communities on pelvic floor concerns in dancers. Dr. Winder holds a doctor of physical therapy degree from the University of Southern California and a bachelor of fine arts degree in dance from Chapman University, and she is a certified Pilates instructor through Body Arts and Science International (BASI).

Elaine Winslow-Redmond, MS, ATC, transitioned from a successful career performing as a Radio City Rockette to becoming the head athletic trainer and director of athletic training and wellness for the Rockettes. She pioneered the first in-house health care program for Madison Square Garden Entertainment at Radio City Music Hall. She specializes in dance medicine, holding a master's degree in applied physiology and nutrition from Columbia University and a bachelor's degree in dance from the University of Massachusetts, Amherst. She has been a consultant with many performing arts companies, including Blue Man Group, Norwegian Cruise Lines, Knicks City Dancers, Troika Entertainment, and the Museum of Modern Art, designing in-house injury risk reduction programs. She is passionate about bringing a level of health care to the performing arts industry that is similar to what professional athletes have been afforded.